PEDIATRIC PRACTICE

Neurology

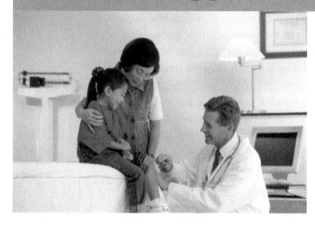

NOTICE

Medicine is an ever-changing science. As new research and clinical experience broaden our knowledge, changes in treatment and drug therapy are required. The authors and the publisher of this work have checked with sources believed to be reliable in their efforts to provide information that is complete and generally in accord with the standards accepted at the time of publication. However, in view of the possibility of human error or changes in medical sciences, neither the authors nor the publisher nor any other party who has been involved in the preparation or publication of this work warrants that the information contained herein is in every respect accurate or complete, and they disclaim all responsibility for any errors or omissions or for the results obtained from use of the information contained in this work. Readers are encouraged to confirm the information contained herein with other sources. For example and in particular, readers are advised to check the product information sheet included in the package of each drug they plan to administer to be certain that the information contained in this work is accurate and that changes have not been made in the recommended dose or in the contraindications for administration. This recommendation is of particular importance in connection with new or infrequently used drugs.

PEDIATRIC PRACTICE

Neurology

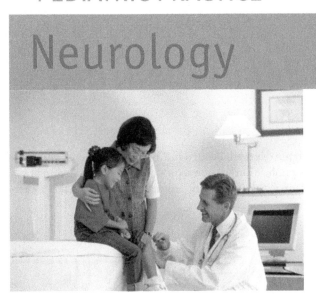

EDITORS

Paul R. Carney, MD
Wilder Chair Professor and Chief
Division of Pediatric Neurology
Departments of Pediatrics, Neurology,
  Neuroscience and Biomedical Engineering
University of Florida McKnight Brain Institute
Gainesville, Florida
USA

James D. Geyer, MD
Clinical Associate Professor
Neurology and Sleep Medicine
College of Community Health Sciences
The University of Alabama
Tuscaloosa, Alabama
USA

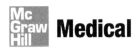 **Medical**

New York Chicago San Francisco Lisbon London Madrid Mexico City
Milan New Delhi San Juan Seoul Singapore Sydney Toronto

Pediatric Practice: Neurology

1 2 3 4 5 6 7 8 9 0   CTP/CTP   12 11 10 9

ISBN 978-0-07-148925-6
MHID 0-07-148925-8

This book was set in Minion by Glyph International.
The editors were Alyssa K. Fried and Christie Naglieri.
The production supervisor was Sherri Souffrance.
Project management was provided by Rajni Pisharody, Glyph International.
The text designer was Janice Bielawa; the cover designer was David Dell'Accio.
China Translation & Printing Services, Ltd. was printer and binder.

This book is printed on acid-free paper.

Photo Credits:
Sections 1, 2, 3: © Getty Images

Library of Congress Cataloging-in-Publication Data

Pediatric practice. Neurology / editors, Paul R. Carney, James D. Geyer.
    p. ; cm.
   Includes bibliographical references and index.
   ISBN-13: 978-0-07-148925-6 (hardcover : alk. paper)
   ISBN-10: 0-07-148925-8 (hardcover : alk. paper) 1. Pediatric neurology.   I. Carney, Paul R.   II. Geyer, James D.
III. Title: Neurology.
   [DNLM: 1. Nervous System Diseases—diagnosis.   2. Nervous System Diseases—therapy.   3. Child.
4. Infant. WS 340 P3718 2009]
   RJ486.P435 2009
   618.92'8—dc22

                                                                    2009023140

McGraw-Hill books are available at special quantity discounts to use as premiums and sales promotions, or for use in corporate training programs. To contact a representative please e-mail us at bulksales@mcgraw-hill.com.

To my lovely wife, Lucia, and to my children, Paulina and Constanza. They are my greatest joy. I also dedicate the book to the loving memory of my mother.

—**PRC**

Dedicated to my beautiful daughters, Sydney and Emery, and to my wife, Stephenie, for her support and assistance. A special thanks to my parents.

—**JDG**

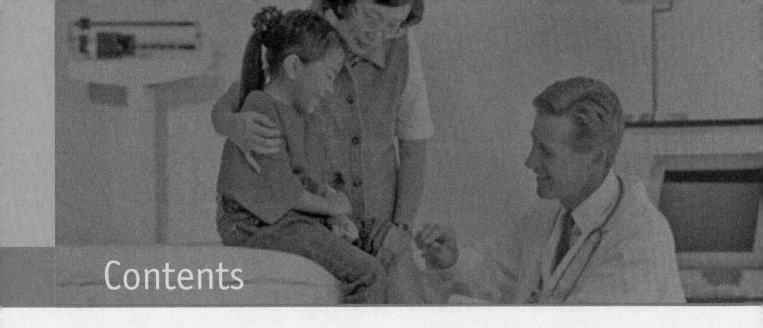

Contents

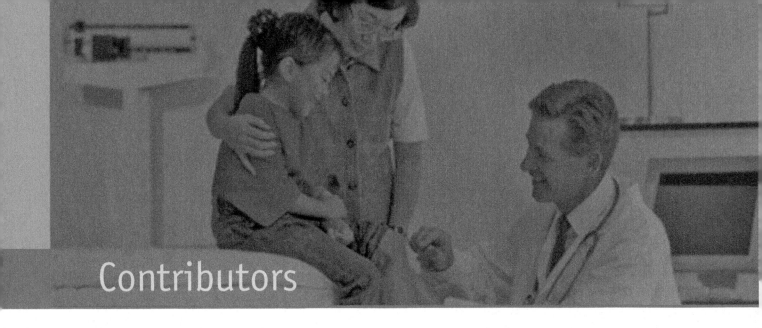

Contributors

Edgard Andrade, MD
Assistant Professor
Division of Pediatric Neurology
Departments of Pediatrics and Neurology
University of Florida
Gainesville, Florida
USA

Khurram Bashir, MD, MPH
Associate Professor
Neurology
University of Alabama at Birmingham
Birmingham, Alabama
USA

M. Tariq Bhatti, MD
Associate Professor
Ophthalmology and Medicine (Division of Neurology)
Duke Eye Center and Duke University Medical Center
Durham, North Carolina
USA

Sharatchandra Bidari, MD
Lecturer
Radiology
University of Florida
Gainesville, Florida
USA

Cynthia J. Campen, MD
Fellow
Child Neurology
Children's Hospital of Philadelphia
Philadelphia, Pennsylvania
USA

Paul R. Carney, MD
Wilder Chair Professor and Chief
Division of Pediatric Neurology
Departments of Pediatrics, Neurology, Neuroscience
   and Biomedical Engineering

University of Florida McKnight Brain Institute
Gainesville, Florida
USA

Carolyn G. Carter, MD
Assistant Professor
Pediatrics
College of Medicine
Gainesville, Florida
USA

Anna Liza Co-Angeles, MD
Resident Physician
Radiology
University of Florida
Gainesville, Florida
USA

Aditi Dagli, MD
Resident Physician
Pediatric Endocrinology
University of Florida
Gainseville, Florida
USA

Stephenie C. Dillard, MD
Clinical Assistant Professor
College of Community Health Science
The University of Alabama
Tuscaloosa, Alabama
USA

Leon S. Dure, MD
Professor and Chief
Pediatrics and Neurology
The University of Alabama at Birmingham
Birmingham, Alabama
USA

Mays El-Dairi, MD
Assistant Professor
Ophthalmology
Duke Eye Center and Duke University Medical Center
Durham, Noth Carolina
USA

Jonathan Etter, MD
Resident Physician
Ophthalmology
Duke Eye Center and Duke University Medical Center
Durham, Noth Carolina
USA

Farjam Farzam, MD
Assistant Professor
Neurology and Pediatrics
University of Kentucky
Lexington, Kentucky
USA

Eileen B. Fennell, PhD
Professor
Clinical and Health Psychology and Neurology
University of Florida
Gainesville, Florida
USA

Laura Flores-Sarnat, MD
Division of Paediatric Neurology
Alberta Children's Hospital
Calgary, Alberta
Canada

Richard E. Frye, MD, PhD
Assistant Professor
Pediatrics and Neurology
University of Texas Health Science Center
Houston, Texas
USA

James D. Geyer, MD
Clinical Associate Professor
Neurology and Sleep Medicine, College of Community
  Health Sciences
The University of Alabama
Tuscaloosa, Alabama
USA

Camilo R. Gomez, MD
Neurologist
Alabama Neurological Institute
Birmingham, Alabama
USA

Mark P. Gorman, MD
Instructor
Neurology
Harvard Medical School
Boston, Massachusetts
USA

Ikram Ul Haque, MD
Associate Professor and Division Head
Pediatric Critical Care Medicine
University of Texas Health Science Center at Houston
Houston, Texas
USA

Marvin B. Harper
Associate Professor
Pediatrics
Harvard Medical School
Boston, Massachusetts
USA

Juan Idiaquez, MD
Professor of Neurology
Neurology
Universidad de Valparaiso
Valparaiso
Chile

Sarah M. Kranick, MD
Instructor
Neurology
University of Pennsylvania
Philadelphia, Pennsylvania
USA

Jeffrey R. Leonard, MD
Assistant Professor
Neurological Surgery
Washington University
St. Louis, Missouri
USA

Daniel J. Licht, MD
Assistant Professor
Pediatrics, Division of Neurology
The Children's Hospital of Philadelphia
Philadelphia, Pennsylvania
USA

Zhao Liu, MD, PhD
Assistant Professor
Division of Pediatric Neurology
Departments of Pediatrics and Neurology
University of Florida College of Medicine
Gainesville, Florida
USA

Michael Lynn, MD
Resident Physician
Neurological Surgery
University of Florida
Gainesville, Florida
USA

Thomas H. Mareci, PhD
Professor
Department of Biochemistry and Molecular Biology
University of Florida McKnight Brain Institute
Gainesville, Florida
USA

Gregory J. A. Murad, MD
Assistant Professor
Department of Neurosurgery
University of Florida
Gainesville, Florida
USA

Troy Payne, MD
Director of Sleep Medicine
Sleep Medicine
CentraCare Health System
St. Cloud, Minnesota
USA

Alan K. Percy, MD
Professor
Pediatrics, Neurology, Neurobiology, and Genetics
University of Alabama at Birmingham
Birmingham, Alabama
USA

David W. Pincus, MD, PhD
Associate Professor
Neurosurgery
University of Florida
Gainesville, Florida
USA

Jose A. Pineda, MD
Assistant Professor
Pediatrics and Neurology
Washington University School of Medicine
St. Louis, Missouri
USA

Scott L. Pomeroy, MD, PhD
Bronson Crothers Professor
Neurology
Harvard Medical School
Boston, Massachusetts
USA

Daniel C. Potts, MD
Assistant Professor
Neurology
The University of Alabama School of Medicine,
  College of Community Health Sciences
Tuscaloosa, Alabama
USA

Deborah M. Ringdahl, ARNP, MSN
Clinical Case Manager
Nursing
Shands Children's Hospital
Gainesville, Florida
USA

Ronald C. Sanders Jr., MD, MS
Associate Professor
Pediatrics
UAMS/Arkansas Children's Hospital
Little Rock, Arkansas
USA

Harvey B. Sarnat, MS, MD, FRCPC
Professor
Pediatrics, Pathology (Neuropathology), Clinical
  Neurosciences
University of Calgary Faculty of Medicine
Calgary, Alberta
Canada

Matthew Saxonhouse, MD
Assistant Professor
Division of Neonatology
Department of Pediatrics
University of Florida College of Medicine
Gainesville, Florida
USA

Anne-Marie Slinger-Constant, MD, FAAP
Clinical Assistant Professor
Multidiciplinary Teaching Program
Division of Pediatric Neurology
Department of Pediatrics
University of Florida College of Medicine
Gainesville, Florida
USA

Amy A. Smith, MD
Assistant Professor and Program Director
Pediatric Hematology
University of Florida
Gainesville, Florida
USA

David V. Smullen, MD
Attending
Radiology and Neuroradiology
University of Florida
Gainesville, Florida
USA

Christie Garzon Snively, ARNP
Nurse Practitioner
Pediatric Neurology
Shands at the University of Florida
Gainesville, Florida
USA

Sachin S. Talathi, PhD
Research Assistant Professor
Department of Biomedical Engineering
University of Florida College of Engineering
Gainesville, Florida
USA

Harrison C. Walker, MD
Assistant Professor
Neurology
University of Alabama at Birmingham
Birmingham, Alabama
USA

David K. Wallace, MD, MPH
Associate Professor
Ophthalmology and Pediatrics
Duke University Medical Center
Durham, North Carolina
USA

Ray L. Watts, MD
John N.Whitaker Professor and Chairman
Neurology
University of Alabama at Birmingham
Birmingham, Alabama
USA

Michael Weiss, MD
Associate Professor
Pediatrics
University of Florida
Gainesville, Florida
USA

Charles A. Williams, MD
Professor
Pediatrics
University of Florida College of Medicine
Gainesville, Florida
USA

Maria Wojtalewicz, PhD.
Assistant Scholar
Pediatrics
University of Florida
Gainesville, Florida
USA

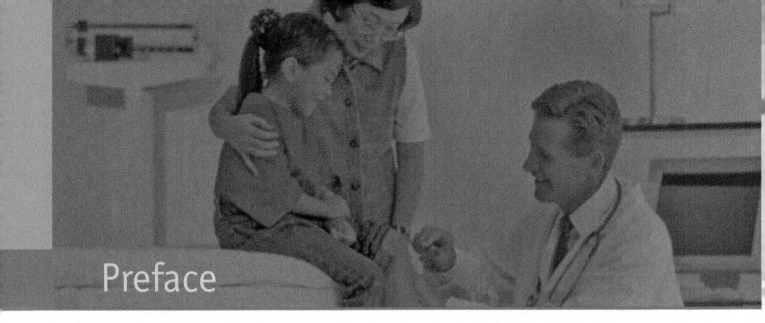

Preface

Neurological, developmental, behavioral, and psychiatric disorders during infancy, childhood, and adolescence are some of the most frequent and challenging problems seen in clinical practice; however, house staff, pediatricians, neurologists, psychiatrists, family physicians, nurses, and psychologists report considerable difficulty in managing the most common child neurological conditions, and promptly refer patients to the pediatric neurologist. In the last decade, significant diagnostic and therapeutic advances have been made for a number of conditions such as epilepsy, sleep disorders, headache, learning disorders, metabolic disorders, brain tumors, autism, tics, and movement disorders. Since office practice is demanding and fast-paced, practitioners must have access to current evaluations and treatment recommendations in a format that lends itself to speedy review and retention, and increases their confidence as principal care providers.

The goal of *Pediatric Practice: Neurology* is to write a comprehensive and current text, and provide primary care providers and neurologists with succinct authoritative reviews on the evaluation and treatment of a complete list of common and less common child brain disorders. The book is designed to meet the busy demands of a wide range of readers, including physicians from all pediatric specialties, resident house staff, child and adult neurologists, clinical laboratory technicians, and students.

The first section of the book, Evaluation, reviews the pediatric neurology history and neurological examination and neuroimaging in the management of pediatric neurological disease. The second section of the book, Common Pediatric Neurologic Problems, reviews seizures and epilepsy, febrile seizures, paroxysmal disorders, pediatric headache, ataxia, abnormalities of head size, attention-deficit/hyperactivity disorder, learning and language disorders, cerebral palsy, and pediatric sleep medicine. In the third section, General Neurologic Disorders, we review the evaluation and treatment of movement and balance disorders, neuropathy, disorders of muscle and motor function, neuroinfectious diseases, multiple sclerosis and white matter disorders, stroke, traumatic brain injury, toxic and metabolic encephalopathies, genetic testing for neurological disorders, metabolic disorders, inherited neurodegenerative disorders, brain tumors, malformations of the nervous system in relation to ontogenesis, autism, newborn neurology, disorders of vision and ocular motility, the floppy infant syndrome, and coma. In summary, this book strives to efficiently provide practical state-of-the-art pediatric neurological advice to the busy physician.

Paul R. Carney and James D. Geyer

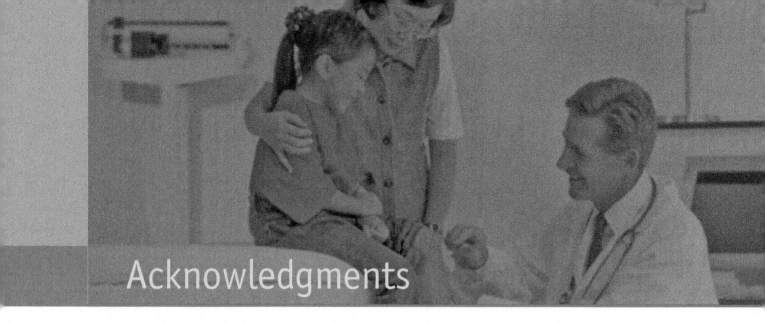

Acknowledgments

The editors would like to thank the patients and their families who helped make this book possible. We would also like to thank Anne Sydor and Alyssa Fried of McGraw Hill for their excellent editorial support and guidance on this project. We extend our gratitude to the authors for their willingness to share their knowledge and expertise. Finally, a special thanks to Senior Project Manager Rajni Pisharody for her superb editing of the book and patient guidance throughout the project.

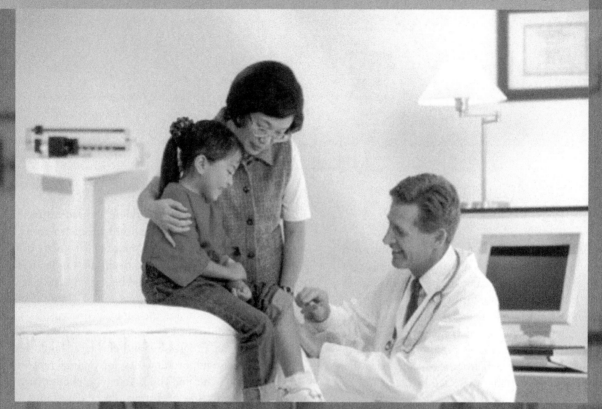

Evaluation

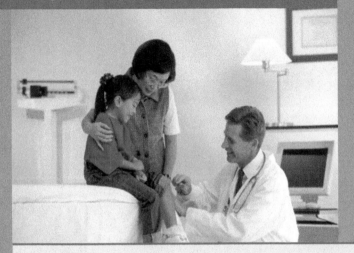

CHAPTER 1

History and Examination

Paul R. Carney and James D. Geyer

HISTORY

Children who present with neurological problems or developmental abnormalities on general physical examination should undergo a complete neurological assessment.[1,2] Initially, as much information as possible from the parents or caregivers should be obtained during the first visit. During the initial clinical encounter, the examiner should formulate an opinion regarding possible causes (Table 1-1). A *diagnostic hypothesis* can then be confirmed, supported, or rejected by the neurological and physical examinations, laboratory tests, and other tests. A clear *chief complaint* is probably one of the most important first steps, and is best elicited from the child, parents, or caretakers. It is common that school-age children may often provide their own chief complaint. The chief complaint should represent the exact words or expression of the child or parent and not a reinterpretation of the symptoms by the physician.

Ideally, the child or parent should be allowed to freely tell the story without interruption or distractions. However, brief directed questions can help focus the interview, especially if the history begins to wander. It is important to note that one should be certain that interrupting will not result in suppression or skewing of important information and the parent's concerns.

Information related to the timing of the onset of symptoms (acute, progressive, and chronic) should be obtained. It is also important to develop optimal *rapport* with both the parents and child. An environment that is both child friendly, free of distractions, and age appropriate will help to facilitate an ambience of ease for both child and parent. Parents are quick to pick up on a hurried care-provider, so allowing at least 1 hour or more for a new consultation and at least 30 minutes for follow-up visits is important to keep in mind. Additional questions such as precipitating factors or triggers, past or concurrent illnesses, toxic exposures, sick contacts,

Table 1-2.	
Tips for Examining Poorly Cooperative Children[3]	
During history taking	Keep the child next to the parent. Observe the child carefully. Smile, be friendly, and maintain eye contact. Avoid wearing the white laboratory coat. Start interacting with the child
Beginning of interaction	Present a toy or a lollipop. Keep hands off; use observation. Keep the younger child in the mother's lap. Let the parents do the undressing. Try not to show all your tools
During examination	Start with the most relevant system. Be focused. Use your observational skills, starting with gait. Demonstrate some testing on the parents. Leave threatening or painful tests to the end
During procedures	Invite parents to attend. Prepare child and parent for their roles. Use the treatment room, with adequate pain control. Position the child in a comfortable manner. Maintain a calm and positive atmosphere.

From Jan MMS, *Neurological examination of difficult and poorly cooperative children. J Child Neurol. 2007;22:1209-1213.*

travel history, and changes in mood or appetite are just some of the other pertinent items that should be obtained. In most cases at this point, the examiner should be able to attempt to develop an initial interpretation of the most likely diagnoses before proceeding to gather more details.

A complete birth history is probably the most important item in the past medical history. Information about the length of pregnancy, complications, use of medication or drugs, and details about the immediate and first days and weeks following birth should be obtained. Prenatal and perinatal events—including duration of labor, route and means of delivery, and Apgar scores—should be obtained. Obtaining developmental milestones is an important reflection of the maturation of the child's nervous system, and assessing development is an essential part of the pediatric neurological assessment. In assessing the child's developmental level, the examiner must know the age when key social, motor, and language skills are normally acquired. There are several screening tools that can be useful for this, such as the Denver Developmental Screening Test II. Delay in obtaining developmental milestones and abnormal patterns of development are important indicators of underlying neurological disease.

When taking a developmental history, key principles of neurodevelopment should be kept in mind. The development of motor control proceeds in a head-to-toe fashion. Head control develops first, then trunk control (sitting), and finally control of the lower extremities (walking). Primitive reflexes (such as the Moro, grasp, and Galant reflexes) are normally present in the term infant and diminish over the next 4 to 6 months of life. The postural reflexes (such as the positive support, Landau, lateral propping, and parachute reflexes) emerge at 3 to 8 months of age. Persistence of primitive reflexes and the lack of development of the postural reflexes are the hallmark of an upper motor neuron abnormality in the infant and should be further investigated.

PHYSICAL EXAMINATION

During the general physical examination (Table 1-2), certain characteristics of the general examination are particularly important to note:

Somatic growth. Measure height and weight, and compare percentiles with head circumference.

Skin. A careful complete skin search is important. Look for the stigmata of the neurocutaneous syndromes such as café au lait or ash leaf lesions, hypopigmentation, or port wine stains.

Dysmorphic features. Carefully make note of the face especially the midface, ears, eye separation, head shape, neck, and extremities.

Eye examination. This part of the exam is often left for last, as children are often uncooperative and it is difficult to clearly observe eye grounds when the child is moving or fails to focus on a distant object.

Abdomen. Palpate for organomegaly, which can indicate the presence of one of the storage diseases or neuroblastoma, for example.

Spine. Look for scoliosis, any sacral anomalies, clefts, dimples, or tufts of hair.

NEUROLOGICAL EXAMINATION

Examination of the nervous system is often deemed by many physicians as one of the most difficult parts of the physical examination. Often, the infant and young child are unable to fully cooperate for the formal neurological examination. Therefore, the examiner must be able to accommodate to the child and his or her developmental level and mood. The first part of the examination is observational, making note of the child's spontaneous movements, how he or she interacts with the parents or caregivers, and spontaneous speech. Initial hands-off careful observation allows for assessment of mental status, cranial nerves, coordination, and motor status. The second part of the examination requires hands-on assessment of cranial nerves, motor and sensory systems, reflexes, and gait. The neurological examination is usually best accomplished if one makes it into a game that engages the child's curiosity and is fun for both the child and examiner. The use of toys can be of great assistance, as these will stimulate the child's imagination and make for a more rewarding experience and accurate exam. The use of finger puppets for coordination testing and saccades, as well as cups, balls, bells, lights, crayons and paper, cubes, and rattles are just a few examples. The last part of the examination is usually reserved for those things that are the most threatening and uncomfortable for the child, such as fundoscopy, otoscopy, undressing the child for a complete examination, or measuring the head circumference.

Head Circumference

An important part of evaluating brain development is measuring the growth of the brain by measuring the head circumference. The head circumference is obtained by placing the measuring tape around the most prominent aspect of the frontal and occipital bones, which forms the occipital-frontal circumference (OFC) measurement. The most accurate measurements are obtained with a plastic tape measure rather than a paper tape measure because the paper can stretch. The brain grows

Table 1-2.

History and Physical Exam

I. History
1. Chief Complaint
   a. Brief statement of primary problem (including duration) that caused family to seek medical attention
2. History of Present Illness
   a. Initial statement identifying the historian, that person's relationship to patient, and their reliability
   b. Age, sex, race, and other important identifying information about patient
   c. Concise chronological account of the illness, including any previous treatment with full description of symptoms (pertinent positives and pertinent negatives). Information relevant to the differential diagnosis of the chief complaint belongs here
3. Past Medical History
   a. Major medical illnesses
   b. Major surgical illnesses: list operations and dates
   c. Trauma: fractures, lacerations
   d. Previous hospital admissions with dates and diagnoses
   e. Current medications
   f. Known allergies (not just drugs)
   g. Immunization status: be specific, not just "up to date"
4. Pregnancy and Birth History
   a. Maternal health during pregnancy: bleeding, trauma, hypertension, fevers, infectious illnesses, medications, drugs, alcohol, smoking, rupture of membranes
   b. Gestational age at delivery
   c. Labor and delivery: length of labor, fetal distress, type of delivery (vaginal, cesarean section), use of forceps, anesthesia, breech delivery
   d. Neonatal period: Apgar scores, breathing problems, use of oxygen, need for intensive care, hyperbilirubinemia, birth injuries, feeding problems, length of stay, birth weight
5. Developmental History
   a. Ages at which milestones were achieved and current developmental abilities: smiling, rolling, sitting alone, crawling, walking, running, first word, toilet training, riding tricycle, etc.
   b. School: present grade, specific problems, interaction with peers
   c. Behavior: enuresis, temper tantrums, thumb sucking, pica, nightmares, etc.
   d. Feeding history
6. Review of Systems
7. Family History
   a. Illnesses: cardiac disease, hypertension, stroke, diabetes, cancer, abnormal bleeding, allergy and asthma, epilepsy
   b. Mental retardation, congenital anomalies, chromosomal problems, growth problems, consanguinity, ethnic background
8. Social environment
   a. Living situation and conditions: daycare, safety issues
   b. Composition of family
   c. Occupation of parents

II. Physical Examination
1. General Approach
   a. Gather as much data as possible by observation first
   b. Position of child: parent's lap vs. exam table
   c. Stay at the child's level as much as possible. Do not tower!
   d. Order of exam: least distressing to most distressing
   e. Rapport with child
   f. Include child: explain to the child's level
   g. Distraction is a valuable tool
   h. Examine painful area last: get general impression of overall attitude
   i. Understand impact of developmental stage on child's response
   j. Assess level of consciousness, mental status, and ability to cooperate; nutritional and hydration status, and signs of toxicity
2. Vital signs (resting heart rate, respirations, blood pressure, temperature, body weight, length or height, and head circumference)
   a. Obtain accurate weight, height, and OFC
3. Skin and Lymphatics
   a. Birthmarks: nevi, hemangiomas, mongolian spots, rashes, petechiae, desquamation, pigmentation, jaundice, texture, turgor

(continued)

Table 1-2. (*Continued*)

History and Physical Exam

4. Head
   a. Size and shape
   b. Fontanelle(s)
   c. Tension: supine and sitting up
   d. Sutures: overriding
   e. Scalp and hair
5. Eyes: stabismus, slant of palpebral fissure, hypertelorism or telecanthus, EOM, pupils, conjunctiva, sclera, cornea, red reflex, visual fields
6. Ears: position of ears, hearing
7. Nose: nasal septum, discharge, sinus tenderness
8. Mouth, throat, neck: lips (color, fissures), gag reflex, tonsils (size, color, exudates), palate (intact, arch), teeth and gums (number, condition), posterior pharyngeal wall (color, bulging)
9. Lungs and thorax: intercostal retractions, breathing pattern, hyper/hypoventilation and breathing regularity, stridor, air exchange, rales
10. Cardiovascular: heart rate and rhythm, murmurs, thrills, and bruits
11. Abdomen: tenderness and pain, bowel sounds, masses, fluid collections and tumors, hepatomegaly and spelenomegaly
12. Musculoskeletal: joint tenderness or erythema, increased or decreased tone, axial slippage to ventral and vertical suspension, atrophy, hypertrophy especially of calf, hammer toes, high arches, Gower sign, strength, pronator drift, scoliosis, and spine dimples or lumbar hair tufts
13. Back
    a. Sacral dimple
    b. Kyphosis, lordosis, or scoliosis
    c. Joints: motion, stability, swelling, tenderness
    d. Muscles
    e. Extremities
       ■ Deformity
       ■ Symmetry
       ■ Edema
       ■ Clubbing
14. Gait
    a. In-toeing, out-toeing
    b. Bow legs, knock knee
    c. "Physiologic" bowing is frequently seen under 2 years of age and will spontaneously resolve
    d. Limp
    e. Hips
    f. Ortolani and Barlow signs

III. Neurological Examination
1. Mental status
2. Cranial nerves
3. Muscle tone and strength
4. Sensation
5. Cerebellum
6. Infant reflexes
7. Deep tendon reflexes

to 80% of its adult volume during the first 2 years of life, so many neurological diseases that occur early in life will impact the growth of the brain. A small head (microcephaly) or a large head (macrocephaly or hydrocephalus) can be key findings in explaining neurological abnormalities of a child. It is essential to plot head circumference for girls and boys on a standardized head growth chart for the appropriate sex (Figures 1-1 and 1-2).[4] Also, palpate the sutures and outline the anterior and posterior fontanels. Posterior fontanels close by 6 weeks. Anterior fontanels close by 12 to 14 months, and sutures close by 3 to 4 years.[5–7]

CDC Growth Charts: United States

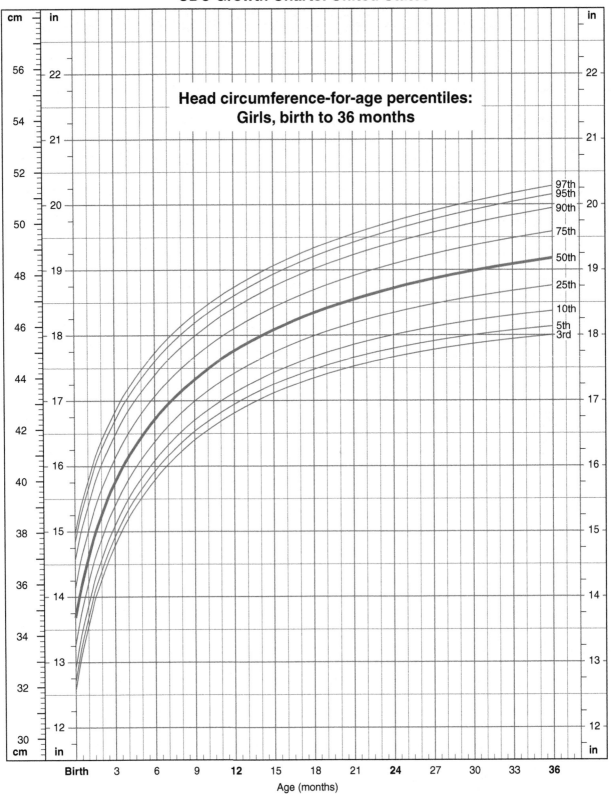

FIGURE 1-1 ■ Head circumference-for-age percentiles: Girls, birth to 36 months. *(From CDC Growth Charts: United States.)*

CDC Growth Charts: United States

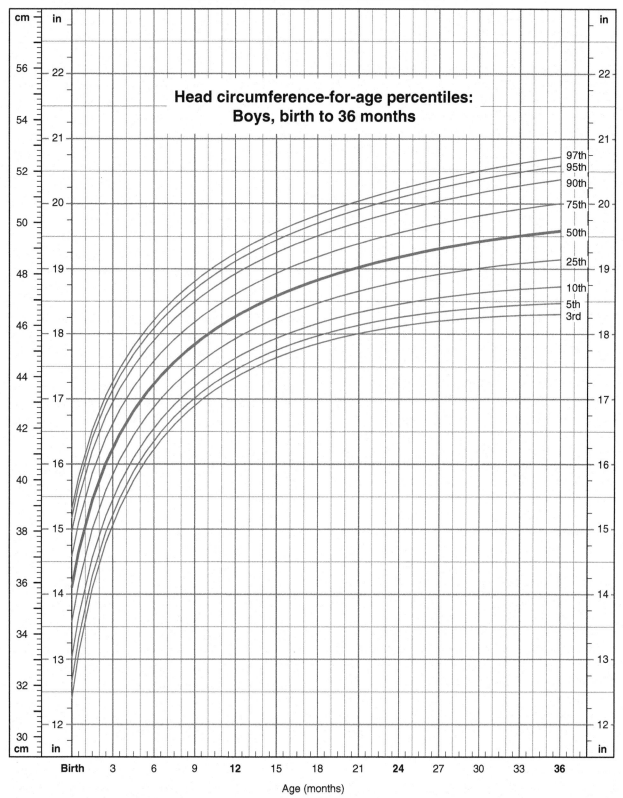

**Head circumference-for-age percentiles:
Boys, birth to 36 months**

Age (months)

FIGURE 1-2 ■ Head circumference-for-age percentiles: Boys, birth to 36 months. *(From CDC Growth Charts: United States.)*

Mental Status

In the acutely ill child, the level of consciousness is the most important part of the neurological examination. Alterations in the level of consciousness, as during an infectious process such as meningitis or encephalitis, will often be the first manifestation of illness. The mental status can be assessed by noting the child's spontaneous activities as you enter the room, such as talking or sleeping. Sometimes a stimulus is required to awaken the patient, such as calling his or her name, or gently pinching the arm. Seeing how the child reacts once you stop stimulation should be taken into account. The child may be observed for clear speech and making sense while talking. Orientation to person, place, and time should be determined, and age-appropriate tests for memory might include immediate (digit span forwards and backwards), short-term (food for breakfast), and long-term (name of teacher, friend, or school) memory. One of the best times to examine a baby is between feeds. If interrupted during a feed, the baby may cry excessively, limiting the examination. If examined immediately after a feed, the baby may be too sleepy to obtain an optimal examination. Observation of the newborn's spontaneous eye opening, movements of the face and extremities, and response to stimulation are essential for the mental status examination. Arousal is defined by the duration of eye opening and spontaneous movement of the face and extremities. Before 28 weeks gestation, the newborn states of wakefulness and sleep are difficult to distinguish. As the newborn matures, there is increasing duration, frequency, and quality of alertness.

At 12 months of age, most children imitate activities, wave bye-bye, and play pat-a-cake. They can follow simple commands, especially if the desired action is demonstrated. They feed themselves finger foods. They usually have one or two meaningful words, usually "mama" and "dada." At 18 months, most children have a vocabulary of 10 or more words and will use single words to indicate wants. They should be able to point to at least two of the pictures from the Denver II assessment tool, and can name at least two body parts. Between 18 and 30 months the toddler should learn to identify 6 to 8 body parts, and at 2.5 years of age, the child should be able to build a tower six to eight blocks high. By 3 years of age, a child should be able to draw a circle, and at 4 years of age, copy a cross.

Cranial Nerves

The cranial nerves (CN) can usually be reliably tested provided that the child is cooperative and at ease. The evaluation of CN I (olfactory nerve) can be reliably tested only if the nasal cavity is unobstructed and free of mucus. The common cold is usually the most frequent cause of impaired olfaction. Each nostril should be tested separately by presenting a non-irritating odor such as cinnamon, cloves, or lavender. Cranial nerves II and III can be tested by the pupillary reflex, which appears consistently at 32 to 35 weeks gestation. A 28-week infant will blink to light shone into the eyes, testing CN II and VII. Beginning at 34 weeks of gestation, an infant will be able to fix and follow on an object, thus testing CN II, III, IV, and VI. Spontaneous roving eye movements and dysconjugate eye movements not fixing on an object are common in the term infant. Another maneuver to test eye movements is to hold the baby by the axillae and rotate the infant from side to side to test the oculovestibular reflex. Not only does this test acuity in the duration of the postrotational nystagmus, but also the integrity of the vestibular system.

The key to seeing the optic disc is the child's visual fixation at a point straight ahead and 15 degrees up. Have the young child fixate on the mother, who often needs to be exceptionally animated in order to get the child's attention. The optic discs and macula and general appearance of the retina and retinal vessels should be evaluated. Disc sharpness refers to the sharpness of the distinction between the yellow optic disc and the pink retina. Disc flatness refers to whether or not the optic disc is mounded up where it comes out of the retina. When the disc is elevated, the vessels may be noted to course downwards as they traverse over the optic disc. While acute papilledema may take 48 hours or more to manifest itself, the first sign is usually loss of spontaneous venous pulsations. Their presence is reassuring that there is probably no significant elevation of intracranial pressure at this moment. This does not mean that there is no serious intracranial pathology, or that there will not be signs and symptoms of raised pressure later. Note that spontaneous venous pulsations may not be detected in many normal patients. One should be aware that multiple small areas of retinal hemorrhages can be present in 20% to 40% of normal vaginally delivered infants, which generally resolve within 1 to 2 weeks.

Facial sensation (CN V) is tested with light pinprick and by observing facial grimace or change in sucking. Facial symmetry and movement should be observed in both the quiet state and during active movement (such as crying). Hearing (CN VIII) can be grossly tested with a bell, keeping in mind that a ringing bell within an isolette can be quite loud and generate 90 dB. If a hearing deficit is suspected, then formal audiometric or brainstem evoked potentials should be performed by a specialist. Often, the newborn may have a very subtle response to auditory stimuli and respond with only a blink. To test CN V, VII, and XII, the newborn can be observed sucking on a pacifier. This can also be used to evaluate CN IX and X, which are tested when the child swallows. As the brainstem matures, coordination improves by the 32nd to 34th week. Palpation of the sternocleidomastoid (CN XI) may be difficult in the newborn or young child, but may be facilitated by extending the head on the side of the bed with the infant in a supine position. Now the bulk of the muscle can be palpated as the head is turned to the side. Cranial nerve XII is mainly responsible for movement of the tongue and may be tested by having the child stick out the tongue and speak.

Motor Examination and Balance

Evaluation of the motor system includes assessment of muscle bulk, tone, strength, stretch reflexes, and whether a plantar response (Babinski sign) is extensor or flexor (Table 1-3). They should always be symmetric, but can be present or absent up to 1 year of age. Assessment of the muscle strength of infants is primarily limited to inspection. Observation of the resting posture can reveal the symmetry and maturity of the passive tone. It is important to keep the head midline to avoid asymmetries in tone related to the asymmetric tonic neck reflex (Table 1-4).

Flexor tone or resistance to passive movement usually develops first in the lower extremities and proceeds cephalad. A 28-week infant will lie with minimally flexed limbs and have minimal resistance to passive movement of all extremities. At 32 weeks, the newborn develops flexor tone at the hips and knees, with some resistance to manipulation of the lower extremities. This progression correlates with increasing myelination of the subcortical motor pathways originating in the brainstem. By 36 weeks, the infant develops flexion at the elbows, and by term, the infant is flexed in all extremities.

For a term newborn, the resting posture is flexion of the extremities with the extremities closely adducted to the trunk. After the first few days of life, the extremities are still predominantly in the flexed position, but they are not as tightly adducted as they are in the first 48 hours of life. The tone of the shoulder girdle is assessed by taking the baby's hand and pulling the hand to the opposite shoulder like a scarf. The hand should not go past the shoulder, and the elbow should not cross the midline of the chest. Arm recoil tests tone and action of the biceps. The arms are held in flexion against the chest for a few seconds, and then are quickly extended and released. The arms should spring back to the flexed position. The hypotonic infant will have slow incomplete recoil. Asymmetry to this response with lack of recoil would be seen with Erb or brachial plexus palsy. Arm traction is done with the baby in the supine position. The wrist is grasped and the arm is pulled until the shoulder is slightly off the mat. There should be some flexion maintained at the elbow. Full extension at the elbow is seen in hypotonia. Assessing motor function of the upper extremities begins with passive range of motion. Each extremity is rotated at the shoulder, elbow, and wrist, feeling for resistance and the range of movement. Too much resistance reflects hypertonia, while too little resistance indicates hypotonia.

Rubbing the ulnar aspect of the hand or touching the dorsum of the hand will often cause extension of the fingers. A newborn infant's hand is held in a fisted position with the fingers flexed over the thumb. The hand should open intermittently and should not always be held in a tight-fisted position. Over the first 1 to 2 months of life, the infant's hand becomes more open. Persistence of a fisted hand is a sign of an upper

Table 1-3.

Normal Major Developmental Milestones

Age (months)	Motor Development	Language	Adaptive Behavior
4–6	Head lift from prone position	Cries	Smiles
4	No head lag when pulled to sitting position	Sounds of pleasure	Smiles, laughs aloud
5	Voluntary grasp with both hands	"Ah, goo"	Smiles at self
6	Grasps with one hand; rolls, sits with support	Increasing sounds	Food preference
8	Sits with support; transfers objects with hands; rolls from supine to prone positions	Combines syllables	Responds to "no"
10	Creeps, stands holding, finger-thumb apposition in picking up objects	Increasing sounds	Waves "bye-bye," plays "peek-a-boo"
12	Stands holding, walks with support	Says 2 to 3 words with cueing	Acknowledges names of objects
15	Walks alone	Several words	Points, imitates
18	Walks up and down stairs	Many well-understood words	Follows simple commands
24	Runs	2- to 3-word phrases	Points to body parts

	28 Weeks	32 Weeks	34 Weeks	40 Weeks	Red Flags
Mental status	Needs gentle rousing to awaken	Opens eyes spontaneously; sleep-wake cycles apparent	N/A	At 36 wk ↑alertness, cries when awake	Irritable or lethargic infant
Cranial nerves					
Pupils	Blinks to light	Consistent pupillary reflex	Fix and follow	N/A	N/A
Hearing	Pauses, no orientation to sound	N/A	N/A	Head + eyes turn to sound	No response to auditory stimulus
Suck + swallow	Weak suck, no synchrony with swallow	Stronger suck, better synchrony with swallow		Coordinated suck + swallow at 37 wk	"Chomp suck" clamps down on pacifier but no suck (bulbar dysfunction)
Motor	Minimally flexed	Flexed hips and knees	↑ Flexion at hips + knees	Flexed in all extremities	Hypotonia Hypertonia 28-wk infant with jerky movements Full-term infant with writhing movements
Reflexes					
Moro	Weak, incomplete hand opening	Complete extension + abduction	N/A	Full Moro (with ant. flexion)	Asymmetry
ATNR*	N/A	N/A	N/A	ATNR appears at 35 wk.	If obligatory or sustained, suggests pyramidal or extrapyramidal motor abnormal
Palmar grasp	Present but weak	N/A	Grasp stronger	Strong grasp, able to be lifted out of bed	Fixed obligate grasp (suggests B hemispheric dysfunction)

Table 1-4.

Neurological Examination Summary with Respect to Gestational Age.

*ATNR = asymmetric tonic neck reflex

motor neuron lesion in an infant and is often referred to as a "cortical thumb." The popliteal angle is an assessment of the tone of the hamstring muscles. It is done one leg at a time. The thigh is flexed on the abdomen with one hand and then the other hand straightens the leg by pushing on the back of the ankle until there is firm resistance to the movement. The angle between the thigh and the leg is typically about 90 degrees. Extension of the leg beyond 90 to 120 degrees is seen in hypotonia. The strength and tone of the neck extensors can be tested by having the infant in sitting position and neck flexed so the baby's chin is on the chest. The infant should be able to bring the head to the upright position. The neck flexors can be tested by having the head in extension while in the sitting position. The infant should be able to bring the head to the upright position. These tests are an extension of the test for head lag, and are done at the same time. In the prone position, the baby should be able to extend the neck to the point where the head can be turned side to side. When the arms are extended by the side of the trunk, the baby should be able to bring them forward into a flexed position. Ventral suspension is a good way to assess a baby's neck and trunk tone. The infant is placed in the prone position, suspended in the air by the hand placed under the chest. The infant's head position, back, and extremities are observed. The head should stay in the same plane as the back. The back should show some resistance to gravity and not be simply draped over the hand on the chest. Finally, for the vertical suspension maneuver, the examiner holds the infant in the upright position with feet off the ground by placing the hands under the arms and around the chest. The infant should be suspended in this position without slipping through the hands of the examiner.

In toddlers and older children, strength may be tested by having the child push and pull against the physician's hands with his or her arms and legs. The child may be asked to squeeze fingers or hop, skip, or jump. Pronator drift is a sensitive test for upper motor neuron weakness, which can detect weakness missed on manual motor testing. The child extends the arms palms down with eyes closed, and a few seconds later, the child turns the arms palms up. During this turning maneuver, a child with upper motor neuron weakness may pull the elbow down and in, or drift toward a pronator position. Finally, observe the arm position when the palms are up. During this maneuver, the eyes should remain closed. Observe for any asymmetric pronation, drift, or finger flexion. Mild symptoms may be provoked by asking the patient to shake the head "no." Manual motor testing can usually be done with children starting around 5 years of age. Test flexion and extension at each joint. In a central lesion, the weakest muscles will be the extensors in the upper extremities and the flexors in the lower extremities. For the lower extremities, the great toe extensor and ankle dorsiflexors are the best screening tests for upper motor neuron lesions. Muscle weakness can best be detected if the muscles are tested at mechanical disadvantage. For example, test the triceps starting with the elbow flexed, and then asking the patient to push away. Functional motor tests, such as getting up from the ground, using stairs, and gait testing, have several uses. First, they may be the best way to pick up proximal weakness, as seen in myopathies. Second, they may be the only way to gain the cooperation of younger children. Third, functional tests can often be used as developmental landmarks. These include the parachute (child puts arms out when tilted forward by 12 months age), and then the wheelbarrow. Asymmetry of these reflexes may indicate focal weakness.

Balance is evaluated by having the older child stand with eyes closed while being gently pushed to one side or the other. Joints may also be checked simply by passive (performed by the physician) and active (performed by the child) movement. In younger children, balance is assessed by having the infant or young child reach out and pick up an object and bring it to his or her mouth.

Right versus left hand preference before 1 year of age is always abnormal and indicates a motor deficit in the nonpreferred hand. At 5 to 6 months, the child should be able to transfer an object from hand to hand, and grasp objects that are the size of a one-inch cube. A thumb-finger pincer grasp develops at 7 to 9 months. Independent sitting is usually accomplished by 6 to 8 months, and independent walking is achieved between 11 and 15 months of age. An infant is delayed if he or she is not walking by 16 months.

Sensory Examination

The sensory examination is performed using light touch and mild pinprick. Emphasis should be placed on dermatomal evaluation of the lower extremities—for example, the sacral region in a child with a neural tube defect. Assessment of sensation can be made by using the sharp end of a wooden cotton applicator on the face and observing the facial grimace or change in state of the infant. In older children, touch the child's legs, arms, or other parts of the body and have him or her identify the sensation (eg, hot/cold, sharp/dull).

Reflexes

Reflexes in the older child can be easily elicited in the biceps, triceps, brachioradialis, knees, and ankles. Cross adductor responses and unsustained clonus are common and normal in the newborn and infant up until 1 year of age.

Infant reflexes

In newborns and infants, reflexes called infant reflexes or primitive reflexes are good indicators of normal or abnormal brain development. Each of these reflexes appears and disappears at a certain age as the infant develops. Examples of infant primitive reflexes are as follows:

1. *Blinking.* The infant will close the eyes in response to bright lights.
2. *Babinski reflex.* As the infant's foot is stroked, the toes will extend upward.
3. *Moro reflex.* Best elicited by dropping the head in relation to the body, into the examiner's hands. A quick change in the infant's position will cause the infant to throw the arms outward, open the hands, and throw back the head.
4. *Asymmetric tonic neck reflex.* Elicited by rotating the head to one side, with subsequent elbow extension to the side the head is turned, and elbow flexion on the side of the occiput. At 6 months of age most infants lose the Moro reflex and the asymmetric tonic neck reflex. Persistence of either one of these primitive reflexes would be abnormal.
5. *Galant reflex.* Obtained by placing the baby in ventral suspension, then stroking the skin on one side of the back. The baby's trunk and hips should swing towards the side of the stimulus.
6. *Palmar and plantar grasp.* Elicited by stimulating the palm with an object. The palmar grasp is present at 28 weeks gestation, strong at 32 weeks, and is strong enough at 37 weeks to lift the baby off the bed. This reflex disappears at 2 months of age with the development of a voluntary grasp.

7. *Startle reflex.* A loud noise will cause the infant to extend and flex the arms while the hands remain in a fist.

8. *Placing reflex.* The infant is held under the axilla in an upright position, and the dorsal aspect of the foot is brushed against a tabletop. The infant's hip and knee will flex, and the infant will appear to take a step. This reflex is useful if asymmetry occurs and may indicate a lesion in the basal ganglia, brainstem, or spinal cord. However, performing this reflex can be limited by the constraints of the isolette, endotracheal tube, or multiple lines.

9. *Landau reflex.* When the infant is suspended by the examiner's hand in the prone position, the head will extend above the plane of the trunk. The Landau reflex is an important postural reflex and should develop by 4 to 5 months of age. The development of postural reflexes is essential for independent sitting and walking.

10. *Parachute reflex.* When the baby is turned face down towards the mat, the arms will extend as if the baby is trying to catch himself or herself. The parachute reflex is the last of the postural reflexes to develop. It usually appears at 8 to 9 months of age.

Cerebellar functions and gait

Rapid alternating movements may be clumsy with either cerebellar or upper motor neuron disorders. Each side should be tested independently. Cerebellar functions should be assessed with finger to nose, heel to shin, and Rhomberg maneuvers. Casual walking and heel-to-toe walking are best performed if the child is asked to walk towards the parent or caregiver. If the parent extends arms out, then the child will also put out his or her arms, eliciting a type of drift test.

REFERENCES

1. Fishman MA. *Pediatric Neurology.* Orlando: Grune & Strutton; 1986:1.

2. Swaiman KF, Ashwal S, Ferriero DM. *Pediatric Neurology: Principles and Practice.* 4th ed. St. Louis, MI: Mosby; 2006.

3. Jan MMS. Neurological examination of difficult and poorly cooperative children. *J Child Neurol.* 2007;22:1209-1213.

4. Nellhaus G. Head circumference from birth to eighteen years: practical composite international and interracial graphs. *Pediatrics.* 1968;41:106-114.

5. Schott JM, Rossor MN. The grasp and other primitive reflexes. *J Neurol Neurosurg Psychiatry.* 2003;74:558.

6. Volpe JJ. Neurological evaluation. In: Volpe JJ, ed. *Neurology of the Newborn.* 4th ed. Philadelphia: Saunders; 2001: 103-133.

7. Painter MJ. Neurological evaluation of newborns, infants, and older children. In: Albright AL, Pollack IF, Adelson PD, eds. *Principles and Practice of Pediatric Neurosurgery.* New York: Thieme; 1999:3-19.

CHAPTER 2

Neuroimaging in the Management of Neurological Disease

James D. Geyer, Camilo R. Gomez, Daniel C. Potts, Thomas Mareci, and Paul R. Carney

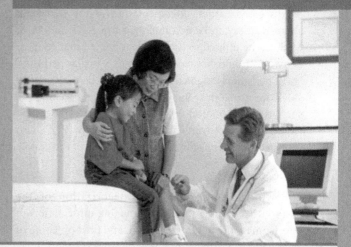

BACKGROUND AND RATIONALE

Advances in imaging technology have played a key role in the progress made over the last two decades in the treatment of patients with neurological disease, facilitating the identification, classification, and documentation of the different pathologic processes that constitute the subspecialty fields of neurology. As such, neuroimaging is an integral part of both the training and practice of this specialty, with many subspecialists spending a considerable portion of their time in the application of imaging techniques for the diagnosis and treatment of their patients.

Purpose of Imaging: Task-Oriented Choices

The most practical approach to a discussion of the application of neuroimaging techniques in neurological care is to first address the tasks, diagnostic or therapeutic, that require their utilization. From this perspective, the clinical scenarios in which imaging techniques are likely to be needed must be assessed along the following lines:

- What information is being sought, and how quickly is it needed?
- Which of the available imaging techniques is most likely to answer the question being asked?
- How will the information obtained by imaging impact further diagnostic algorithms, the treatment, and the prognosis of the patient?

Based on these considerations, the tasks that require the utilization of imaging during clinical care include initial diagnosis, categorization and therapeutic allocation, imaging of the brain blood vessels, characterization of the pathologic process and its consequences (edema, mass effect, etc.), and assessment of prognosis.

Initial diagnosis

Direct imaging of the brain is necessary in order to assess the status of the tissue. The techniques available to complete this task include computed tomography (CT) and magnetic resonance imaging (MRI). As it will be discussed below, choosing one or the other involves considerations of speed, sensitivity, type of lesion, resource availability, and temporal profile of the event.

Categorization and therapeutic allocation

Once the diagnosis is made, a more precise definition of the condition has enormous therapeutic implications, both immediate and long-term. The same technologic advances described above have extended to improvements in image resolution, with better signal-noise ratios, and a superior definition of the pathologic processes. Furthermore, since the cerebral vasculature is so often implicated in the pathogenic process, imaging of the cerebral arteries and veins becomes an additional dimension in the categorization of these patients.

Imaging of the brain vessels

Imaging of the brain blood vessels is an integral component of the evaluation of stroke, vascular anomalies and in some cases, tumor evaluation (especially in the surgical planning stage). In general, the tests that are available for the completion of this task are divided into two groups: (1) those that are non-invasive (ultrasonic, radiotomographic, and magnetic-based techniques) and (2) those that are invasive (catheterization and angiography). In addition to its diagnostic capabilities, the latter also allows the application of endovascular therapeutic techniques.

Characterization of the process

As discussed earlier, documentation of the structural abnormalities can be accomplished using CT and MRI. MRI can be utilized to further identify the brain connectivity (MRI diffusion tensor imaging), vascular perfusion (MRI perfusion-weighted imaging), and chemical activity (MRI spectroscopy). Nuclear-based imaging techniques, such as single photon emission computed tomography (SPECT) and positron emission tomography (PET), also provide mechanisms for functional imaging of the brain.

Assessment of prognosis

Following identification and categorization of the lesion, it is possible to use the imaging information to approximate the potential outlook and final outcome of each patient. Furthermore, it is often possible to make predictions about the potential benefit of a specific treatment strategy. Clearly, this characteristic of imaging relates to the fact that the existing techniques represent the equivalent of "bedside neuropathology."

NEUROIMAGING TECHNIQUES

Computed Tomography

Every discussion about modern neuroimaging techniques must begin with computed tomography (CT). Its introduction in the 1970s changed the way all neurological diseases are diagnosed and treated. With CT, it became possible to directly look at the brain tissue, and document the damage from a particular lesion. The principles of CT are relatively simple: narrow beams of X-rays are used to rotationally acquire tissue density information in one of several tomographic planes. The raw data acquired over a period of a few minutes is then entered into a computer that reconstructs the tissue sample in two-dimensional tomographic images. At present, fast helical scanning techniques, and powerful reconstruction algorithms, allow even three-dimensional reconstruction of the brain tissue and the brain blood vessels. The images obtained represent a map of the density of tissue in a scale of Hounsfield units (HU, Figure 2-1) that spans between −1000 (the green corresponding to air) and +1000 (the white corresponding to calcium). CT is particularly useful in the urgent evaluation of stroke, trauma, monitoring edema, and the evaluation of calcifications.

CT Angiography

CT angiography is a relatively noninvasive technique that couples helical CT scanning with contrast enhancement to obtain vascular images. It is performed by first obtaining a series of helical axial images following the injection

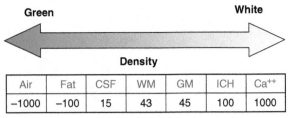

Air	Fat	CSF	WM	GM	ICH	Ca^{++}
−1000	−100	15	43	45	100	1000

Hounsfield units

FIGURE 2-1 ■ Relationship between the various tissues and their corresponding Hounsfield units (HU) in computed tomography (CT). Density increases as HU increases. Note that the HU (and the density of intracranial hemorrhage, ICH) is greater than white matter (WM) and of gray matter (GM). (CSF, cerebrospinal fluid.) *(Reproduced with permission from Geyer J, Potts D, Dillard S, Gomez C. Neuroimaging in the management of stroke patients. In: Geyer J, Gomez CR, eds. Stroke: A Practical Approach. Philadelphia: Lippincott Williams & Wilkins; 2009:167.)*

of iodinated contrast. These are then reconstructed using 1.25-mm thick slices and 0.5- to 1.0-mm increments. This protocol allows three-dimensional rendering of the angiographic images (Figure 2-2). The development of this technique required the introduction of a scanner that allowed the patients to be translated through a continuously rotating gantry, with very rapid data acquisition. The operator controls several variables that determine the protocol to be utilized for each region of interest to be imaged, including duration of the scan, speed of movement of the table, and collimation. As with any other technique, CT angiography has advantages and disadvantages. On one hand, it is not susceptible to flow perturbations and complex flow patterns like magnetic angiography. On the other hand, it utilizes ionizing radiation and iodinated contrast administration, which limits its use in patients with azotemia and contrast allergy, while resulting in a more limited field of view (FOV) per study. The latter is very important, for it requires that the planning and post-processing of the study take into consideration the question being asked. Furthermore, post-processing and three-dimensional rendering typically involve "sculpting out" some of the tissue that surrounds the vessels, based on its density. This process, when not carefully carried out, can conceivably lead to the exclusion of important structures or pathologic findings. Its best application appears to be in the definition of intracranial aneurysms prior to their treatment (Figure 2-3).

Magnetic Resonance Imaging

The utilization of magnetic resonance imaging (MRI) in clinical medicine became widespread during the 1980s. The increased sensitivity of this technique, as compared with CT, for the detection of abnormalities in brain structure made it an immediate candidate for the imaging modality of choice. MRI has allowed the documentation of brain lesions earlier and more precisely, particularly in regions

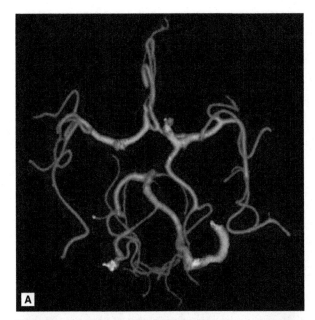

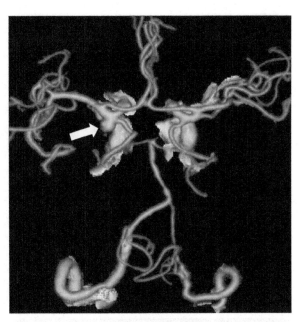

FIGURE 2-3 ■ Use of computed tomographic angiography (CTA) to diagnose aneurysms. Three-dimensional rendering of the CTA clearly identifies a left posterior communicating artery aneurysm (arrow). (Reproduced with permission from Geyer J, Potts D, Dillard S, Gomez C. Neuroimaging in the management of stroke patients. In: Geyer J, Gomez CR, eds. Stroke: A Practical Approach. Philadelphia: Lippincott Williams & Wilkins; 2009:168.)

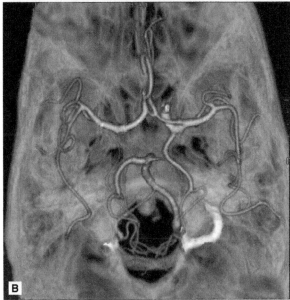

FIGURE 2-2 ■ Three-dimensional rendering of the intracranial arteries using computed tomographic angiography (CTA). The arteries are displayed by themselves in the axial plane (A). It is also possible to display them in the context of the surrounding bony environment (B). (Reproduced with permission from Geyer J, Potts D, Dillard S, Gomez C. Neuroimaging in the management of stroke patients. In: Geyer J, Gomez CR, eds. Stroke: A Practical Approach. Philadelphia: Lippincott Williams & Wilkins; 2009:168.)

that had remained relatively poorly visualized by CT, such as the brainstem. More recently, the introduction of additional MRI sequences has resulted in the ability to image the brain vessels, as well as to study the chemical composition of the tissues being imaged and viability of the tissue.

MRI is particularly well suited to the identification of cerebral edema (increased water content, whether related to tumor, injury, or infarction). Increased tissue signal on T2-weighted, proton density, and fluid-attentuated inversion recovery (FLAIR) images, as well as a less

pronounced drop in signal on T1-weighted sequences, accompanies this pathophysiologic process. These findings are evident in MRI of the chronic infarction shown in Figure 2-4. As opposed to the flow-related findings noted earlier, the parenchymal changes evolve over a period of hours to days.

The MRI appearance of intracranial hemorrhages over time is one of the most interesting subjects in neuroimaging, for it largely depends upon the natural evolution of hemoglobin degradation within the tissue and the strength of the magnetic field (Figure 2-5). Typically, the sequence of conversion from oxyhemoglobin to deoxyhemoglobin, followed by that from deoxyhemoglobin to methemoglobin (first intracellular and then extracellular, as the erythrocytes disappear), and finally to hemosiderin, occur as parts of a continuum that evolves over weeks to months.[1] Hyperacute hemorrhage (ie, a few hours), in the form the oxyhemoglobin, is isointense with the brain parenchyma on T1-weighted spin echo (SE) images, and hyperintense on T2-weighted SE images. After a few hours, the oxyhemoglobin evolves into deoxyhemoglobin within the hematoma (Figure 2-5). The latter predominantly shortens T2, and this leads to low signal on T2-weighted images. After 3 to 4 days, deoxyhemoglobin is progressively converted to methemoglobin, which is a paramagnetic substance that shortens both T1 and T2, although its predominant effect is shortening T1 (Figure 2-5). As a result, at this stage, hematomas display high signal in both

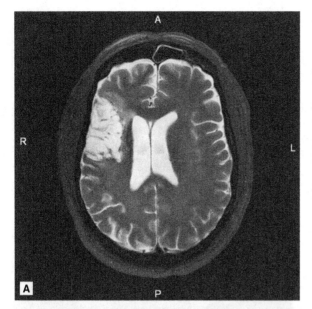

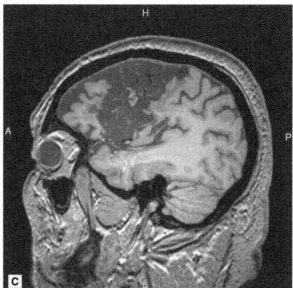

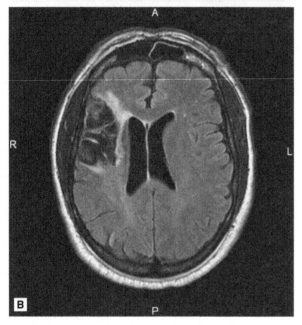

FIGURE 2-4 ■ Appearance of a chronic infarction of a large portion of the right middle cerebral artery on magnetic resonance imaging, using spin-echo (SE) sequences. T2-weighted imaging shows the entire area of infarction as hyperintense **(A)**. Fluid-attenuated inversion recovery (FLAIR) images display a core of low intensity with a margin of high intensity **(B)**. The cystic transformation of the damaged tissue can be greatly appreciated. T1-weighted images show the area as hypointense **(C)**. *(Reproduced with permission from Geyer J, Potts D, Dillard S, Gomez C. Neuroimaging in the management of stroke patients. In: Geyer J, Gomez CR, eds.* Stroke: A Practical Approach. *Philadelphia: Lippincott Williams & Wilkins; 2009:169.)*

T1- and T2-weighted images. Over the next few months, the methemoglobin is slowly broken down into hemichromes that produce only mild T1 shortening. Hematomas at this end stage have a slightly high signal on T1-weighted images, but retain a high signal on the T2-weighted images. Finally, around the periphery of hematomas, macrophage activity results in degradation of the methemoglobin and conversion of the iron moiety to hemosiderin, which shortens T2 and produces a black ring around the hematoma on T2-weighted images. This can be observed within 2 weeks after hemorrhage, and it has a tendency to become thicker over time. In small hematomas (less than 1 cm), the low signal intensity from hemosiderin may essentially occupy the entire ultimate volume of the cavity. The length of time that the

hemosiderin will remain in the area of a hematoma mimics autopsy findings many years after an intracerebral hemorrhage, and it is suspected, using high-field MRI, the hemorrhage can be readily identified over the lifetime of the patient.

Gradient Refocused Echo MRI Techniques

Our discussion above is largely applicable to spin echo (SE) techniques. However, over the last decade, as more knowledge has accumulated about the various methods of applying MRI to clinical practice, sequences that are more sensitive to intracranial hemorrhages have been introduced. In general, different materials vary in their

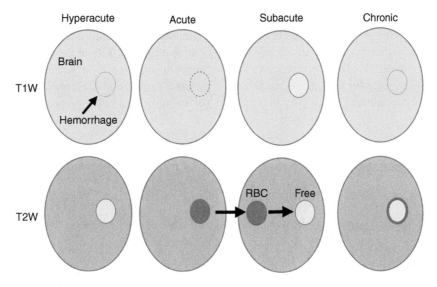

Stage	Hgb	T1W	T2W	Time
Hyperacute	Oxy Hgb	Isointense	Hyperintense	<12 Hours
Acute	Deoxy Hgb	Isointense	Hypointense	1–3 Days
Subacute (Early)	Met Hgb (RBC)	Hyperintense	Hypointense	3–7 Days
Subacute (Late)	Met Hgb (Free)	Hyperintense	Hyperintense	>7 Days
Chronic (Rim)	Hemosiderin	Isointense	Hypointense	>14 Days
Chronic (Center)	Hemichromes	Isointense	Hyperintense	>14 Days
Edema	Not applicable	Hypointense	Hyperintense	1–14 Days

FIGURE 2-5 ■ Schematic representation of the appearance of intracranial hemorrhages at their various stages, when using spin-echo magnetic resonance imaging (MRI) techniques, in terms of their intensity in the images. See the text for an explanation. (T1W, T1 weighted; T2W, T2 weighted; RBC, red blood cells; Hgb, hemoglobin.) *(Reproduced with permission from Geyer J, Potts D, Dillard S, Gomez C. Neuroimaging in the management of stroke patients. In: Geyer J, Gomez CR, eds. Stroke: A Practical Approach. Philadelphia: Lippincott Williams & Wilkins; 2009:170.)*

ability to support magnetic fields within them. This property, known as magnetic susceptibility, is significantly different between some of the hemoglobin breakdown products (deoxyhemoglobin and methemoglobin) and the surrounding brain tissue. Such differences exist because the substances in question have unpaired electrons that superimpose their own magnetic field on the external field. This creates field inhomogeneities that increase magnetic susceptibility artifacts and make these substances stand out against the background tissue.

The presence of magnetic susceptibility artifacts can be emphasized by using techniques that are T2-star (T2*) weighted. As an MRI parameter, T2* is the time constant that describes the decay of transverse magnetization,

taking into account both the inhomogeneities of the static magnetic field, and the spin-spin relaxation of protons in the human body.[2] This interaction results in rapid loss of phase coherence, causing the MRI signal to decrease. The T2* is always less than the T2 time, which is the time of spin-spin relaxation mentioned above, and T2* is a characteristic that will be of benefit when studying intracranial hemorrhage. Because the SE technique uses a refocusing 180-degree RF pulse, the effect of susceptibility on transverse magnetization is removed and the MRI signal is only T2 weighted. However, because the gradient refocused echo (GRE) imaging sequences do not use a refocusing RF pulse, the technique is sensitive to susceptibility differences, which can be controlled by the selection of the echo time. These GRE sequences can be identified by various acronyms used by the different companies to identify them, but fundamentally all rely on the increased susceptibility artifact displayed by intracerebral hemorrhages at nearly any stage, for their rapid detection due to their low signal appearance (Figure 2-6). Indeed, the literature describing the increased sensitivity of GRE techniques for detecting acute intracranial hemorrhages continues to grow, both in the acute and chronic care settings. The latter relates to the ability to detect microhemorrhages in patients with conditions that place them at risk for additional future hemorrhages.

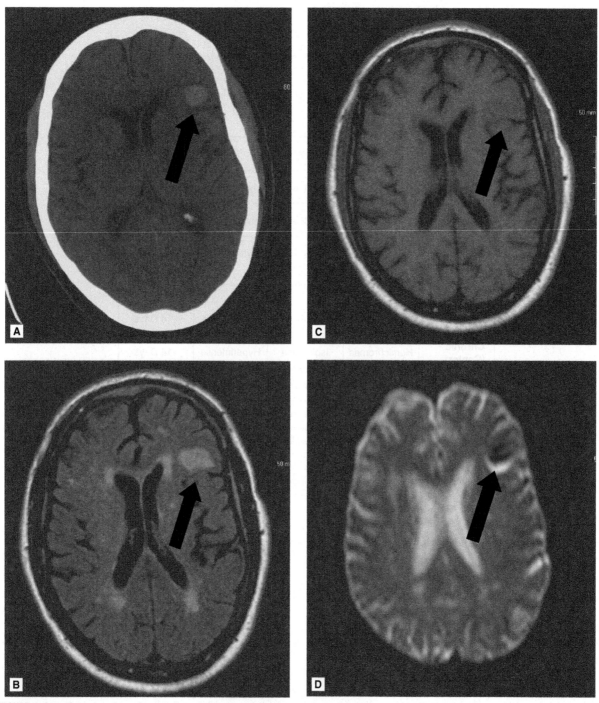

FIGURE 2-6 ■ The appearance of an acute cortical hemorrhage using various types of images. **(A)** Computed tomography (CT) clearly shows the hemorrhage as an area of increased density (*arrow*). **(B)** Magnetic resonance imaging (MRI) using a FLAIR sequence clearly shows the hemorrhage (*arrow*) but does not allow its differentiation from other chronic ischemic lesions. **(C)** T1-weighted SE imaging does not clearly show the lesion, which is isointense (*arrow*). **(D)** T2-star (T2*) weighted sequence using gradient refocused echo clearly shows the lesion as hypointense (*arrow*). *(Reproduced with permission from Geyer J, Potts D, Dillard S, Gomez C. Neuroimaging in the management of stroke patients. In: Geyer J, Gomez CR, eds.* Stroke: A Practical Approach. *Philadelphia: Lippincott Williams & Wilkins; 2009:171.)*

Diffusion-weighted MRI

Ischemia of brain tissue results in disruption of oxidative phosphorylation due to impaired oxygen delivery to tissue. The brain cells resort to anaerobic glycolysis, a more inefficient form of energy production. These changes lead to impaired function of the Na-K pump function of the cell membrane, with consequent accumulation of intracellular sodium. Other high-energy phosphates are depleted, with accumulation of inorganic phosphate and lactic acid within the tissue. The osmotic gradient created by the accumulation of intracellular sodium facilitates the influx of water into the cells with the production of cytotoxic edema.

Signal intensity on diffusion-weighted MRI (DW-MRI) is related to the random microscopic motion of water (Brownian motion), while conventional MRI sequences depend upon the density of water and other proton-containing molecules within the tissue.[3] It is thus possible to detect slower water motion within the ischemic tissue, with lower diffusion coefficients, as early as minutes following the onset of ischemia. Regardless of the exact cause of these findings, it is apparent that DW-MRI findings represent the earliest sign of ischemic injury, perhaps at a stage in which the tissue can still be recovered. Regions of ischemia have a decreased apparent diffusion coefficient (ADC) and high signal intensity on DW-MRI, reflecting restricted diffusion of water relative to normal brain (Figure 2-7). Further research is currently being conducted in this area and the future utilization of this technique in the algorithms for imaging cerebrovascular disorders is yet to be uniformly defined.

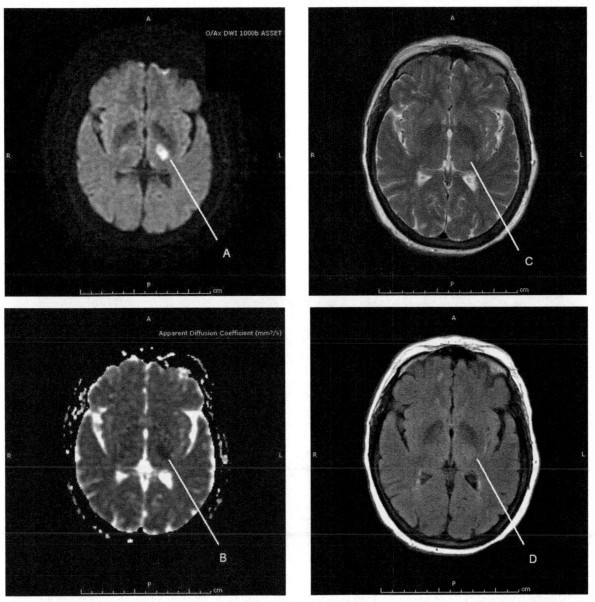

FIGURE 2-7 ▪ MRI appearance of an acute thalamic infarction. The diffusion weighted imaging (DWI) sequence clearly shows the lesion as a hyperintense region (A). The apparent diffusion coefficient (ADC) sequence shows the same lesion as a hypointense (black) region (B). The area is barely visible on the more commonplace T2 (C) and flair (D) sequences.

As methods and applications mature, DW-MRI should be able to provide information about the fiber structure of the brain, which may aid in clinical diagnosis. In addition to information about the rate of water diffusion, DW-MRI also provides information about the direction of water diffusion.[4] Tissue boundaries (eg, myelin and membranes) restrict the direction of water diffusion. In particular, white matter fiber bundles effectively "channel" water diffusion. In the brain, this directional information can be used to image white-matter fiber structure, as shown for a normal brain in Figure 2-8. To produce this image, diffusion-weighted images were measured repeated in a range of diffusion-weighting directions uniformly spaced over a hemisphere. Then the series of images are used to model the diffusion as a rank-2 tensor, which results in a 3×3 diffusion tensor at each image voxel position. The images in Figure 2-8 are colored (directions indicated by the reference color spheres) according to the direction of the highest rate of diffusion, and the image intensity is scaled so that the highest spatial anisotropy of diffusion is the most intense. A loss of structural organization due to pathology would then appear as lower image intensity in this type of image.

Using the diffusion tensor image, the fibrous structure of white matter can be mapped by following the dominant direction of diffusion from voxel to voxel, as shown in Figure 2-9. This image was produced by following the direction of diffusion from all the voxels in the corpus callosum within the mid-sagittal image in Figure 2-8 (shown in red). For this image, the fibers are followed until the tissue appears unstructured (low anisotropy). This visualization approach may allow the identification of white-matter pathology from a three-dimensional perspective. But before this structural information can be used routinely, the results must be validated to ensure the potential and understand limitations of this method fully understood.

Perfusion-weighted MRI

The ability to induce enhancement of MRI with magnetic susceptibility agents that facilitate T2* relaxation provides a method for assessing cerebral blood volume and tissue perfusion.[5] These agents, dysprosium or gadolinium DTPA-BMA (DyDTPA-BMA and GdDTPA-BMA, respectively) are confined to the intravascular space by the intact blood–brain barrier. A field gradient is created at the capillary level, resulting in significant signal loss in regions with normal blood flow. In contrast, nonperfused areas appear relatively hyperintense. This technique has been shown to significantly advance the time of detection of focal brain ischemia and reveal small infarctions not shown by conventional MRI sequences. In addition, ultrafast MRI techniques allow resolution of the passage of contrast through the vascular bed, with kinetic modeling of regional blood flow and volume (Figures 2-10 and 2-11).

MR Spectroscopy

In addition to the structural information provided by MRI, the same MR scanner can be used to acquire functional information about underlying biochemical

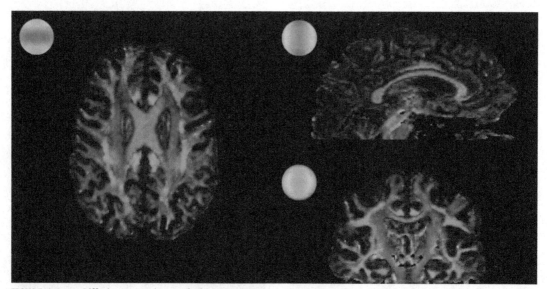

FIGURE 2-8 ■ Diffusion tensor image of white matter in the normal human brain with isotropic resolution (2 mm). This three-dimensional data was acquired in about 16 minutes using diffusion-weighted echo planar acquisition. The direction of diffusion is indicated by the reference color sphere in each image. The image on the left shows a transverse slice though the top of the corpus callosum (red "X" in the center of the brain). The upper right image is a mid-sagittal plane (note the corpus callosum in red) and the lower right image is from a coronal plane centered in the anterior-posterior direction.

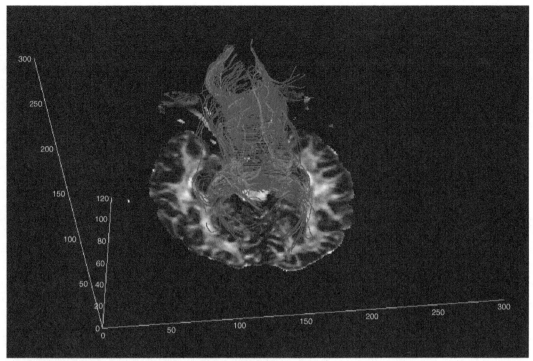

FIGURE 2-9 ■ Three-dimensional white-matter fiber pathways through the corpus callosum. Using water diffusion directional information from DW-MRI (see Figure. 2-8), the implied white-matter fibers, though the region of interest defined by the corpus callosum in the mid-sagittal image in Figure 2-8 (central red-colored structure), were followed until the tissue appears unstructured (low diffusion anisotropy). The fibers are shown in red along with a gray-scale reference image of diffusion anisotropy (highest anisotropy appears most intense) at the level of the optical nerves.

processes in tissue. Since tissue contains many proton-continuing molecules, in addition to water, an MR signal can be measured from the most concentrated molecular constituents.

Although the differences are small (of the order of parts per million), protons in different molecular environments resonance at different frequencies (for example, see Figure 2-11D and 2-11E). Using techniques similar to imaging sequences, these frequencies can be discriminated into a spectrum representing parts of molecules, where the spectrum is localized to distinct volume at low spatial resolution. In this way, a localized MR spectrum may be measured, from specific regions of the brain, with distinct resonances in the spectrum from major metabolites,[6] like choline (Cho), creatine (Cr), and the neuronal marker, N-acetylaspartate (NAA) shown in Figure 2-11. In the case of severe internal carotid artery stenosis shown in Figure 2-11, an elevated level of lactate is detected in the border zone of the right internal carotid artery (indicated by the arrow in Figure 2-11D), which suggests ischemic metabolism.

Magnetic Resonance Angiography

In general, magnetic resonance angiography (MRA) allows for the identification of vascular anomalies, either congenital or acquired, that may be causally related to the cerebrovascular process (eg, stenoses, vascular malformations, aneurysms). Originally, the use of SE MRI sequences produced images in which there was "negative" visualization of the cerebral blood vessels, due to their characteristic signal-void relative to the speed of flowing blood. This was recognized early in the utilization of MRI but did not seem to provide a reliable method for studying the cerebral vasculature. The advent of fast scanning MRI pulse sequencing, particularly GRE and bipolar flow-encoding gradient, has allowed direct vascular imaging and the widespread utilization of MRA.[7]

At present, and specifically for imaging intracranial vessels, either time-of-flight (TOF) or phase-contrast (PC) techniques can be applied. The technique of TOF angiography is based upon the phenomenon of flow-related enhancement, and it can be performed with either two- or three-dimensional volume acquisitions. It utilizes flip angles of less than 60 degrees and no refocusing 180-degree pulse (the echo is refocused by reversing the readout gradient). On the other hand, PC angiography is based upon the detection of velocity-induced phase shifts to distinguish flowing blood from the surrounding stationary tissue. By using bipolar flow-sensitized gradients it is possible to subtract the two acquisitions of opposite polarity and no net phase

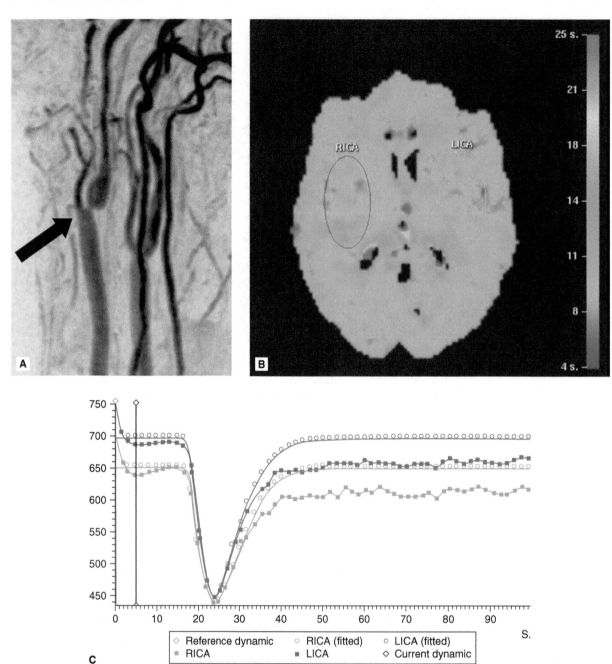

FIGURE 2-10 ■ The hemodynamic effects of a moderate degree of internal carotid artery stenosis. The MRA shows a stenosis of the origin of the right internal carotid artery *(arrow, **A**)*. Perfusion MRI shows a graphic representation of the mean transit time (MTT) of the flow in both regions of interest **(B)**, as well as a direct measurement with graphic plot **(C)**. No significant side-to-side differences are found. *(Reproduced with permission from Geyer J, Potts D, Dillard S, Gomez C. Neuroimaging in the management of stroke patients. In: Geyer J, Gomez CR, eds. Stroke: A Practical Approach. Philadelphia: Lippincott Williams & Wilkins; 2009:173.)*

(stationary tissue) from one another. The data that remains reflect the phase shift induced by flowing blood. The use of cardiac gating helps overcome the sensitivity of PC angiography to pulsatile and non-uniform flow.

The advantages of MRA are obvious; it can be carried out as part of the entire MRI evaluation of the patient and, for the intracranial circulation, it does not require contrast administration. Furthermore, in the

context of using very high field instruments (eg. 3.0 Tesla), the vascular detail is simply exquisite, with an ability to resolve very small pathologic structures (Figure 2-12). The main disadvantage is the fact that it is not widely understood that MRA represents an anatomic rendering of flow dynamics, not vessel anatomy! This results in common misinterpretations of the images due to wrongful expectations and assumptions.

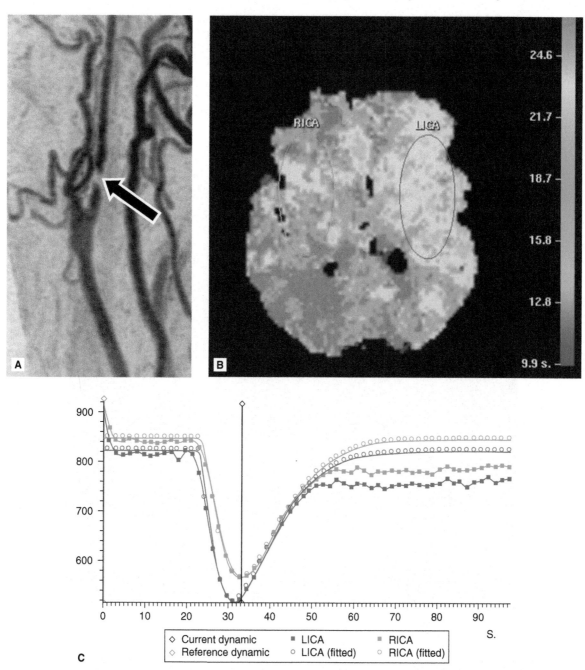

FIGURE 2-11 ■ Hemodynamic and metabolic consequences of a severe internal carotid artery stenosis. The MRA shows a signal gap in the proximal right internal carotid artery (*arrow*, **A**). Perfusion MRI shows the imaging (**B**) and mathematic/graphic (**C**) representation of the mean transit times (MTT) of both regions of interest. There is clear delay in the right internal carotid artery territory. In addition, MR spectroscopy analysis of the arterial borderzones of the right (**D**) and left (**E**) internal carotid arteries also show a difference. On the right side, a tall peak consistent with lactate accumulation (*arrow*, **D**) is suggestive of ischemic metabolism. *(Reproduced with permission from Geyer J, Potts D, Dillard S, Gomez C. Neuroimaging in the management of stroke patients. In: Geyer J, Gomez CR, eds. Stroke: A Practical Approach. Philadelphia: Lippincott Williams & Wilkins; 2009:174.)*

Neurovascular Ultrasonography: Noninvasive Flexibility

Ultrasound provides noninvasive methods by which it is possible to obtain diagnostic information, both anatomic and physiologic. All of these methods are based upon the interaction of ultrasound waves transmitted into the tissues, and the echoes generated and returning from the tissues. The domain of vascular ultrasonography includes all the ultrasonic methods that are primarily utilized for the study of blood vessels and blood flow. It is possible to apply the principles of vascular ultrasonography to the evaluation of patients with disorders of the cerebral circulation.

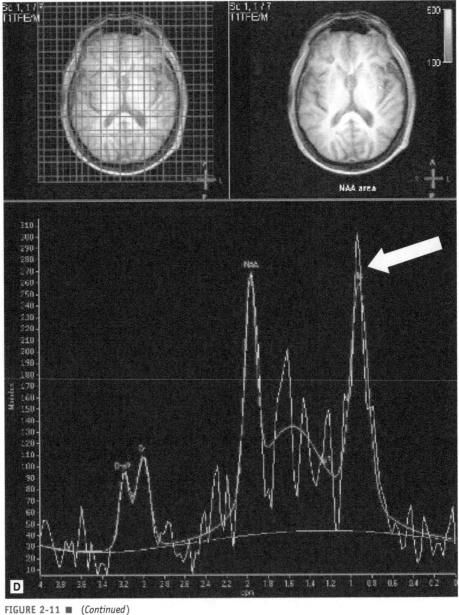

FIGURE 2-11 ■ *(Continued)*

Transcranial Doppler

Transcranial Doppler (TCD) ultrasound is a diagnostic technique based upon the use of a range-gated pulse-Doppler ultrasonic beam of 2 MHz frequency to assess the hemodynamic characteristics of the major cerebral arteries. The ultrasonic beam crosses the intact adult skull at points known as *windows*, bounces off the erythrocytes flowing within the basal brain arteries, and allows the determination of blood flow velocity, direction of flow, collateral patterns, and state of cerebral vasoreactivity. Sampling of multiple cerebral blood vessels using TCD, it is possible to identify patterns pointing to lesions localized intra- or extracranially; follow-up their natural history over time; and even monitor the effects of therapeutic strategies. Although certainly having its own inherent limitations, TCD

provides physiologic information about the brain circulation that cannot be obtained by any other means. In addition of the uniqueness of the information gathered by TCD, other attractive characteristics are that it is noninvasive (safe), reproducible, versatile, and dynamic.

The utilization of TCD in clinical practice over the last decade has made us change somewhat our concept of the role that it plays. The technique, rather an ancillary procedure, is best conceived as a specialized "stethoscope" that allows clinicians to "listen" to the hemodynamic changes of the brain blood vessels, and to compare the findings over time. Indeed, the best approach to TCD is to consider it an extension of the clinical examination, analogous to the way in which electromyography has been regarded for many years. From the clinical point of view, TCD is an

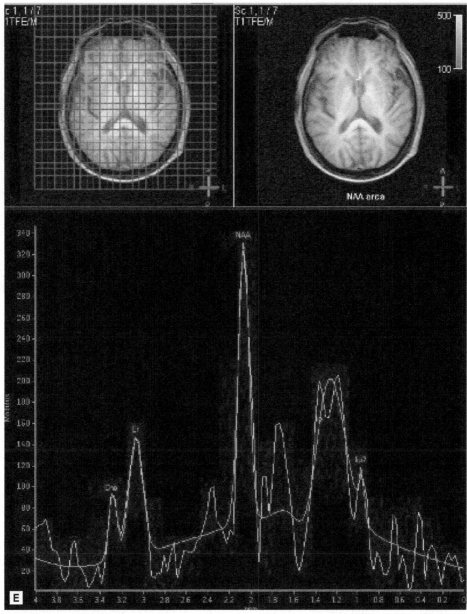

FIGURE 2-11 ■ (*Continued*)

ideal tool not only for diagnosis, but also for follow-up. Just as cardiologists have previously performed sequential auscultatory examinations of patients looking for new murmurs which would alert to the development of valvular dysfunction, it is also possible to use TCD to alert us about the presence of hemodynamic disturbances representative of cerebrovascular pathology. This is especially useful in the patient with sickle cell disease.

APPLICATION SCENARIOS: DIMENSIONS OF PRACTICE

The tasks noted above must also be placed in the practical context of three distinct clinical scenarios: (1) emergency care, (2) monitoring, and (3) non-emergent evaluation.

Depending upon the scenario, the choice of imaging technique is then guided by the question being asked, the diagnostic characteristics inherent to each imaging modality, and the expectations of results based upon the natural history of the process being investigated.

Imaging in Emergency Care

The majority of patients with acute neurological changes are initially evaluated in emergency departments, following algorithms with priorities that include answering specific questions with direct relevance to the management of the patient, both immediate and within the days that follow. At the bedside, the first set of clinical questions confronted by stroke specialists is:

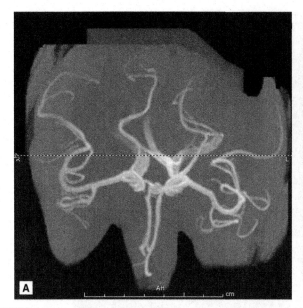
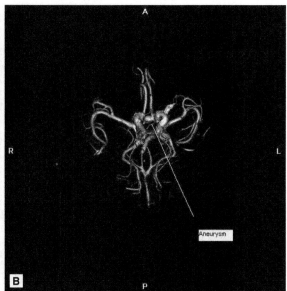

FIGURE 2-12 ■ Ability of MRA and CTA to resolve small structures such as aneurysms. A left anterior cerebral artery aneurysm is easily visualized by MRA (A) and CTA (B).

- Does the patient have a stroke?
- Is it an ischemic or a hemorrhagic stroke?
- Is there a tumor?
- What is the likelihood of neurological deterioration?
- Is there cerebral edema?

It is important to know whether (1) there is an identifiable cause of the event, (2) the brain has already undergone damage, and (3) there is any alternative diagnostic possibility.

In the urgent evaluation of patients with neurological complaints, all possible neuroimaging findings can be allocated into one of the following categories:

- *Normal brain tissue.* A large number of patients presenting acute neurological processes have normal CT scans. This results from the low sensitivity of the test for the detection of small lesions and acute ischemic tissue. A normal CT scan in the context of a patient with an acute focal neurologic deficit by no means excludes the diagnosis of a central nervous system lesion such as an ischemic stroke. Clearly, for patients suspected of having hemorrhagic stroke, a normal CT scan almost completely excludes the diagnosis. In regards to MRI, on the other hand, a perfectly normal, high-quality MRI-DWI study almost unequivocally implies the absence of any type of stroke.
- *Abnormal, demonstrating a lesion consistent with the symptoms.* Diagnosis of a lesion appearing on CT depends upon the size and location of the affected tissue. The findings on MRI are often more helpful in diagnosis given the increased sensitivity of MRI as compared to CT.

- *Abnormal, with findings related to the lesion.* Frequently, CT scans show abnormalities that bear a relationship with the lesion itself. For example, in patients with a small tumor, the CT may reveal edema with midline shift. The tumor itself may be difficult to visualize with contrast administration. Using MRI, the same is true, but to even a greater extent since the MRI is much more informative due to the various other sequences that can be utilized concurrently.
- *Abnormal, displaying an alternative diagnostic process.* Not every patient who presents with a clinical syndrome suggestive of a particular diagnosis has it. CT and MRI are helpful in uncovering other conditions that mimic various diagnoses and require alternative treatment (tumor versus stroke).
- *Abnormal, showing a combination of the various above.* The routine utilization of contrast during CT examination of the emergency neurological patient is unwarranted. There are risks associated with contrast administration such as renal insufficiency and allergic reaction. Furthermore, the intense nausea that can be produced by intravenous contrast administration can jeopardize the fate of patients with ruptured aneurysms.

Monitoring of Lesion Evolution

Regardless of how the patient is being treated, the time continuum that follows initial evaluation and treatment demands that the clinical team follows the evolution of the patient in order to make decisions about which aspects of treatment to continue, and which ones to change. In certain situations, such as in the intensive care unit (ICU), when clinical assessment may not be easy or feasible due to the need for deep sedation, imaging becomes of paramount importance to assess changes and guide therapy. An example of this is the resolution of hydrocephalus in a patient who requires a ventriculostomy following an intraventricular hemorrhage. Patients in a less intensive setting also need follow-up imaging to allow the physician to monitor the lesion and the patient's response to therapy.

Imaging and Risk Stratification Algorithms

The diagnostic perspective of patients with neurological conditions revolves around defining the lesion and its structural consequences. In this context, the importance of imaging techniques cannot be overemphasized. The patient presenting with a focal seizure should be evaluated with MRI and seizure focus protocol. The MRI may be normal in this case, but there may be mesial temporal sclerosis, evidence of a remote injury, a vascular anomaly, or a mass lesion.

The practical aspects of choosing one imaging modality or another depends largely on the following variables: (1) the type of pathology being evaluated, (2) the timing of the evaluation, (3) the availability and technical quality of the diagnostic resources, and (4) the practitioner's experience and judgment.

CONCLUSION

The utilization of imaging techniques for the evaluation of patients with neurological disease must be guided by the specific needs of the clinical situation. Newer tests being introduced will not necessarily replace the old ones, but rather will provide additional dimensions to our ability to diagnose and treat different conditions capable of causing neurological disease. It is important to keep in mind that every one of these diagnostic techniques is operator-dependent, even if to different degrees. As such, another aspect of choosing the appropriate diagnostic technique requires the recognition of the quality of the resources available.

REFERENCES

1. Young RJ, Destian S. Imaging of traumatic intracranial hemorrhage. *Neuroimaging Clin N Am.* 2002;12:189-204.
2. Imaizumi T, Horita Y, Hashimoto Y, Niwa J. Dotlike hemosiderin spots on T2*-weighted magnetic resonance imaging as a predictor of stroke recurrence: a prospective study. *J Neurosurg.* 2004;101(6):915-920.
3. Augustin M, Bammer R, Simbrunner J, Stollberger R, Hartung HP, Fazekas F. Diffusion-weighted imaging of patients with subacute cerebral ischemia: comparison with conventional and contrast-enhanced MR imaging. *AJNR Am J Neuroradiol.* 2000;21:1596-1602.
4. Le Bihan D. Looking into the functional architecture of the brain with diffusion MRI. *Nat Rev Neurosci.* 2003;4:469-480.
5. Nasel C, Kronsteiner N, Schindler E, Kreuzer S, Gentzsch S. Standardized time to peak in ischemic and regular cerebral tissue measured with perfusion MR imaging. *AJNR Am J Neuroradiol.* 2004;25:945-950.
6. Burtscher IM, Holtas S. Proton MR spectroscopy in clinical routine. *J Magn Reson Imaging.* 2001;13:560-567.
7. Westerlaan HE, van der Vliet AM, Hew JM, Metzemaekers JD, Mooij JJ, Oudkerk M. Magnetic resonance angiography in the selection of patients suitable for neurosurgical intervention of ruptured intracranial aneurysms. *Neuroradiology.* 2004;46(11):867-875. Epub 2004 Oct 20.
8. Geyer J, Potts D, Dillard S, Gomez C. Neuroimaging in the management of stroke patients. In: Geyer J, Gomez CR, eds. *Stroke: A Practical Approach.* Philadelphia: Lippincott Williams & Wilkins; 2009.

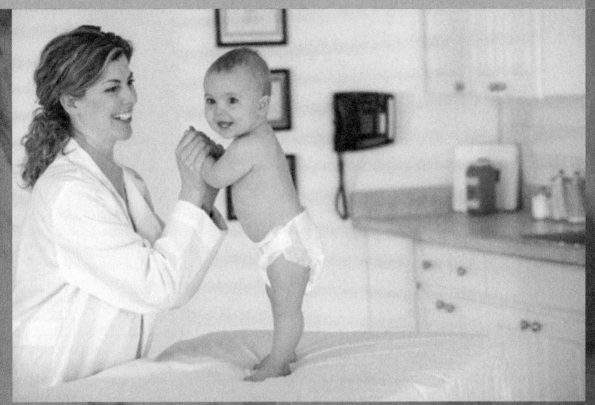

Common Pediatric Neurologic Problems

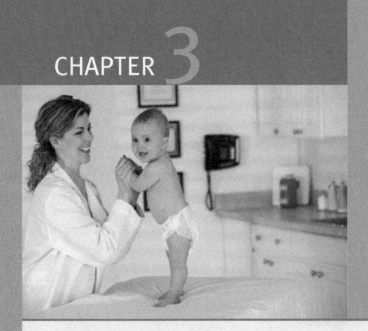

CHAPTER 3

Seizures and Epilepsy

Paul R. Carney and James D. Geyer

DEFINITIONS AND EPIDEMIOLOGY

A general simplified definition of a seizure is a sudden temporary change in brain function caused by an abnormal rhythmic electrical discharge. Epilepsy is, simply put, a state of recurrent seizure activity. The mechanism whereby a seizure turns into epilepsy, a process known as epileptogenesis, is controversial.

Seizures are common in humans, with an incidence of approximately 80/100,000 per year and an overall risk of epilepsy of 1% to 3%.[1] Status epilepticus is a less common form of severe prolonged seizure activity with a high morbidity and mortality.

PATHOGENESIS

Seizures arise secondary to a number of etiologies. Idiopathic seizures, or "cryptogenic" seizures, are fairly common. Contrary to what many patients and families might think, the inability to find a cause for the seizure is not necessary "bad." In fact, this may portend a somewhat better prognosis for long-term seizure control. Febrile seizures are common in children and are covered in detail in Chapter 4.

Trauma contributes to the risk of seizures in two fairly distinct fashions. Early posttraumatic seizures are typically associated with intracranial hemorrhage, focal neurological deficits, posttraumatic amnesia exceeding 24 hours, and linear skull fractures. Late posttraumatic seizures are also associated with intracranial hemorrhage and posttraumatic amnesia exceeding 24 hours, but are usually seen in patients with depressed skull fractures and with the injury after age 16 years.[2–4]

A number of congenital malformations increase the risk for epilepsy. Disorders associated with migrational disorders and structural anomalies often increase the risk of subsequent seizures. The genetic diseases listed in Table 3-1 also increase the risk of epilepsy whether or not they are associated with structural malformations.[5–7]

Infections are also common causes of seizure activity in the pediatric population. Meningitis and encephalitis can result in seizures either related to the fever or to the direct effects of the infection. These are covered in detail in the chapters on infectious disease. Bacterial infections can result in meningitis, encephalitis, and abscess formation. Herpes simplex virus (HSV) is a well known cause of seizures and can be catastrophic.[8] Other viral infections including cytomegalovirus (CMV) infection and various viral encephalitides can result in seizures. Fungal infections and toxoplasmosis also raise the risk of developing seizures.

A wide array of toxic and metabolic disorders can result in seizures. These derangements can cause seizures to occur de novo but can also worsen a pre-existing epilepsy. The common metabolic and toxic causes of seizures are listed in Table 3-2.

Table 3-1.

Genetic Causes of Epilepsy

Amino acidurias
Channelopathies
Lysosomal storage diseases
Phakomatoses—tuberous sclerosis, von Hippel–Lindau disease, neurofibromatosis
Phenylketonuria (PKU)
Sturge–Weber syndrome

Table 3-2.

Toxic/Metabolic Causes of Seizures

Drug Intoxication
  Amphetamines
  Cocaine
  Lidocaine
  Theophylline
  Tricyclic antidepressants
Drug withdrawal
  Antiepileptic drugs (AEDs)
  Barbiturates
  Benzodiazepines
  Ethanol
Electrolyte—hypo/hypernatremia, hypo/hyperglycemia,
  hypocalcemia, hypomagnesemia
Heavy metals—lead, mercury
Hyperosmolarity
Hypoxia
Liver failure
Porphyria
Pyridoxine deficiency
Thyroid storm
Uremia (usually following 3 days of anuria)

Cerebral ischemia is a common cause of seizures in the neonate and in the older adult but is relatively uncommon in the older pediatric population.

Seizures usually occur in the more slowly growing tumors. Tumors located in the supratentorial region cause seizures more frequently than do cerebellar or brainstem tumors.

CLINICAL PRESENTATION

Epilepsy is divided into several categories with significant differences in the characteristics of the electrical discharges as well as the clinical manifestations. Localization-related epilepsy or partial epilepsy has a primary focus from which the electrical discharges arise. Complex partial seizures occur with alteration of awareness while simple partial seizures have no alteration of awareness. Jacksonian motor seizures, Rolandic epilepsy, temporal lobe epilepsy, and frontal lobe epilepsy are all examples of partial epilepsy.

The Revised International Classification of Epilepsies, Epileptic Syndromes and Related Seizure Disorders divides the localization-related epilepsies as follows:[10]

> Idiopathic localization-related epilepsy
> Symptomatic or secondary localization-related epilepsy
> Cryptogenic localization-related epilepsy

Generalized seizures are the other major seizure type. In this category of epilepsy, the seizure affects the entire cortex electrically. Several subtypes of generalized seizures have also been identified, including absence epilepsy with 3-Hz spike and wave activity, generalized tonic-clonic seizures, juvenile myoclonic epilepsy, and progressive myoclonic epilepsy.

The Revised International Classification of Epilepsies, Epileptic Syndromes and Related Seizure Disorders divides the generalized epilepsies as follows[10]:

> Primary generalized epilepsy
> Symptomatic generalized epilepsy
> Cryptogenic epilepsy

A number of seizures and epilepsies may be very difficult to categorize. The Revised International Classification of Epilepsies, Epileptic Syndromes and Related Seizure Disorders groups these disorders in the "undetermined" category. These seizures may be divided as follows[10]:

> Both focal and generalized
> Situation-related epilepsy
> Febrile convulsions
> Isolated seizure
> Isolated status epilepticus
> Toxic/metabolic

In each of these cases, the electroencephalographic (EEG) findings may be different. The EEG serves as a vitally important tool in the correct diagnosis of the various epilepsy subtypes and syndromes.

DIAGNOSIS

Seizure Types

Generalized tonic-clonic seizures

Generalized tonic-clonic seizures typically have no preceding aura but may have a prodrome of apathy or irritability. During the tonic phase, the jaw snaps shut followed by 10 to 15 seconds or longer of tonic spasms, apnea, and cyanosis. The clonic phase usually consists of 1 to 2 minutes of rhythmic generalized muscle contractions and increased blood pressure. The postictal phase lasts for minutes to hours, with confusion, somnolence, and possibly agitation.

The ictal EEG usually consists of generalized spike and wave or polyspike activity. The interictal EEG is highly variable with a normal background in some patients and slowing present in others.

Generalized seizures are rare in newborns. Generalized seizures occur most frequently in children secondary to fevers and metabolic derangements.

Absence seizures

Absence seizures typically have no preceding aura or prodrome. An absence seizure usually lasts for only several seconds to minutes. There is a sudden interruption of consciousness, staring, 3-Hz blinking, and less frequently automatisms. There is no postictal confusion.[11]

The ictal EEG usually consists of 3-Hz generalized spike and wave activity with some slowing of the discharge frequency during the seizure. The interictal EEG usually has a normal background. Atypical absence seizures have generalized spike and wave activity but usually have a frequency less than 3 Hz.[12]

Absence seizures typically start between ages 4 and 10 years and resolve by age 20 years. Atypical absence epilepsy usually occurs in children who are neurologically or developmentally abnormal.[13]

Febrile seizures

Febrile seizures occur with a prodromal fever. A simple febrile seizure occurs as a brief generalized tonic clonic seizure occurring after the onset of fever. A complicated febrile seizure has prolonged seizure activity or focal seizure activity. Febrile seizures are covered in detail in Chapter 4.

Juvenile myoclonic epilepsy

The seizures associated with juvenile myoclonic epilepsy typically have no preceding aura but may have a prodrome of morning myoclonus. The seizures may consist of generalized tonic-clonic activity; however, absence seizures may also occur. The postictal phase is variable depending on the seizure type.[11]

The ictal EEG usually consists of generalized polyspike and slow wave activity. The interictal EEG is typically unremarkable.[12]

The age of onset of juvenile myoclonic epilepsy is typically 10 to 20 years. Patients are usually developmentally and neurologically normal.[13]

Progressive myoclonic epilepsy

The family of disorders known as the progressive myoclonic epilepsies (Table 3-3) consists of a number of loosely related disorders. These epilepsy subtypes are quite rare and have complex presentations and diagnostic findings. Most of these disorders have a genetic basis, though sporadic cases have occurred in some cases (Table 3-4). The EEG associated with these disorders is variable. The background is often slow. The seizures are typically generalized.[11]

Infantile spasms

West syndrome typically begins between 3 months and 3 years of age.[14–16] The seizures associated with West syndrome consist of a jack-knifing movement and myoclonus. The EEG consists of a hypsarrhythmia pattern with bursts of asynchronous slow waves; spikes and

Table 3-3.

Progressive Myoclonic Epilepsies

Dentorubral-pallidoluysian atrophy
Juvenile neuroaxonal atrophy
Lafora disease
Late infantile and juvenile GM2 gangliosidosis
Myoclonic epilepsy and ragged red fibers (MERRF)
Neuronal ceroid lipofuscinosis (NCL) (also known as Batten disease)
Noninfantile Gaucher disease
Sialidosis
Unverricht–Lundborg disease (Baltic myoclonus)

sharp waves alternate with a suppressed EEG.[17] The clinical features of West syndrome include infantile spasms and mental retardation, which varies according to the etiology of the spasms.

Aicardi syndrome is an X-linked disorder present from birth that is associated with infantile spasms. The seizures are described as infantile spasms, but alternating hemiconvulsions may also be seen. The clinical features of Aicardi syndrome include coloboma, chorioretinal lacunae, agenesis of the corpus callosum, vertebral anomalies, and seizures.[18]

Lennox–Gastaut syndrome

Lennox–Gastaut syndrome typically begins between 1 and 10 years of age. There are multiple seizure types, associated with variable degrees of mental retardation.

The EEG reveals a slow spike wave complex with a frequency of 1 to 2.5 Hz, multifocal spikes, and generalized paroxysmal fast activity (GPFA).[19]

Partial seizures: localization-related epilepsy

Jacksonian motor seizures are simple partial seizures with no alteration of consciousness. These seizures begin with tonic contractions of the face, fingers, or feet and transform into clonic movements that march to other muscle groups on the ipsilateral hemibody. There is no alteration in consciousness, but postictal aphasia may occur if the primary epileptogenic zone involves the dominant hemisphere. Simple partial seizures may involve autonomic (Table 3-5), sensory, motor, or psychic functions.

Complex partial seizures

Benign Rolandic epilepsy. Benign Rolandic epilepsy usually begins between ages 5 and 10 years and is transmitted in an autosomal dominant pattern with variable penetrance. It is fairly common, with an incidence of

Table 3-4.

Distinguishing Characteristics of the Progressive Myoclonic Epilepsies

Clinical Features

Chorea
Dentorubral-pallidoluysian atrophy
Juvenile neuroaxonal dystrophy
Juvenile Gaucher disease

Deafness
Biotin-responsive encephalopathy
MERRF
Sialidosis type II

Focal Occipital Spikes
MERRF
Unverricht–Lundborg disease

Little or No Dementia
Biotin-responsive encephalopathy
Noninfantile Gaucher disease
Myoclonus—nal failure
Sialidosis type I
Unverricht–Lundborg disease

Severe Dementia
GM2 gangliosidosis
Juvenile neuroaxonal dystrophy
Lafora disease
Late infantile NCL

Severe Myoclonus
Lafora's disease
MERRF
Sialidosis

Genetics

Autosomal Dominant
Dentatorubral-pallidoluysian atrophy
Kuf disease

Geography

Canada
Myoclonus—renal failure

Finland
Santavori disease
Unverricht–Lundborg disease

Japan
Dentatorubral pallidoluysian atrophy
Sialidosis type II

Sweden
Gaucher disease

Maternal Inheritance
MERRF

21/100,000 children.[20] The clinical features include a single nocturnal seizure with clonic movement of the mouth and gurgling. Secondary generalization is common. Alteration in consciousness, aura, and postictal confusion are rare. The seizures resolve by age 16 years.[21, 22]

Table 3-5.

Possible Autonomic Seizure Clinical Features

Abdominal sensations
Apnea
Arrhythmia
Chest pain
Cyanosis
Erythema
Flushing
Genital sensations
Hyperventilation
Incontinence
Miosis
Perspiration
Vomiting

The interictal EEG consists of central and mid-temporal high-amplitude spike and wave with a characteristic dipole. The ictal EEG usually consists of a focal central or mid-temporal ictal onset, with the possibility of secondary generalization.[23,24]

Temporal lobe epilepsy. Temporal lobe epilepsy accounts for approximately 70% of partial seizures. Many patients have a prior history of febrile seizures or head trauma. A prodrome consisting of lethargy is common. Auras are also common but not universal and include an array of findings such as déjà vu. The ictal findings or semiology include oral or motor automatisms, alteration of consciousness, head and eye deviation, contralateral twitching or tonic–clonic movements, and posturing. Right temporal lobe seizures are often hypermobile. Left temporal lobe seizures often result in behavior arrest. Versive head movements are relatively common, and 90% of patients with versive head movements had a primary epileptogenic zone in the contralateral hemisphere. Ipsiversive movements are less common but occur most commonly in patients with temporal foci. The postictal phase consists of minutes to hours of confusion and somnolence.[24–30]

Frontal lobe epilepsy. Frontal lobe epilepsy accounts for approximately 20% of partial seizures. A prodrome is rare. Auras are unusual. The seizures typically consist of combinations of behavior alteration and automatisms of very brief duration. Frontal seizures often have atypical presentations and vary widely depending on the region of the frontal lobe from which the seizures arise (Table 3-6). Postictal confusion is rare.[31–36]

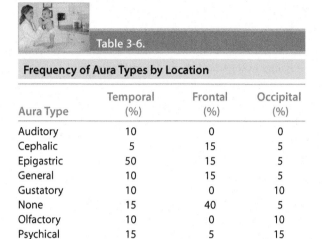

Table 3-6.

Frequency of Aura Types by Location

Aura Type	Temporal (%)	Frontal (%)	Occipital (%)
Auditory	10	0	0
Cephalic	5	15	5
Epigastric	50	15	5
General	10	15	5
Gustatory	10	0	10
None	15	40	5
Olfactory	10	0	10
Psychical	15	5	15
Somatosensory	5	15	0
Visual	10	5	50
Vertiginous	10	2	0

Occipital lobe epilepsy. Occipital lobe epilepsy is rare, accounting for less than 10% of partial seizures. Prodromes are rare with occipital lobe seizures and auras are unusual. As with the frontal lobe seizures, the seizure characteristics are dependent on the area of the occipital lobe involved. When the striate cortex is involved, there are typically elemental visual hallucinations. Involvement of the lateral occipital lobe results in twinkling, pulsing lights. Seizures arising from the temporo-occipital are usually associated with formed visual hallucinations.[37-39]

Parietal lobe epilepsy. Parietal lobe seizures are also relatively uncommon. The may be seen as simple partial seizures but they will often propagate. The initial features can include contralateral paresthesias, contralateral pain, idiomotor apraxia, and limb movement sensations. As the seizure progresses and propagates, asymmetric tonic posturing and automatisms may develop.[40-42]

Landau–Kleffner syndrome. Landau–Kleffner syndrome is a rare, invariably progressive, idiopathic acquired aphasia related to a focal epileptic disturbance in the area of the brain responsible for verbal processing.[43] The syndrome begins between ages 3 and 10 in a child with normally acquired language abilities. The child then develops a verbal auditory agnosia and infrequent nocturnal partial or secondarily generalized seizures. The syndrome has a pathognomonic EEG pattern consisting of high-voltage multifocal spikes, predominating in the temporal lobes.[44] Treatment is usually with valproic acid and benzodiazepines.[45] Sometimes corticosteroids and IV Ig or even surgery with subpial transection[46] are used in refractory

cases. The outcome for overall language and cognitive function depends in part on how early the syndrome is recognized and treated, but over 2/3 of children are left with significant language or behavioral deficits.[47]

Rasmussen encephalitis. Rasmussen encephalitis is a syndrome of diffuse lymphocytic infiltration of the brain associated with partial seizures and progressive neurological deterioration with hemiparesis. This disorder typically affects children 1 to 14 years old. The syndrome is associated with perivascular cuffing on pathologic sections, and antibodies to the glutamate subunit GluR3 are commonly identified. The disorder is usually unilateral. Rasmussen encephalitis is very difficult to treat and frequently requires surgical management with hemispherectomy.

EVALUATION

As with many facets of neurology, the history is the most important diagnostic tool and should include information on each of the items in Table 3-7. The history should be obtained from family and eyewitnesses, if possible. Many patients are unable to provide accurate descriptions of the seizure and the postictal period.

MRI of the head with temporal lobe protocol (thin coronal slices through hippocampi) is the preferred imaging modality for most patients. The MRI sequences are much more sensitive to the causes of epilepsy than is CT imaging. CT can, however, be of help in the emergency department setting. EEG is a vital component of the evaluation to categorize the seizure type and assist with planning of the treatment strategy. The need for laboratory testing is highly variable depending on the history. Initial evaluation with fluid balance profile (FBP), Ca++,

Table 3-7.

Aura Types

Psychical Auras	Illusion	Hallucination
Memory	Déjà vu, jamais vu, strangeness	Flashbacks
Sound	Advancing, receding, louder, softer, clearer	Voices, music
Self-image	Depersonalization, remoteness	Autoscopy
Time	Stand-still, rushing, slowing	
Vision	Macropsia, micropsia, near, far, blurred	Objects, faces, scenes

Mg++, and liver function tests (LFTs) is important for both the search for a potential cause of the seizures and for medication selection. Urine drug screening should be obtained for patients with new-onset seizures.

TREATMENT

Physicians and families often agonize over the decision about whether to initiate therapy after a single seizure. In the absence of a structural cause for the seizures or a typical syndrome of epilepsy, most patients do not require long-term treatment with an antiepileptic medication. The patient selection criteria for treatment after a single seizure are listed in Table 3-8.[48,49]

Stopping the antiepileptic medication can also be a challenge. The prognostic factors used for making the decision regarding discontinuation are listed in Table 3-9.[49]

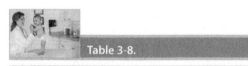

Table 3-8.

Characteristics of Frontal Lobe Seizures by Region of Onset

Anteromedial Frontal
Contralateral eye and head version
Frequent generalization
Somatosensory aura
Tonic posture

Cingular
Amnesia
Facial expressions of fear and anger
"Psychotic" appearance

Dorsolateral frontal
Simple partial
Tonic eye and head contraversion

Frontopolar
Loss of tone
Rapid generalization

Opercular/Insular
Complex seizures include gagging, swallowing, chewing, amnesia, genital manipulation
Seizures include gustatory sensation, salivation, gagging

Orbitofrontal
Blinking or staring
Complex automatisms

Supplementary Motor Area
Contralateral tonic posture
Simple motor seizure
Somatosensory aura
Tonic eye and head contraversion
Vocalizes

Table 3-9.

Components of a Seizure History

Aura
Birth and developmental history
CNS infections
Exacerbating factors (sleep, emotion, stress, menstrual cycle, substance abuse)
Family history of epilepsy
Head trauma
Postictal state
Seizure description by an eyewitness

The selection of a particular antiepileptic medication for a given subtype of epilepsy has long been the subject of controversy. When selecting a given drug, the concomitant medical disorders such as headache, bone marrow dysfunction, and liver insufficiency should be considered. Guidelines for the selection of antiepileptic drugs, the pharmacology of the common antiepileptic drugs, and potential interactions are reviewed in Tables 3-10 to 3-13.[50-53]

Surgery for epilepsy is an important but often underutilized treatment option. The surgical option provides an opportunity for some patients to become seizure free. However, this is a complex discussion and beyond the scope of this book.

Table 3-10.

Patient Selection Criteria for Treatment After a Single Seizure

Probably
AVM
Brain tumor
CNS infection
Immediate family history of epilepsy

Probably Not
Acute febrile illness
Drug withdrawal or intoxication
Electrolye imbalance
EtOH withdrawal
Hyper/hypoglycemia
Immediate posttraumatic seizure
Severe sleep deprivation–related seizure

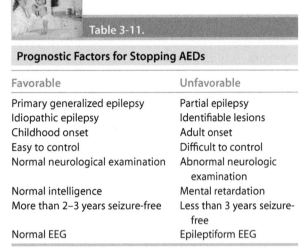

Table 3-11.

Prognostic Factors for Stopping AEDs

Favorable	Unfavorable
Primary generalized epilepsy	Partial epilepsy
Idiopathic epilepsy	Identifiable lesions
Childhood onset	Adult onset
Easy to control	Difficult to control
Normal neurological examination	Abnormal neurologic examination
Normal intelligence	Mental retardation
More than 2–3 years seizure-free	Less than 3 years seizure-free
Normal EEG	Epileptiform EEG

From Geyer J, Keating J, Potts D, Carney P, eds. Neurology for the Boards. 3rd ed. Philadelphia: Lippincott Williams & Wilkins; 2006.

Non-epileptic Events

Non-epileptic events are unusual in the pediatric population, especially in the younger child. Several categories of non-epileptic events (thrashing, staring, etc.) have different natural histories and variable prognosis. Etiologies include conversion disorder, malingering, and medical conditions, especially cardiac disorders. Symptoms suggesting non-epileptic events include closed eyes, resisted eyelid opening, non-physiologic progression, pelvic thrusting, lack of cyanosis, lack of tongue biting, variable semiology, crying, and rapid reorientation following the event.[54-56]

Neonatal Seizures

Neonatal seizures are poorly classified, under-recognized, especially in sick neonates, and often difficult to treat.

Neonatal seizures are often the presenting clinical manifestation of underlying neurological conditions such as hypoxic-ischemic encephalopathy, stroke, intraventricular or intraparenchymal hemorrhages, meningitis, sepsis, or metabolic disorders. Of these, hypoxic ischemic encephalopathy is the most common etiology, accounting for 50% to 60% of patients with neonatal seizures.[57]

The neonatal brain is particularly vulnerable to seizure activity as a result of an imbalance of excitatory to inhibitory circuitry. The imbalance favors excitation, and does so to facilitate important developmental processes that occur during the neonatal period (synaptogenesis, apoptosis, progressive integration of circuitry, synaptic pruning). The imbalance occurs anatomically and physiologically by an overexpression of NMDA receptor in the hippocampus and neocortical regions of the neonatal brain, a delay in the maturation of the inhibitory system, and neurons in such regions as the hippocampus are excited rather than inhibited by the neurotransmitter GABA (normally the primary inhibitory neurotransmitter in the brain).

Clinical presentation

Subtle. Subtle seizures are more common in premature infants. As the name suggests, the seizures may be difficult to identify with only tonic horizontal eye movements, sustained eye opening, chewing, or apnea. In some cases there may be "boxing" movements. These seizures may have limited EEG changes correlating with the seizure activity.[58-61]

Clonic. Clonic seizures typically present as rhythmic, slow movements. The movements have a frequency of 1 to 3 Hz. *Focal* clonic seizures involve one side of the body, and the infant is not clearly unconscious.

Table 3-12.

Antiepileptic Drug Selection[a]

Seizure Type	VPA	LTG	TPM	LVT	ETX	ACTH	GBP	CBZ	PHT	PHB
Infantile spasms						1			2	
Absence	2	2			1					
Tonic-clonic	1	2	2	2				3	2	4, 1[b]
Myoclonic	1	2								
Atypical absence	1	2								
Simple partial	3		2	2			2	1	2	1[b]
Complex partial	2	2	2	2			2	1	2	1[b]

[a]Numbers refer to order of preference for use in specific seizure types.
[b]Infants.
From Geyer J, Keating J, Potts D, Carney P, eds. Neurology for the Boards. 3rd ed. Philadelphia: Lippincott Williams & Wilkins; 2006.

Table 3-13.

Drug–Drug Interactions: Effects on Serum Concentration of Adding a Second Antiepileptic Drug to First Antiepileptic Drug

Original Drug	Added Drug	Effects of Added Drug on Serum Concentration of Original Drug
Carbamazepine	Clonazepam	No change
	Phenobarbital	Decrease
	Phenytoin	Decrease
	Primidone	Decrease
Clonazepam	Phenobarbital	Decrease
	Phenytoin	Decrease
	Valproate	No change
Ethosuximide	Carbamazepine	Decrease
	Methylphenobarbital	Increase
	Phenobarbital	No change
	Phenytoin	No change
	Primidone	No change
	Valproate	Increase or no change
Phenobarbital	Carbamazepine	No change
	Clonazepam	Data conflicting
	Methsuximide	Increase
	Phenytoin	Increase
	Valproate	Increase
Phenytoin	Carbamazepine	Increase or decrease
	Clonazepam	Data conflicting
	Ethosuximide	No change
	Methsuximide	Increase
	Phenobarbital	Decrease, increase, or no change
	Primidone	No change
	Valproate	Decrease
Primidone	Carbamazepine	Increased concentration of derived phenobarbital
	Clonazepam	No change
	Ethosuximide	No change
	Phenytoin	Increased concentration of derived phenobarbital
	Valproate	Increase
Valproate	Carbamazepine	Decrease, increase, or no change
	Clonazepam	No change
	Ethosuximide	No change
	Phenobarbital	Decrease
	Phenytoin	Decrease
	Primidone	Decrease

From Geyer J, Keating J, Potts D, Carney P, eds. Neurology for the Boards. *3rd ed. Philadelphia: Lippincott Williams & Wilkins; 2006.*

Multifocal clonic seizures involve several body parts, often in a migrating pattern. *Generalized* clonic seizures are rarely observed in newborn because of the incomplete myelination of the brain.[58–61]

Tonic. *Focal* tonic seizures result in sustained posturing of a limb, the trunk, or the neck. These seizures are usually accompanied by EEG changes. *Generalized* tonic seizures exhibit tonic extension of all limbs (mimicking decorticate posturing) or tonic flexion of upper limbs and tonic extension of lower limbs (mimicking decerebrate posturing). There are no EEG changes in 85% of cases.[58–61]

Myoclonic. *Focal* myoclonic seizures usually involve flexor muscles of an upper extremity. Often, there are no EEG changes. Conversely, *generalized* myoclonic seizures exhibit bilateral jerks of both upper and lower limbs, and may resemble infantile spasms. These generalized seizures are more likely to have EEG changes.[58–61]

Syndromes

Benign familial neonatal seizures

Benign familial neonatal seizures occur as a genetic disorder with an autosomal dominant inheritance pattern associated with chromosome 20q. The seizures typically start on day of life 2 or 3. The neonate may have as many as 10 to 20 seizures per day. The syndrome is usually self-limited and benign, but approximately 10% of cases progress to an antiepileptic drug-requiring seizure disorder. Neurological development is normal.[58–61]

Fifth-day fits

Fifth-day fits usually begin on day of life 4 to 6. The seizures are typically multifocal clonic seizures and are frequently associated with apnea. The seizures usually last for less than 24 hours. Fifth-day fits progress to status epilepticus in 80% of cases.[58–61]

Benign neonatal sleep myoclonus

Benign neonatal sleep myoclonus begins during the first week of life. The seizures are usually bilateral myoclonic jerks that last for several minutes and occur only during NREM sleep. The EEG is normal or slow. The seizures worsen with the administration of benzodiazepines. The seizures usually resolve within 2 months and neurological outcome is normal.[58–61]

Benign myoclonus of early infancy

Benign myoclonus of early infancy has an onset at age 3 to 9 months but it can be much earlier. The seizures resemble infantile spasms but the EEG is normal. The seizures usually occur while the patient is awake. The seizures disorder may continue for 1 to 2 years but neurological outcome is normal.[58–61]

Treatment

The clinician should first search for underlying etiologies producing the seizures and treat (hypoglycemia, hypocalcemia, sepsis). If the clinician cannot find a readily identifiable and treatable etiology, the frontline agent of choice for treating seizures is phenobarbital (see Table 3-14 for dosing suggestions).[62] Phenobarbital as a single agent will stop seizure activity in 42% of patients. When the seizure does not respond to a single agent, phenytoin is added with an increase in efficacy to 65%. Currently, fosphenytoin, the salt ester of phenytoin, is preferred in the neonate because it is an aqueous solution that is soluble in glucose-containing solutions, can be administered more quickly than phenytoin, and will not cause "purple glove syndrome."[62] Purple glove syndrome is necrosis or injury of the soft tissue that can

Table 3-14.
Neonatal AED Dosing Suggestions

Phenobarbital—20 mg/kg load over 10 to 15 min.
If necessary add more phenobarbital in 5-mg/kg boluses
Fosphenytoin—20 mg/kg at 1 mg/kg/min
Ativan—0.1 mg/kg

From Rennie J, Boylan G. Treatment of neonatal seizures. Arch Dis Child Fetal Neonatal 2007;92:F148–F150.

occur with intravenous infusion of the highly alkaline phenytoin. The drug of choice for neonates in status is lorazepam. This agent has several properties that make it ideal—a long half-life and a small volume of distribution, which prolongs its retention at high levels in the brain.

REFERENCES

1. Hauser WA, Beghi E. First seizure definitions and worldwide incidence and mortality. *Epilepsia.* 2008; 49(suppl 1): 8-12.
2. Teasell R, Bayona N, Lippert C, Villamere J, Hellings C. Post-traumatic seizure disorder following acquired brain injury. *Brain Inj.* 2007;21:201-214.
3. Statler KD. Pediatric posttraumatic seizures: epidemiology, putative mechanisms of epileptogenesis and promising investigational progress. *Dev Neurosci.* 2006;28: 354-363.
4. Agrawal A, Timothy J, Pandit L, Manju M. Post-traumatic epilepsy: an overview. *Clin Neurol Neurosurg.* 2006; 108:433-439.
5. Weber YG, Lerche H. Genetic mechanisms in idiopathic epilepsies. *Dev Med Child Neurol.* 2008;50:648-654.
6. Leventer RJ, Guerrini R, Dobyns WB. Malformations of cortical development and epilepsy. *Dialogues Clin Neurosci.* 2008;10:47-62.
7. Steinlein OK. Genetics and epilepsy. *Dialogues Clin Neurosci.* 2008;10:29-38.
8. Griffith JF, Ch'ien LT. Herpes simplex virus encephalitis. Diagnostic and treatment considerations. *Med Clin North Am.* 1983;67:991-1008.
9. Geyer J, Keating J, Potts D, Carney P, eds. *Neurology for the Boards.* 3rd ed. Philadelphia: Lippincott Williams & Wilkins;2006.
10. Riviello JJ. Classification of seizures and epilepsy. *Curr Neurol Neurosci Rep.* 2003;3:325-331.
11. Durón RM, Medina MT, Martínez-Juárez IE, et al. Seizures of idiopathic generalized epilepsies. *Epilepsia.* 2005;46:34-47.
12. Gardiner M. Genetics of idiopathic generalized epilepsies. *Epilepsia.* 2005;46(suppl 9):15-20.
13. Jallon P, Latour P. Epidemiology of idiopathic generalized epilepsies. *Epilepsia.* 2005;46(suppl 9):10-14.

14. West WJ. On a peculiar form of infantile convulsions. *Lancet.* 1841;1:724-725.

15. Wong M, Trevanthan E. Infantile spasms *Pediatr Neurol.* 2001;24:89-98.

16. Riikonen R. The latest on infantile spasms. *Curr Opin Neurol.* 2005;18:91-95.

17. Hrachovy RA, Frost JD Jr. Infantile epileptic encephalopathy with hypsarrhythmia (infantile spasms/West syndrome). *J Clin Neurophysiol.* 2003;20:408-425.

18. Aicardi J. Aicardi syndrome. *Brain Dev.* 2005;27:164-171.

19. Markand ON. Lennox–Gastaut syndrome (childhood epileptic encephalopathy). *J Clin Neurophysiol.* 2003;20:426-441.

20. Neubauer BA, Hahn A, Stephani U, Doose H. Clinical spectrum and genetics of Rolandic epilepsy. *Adv Neurol.* 2002;89:475-479.

21. Camfield P, Camfield C. Epileptic syndromes in childhood: clinical features, outcomes, and treatment. *Epilepsia.* 2002;43(suppl 3):27-32.

22. Saint-Martin AD, Carcangiu R, Arzimanoglou A, et al. Semiology of typical and atypical Rolandic epilepsy: a video-EEG analysis. *Epileptic Disord.* 2001;3:173-182.

23. Kellaway P. The electroencephalographic features of benign centrotemporal (rolandic) epilepsy of childhood. *Epilepsia.* 2000;41:1053-1056.

24. Rodriguez AJ, Buechler RD, Lahr BD, So EL. Temporal lobe seizure semiology during wakefulness and sleep. *Epilepsy Res.* 2007;74:211-214.

25. Maillard L, Vignal JP, Gavaret M, et al. Semiologic and electrophysiologic correlations in temporal lobe seizure subtypes. *Epilepsia.* 2004;45:1590-1599.

26. Hoffmann JM, Elger CE, Kleefuss-Lie AA. Lateralizing value of behavioral arrest in patients with temporal lobe epilepsy. *Epilepsy Behav.* 2008;13(4):634-636.

27. Marks WJ Jr, Laxer KD. Semiology of temporal lobe seizures: value in lateralizing the seizure focus. *Epilepsia.* 1998;39:721-726.

28. Geyer JD, Payne TA, Faught E, Drury I. Postictal nose-rubbing in the diagnosis, lateralization, and localization of seizures. *Neurology.* 1999;52:743-745.

29. French JA, Williamson PD, Thadani VM, et al. Characteristics of mesial temporal lobe epilepsy. I. Results of history and physical examination. *Ann Neurol.* 1983;34:374-380.

30. Geyer JD, Bilir E, Faught RE, et al. Significance of interictal temporal lobe delta activity for localization of the primary epileptogenic region. *Neurology.*1999;52:202-205.

31. O'Brien TJ, Mosewich RK, Britton JW, Cascino GD, So EL. History and seizure semiology in distinguishing frontal lobe seizures and temporal lobe seizures. *Epilepsy Res.* 2008;82(2-3):177-182.

32. Battaglia D, Lettori D, Contaldo I, et al. Seizure semiology of lesional frontal lobe epilepsies in children. *Neuropediatrics.* 2007;38:287-291.

33. Lee JJ, Lee SK, Lee SY, et al. Frontal lobe epilepsy: clinical characteristics, surgical outcomes and diagnostic modalities. *Seizure.* 2008;17:514-523.

34. Bonelli SB, Lurger S, Zimprich F, Stogmann E, Assem-Hilger E, Baumgartner C. Clinical seizure lateralization in frontal lobe epilepsy. *Epilepsia.* 2007;48:517-523.

35. Bleasel A, Kotagal P, Kankirawatana P, Rybicki L. Lateralizing value and semiology of ictal limb posturing and version in temporal lobe and extratemporal epilepsy. *Epilepsia.* 1997;38:168-174.

36. Gardella E, Rubboli G, Tassinari CA. Ictal grasping: prevalence and characteristics in seizures with different semiology. *Epilepsia.* 2006;47(suppl 5):59-63.

37. Taylor I, Berkovic SF, Kivity S, Scheffer IE. Benign occipital epilepsies of childhood: clinical features and genetics. *Brain.* 2008;131:2287-2294.

38. Ludwig, BI, Ajmone-Marsan C. Clincial ictal patterns in epileptic patients with occipital electroencephalographic foci. *Neurology.* 1975;25:463-471.

39. Blume WT, Wiebe S, Tapsell LM. Occipital epilepsy: lateral versus mesial. *Brain.* 2005;128:1209-1225.

40. Kim DW, Lee SK, Yun CH, et al. Parietal lobe epilepsy: the semiology, yield of diagnostic workup, and surgical outcome. *Epilepsia.* 2004;45:641-649.

41. Cascino GD, Hulihan JF, Sharborough FW, Kelly PJ. Parietal lobe lesional epilepsy: electroclinical correlation and operative outcome. *Epilepsia.* 1993;34:522-527.

42. Williamson PD, Boon PA, Thadani VM, et al. Parietal lobe epilepsy: diagnostic considerations and results of surgery. *Ann Neurol.* 1992;31:193-201.

43. Hirsh E, Valenti MP, Rudolf G, et al. Landau–Kleffner syndrome is not an eponymic badge of ignorance. *Epilepsy Res.* 2006;70:S239-S247.

44. Landau WM, Kleffner FR. Syndrome of acquired aphasia with convulsive disorder in children. *Neurology.* 1957;7:523-530.

45. Mikati MA, Shamseddine AN. Management of Landau–Kleffner syndrome. *Pediatric Drugs.* 2005;7:377-389.

46. Morrell F, Whisler WW, Smith MC, et al. Landau–Kleffner syndrome: treatment with subpial intracortical transaction. *Brain.* 1995;118:1529-1546.

47. Beaumanoir A. The Landau–Kleffner syndrome. In : Roger J, Bureau M, Dravet C, et al., eds. *Epileptic Syndromes in Infancy, Childhood and Adolescence.* London; John Libbey;1992:231-243.

48. Berg AT, Shinnar S. The risk of seizure recurrence following a first unprovoked seizure: a quantitative review. *Neurology.* 1991;41:965-972.

49. Hughes JR, Fino JJ. Focal seizures and EEG: prognostic considerations. *Clin Electroencephalogr.* 2003;34:174-181.

50. Riikonen R. Infantile spasms: therapy and outcome. *J Child Neurol.* 2004;19:401-404.

51. Mackay MT, Weiss SK, Adams-Webber T, et al., for the American Academy of Neurology; Child Neurology Society. Practice parameter: medical treatment of infantile spasms: report of the American Academy of Neurology and the Child Neurology Society. *Neurology.* 2004;62:1668-1681.

52. Sato S, White BG, Penry JK, et al. Valproic acid vs ethosuximide in the treatment of absence seizures. *Neurology.* 1982;32(2):157-163.

54. Selwa LM, Geyer J, Nikakhtar N, Brown MB, Schuh LA, Drury I. Nonepileptic seizure outcome varies by type of spell and duration of illness. *Epilepsia.* 2000;41:1330-1334.

55. Geyer JD, Payne TA, Drury I. The value of pelvic thrusting in the diagnosis of seizures and pseudoseizures. *Neurology.* 2000;54:227-229.

56. Duncan R, Oto M, Russell AJ, Conway P. Pseudosleep events in patients with psychogenic non-epileptic seizures: prevalence and associations. *J Neurol Neurosurg Psychiatry.* 2004;75:1009-1012.

57. Tuxhorn I, Kotagal P. Classification. *Semin Neurol.* 2008;28:277-288.

58. Nabbout R, Dulac O. Epileptic syndromes in infancy and childhood. *Curr Opin Neurol.* 2008;21:161-166.

59. Tich SN, d'Allest AM, Villepin AT, et al. Pathological features of neonatal EEG in preterm babies born before 30 weeks of gestational age. *Neurophysiol Clin.* 2007;37: 325-370.

60. Silverstein FS, Jensen FE. Neonatal seizures. *Ann Neurol.* 2007;62:112-120.

61. Specchio N, Vigevano F. The spectrum of benign infantile seizures. *Epilepsy Res.* 2006;70(suppl 1):S156-S167.

62. Rennie J, Boylan G. Treatment of neonatal seizures. *Arch Dis Child Fetal Neonatal Ed.* 2007;92:F148-F150.

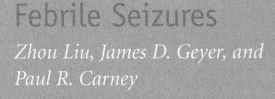

CHAPTER 4

Febrile Seizures

Zhou Liu, James D. Geyer, and Paul R. Carney

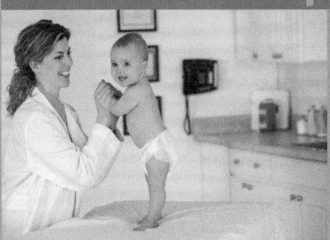

DEFINITIONS AND EPIDEMIOLOGY

Febrile seizures are convulsions induced by a fever in infants or young children. They are the most common type of seizure during childhood. While febrile seizures are usually benign, they are often very upsetting to parents. There are several operational definitions of febrile seizures

1. American Academy of Pediatrics Practice Parameter: "A simple febrile seizure is a generalized seizure occurring in an infant or child between the ages of six months and five years, lasting less than 15 minutes and occurring only once in 24 hours. The child should not have an intracranial infection or a severe metabolic disturbance."[1]
2. The International League Against Epilepsy (ILAE): "A seizure occurring in childhood after one month of age, associated with a febrile illness not caused by an infection of the central nervous system, without previous neonatal seizures or a previous unprovoked seizure, and not meeting criteria for other acute symptomatic seizures."[2]

Both definitions exclude seizures with fever in children who have previously had seizures unrelated to fever and do not exclude children with prior neurological impairment. Although these two definitions are similar, there is a discrepancy regarding the lower age limit of first seizure onset (3 months versus 1 month). The three critical elements of febrile seizures are shown in Table 4-1.

Epidemiologic studies show that approximately 3% to 4% of children have at least one febrile seizure by 7 years of age.[3] There is a regional variation of the cumulative incidence of febrile seizures in different countries (Table 4-2). Febrile seizures are slightly more common in boys than girls. In the United States, the prevalence of febrile seizures in African American children is 4.2% versus 3.5% in Caucasian children.[3]

PATHOGENESIS AND PATHOPHYSIOLOGY

The pathophysiology of febrile seizures is unknown. It is possible that the following three features interact, resulting in a febrile seizure:

- Immature brain
- Fever
- Genetic predisposition

Immature Brain

Febrile seizures rarely occur before ages 1 to 3 months, suggesting that a certain degree of myelination or network maturation is required for the clinical expression of febrile seizures. Animal studies have shown that immature neuronal networks tend to generate periodic discharge and this facilitates the generation of pathologic and pathogenic oscillations.[4]

Febrile seizures rarely occur after ages 5 to 6 years, so there is a clear relationship between febrile seizures and brain maturation. Several studies have suggested that there is enhanced neuronal excitability during normal brain maturation.[5] It is well established that many factors contribute the increased excitability of the immature brain. The tendency of immature neurons to oscillate is due to their high input resistance, which helps the generation of

Table 4-1.

Three Critical Elements of Febrile Seizures

Age of first seizure onset	■ Typically between 6 months and 5 years with the peak incidence at 18 months[1]
	■ Febrile seizures occuring after 4 years account for 6-15%[20]
	■ Febrile seizure occurring before 3 months or after 6 years are atypical and the outcome of these febrile seizures may not be as benign as typical febrile seizures
Temperature of a fever	■ Both AAP and ILAE definitions do not provide a specific temperature criterion for its diagnosis
	■ An axillary temperature of either >38.5°C or >37.8°C as a simple cutoff level has been proposed to diagnose febrile seizures, but consensus is lacking
	■ The majority of children with febrile seizures have rectal temperatures greater than 102°F or 38.5°C and most febrile seizures occur during the first day of fever
	■ There are no data to support the rate of temperature rise as being more important than the peak temperature achieved[8]
Seizures	■ Seizures are caused by paroxysmal synchronous firing of large neuronal networks in the brain, resulting in an alteration in mental status, tonic or clonic convulsions, and various other associated symptoms
	■ Most common type of febrile seizures are generalized seizures involving both sides of the body
	■ Simple partial seizures or complex partial seizures may occur, and these seizures might become generalized after a partial onset
	■ Febrile seizures with partial onset are usually less benign than generalized febrile seizures

action potentials and increases excitability. In addition, during the early postnatal period GABA exerts a paradoxical excitatory effect in all animal species including primates.[6,7] The lack of efficient GABAergic inhibition increases excitability and can facilitate synchronicity.[4] The delayed maturation of postsynaptic G protein mediated $GABA_B$-mediated inhibition will also contribute to augment neuronal excitability. The prolonged NMDA-mediated excitatory postsynaptic currents in immature versus adult neurons promotes the generation of network-driven events. These properties also underscore the propensity of immature networks to generate early network-driven patterns such as giant depolarizing potentials.[8] The transient exuberant formation of excitatory synapses may also contribute to increased excitability in more developed stages.[9]

Table 4-2.

Cumulative Incidence of Febrile Seizures by Geographic Regions

United States	2-5%
South America	2-5%
Western Europe	2-5%
India	5-10%
Japan	8.8%
Guam	14%

From Hauser WA. The prevalence and incidence of convulsive disorders in children. Epilepsia. 1994;35(suppl):S1–S6.

Fever

Fever is associated with cytokine release. Activation of the cytokine network may increase the susceptibility to febrile seizures.[10–12] It is also possible that circulating toxins and immune reaction products modulate neuronal excitability. Previous studies have suggested that interleukin-1β, a pyrogenic pro-inflammatory cytokine, and hyperpolarization-activated cyclic nucleotide-gated cation channels are involved in the generation of febrile seizures or enhanced seizure susceptibility in animals. Conversely, neuropeptide Y could prevent febrile seizures by increasing the seizure threshold.[13]

Variations in temperature have effects on most cellular events, and several neurological disorders are provoked by elevated temperature, including febrile seizures and febrile episodic ataxia (calcium channels, CACN1A).[14] Temperature changes have been shown to affect plasma membrane states[15] and synaptic transmission.[16] Synaptic vesicle recycling has been shown to be temperature dependent. The size of recycling vesicles is twice as large, and the speed of both endocytosis and exocytosis are faster at physiologic temperature than at room temperature.[17] Although the dynamic temperature dependence of turnover of $GABA_A$ receptors is unclear, there is evidence that inhibitory synaptic strength can be modulated within 10 minutes through recruiting more functional $GABA_A$ receptor to the postsynaptic plasma membrane.[18] Kang and associates[19] discovered recently that $GABA_A$ receptors containing mutant gamma subunits were not as good at getting to the neuronal cell surface when they were exposed to high temperatures. When exposing cells expressing the mutant receptors to 40°C, simulating a "fever" of 104°F, the receptors disappeared from the cell surface. Fewer inhibitory GABA$_A$ receptors on the cell membrane could leave a neuron open to the excitation and repetitive firing that characterizes seizures. The investigators are currently studying where the receptors go when the temperature is raised. Are they taken inside the cell more quickly, degraded, or is their forward insertion into the cell membrane slowed?

Genetic Factors

Although the mode of inheritance is unknown, genetic factors are clearly important. These factors may be either causative or protective against febrile seizures. The literature describing the genetics of febrile seizures is extensive, continually expanding, and complicated, reflecting the complexity of the disorder. The risk of developing febrile seizures is higher in some families than in others. A positive family history for febrile seizures can be elicited in 25% to 40% of patients with febrile seizures, and the reported frequency in siblings of children with febrile seizures has ranged from 9% to 22%. Studies showing a higher concordance rate in monozygotic rather than in dizygotic twins also support a genetic contribution. Familial clustering studies indicate a doubling of risk in children when both parents, rather than one parent, had febrile seizures.[20]

While there is clear evidence for a genetic basis of febrile seizures, the mode of inheritance is unclear. The mode of inheritance is more likely polygenic or autosomal dominant with reduced penetration.[21] The most convincing evidence has emerged from linkage studies with reported linkages on numerous chromosomes (Table 4-3) with the strongest linkage on chromosome 2q and specifically, linkage to the genes responsible for sodium channel receptors and specifically a mutation in the alpha (α) subunit of the first neuronal sodium channel gene (*SCN1A*). The linkage on chromosomes 2q and 19q associated with the phenotype of febrile seizures, generalized epilepsy (tonic-clonic, absence, and myoclonic) (GEFS+), shows evidence of sodium channel involvement. Clearly, febrile seizures are an extremely heterogeneous condition with a complicated and, as yet, unclear pathophysiologic and genetic basis. More than seven chromosome linkage sites have been associated with febrile seizures, suggesting locus heterogeneity. In addition, at least 5 genes have been identified as causal for epilepsy syndromes that include febrile seizures.[22] This includes the unique syndrome of generalized epilepsy with febrile seizure plus (GEFS+), which is caused in most cases by an autosomal dominant defect in cerebral voltage-gated sodium channels subunits (SCN1B, SCN1A, and SCN2A) or a defect in the gamma 2 subunit of the GABAA receptor.[23] Although GEFS+ includes seizure types other than febrile seizures, it may give insight into the biology of age-limited temperature-dependent seizure susceptibility. In these patients with genetic predisposition, a low-grade fever can cause febrile seizures.

CLINICAL PRESENTATION

Febrile seizures typically begin with a sudden contraction of muscles involving the face, trunk, arms, or legs on both sides of the body. The force of the muscle contraction may cause the child to emit an involuntary cry or moan. The seizures may be accompanied with loss of consciousness, tongue biting, urinary/bowel incontinence, fall, vomiting, and apnea; and followed by postictal sleepiness, confusion, or feelings of fear.

In some cases, the febrile seizure is the first clear symptom of illness, but the study by Berg and colleagues in 1997[24] found that only 21% of children experienced febrile seizures before or within an hour of recognized fever onset. Most patients (57%) had a seizure after 1 to 24 hours of recognized fever, and 22% had seizures more than 24 hours after the onset of fever.

The common causes of fever associated with febrile seizures are shown in Table 4-4. There are no recent studies of the nature of inciting infections preferably

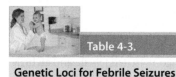

Table 4-3.

Genetic Loci for Febrile Seizures

- 8q13-q21
- 19p
- 2q23-24
- 6q22-24
- 5q14-q15

Table 4-4.[25]

Causes of Fever in Febrile Seizure

- Upper respiratory tract infection or pharyngitis (38%)
- Otitis media (23%)
- Pneumonia (15%)
- Gastroenteritis (7%
- Roseola infantum (5%)
- Noninfectious illness (12%)

causing febrile seizures. While the widespread use of vaccines against *Haemophilus influenzae*, varicella, *pneumococcus*, and *meningococcus* have changed the background of infections in the pediatric population, the incidence of febrile seizures has not significantly changed, suggesting the specific inciting infectious pathogens are not responsible for febrile seizures. Only documented pathogen associated with febrile seizures is human herpes virus type 6 (HHV6).[26] HHV6 causes infant roseola, a common infection of infants and toddlers that is usually associated with fever ≥ 103°F. It is postulated that direct viral invasion of the brain, combined with fever, causes the initial febrile seizure, and that the virus might be reactivated by fever during subsequent illnesses, causing recurrent febrile seizures.

Seizures occurring soon after vaccinations should not be regarded as a direct adverse effect of the vaccine.[27] Such seizures are believed to be triggered by fever induced by the vaccine. Their subsequent clinical course is identical to other febrile seizures,[28] with no increased risk for subsequent afebrile seizures or abnormal neurological development.[29] The frequency of febrile seizures after diphtheria-pertussis-tetanus or measles vaccination is 6 to 9 and 24 to 25 per 100,000 children vaccinated, respectively. The newer acellular pertussis vaccines rarely induce a febrile reaction, and therefore fewer febrile seizures currently result from this immunization.[30]

Types of Febrile Seizures

Febrile seizures can be divided into simple or complex febrile seizures depending on the duration of seizure, seizure type, and number of seizures during a 24-hour period (Table 4-5).

Simple febrile seizures are relatively brief (< 10 to 15 min) generalized seizures that do not recur during the same febrile illness. Complex febrile seizures are characterized by one of the following features: prolonged duration (> 10 to 15 min), partial onset, or multiple recurrences within 24 hours. If a careful history is taken,

approximately one-third of all febrile seizures presenting to the emergency room have complex features.

Seizures in the context of a febrile illness occurring in a neurologically abnormal child are still considered simple or complex according to the above criteria. Although children who have preexisting neurological abnormalities are more likely to present with complex febrile seizures and are more likely to develop subsequent epilepsy, they can still have simple febrile seizures.

In the National Collaborative Perinatal Project study of 55,000 infants, 1706 experienced a first febrile seizure and were followed to age 7 years[20]

- 74% of initial febrile seizures were "simple."
- 26% of the initial febrile seizures were "complex."
  - 4% focal
  - 8% prolonged greater than 15 minutes
  - 16% with recurrence within 24 hours
  - 0.4% with Todd paresis

In another prospective cohort study of first febrile seizures, 35% of 428 children had one or more features of a complex febrile seizure.[31] A retrospective study from Singapore reported similar findings.[32] Prolonged (greater than 30 minutes) postictal unconsciousness, while rare, has been associated with seizures that are focal or last longer than 5 minutes.[33] About 75% of febrile convulsions are "simple" febrile seizures, and first febrile seizure is complex in approximately 25% of cases. For 7 years after a first "simple" febrile seizure, children have the same health care utilization as age-matched febrile and afebrile controls, except for a minor increase in referrals to ear, nose, and throat services shortly after the febrile seizure.[34] Children with febrile seizures do not seem to be more vulnerable to illness and their parents do not excessively consult a physician.

If the febrile seizure lasts longer than 30 minutes (whether as a single seizure or as a series of seizures) without full recovery between seizures, it is classified as febrile status epilepticus. Febrile status epilepticus accounts for approximately 5% of all febrile seizures. However, because of the frequency with which febrile seizures occur, it accounts for approximately one-quarter of all cases of status epilepticus in childhood and for two-thirds of cases of status epilepticus in the second year of life.

Risk Factors for First Febrile Seizure

Risk factors for a first febrile convulsion have been studied in comparison with age-matched febrile and afebrile controls.[35] The risk of a first febrile seizure is about 30% if a child has two or more of the independent risk factors listed in Table 4-6. It may be reasonable to offer anticipatory guidance (familiarization with febrile seizures, first aid, and types of management) to families at high risk.

Table 4-5.

Simple and Complex Febrile Seizures

Simple Febrile Seizures	Complex Febrile Seizures
■ Generalized tonic-clonic	■ Focal
■ Duration less than 15 minutes	■ Duration more than 15 minutes
■ Without recurrence within the next 24 hours	■ Occurring in a cluster of 2 or more convulsions within 24 hours

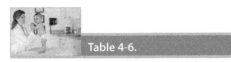

Table 4-6.

Risk Factors for First Febrile Seizures

- A first- or second-degree relative with febrile seizures
- Delayed neonatal discharge of greater than 28 days of age
- Parental report of slow development
- Day care attendance

DIAGNOSIS

The initial workup of a febrile seizure should include a thorough history from a reliable witness and a careful pediatric and neurological examination. Meningitis, encephalitis, accidental poisoning, trauma or abuse, electrolyte imbalance, and acute symptomatic seizures must be excluded first. Examination looking for evidence of meningitis, underlying neurological deficit, asymmetry, or stigmata of a neurocutaneous or metabolic

disorder, and signs of developmental delay are important. A number of questions need to be addressed when faced with a child who has had the first or subsequent febrile seizures using Table 4-7.

DIAGNOSTIC EVALUATION

If the cause of fever can be identified and if the child presents no disturbance of consciousness, it is usually not necessary to obtain further laboratory evaluation (Table 4-7).

DIFFERENTIAL DIAGNOSIS

When considering febrile seizures, it is important to differentiate them from other paroxysmal and non-epileptic events that may mimic epileptic seizures. These seizure-like events are rigors, syncope, reflex anoxic seizures, breath-holding spells, impaired consciousness, and apnea, and may also be associated with any febrile illness (Table 4-8).

Table 4-7.

Evaluation of Febrile Seizures

Lab Studies	■ Routine laboratory studies usually are not indicated unless they are performed as part of a search for the source of a fever.
	■ Serum electrolytes (particularly sodium), glucose, blood urea nitrogen, calcium, and phosphorus levels should be reserved for children for whom there is a reasonable suspicion that one or more may be abnormal.
	■ Patients with febrile seizures have an incidence of bacteremia similar to patients with fever alone; therefore, blood cultures and complete blood count are not routinely necessary.
Imaging Studies	■ Neuroimaging should not be performed in the routine evaluation of child with a first simple febrile seizure.
	■ A CT or MRI should be performed only when an underlying structural lesion is suspected.
	■ A CT or MRI should be considered in patients with complex febrile seizures.
	■ Neuroimaging might be considered when the child has significant focal neurological abnormalities, developmental abnormalities, neurocutaneous lesions, or abnormal head size.
EEG	■ An EEG should not be routinely performed in the evaluation of a neurologically healthy child with a first simple febrile seizure, either at the time of presentation or within the following month.
Lumbar Puncture	■ In 1996, the American Academy of Pediatrics (AAP) recommended that a lumbar puncture be strongly considered in patients younger than 12 months presenting with fever and seizure. The AAP also recommended that a lumbar puncture be considered in patients aged 12-18 months. A lumber puncture is not routinely necessary in patients older than 18 months. This recommendation takes into account the difficulty in recognizing meningitis in infants and young children and the range of experience in the evaluation of pediatric patients among health care providers.
	■ The incidence of meningitis in children with first seizures associated with fever is 2-5%.
	■ Patients who have a first-time febrile seizure and do not have a rapidly improving mental status should be evaluated for meningitis.
	■ Risk factors for meningitis in patients presenting with seizure and fever include the following:
	■ A physician visit within 48 hours
	■ Seizure activity at the time of arrival in the ED
	■ Focal seizure, suspicious physical examination findings (rash, petechiae), cyanosis, hypotension, or grunting
	■ Abnormal neurological examination

Table 4-8.

Paroxysmal Events That Mimic Seizures

- Rigors
- Febrile myoclonus
- Syncope
- Breath-holding spells (reflex anoxic seizures)
- GE reflux
- Apnea
- An acute and transient confusion state associated with high fever

PROGNOSIS AND COMPLICATIONS

There are two significant risks associated with febrile seizures: recurrent febrile seizures and later epilepsy.[36]

Risk Factors for Recurrent Febrile Seizures

About one-third of all children with a first febrile seizure experience recurrent seizures. Recurrent febrile seizures occur in about 30% to 40% of patients, usually within a year of the first seizure.[31,32] Predictors of recurrence include age, family history, duration of illness, and temperature at the time of the seizure (Table 4-9).

Risk factors can be combined to provide a useful prediction scheme. The recurrence risk for patients with none of the four risk factors (age less than 18 months, family history of febrile seizures, low temperature at the time of the seizure, and short duration of illness) was

4%; with one factor, 23%; with two, 32%; with three, 62%; and with all four, 76%.

Risk Factors for Epilepsy

Febrile seizures are now known to be benign and only 2% to 3% of children will later develop epilepsy.[3] The risk of epilepsy following a simple febrile seizure is about 2%, and following a complex febrile seizure still only 5% to 10% (Table 4-10). Therefore, febrile seizures can be viewed as a syndrome of reactive seizures, and not as a true epileptic syndrome.[37]

Risk factors for later epilepsy include:

- Abnormal neurological or developmental status prior to the first febrile seizure
- Family history of afebrile seizures
- Complex febrile seizure

In addition, children having the onset of febrile seizures after the age of 5 years do not have an increased risk of epilepsy.[38] Therefore, risk factors in the individual child are not useful clinical predictors of epilepsy. When epilepsy does develop, the seizures can be of virtually any type, although the highest association is with generalized, rather than partial, seizures.[39,40]

Approximately 15% of children with epilepsy have one or more preceding febrile seizures, regardless of the cause of the epilepsy.[38] This observation suggests that the tendency for febrile seizures plays an important role in the creation of an individual person's seizure threshold. However, there is no evidence that one or multiple febrile seizures cause epilepsy.

A family history of seizures, preexisting brain damage, or birth complications may modify the long-term risk of epilepsy after febrile seizures. Recently, Vestergaard

Table 4-9.

Risk Factors for Recurrent Febrile Seizures

Young age at time of first febrile seizure	■ The earlier the age of onset, the greater is the risk of recurrence.
	■ 50% chance of recurrence if first febrile seizure before 1 year of age.
	■ 20% chance of recurrence if the first seizure is after age 3 years.
Relatively low fever at time of first seizure	■ A lower temperature at the time of the first seizure increases the chance of recurrence.
	■ A meta-analysis by Berg has shown that young age of onset and family history of febrile seizures are the strongest predictors of another seizure.
Family history of a febrile seizure in a first-degree relative	■ A family history of febrile seizures is consistently associated with recurrences.
	■ A family history of afebrile seizures has inconsistently demonstrated this relationship.
	■ Complex febrile seizures are not more frequently associated with recurrences.
Brief duration between fever onset and initial seizure	■ A shorter duration of fever before the febrile seizure onset increases the chance of recurrence.

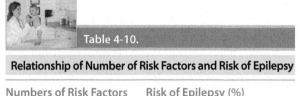

Table 4-10.	
Relationship of Number of Risk Factors and Risk of Epilepsy	
Numbers of Risk Factors	Risk of Epilepsy (%)
0	0.9
1	2
2 or more	10

and associates[41] evaluated the association between febrile seizures and epilepsy in a population-based cohort of 1.54 million persons born in Denmark (1978–2002), including 49,857 persons with febrile seizures and 16,481 persons with epilepsy. Overall, for children with febrile seizures compared with those without such seizures, the rate ratio for epilepsy was 5.43 (95% confidence interval: 5.19, 5.69). The risk remained high during the entire follow-up but was particularly high shortly after the first febrile seizure, especially in children who experienced early (< 1 year of age) or late (> 3 years of age) onset of febrile seizures. At 23 years of follow-up, the overall cumulative incidence of epilepsy after febrile seizures was 6.9% (95% confidence interval: 6.5, 7.3). In conclusion, persons with a history of febrile seizures had a higher rate of epilepsy that lasted into adult life, but less than 7% of children with febrile seizures developed epilepsy. The risk was higher for those who had a family history of epilepsy, cerebral palsy, or low Apgar scores at 5 minutes.[41]

MANAGEMENT

The management of febrile seizures should focus on seizure first aid and parental counseling.

Febrile seizures are usually brief and self-limited and no treatment is necessary in most cases. When the seizure occurs, the child should be placed on his or her side on a protected surface and observed carefully. If the seizure lasts longer than 10 minutes, intravenous diazepam (0.2-0.5 mg/kg of body weight) or rectal diazepam (0.5 mg/kg of body weight) should be given to halt the seizure. If the convulsion is prolonged, the child's airway should be kept clear and oxygenation maintained. In the rare event that seizures continue after the initial treatment with diazepam, a diagnosis of febrile status epilepticus should be made and the standard status epilepticus treatment protocol is indicated. Optimal management of status epilepticus requires admission to a pediatric intensive care unit.

Witnessing a febrile seizure is emotionally traumatic for parents, and many think that their child is dying or their child's brain is being damaged. After an initial

febrile seizure, parents can develop persistent fear of fever, recurrence of febrile seizure, and future epilepsy. These concerns could negatively affect the family routines and often parents worry about the potential association of febrile seizures and sudden infant death. Therefore, reassuring and counseling parents is one of the most important aspects of management of febrile seizures. Parental counseling aims at educating the parents regarding the common concerns described in the next sections.

There is no increased risk of mortality in febrile seizures. Vestergaard and colleagues[42] compared the risk of sudden infant death syndrome in 9,977 siblings of children with a febrile seizure and 20,177 siblings who never had febrile seizures. These data did not support a shared susceptibility hypothesis. Several studies have documented that there is no increased risk or incidence of death in children with febrile seizures including febrile status epilepticus.

There is no evidence that febrile seizures can cause brain damage or cognitive impairment. The National Collaborative Perinatal Project study included 431 sibling pairs discordant for febrile seizures.[43] Psychometric testing at age 7 years included the Wechsler Intelligence Scale for Children as a measure of overall intelligence and the Wide Range Achievement Test as a measure of academic achievement. For those known to be normal before the first febrile seizure, there was no difference in intelligence or school achievement between sibling pairs, even in the 27 with febrile seizures lasting more than 30 minutes. Chang and colleagues[44] conducted another study utilizing a prospective, population-based, case-control method to assess the learning, spatial, and sequential working memory of 87 school-aged children with a previous febrile seizure and 87 randomly selected age-matched control subjects. The febrile seizure group performed significantly and consistently better than control subjects on mnemonic capacity and had more flexible mental processing abilities than their age-matched controls.

There is controversy regarding prolonged febrile seizures causing temporal lobe epilepsy. Data from large cohorts of children with febrile seizures indicate that in 2% to 10% of children who have febrile seizures, unprovoked seizures or epilepsy will subsequently develop. In most studies, the risk of developing epilepsy after *simple* febrile seizures is only mildly elevated compared with the risk for the general population. *Complex* febrile seizures, however, are clearly associated with an increased risk of subsequent epilepsy. Prolonged febrile seizures, particularly very prolonged febrile seizures and febrile status epilepticus, are associated with a substantially elevated risk for future epilepsy. However, not all children with febrile seizures in whom epilepsy develops will have temporal lobe epilepsy (TLE). Typically, in those patients with generalized febrile seizures, generalized epilepsies will develop, whereas in those individuals with focal febrile seizures, focal epilepsies will develop, suggesting that febrile seizures may be an age-specific expression of seizure susceptibility in patients with an underlying seizure predisposition. The types of epilepsy that occur in children with prior febrile seizures are varied and not very different from those that occur in children without such a history of febrile seizures. There are no prospective studies that document a normal MRI, followed by a prolonged febrile seizure, then followed by unilateral hippocampal swelling, followed by mesial temporal sclerosis (MTS) and intractable TLE. Additional prospective studies are needed.

Key questions left to be answered include the following: How often does seizure-induced damage occur? What are the risk factors? How often does MTS result?

Antiepileptic Medications

There is no compelling reason to treat children with daily prophylactic medication after one or more simple febrile seizures.[1] The potential side effects of drugs outweigh the benefits.

Antipyretic Medications

There is no evidence that rigorous use of antipyretic medication could prevent febrile seizures or recurrent febrile seizures. A Finnish study randomized children to receive placebo or acetaminophen (10 mg/kg) at the time of illness for 2 years following a first febrile seizure.[45] Those receiving placebo had recurrent febrile seizures during 8.2% of febrile illnesses, compared with 5.2% for those receiving acetaminophen. A similar randomized study showed that administration of ibuprofen syrup during a febrile illness does not prevent febrile seizure recurrences.[46] Therefore, the compulsive use of antipyretics for prevention of febrile seizures is not recommended.

SUMMARY

Febrile seizures are fever-induced convulsions in children aged 6 months to 5 years. They are the most common type of childhood seizure and usually benign.

There is no evidence that febrile seizures are associated with an increased risk of sudden infant death syndrome, brain damage, cognitive impairment, or in most cases, epilepsy. There is controversy regarding prolonged febrile seizures and subsequent temporal lobe epilepsy. No specific treatment is necessary in most cases of febrile seizures since it is usually brief and self-limited. The management of febrile seizures is focused on seizure first aid and parental counseling. This chapter is aimed at helping physicians understand the natural history and prognosis of febrile seizures and to choose the appropriate management plans while avoiding unnecessary diagnostic procedures and therapies.

REFERENCES

1. Anonymous. Practice parameter: long-term treatment of the child with simple febrile seizures. American Academy of Pediatrics. Committee on Quality Improvement, Subcommittee on Febrile Seizures. *Pediatrics*. 1999;103:1307-1309.
2. ILAE. Guidelines for epidemiologic studies on epilepsy. *Epilepsia*. 1993;34:592-596.
3. Nelson KB, Ellenberg JH. Predictors of epilepsy in children who have experienced febrile seizures. *N Engl J Med*. 1976;295:1029-1033.
4. Khazipov R, Khalilov I, Tyzio R, Morozova E, Ben-Ari Y, Holmes GL. Developmental changes in GABAergic actions and seizure susceptibility in the rat hippocampus. *Eur J Neurosci*. 2004;19:590-600.
5. Jenssen FE, Sanchez RM. Why does the developing brain demonstrate heightened susceptibility to febrile and other provoked seizures? In: Baran TZ, Shinnar S, eds. *Febrile Seizures*. San Diego: Academic Press; 2002:153-168.
6. Jensen FE, Baram TZ. Developmental seizures induced by common early-life insults: short- and long-term effects on seizure susceptibility. *Ment Retard Dev Disabil Res Rev*. 2000;6:253-257.
7. Khazipov R, Esclapez M, Caillard O, et al. Early development of neuronal activity in the primate hippocampus in utero. *J Neurosci*. 2001;21:9770-9781.
8. Ben-Ari Y. Excitatory actions of GABA during development: the nature of the nurture. *Nat Rev Neurosci*. 2002;3:728-739.
9. McDonald JW, Johnston MV, Young AB. Differential ontogenic development of three receptors comprising the NMDA receptor/channel complex in the rat hippocampus. *Exp Neurol*.1990;110:237-247.
10. Kira R, Torisu H, Takemoto M, et al. Genetic susceptibility to simple febrile seizures: interleukin-1beta promoter polymorphisms are associated with sporadic cases. *Neurosci Lett*. 2005;384:239-244.
11. Tsai FJ, Hsieh YY, Chang CC, Lin CC, Tsai CH. Polymorphisms for interleukin 1 beta exon 5 and interleukin 1 receptor antagonist in Taiwanese children with febrile convulsions. *Arch Pediatr Adolesc Med*. 2002;156:545-548.
12. Virta M, Hurme M, Helminen M. Increased plasma levels of pro- and anti-inflammatory cytokines in patients with febrile seizures. *Epilepsia*. 2002;43:920-923.

13. Bender RA, Soleymani SV, Brewster AL, et al. Enhanced expression of a specific hyperpolarization-activated cyclic nucleotide-gated cation channel (HCN) in surviving dentate gyrus granule cells of human and experimental epileptic hippocampus. *J Neurosci.* 2003;23:6826-6836.

14. Subramony SH, Schott K, Raike RS, et al. Novel CACNA1A mutation causes febrile episodic ataxia with interictal cerebellar deficits. *Ann Neurol.* 2003;54:725-731.

15. Thompson SM, Masukawa LM, Prince DA. Temperature dependence of intrinsic membrane properties and synaptic potentials in hippocampal CA1 neurons in vitro. *J Neurosci.* 1985;5:817-824.

16. Volgushev M, Vidyasagar TR, Chistiakova M, Eysel UT. Synaptic transmission in the neocortex during reversible cooling. *Neuroscience.* 2000;98:9-22.

17. Micheva KD, Smith SJ. Strong effects of subphysiological temperature on the function and plasticity of mammalian presynaptic terminals. *J Neurosci.* 2005;25:7481-7488.

18. Wan Q, Xiong ZG, Man HY, et al. Recruitment of functional GABA(A) receptors to postsynaptic domains by insulin. *Nature.* 1997;388:686-690.

19. Kang JQ, Shen W, Macdonald RL. Why does fever trigger febrile seizures? GABAA receptor gamma2 subunit mutations associated with idiopathic generalized epilepsies have temperature-dependent trafficking deficiencies. *J Neurosci.* 2006;26:2590-2597.

20. Nelson KB, Ellenberg JH. Prognosis in children with febrile seizures. *Pediatrics.* 1978;61:720-777.

21. Tsuboi T, Endo S. Genetic studies of febrile convulsions: analysis of twin and family data. *Epilepsy Res.* 1991;4(suppl): 119-128.

22. Winawer M, Hesdorffer D. Turning on the heat: the search for febrile seizure genes. *Neurology.* 2004;63:1770-1771.

23. Berkovic SF, Scheffer IE. Febrile seizures: genetics and relationship to other epilepsy syndromes. *Curr Opin Neurol.* 1998;11:129-134.

24. Berg AT, Shinnar S, Darefsky AS, et al. Predictors of recurrent febrile seizures: a prospective cohort study. *Arch Pediatr Adolesc Med.* 1997;151:371-378.

25. Lewis HM, Parry JV, Parry RP, et al. Role of viruses in febrile convulsions. *Arch Dis Child.* 1979;54:869–876; and Nelson KB, Ellenberg JH. Prognosis in children with febrile seizures. *Pediatrics.* 1978;61:720–777.

26. Suga S, Suzuki K, Ihira M, et al. Clinical characteristics of febrile convulsions during primary HHV-6 infection. *Arch Dis Child.* 2000;82:62-66.

27. Hirtz DG, Nelson KB, Ellenberg JH. Seizures following childhood immunizations. *J Pediatr.* 1983;120:14-18.

28. Hirtz DG, Nelson KB. The natural history of febrile seizures. *Annu Rev Med.* 1983;34:453-471.

29. Barlow WE, Davis RL, Glasser JW, et al. The risk of seizures after receipt of whole cell pertussis or measles, mumps, and rubella vaccine. *N Engl J Med.* 2001;345:656-661.

30. Le Saux, Barrowman N, Moore D, et al. Decrease in hospital admissions for febrile seizures and reports of hypotonic-hyporesonsive episodes presenting to hospital emergency departments since switching to acellular pertussis vaccine in Canada: a report from IMPACT. *Pediatrics.* 2003;112:e348.

31. Berg AT, Shinnar S. Complex febrile seizures. *Epilepsia.* 1996;37:126-133.

32. Lee W, Ong H. Afebrile seizures associated with minor infections: comparison with febrile seizures and unprovoked seizures. *Pediatr Neurol.* 2004;31:157-164.

33. Okumura A, Uemura N, Suzuki M, Itomi K, Watanabe K. Unconsciousness and delirious behavior in children with febrile seizures. *Pediatr Neurol.* 2004;30:316-319.

34. Gordon KE, Camfield PR, Camfield CS, Dooley JM, Bethune P. Children with febrile seizures do not consume excess health care resources. *Arch Pediatr Adolesc Med.* 2000;154:594-597.

35. Bethune P, Gordon KG, Dooley JM, Camfield CS, Camfield PR. Which child will have a febrile seizure? *Am J Dis Child.* 1993;147:35-39.

36. Freeman JM. Febrile seizures: long-term management of children with fever-associated seizures. *Pediatrics.* 1980;66:1009-1012.

37. Engel J Jr. International League Against Epilepsy (ILAE). A proposed diagnostic scheme for people with epileptic seizures and with epilepsy: report of the ILAE Task Force on Classification and Terminology. *Epilepsia.* 2001; 42:796-803.

38. Webb DW, Jones RR, Manzur AY, Farrell K. Retrospective study of late febrile seizures. *Pediatr Neurol.* 1999;20: 270-273.

39. Camfield PR, Camfield CS, Gordon K, Dooley JM. What types of epilepsy are preceded by febrile seizures? A population based study of children. *Dev Med Child Neurol.* 1994;36:887-892.

40. Rocca WA, Sharbrough FW, Hauser WA, Annegers JF, Schoenberg BS. Risk factors for generalized tonic-clonic seizures: a population-based case control study in Rochester, Minnesota. *Neurology.* 1987;37:1315-12322.

41. Vestergaard M, Bocker C, Per Sidenius P, Olsen J, Christensen J. The long-term risk of epilepsy after febrile seizures in susceptible subgroups. *Am J Epidemiol.* 2007; 165(8):911-918.

42. Vestergaard M, Basso, Henriksen TB, Ostergaard J, Olsen J. Febrile convulsions and sudden infant death syndrome. *Arch Dis Child.* 2002;86:125-126.

43. Ellenberg JH, Nelson KB. Febrile seizures and later intellectual performance. *Arch Neurol.* 1978;35:17-21.

44. Chang YC, Guo NW, Wang ST, Huang CC, Tsai JJ. Working memory of school-aged children with a history of febrile convulsions: a population study. *Neurology.* 2001;57:37-42.

45. Uhari M, Rantala H, Vainionpaa, Kurttila BM. Effect of acetaminophen and of low dose intermittent diazepam on prevention of recurrences of febrile seizures. *J Pediatr.* 1995;126:991-995.

46. van Stuijvenberg M, Derksen-Lubsen G, Steyerberg EW, Habbema JD, Moll HA. Randomized, controlled trial of ibuprofen syrup administered during febrile illnesses to prevent febrile seizure recurrences. *Pediatrics.* 1998;102:E51

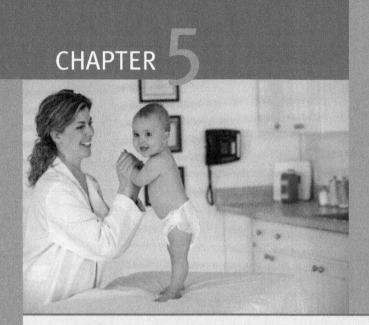

CHAPTER 5

Paroxysmal Disorders

Troy Payne

Three of the most common neurological paroxysmal disorders in childhood are headache, sleep disorders, and epilepsy. As these subjects are examined thoroughly in other chapters in this book, they will not be covered here. Instead, this chapter will cover non-epileptic neonatal events, breath-holding spells, syncope, paroxysmal dyskinesia, episodic ataxia, tics, panic disorder, and psychogenic non-epileptic seizures in children.

NEONATAL AND INFANT NON-EPILEPTIC EVENTS

The following events may appear similar to seizures but are of non-epileptic origin.

Apnea

Definitions and epidemiology

Short pauses in breathing are normal in infants. Apnea in a premature infant is longer than 20 seconds, and in a mature infant is more than 15 seconds. The more premature the infant, the greater the risk of apnea. There is often associated temporary paleness or bluish skin, and decreased muscle tone. In a premature infant, apnea can be associated with bradycardia. There is an increased risk of infant apnea if the infant is male, is of premature birth, has a teenage mother, or is one of multiples (twins or multiple-birth siblings).

Pathophysiology

In the neonate, apnea if often due to respiratory center immaturity. In an infant up to 1 year of age, apnea can be caused by a number of medical conditions. These include stroke, meningitis, hypoglycemia, infection, airway obstruction, gastroesophageal reflux, and medication effect. If apnea is associated with eye deviation or rhythmic jerky eye or body movements, one should consider the possibility of a seizure.

Treatment

Treatment is dependent on the underlying mechanism, if one can be found. Tactile stimulation of the infant during an event can often abort the apnea. An apnea monitor, continuous positive airway pressure (CPAP) machine or an oxygen hood may be used to treat the infant.

Benign Sleep Myoclonus

Definitions and epidemiology

Hypnogogic myoclonic jerks are common in all ages and are commonly called "sleep starts." In infants before 3 months of age, benign myoclonic jerks are seen in non–rapid eye movement (NREM) sleep and are usually symmetric and bilateral. Usually, they involve both arms and legs but can rarely be isolated to a single extremity.

Clinical presentation and differential diagnosis

Electroencephalography during the episode is normal. Movements can happen repetitively every 2 to 3 seconds sounding similar to a seizure.[1] However, they only happen in sleep, and the child's examination and development is usually normal. If the child is awoken during these movements, they stop immediately. If the movements continue after the child is awoken, seizure should be considered. Benign sleep myoclonus is different than the many other causes of non-epileptic myoclonus.

Pathologic focal, multifocal, or generalized myoclonus can be seen during wakefulness or sleep. It is sometimes stimulus induced. Hypoxic-ischemic encephalopathy, metabolic encephalopathy, head trauma, stroke, and medications can all cause myoclonus.

Hyperekplexia

Clinical presentation

As children, people with hyperekplexia have an exaggerated startle response to tactile or auditory stimulation. Upon awakening infants become markedly stiff with forced closure of the eyelids and extension of the extremities and often have a brief apneic episode. This can often be reproduced by gently tapping the infant on the nose. Nocturnal myoclonus may be seen in some infants with hyperekplexia. Abdominal and inguinal hernias and hip dislocations have been noted as a result of the sudden increase in tone.

Pathophysiology

Usually autosomal dominant, this disease has been associated with an abnormality on chromosome $5q^2$ and is thought to be from a defect in a glycine receptor. Autosomal recessive families have been noted.

Treatment

Caregivers can be taught a technique that often helps to overcome a spell by gently flexing the child's legs at the hip. In older children clonazepam, diazepam, phenobarbital, or valproic acid are sometimes useful.

Jitteriness

Common in the neonatal care unit, jitteriness in a neonate or infant is often precipitated by auditory or tactile stimulation. The movement is a tremor and is often associated with irritability. The infant is usually alert and responsive. There may be an exaggerated Moro response or an increased startle response. It can be caused by medications given to the mother before birth or to the infant after birth. It can be observed as an infant is withdrawing off medications the mother took during the pregnancy. Hypoglycemia, hypocalcemia, and hypoxia can cause jitteriness. The tremor stops when the limb is repositioned. Often, holding the baby and rocking suppresses the tremor. This helps differentiate jitteriness from seizures.

Shuddering

Shuddering is a paroxysmal shiver-like movement of the head, shoulder, and trunk that usually lasts 5 to 15 seconds. The elbows are often held close to the trunk. The episodes only happen during wakefulness and are not associated with any alteration of consciousness. Spells can be occasional or occur multiple times a day. Feeding may evoke spells of shuddering. An EEG during the spells is normal. The vast majority of children with even frequent shuddering need no medication. If felt clinically necessary, propranolol may help. There is no increased risk of epilepsy in children who have shuddering spells. Of note, children with frequent shuddering are more commonly seen in families with people manifesting essential tremor.[3]

Stereotypies

Definitions and clinical presentation

Stereotypies are repetitive suppressible stereotypic actions such as finger tapping, blinking, hair pulling, body rocking, and head banging. It is believed that the self-stimulatory action helps relieve some inner anxiety or stress. Body rocking or repetitive limb movements can be seen as the child falls asleep, and requires no specific treatment. This is often called rhythmic movement disorder.

Pathophysiology

Although common in children with autism or mental retardation, children of normal intelligence can have these movements.[4] The underlying cause is unknown. In extreme cases, benzodiazepines, tricyclic antidepressants, and antipsychotic medications may be useful.

Treatment

Behavioral management is sometimes useful if the behavior persists into childhood. An alternative activity that is less harmful can be promoted. For instance, instead of pulling the hair, the child could twist beads on a bracelet. A positive reward system is sometimes helpful.

Gastroesophageal Reflux Disease (GERD)

An infant who has recently been fed can suddenly and temporarily stiffen, stare, and become apneic from gastroesophageal reflux disease. In rare cases, the back can actually arch and the child can have opisthotonic posturing for 1 to 3 minutes (Sandifer syndrome). The child is often referred for possible seizures.[5] The key in diagnosis is that these episodes usually occur within an hour of feeding. EEG during the episode is normal. If the reflux persists, treatment with metaclopramide may be useful.

Spasmus Nutans

Infants with spasmus nutans have repeated episodes of nystagmus, head bobbing, and head tilting, or torticollis. The nystagmus may be horizontal, vertical, or pedular. Consideration should be given to possibly obtaining an MRI of the head to rule out a tumor of the third ventricle or an optic glioma. If the MRI is normal, no specific therapy is needed. EEG is normal during the spells. The symptoms become less as the child grows older and usually disappear before school age.

SYNCOPE

Definitions and Epidemiology

Syncope can be defined as cerebral hypoperfusion sufficient to cause transient loss of consciousness. There are many potential causes, and most are benign. However, there are some life-threatening causes of syncope, and anyone who falls from syncope of any reason could injure themselves. Between 20% and 50% of people say they have had syncope at some point. It appears most commonly in females.

Pathophysiology

Abnormal circulatory control or cardiovascular volume can lead to situational syncope, vasovagal syncope, orthostatic hypotension, or reflex asystolic (pallid) syncope.

There are tachyarrhythmias, bradyarrhythmias, and structural heart defects that can lead to syncope. Toxic or metabolic abnormalities such as hypoglycemia, hypocalcemia, hypomagnesemia, hypoxia, and alcohol/ medication overdose are associated with syncope. Addison disease can cause syncope through volume depletion.

Diagnostic Evaluation

A good history and physical examination are absolutely necessary if the cause of syncope is to be determined. Blood pressures should be checked lying, sitting, and standing. A drop in the systolic blood pressure of more then 20 mm Hg or a significant increase in pulse indicates probable volume loss or abnormal neurocardiac control. Check the pulse in all extremities. Check for a detectable mass in the abdomen. Listen for a heart murmur.

Check the mental status of the patient after the spell is over. An EKG to look for long QT syndrome, heart block, and ventricular hypertrophy should be performed. Cardiac monitoring for an arrhythmia may be indicated depending on the situation. A complete blood count to look for evidence of anemia and infection, electrolytes, glucose, calcium, magnesium, blood urea nitrogen, and creatinine should be checked. If appropriate, a pregnancy test, toxicology screen, or medication blood level should be done. If a seizure is suspected, an EEG should be ordered. An echocardiogram should be performed if there is a cardiac murmur, if the syncope occurred during exercise, or if there is a family history of cardiomyopathy or sudden death. Magnetic resonance imaging of the brain and cerebrovasculature is advised if any focal neurological signs were present at any time during the syncope. Tilt table testing is reasonable if there is suspicion of an inducible arrhythmia or hypotension. The most common finding on tilt table testing is hypotension and bradycardia or hypotension alone. Implanted loop recorders should be considered if syncope is recurrent and the workup is unrevealing. Repeated episodes of syncope that only occur when a certain parent or caregiver is present should raise the possibility of a factitious disorder.

Differential Diagnosis and Management

Vasovagal syncope

This is the most common cause of syncope in childhood. It is often triggered by pain, fear, or the sight of something unpleasant. Diaphoresis, light-headedness, and nausea are common before loss of consciousness but are often of short duration in children. It does not occur while supine, but may. The child will appear still while briefly unresponsive for usually under 1 minute. Occasionally, there may be brief jerks of the extremities for a second or two. The child may even have incontinence. These phenomena often raise the question of the possibility of a seizure. However, the patient with vasovagal syncope usually has no or only very limited jerking, little or no cyanosis, rarely bites the tongue, and usually awakens without much of a postictal state. Afterwards, there may be headache or fatigue.

Vasovagal syncope is caused by involuntary reflex activation of the vasovagal nervous system leading to bradycardia and vasodilation, resulting in a drop in blood pressure and cardiac output. Avoidance of the activity that triggers the response is sometimes helpful. Lying the person down flat is recommended. If a person is prone to vasovagal syncope they should pay particular attention to avoid becoming dehydrated. Fludrocortisone, midodrine, beta-blockers, serotonin reuptake inhibitors, and even pacemakers have been useful.[6]

Situational syncope

A variety of activities can lead to an abnormal vasovagal response in some individuals, resulting in syncope. Coughing, micturation, defecation, and swallowing cold fluids or food have all lead to syncope in susceptible children. This is really just a form of vasovagal syncope caused by certain actions.

Breath-holding spells

A healthy child who has breath-holding spells may become still and stop breathing after an episode of normal crying. It is often accompanied by cyanosis. The apnea usually occurs on expiration. If the apneic episode is long enough, hypoxia will occur. The child may lose consciousness and become limp. Further, the child may have short, limited muscle clonic jerks for a second or two after loss of consciousness. The episode usually lasts less than a minute and often ends with a deep inspiration. It usually starts between 6 and 24 months and disappears by 6 years. The breath holding is involuntary and scolding the child does not help. It is felt to be due to an immature autonomic nervous system. Parents or caregivers should be informed that the child has no control over these spells. Iron deficiency has been reported in some children with breath-holding spells. Treating these children with iron often helps reduce the number of spells.[7] It seems reasonable to check the iron and ferritin level of any child with breath-holding spells. Iron deficiency states should be treated with iron supplementation. In a study by Daoud and colleagues,[8] some children without iron deficiency responded to therapy and some with iron deficiency did not.

Reflex asystolic (pallid) syncope

While reported between ages 3 months and 14 years, reflex asystolic syncope is usually seen in toddlers.[9] These events were once called "pallid" breath-holding spells, but many of these children will not hold their breath during the episodes. The child will suddenly become pale or dizzy following a sudden painful or frightening event. As they lose consciousness and become limp, the child may or may not cry out. If the child is hypoxic long enough, there may be stiffening, twitching, and incontinence. The EEG shows no epileptiform activity during the spell and is usually attenuated. The EKG shows bradycardia or even asystole for several seconds immediately after the stimulus. It is felt to represent an abnormal vagal response to the painful or frightening event. To help the child regain consciousness, the child should be laid down flat and not carried around. Most children do not require any specific medical therapy. Atropine has been used successfully in some cases.

Orthostasis

Orthostatic hypotension occurs when there is insufficient intravascular volume or autonomic nervous system dysfunction. The blood pressure drops when sitting up or standing, leading to cerebral hypoperfusion and syncope. Orthostatic intolerance can easily be tested by having the child stand still for 10 minutes while taking blood pressures every 2 minutes. A child with orthostatic intolerance will have a drop in blood pressure after standing still for a few minutes and will fall. It is recommended to do this test on a padded mat with someone ready to break the child's fall. Increasing the volume of fluids may help. Octreotide and midodrine have been shown to be effective.[10]

Long QT syndrome

There are familial dominant (Romano-Ward syndrome), familial recessive (Jervell Lange-Nielsen syndrome which is associated with deafness), idiopathic nonfamilial, and medication-induced causes of long QT syndrome. Quinidine, procainimide, amiodarone, and cyclic antidepressants have each been associated with long QT syndrome. When terfenadine is taken with macrolide antibiotics (eg, erythromycin) there is an increased chance of developing long QT syndrome. An EKG can detect a long QT interval. There are normal people with a long QT interval and some people with long QT syndrome may have a normal QT interval. This can further complicate obtaining a diagnosis in some people. Genetic testing may help obtain the diagnosis in some. Epinephrine given during a stress test can help with diagnosis in others. Heart palpitations or an irregular heartbeat may occur in some people with long QT syndrome. People with long QT syndrome can develop syncope after an episode of sudden emotion, fright, or during vigorous exercise. Syncope in people with long QT syndrome may be due to a persistent burst of polymorphic ventricular tachycardia in a form called "torsades de pointes" or "twisting of the points" that can lead to ventricular fibrillation. Sudden death can occur if ventricular fibrillation is not treated. An implanted or automated external defibrillator (AED) may correct the abnormal fibrillation. Beta-blockers are sometimes recommended.

Bradyarrhythmias

Sinus node disease can cause severe bradycardia, which decreases cardiac output and cerebral perfusion. It may be seen in children with atrial septal defects or Ebstein anomaly of the tricuspid valve. In children who have a complete heart block and have an escape rhythm that is slow, cardiac output will also be low and syncope can occur. These children may benefit from a pacemaker.

Tachyarrhythmias

Tachycardias can occur that are so fast that diastolic filling and stroke volume are impaired. Syncope can occur with atrial tachycardias such as rapid atrial fibrillation due to the loss of "atrial kick." Occasionally, supraventricular tachycardia can last for a long time and may affect cardiac output. Wolff-Parkinson-White syndrome with atrial fibrillation or exercise-induced supraventricular tachycardia has caused syncope. Syncope occurs in ventricular tachycardia because of decreased stroke volume. When ventricular tachycardia persists and the myocardium becomes desynchronized, ventricular fibrillation can occur. Without cardioversion, persistent ventricular fibrillation will cause death within minutes. Seizures have been associated with atrial and ventricular fibrillation (Figure 5-1).

PAROXYSMAL DYSKINESIAS

Clinical Presentation

Children with paroxysmal dyskinesias have sudden abnormal involuntary movements that may appear irregular and jerky (choreiform) or slow and writhing (athetoid). There is increased muscle tone and dystonic posturing. Ballism is sometimes noted. There is no alteration in consciousness during the episodes. Episodes are often divided into short duration (< 5 min) or long duration (> 5 min). Between the episodes the child usually appears normal.

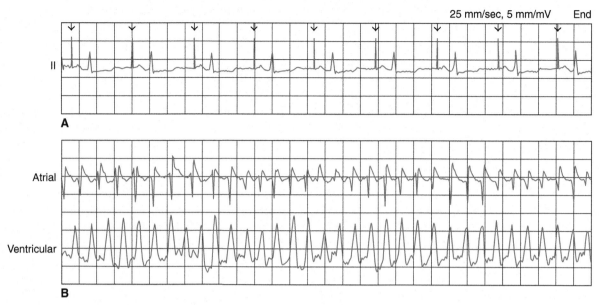

FIGURE 5-1 ■ A. Baseline electrocardiogram recording of lead II in a 12-year-old boy with known sinus node dysfunction. He has an automatic implantable cardioverter/defibrillator (AICD). This recording shows an atrial paced rhythm, with normal atrioventricular node conduction at a rate of 85 bpm (25 mm/sec). **B.** Intracardiac electrograms from the AICD during a seizure in this 12-year-old boy. Simultaneous atrial and ventricular electrograms are demonstrated. Both atria and sentricles are fibrillating with rates greater than 300 bpm in all cardiac chambers. *(Courtesy of Ann Dunnigan, M.D., Central Minnesota Heart Center, St. Cloud, MN.)*

Differential Diagnosis and Treatment

Paroxysmal kinesigenic dyskinesia

In a child with paroxysmal kinesigenic dyskinesia (PKD), a startle or a sudden voluntary movement elicits the dyskinesia. PKD primarily affects the arms and legs but can involve the face, neck, or trunk. Attacks usually are worse on one side of the body. Attacks can cause dysarthria if the face is involved or falling if the legs are affected. Most attacks last from seconds up to 5 minutes, although they can last longer. Many people get a paresthetic warning just before the episode occurs. Most children experience near daily episodes, but the spells can happen only once a month or multiple times per day. With age, the frequency of the episodes often decreases. Familial cases have been reported. The syndrome has been mapped to chromosome 16 (16p11.2-q11.2).[11] In some families, PKD and infantile convulsions coexist. Attacks are often helped by anticonvulsants such as phenytoin or carbamazepine, although the EEG is usually normal. Symptomatic cases secondary to head injury, multiple sclerosis, and other causes have been reported.

Paroxysmal non-kinesiogenic dyskinesia

While the episodes of dyskinesia may be exacerbated by a variety of stressors, the abnormal movements of people with paroxysmal non-kinesiogenic dyskinesia (PNKD) occur without any specific cause. Episodes can be severe enough to cause falling without warning. Similar to PKD, some people get a paresthetic warning before the episode. Others with PNKD find that stress, alcohol, caffeine, and sleep deprivation increase the frequency of attacks. Episodes may be monthly or daily, but the number of attacks is often less than those with PKD. Attacks are often longer than those in people with PKD, lasting 5 minutes to hours in length.

Episodes tend to decrease with age. Familial cases have been noted. Families with PKND have manifested genetic defects mapped to chromosome 2.[12] There are several ion channel genes in this region, suggesting the possibility that PNKD may be a channelopathy. The response to anticonvulsants is not as good in PNKD; however, many do respond to clonazepam. Symptomatic cases due to multiple sclerosis, hypoparathyroidism, diabetes, and other causes have been reported.

Paroxysmal exertion-induced dyskinesia

Children with the rare syndrome of paroxysmal exertion-induced dyskinesia (PED) have the movements only after long exertion. After running or exerting oneself for 5 to 15 minutes the child suddenly develops involuntary twisting, dystonic movements of legs and feet without any warning.

Episodes usually occur weekly but can occur daily. Attacks can last from 5 minutes to half an hour. The frequency of attacks often decreases with age. Familial cases are rare.

Some people have a decrease in attacks with clonazepam or carbamazepine, but anticonvulsants are not as effective as in PKD.

Paroxysmal hypnogenic dyskinesia

A rare condition, paroxysmal hypnogenic dyskinesia (PHD) causes episodes of dyskinetic movements solely in non-REM sleep. There is often an arousal out of non-REM sleep followed by rigidity and twisting of the limbs with ballism, chorea, and athetosis. Episodes are usually under 2 minutes, but may last longer. Often, the patient remembers the episode. Attacks typically occur only a few times per year but may be more frequent in some individuals. Familial cases are rare and are predominantly male. Short duration PHD is now considered a frontal lobe epileptic condition, which is often successfully treated with anticonvulsants such as carbamazepine. In contrast, long duration PHD does not respond as well to anticonvulsant medications.

EPISODIC ATAXIA

Type 1

Patients with episodic ataxia disorder have episodes of cerebellar ataxia following movement, fright, or stress. Episodes usually last less than 2 minutes. Myokymia, particularly in the face, is observed between attacks. Neuromyotonia may be noted. It is most often autosomal dominant, but sporadic cases have been noted. It usually presents in childhood. A defect in the potassium channel (KCNA1) on chromosome 12p has been described.[13] Acetazolamide and valpoic acid have been used successfully. Interestingly, there is an increased prevalence of epilepsy in people with episodic ataxia type 1.

Type 2

Patients with this disorder have episodes of cerebellar ataxia that last much longer, from a few minutes to days. The attacks often occur during times of emotional stress or following alcohol or caffeine ingestion. Nystagmus is noted on exam. Cerebellar signs including dysarthria and dysmetria are often noted between attacks. A defect in a voltage-dependent P/Q type calcium channel (CACNL1A4) on chromosome 19 has been described.[14,15] Acetazolamide has been used successfully. See Table 5-1.

TICS

Simple tics are a product of repetitive activation of one or a few muscle groups. Blinking, facial twitches, grimacing, sniffing, throat clearing, and shoulder jerks are all common tics. Sleep deprivation and stress may make the tics more frequent. Simple tics are more commonly seen in boys. Most of the time the child will outgrow the tic with no medical treatment required.

Table 5-1.

Episodic Ataxias

	Episodic Ataxia 1	Episodic Ataxia 2
Activation	Sudden movement	None
Length of ataxia	Seconds to minutes	Minutes to hours
Mutation	Voltage-gated potassium channel (KCNA1)	Voltage-gated calcium channel (CACN1A)
Chromosome	12p	19
Treatment	Acetazolamide, valproic acid	Acetazolamide

Complex tics involve multiple muscle groups often occurring in rapid succession.

When these persist for over a year and are accompanied by frequent vocal tics, the diagnosis of Tourette syndrome may be made. Symptoms usually begin between 5 and 10 years of age. People with Tourette syndrome can often temporarily suppress the tics, indicating some degree of voluntary control. Caprolalia (spontaneous, foul words), echopraxia (mimicking actions), echolalia (repeating what was just heard), and palilalia (repeating words over again) can all been seen but are not required for the diagnosis. Attention deficit disorder with hyperactivity and obsessive compulsive disorder are frequently seen as well.[16] Haloperidol, risperidone, and clonidine have been used successfully in treating the tics of Tourette syndrome. The tics tend to lessen with age following adolescence.

PANIC DISORDER

Panic attacks are discrete episodes of overpowering fear that can be manifested as palpitations, shortness of breath, trembling, diaphoresis, choking, chest discomfort, nausea, tingling, faintness, and a sense of imminent death. There is often a feeling of needing to flee. Panic attacks can happen during the day or night, but pure nocturnal panic disorder is rare. People with panic disorder have attacks spontaneously without any warning. This is different than social anxiety disorder, where a social situation elicits the panic attack; or posttraumatic stress disorder, where there is a memory of an actual event that triggers panic. As it is episodic, it is sometimes confused with epilepsy. Panic disorder is more common in females, with onset in adolescence or early adulthood. There are serotonergic, noradrenergic, and GABAergic theories as to the cause of panic disorder. The mainstay of treatment is the serotonin reuptake inhibitors such as fluoxetine, paroxetine, and sertraline, all of which are approved by the Food and Drug Administration for treatment of panic disorder. Tricyclic antidepressants are also effective but may be less well tolerated. Two benzodiazepines, clonazepam and alprazolam, have been approved by the Food and Drug Administration to treat panic disorder but need to weaned off slowly to avoid withdrawal. Trials with anticonvulsant medications such as valproic acid, gabapentin, and tiagabine have shown success.

PSYCHOGENIC NON-EPILEPTIC SEIZURES

Definitions and Epidemiology

Psychogenic non-epileptic seizures (PNES) resemble epileptic seizures but are not associated with any EEG change (Table 5-2). Most commonly the event is a symptom of a conversion disorder. The events are not consciously produced. If the event is consciously produced, then it would be malingering. Approximately 20% of patients referred to epilepsy centers for medically refractory seizures are diagnosed with PNES.

Clinical Presentation

Many of these patients have multiple seizure types and do not improve after trying several antiepileptic

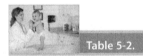

Table 5-2.

Clues Suggesting Psychogenic Non-epileptic Seizures

- Multiple seizure types
- Inadequate response to antiepileptic medication
- Irregular jerking or thrashing
- Movements that are out of phase between the limbs
- Movements that move back and forth between left and right sides
- Abrupt cessation of spells, which then may start up again suddenly
- Foul language during the spell
- Unresponsive spells often lasting for several minutes or even over an hour
- Ability of a bystander to alter the pattern of the movements
- Child resists eye opening during the spell
- History of physical or sexual abuse

medications. If the patient does bite the tongue it is often on the tip, instead of on the side as seen with some epileptic seizures. Incontinence is rare in PNES, but possible. Often people with temporal lobe epilepsy rub their nose after a seizure. In contrast, patients with PNES usually do not.[17] Movements of the extremities are often out of phase. Sometimes there may be movements rarely seen in temporal lobe epilepsy such as pelvic thrusting. However, this can be seen in frontal lobe epilepsy as well.[18] Episodes are often recurrent. In an unresponsive form, the patient may just suddenly stop moving or interacting with the environment for minutes to over an hour. One might think that a history of depression or personality disorder would help distinguish those with PNES; however, these are also commonly seen in patients with epilepsy. Stress from relationships with family and friends, academic stress, drug and alcohol abuse, and sexual abuse all can precipitate PNES in some people. According to Bowman, childhood sexual abuse was noted in half of adults with PNES and one-third of children with PNES.[19] A propensity for a conversion disorder is often seen on the Minnesota Multiphasic Personality Inventory (MMPI), where the patient scores high for hypochondriasis and hysteria but only slightly high or within normal limits for depression.

Diagnosis

The best way to confirm the presence of PNES is to record several typical spells on video-EEG monitoring. One must be careful as some focal seizures do not show on surface EEG. However, most of the time a trained epileptologist can determine if the spells are non-epileptic. Carefully taking a complete history and observing the time-synched video and EEG taken during the events usually results in the correct assessment.

While it is true some patients with PNES also have epilepsy, a study by Martin and colleagues showed that when strict diagnostic criteria were used, only 5.3% of patients had both PNES and epilepsy.[20] Another useful tool is that prolactin is often elevated at least twice the baseline value 10 to 20 minutes after a many generalized seizures and some complex partial seizures and syncopal events, but usually not after PNES.[21]

Treatment

Treatment begins with calm, respectful delivery of the diagnosis. Psychological assessment for sexual abuse, physical abuse, panic attacks, and conflict is required. With proper treatment of the underlying psychological, cause many patients with PNES will stop having events.

REFERENCES

1. Ramelli GP, Sozzo A, Vella S, Bianchetti M. et al. Benign neonatal sleep myoclonus: an under-recognized, non-epileptic condition. *Acta Paediatr.* 2005;94:962-963.

2. Ryan S, Sherman S, Terry J, Sparkes R, Torres M, Mackey R. Startle disease, or hyperekplexia: a response to clonazepam and assignment of the gene (STHE) to chromosome 5q by linkage analysis. *Ann Neurol.* 1992;31: 663-668.

3. Vanase M, Bedard P, Andermann F. Shuddering attacks in children: an early clinical manifestation of essential tremor. *Neurology.* 1976;26:1027-1030.

4. Mahone E, Bridges D, Prahme C, Singer H. Repetitive arm and hand movements (complex motor stereotypies) in children. *J Pediatr.* 2004;145:391-395.

5. Kabakus N, Kurt A. Sandifer syndrome: a continuing problem of misdiagnosis. *Pediatr Int.* 2006;48:622-625.

6. Sheldon R, Morillo C, Krahn A. Management of vaso-vagal syncope. *Expert Rev Cardiovasc Ther.* 2004;2: 915-923.

7. Mocan H, Yildiran A, Orhan F, Enduran E. Breath holding spells in 91 children and response to treatment with iron. *Arch Dis Child.* 1999; 81:261-262.

8. Daoud A, Batieha A, al-Sheyyab M, Abuekteish F, Hijazi S. Effectiveness of iron therapy on breath-holding spells. *J Pediatr.* 1997;130:547-550.

9. DiMario F. Jr. Prospective study of children with cyanotic and pallid breath-holding spells. *Pediatrics.* 2001;107: 265-269.

10. Hoeldtke R, Bryner K, Hoeldtke M, Hobbs G. Treatment of postural tachycardia syndrome: a comparison of octreotide and midodrine. *Clin Auton Res.* 2006;16:390-395.

11. Bennet L, Roach E, Bowcock A. A locus for paroxysmal kinesigenic dyskinesia maps to human chromosome 16. *Neurology.* 2000; 54:125-130.

12. Spacey S, Adams P, Lam P, Materek L, Stoessl A, Snutch T, Hsiung G. Genetic heterogeneity in paroxysmal nonkine-sigenic dyskinesia. *Neurology.* 2006;66:1588-1590.

13. Litt M, Kramer P, Browne D, Gancher S, Brunt E, Root D, et al. A gene for episodic ataxia/myokymia maps to chro-mosome 12p13. *Am J Hum Genet.* 1994;55:702-709.

14. Vahedi K, Joutel A, Van Bogaert P, Ducros A, Maciazeck J, Bach J, et al. A gene for hereditary paroxysmal cerebellar ataxia maps to chromosome 19p. *Ann Neurol.* 1995; 37:289-293.

15. Von Brederlow B, Hahn A, Koopman W, Ebers G, Bulman D. Mapping the gene for acetazolamide responsive heredi-tary paroxysmal cerebellar ataxia to chromosome 19p. *Hum Mol Genet.* 1995;4:279-284.

16. Gaze C, Kepley H, Walkup T. Co-occuring psychiatric dis-orders in children and adolescents with Tourette syn-drome. *J Child Neurol.* 2006;21:657-664.

17. Geyer J, Payne T, Faught E, Drury I. Postictal nose-rub-bing in the diagnosis, lateralization and localization of seizures. *Neurology.* 1999; 52:743-745.

18. Geyer J, Payne T, Drury I. The value of pelvic thrusting in the diagnosis of seizures and pseudoseizures. *Neurology.* 2000;54:227-229.

19. Bowman E. Relationship of remote and recent life events to the onset and course of nonepileptic seizures. In: Gates J, Rowan A, eds. *Nonepileptic Seizures.* 2nd ed. Boston: Butterworth-Heinemann; 2000:269-283.

20. Martin R, Burneo J, Prasad A, Powell T, Faught E, Knowlton R, et al. Frequency of epilepsy in patients with psychogenic seizures monitored by video-EEG. *Neurology.* 2003;61:1791-1792.

21. Chen D, So Y, Fisher R. Use of serum prolactin in diag-nosing epileptic seizures: report of the Therapeutics and Technology Assessment Subcommittee of the American Academy of Neurology. *Neurology.* 2005;65:668-675.

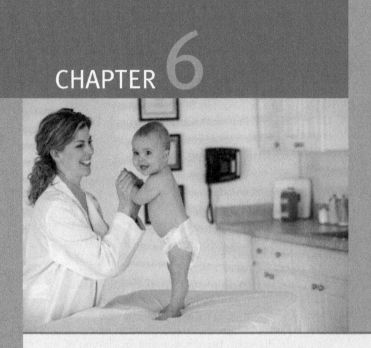

CHAPTER 6

Headache

Paul R. Carney and James D. Geyer

UNDERSTANDING PEDIATRIC HEADACHES

Headaches are common in children, with the average age of onset at 7 for boys and 11 for girls. The frequency of migraine increases through adolescence. An estimated 8% to 23% of children aged 11 to 15 experience headaches. Headaches can be divided into two categories, primary or secondary. Primary refers to headaches that occur on their own and not as the result of some other health problem. Primary headaches (Figure 6-1) include migraine, migraine with aura, tension-type headache, and cluster headache.

Secondary refers to headaches that result from some cause or condition, such as a head injury or concussion, blood vessel problems, medication side effects, infections in the head or elsewhere in the body, sinus disease, or tumors (Figure 6-2). Signs and symptoms of the underlying cause need to be searched for. Headaches associated with infection may represent a systemic reaction to the infection and do not necessarily signify severe disease. For example, strep throat is frequently associated with headaches. There are many different causes for secondary headaches, ranging from rare, serious diseases to easily treated conditions. Sometimes headaches occur almost every day and are called chronic daily headaches.

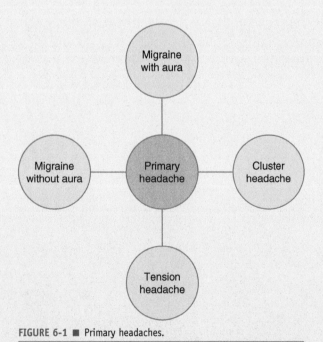

FIGURE 6-1 ■ Primary headaches.

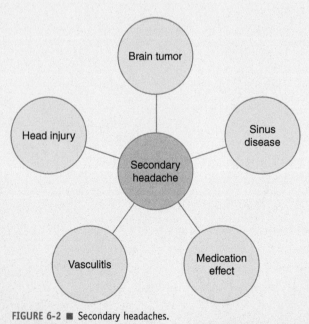

FIGURE 6-2 ■ Secondary headaches.

Migraine is a headache condition that comes back again and again. Ten percent of children get migraines, and an even higher percentage of teenagers have them. These headaches are very painful and throbbing, and children who have them often look ill and pale. Relief is usually linked with sleep. One should focus on ruling out other serious diseases or conditions when first examining migraineurs.

Migraineurs have various signs and symptoms. Typically, a child migraineur has a severe headache located around the eyes, in the front of the head, or in the temples. Some children experience vision changes ("auras") during a headache. A sick feeling in the stomach or vomiting is common. Many children avoid bright lights, loud noises, or strong odors, as these seem to make the headache worse. The severe head pain is often completely relieved by deep sleep. Recurring spells of dizziness may represent another form of migraine in children. An inherited tendency is believed to make some people more likely to have a migraine after some minor trigger (Table 6-1), although no single theory explains how the human body produces all the symptoms of a typical migraine headache. The key to recognizing migraines is identification of a pattern of short but very painful headache episodes that are relieved by sleep and separated by symptom-free intervals.

Although migraine headaches have long been considered a benign (relatively harmless) condition, they can cause a lot of damage to a person's quality of life and ability to take part in normal life activities. The pain is so intense that migraineurs often cannot think or function very well during or right after episodes.

About 65% to 80% of children with migraines interrupt their normal activities because of the symptoms. In one study of 970,000 self-reported migraineurs aged 6 to 18 years, 329,000 school days were lost per month. The burden of migraines may cause emotional changes like anxiety or sadness. Appropriate diagnosis and treatment of migraines can greatly improve quality of life.

Studies suggest that migraine headaches occur in 5% to 10% of school-aged children in the United States, a percentage that constantly increases through adolescence and peaks at about age 44 years. Many people experience spontaneous remission, meaning that the headaches go away on their own for no clear reason.

Migraine headaches begin earlier in boys than in girls. From infancy to 7 years, boys are affected equally or slightly more than girls. The prevalence of migraines increases during the adolescent and young adult years, during which 20% to 30% of young women and 10% to 20% of young men experience migraines. After menarche (the time when the first menstrual period occurs), a female predominance occurs. This continues to increase until middle age. The frequency of migraines declines in both sexes by age 50 years.

Most migraineurs begin to experience attacks before turning 20 years old. Approximately 20% have their first attack before their 5th birthday. Preschool children experiencing a migraine attack usually look ill and have abdominal pain, vomiting, and a strong need to sleep. They may show pain by irritability, crying, rocking, or seeking a dark room in which to sleep.

Migraineurs aged 5 to 10 years experience headache, nausea, abdominal cramping, vomiting, photophobia (sensitivity to light), phonophobia (sensitivity to sound), osmophobia (sensitivity to smells), and a need to sleep. They usually fall asleep within an hour of the time the attack starts. The most common accompanying symptoms include paleness with dark circles under the eyes, tearing, swollen nasal passages, thirst, swelling, excessive sweating, increased urination, and diarrhea. Older children tend to present with headache on one side. Many sinus headaches are really of migrainous origin. The headache location and intensity often changes within or between attacks.

As children grow older, headache intensity and duration increases, and migraines start to happen at more regular intervals. Older children also describe a pulsating

Table 6-1.

Migraine Triggers

Foods
- Ripened cheeses such as cheddar, Gruyere, Stilton, Brie and Camembert
- Chocolate
- Vinegar (except white vinegar)
- Sour cream, yogurt
- Nuts, peanut butter
- Hot fresh breads, raised coffee cakes, and doughnuts
- Lima beans, navy beans, and pea pods
- MSG (monosodium glutamate)
- Canned figs
- Bananas
- Pizza
- Pork
- Fermented sausages, bologna, pepperoni, hotdogs
- Food dyes
- Sauerkraut
- Caffeine

Odors
- Perfume
- Gasoline
- Various food odors

Stresses
- School work
- Excess number of extra-curricular activities
- Relationships, friends, siblings or parents
- Disruption of lifestyle
- Feeling "bummed out" or sad all the time

or throbbing character to their headaches. Headaches often shift to the one-sided temple location that most adult migraineurs report. Childhood migraines often stop for a few years after puberty.

To young children, non-headache symptoms may be more troubling than the headache. Younger children may experience photophobia and phonophobia without accompanying stomachache or headache. Some children have repeated bouts of stomach pain without accompanying headache.

MIGRAINE HEADACHE

Migraine headaches are recurrent headaches that occur at intervals of days, weeks or months.[1] There may or may not be a pattern to the attacks—for example, teenage girls may tend to have attacks at a particular point in their monthly menstrual cycle. Migraines generally have some of the following symptoms and characteristics:

- Untreated, they can last from 2 to 48 hours in children. Sleep or medical treatment can reduce this time period.
- Headache starts on one side of the head. This may vary from headache to headache and in children, they may start in the front or in both temples.
- Throbbing or pounding pain occurs during the headache.
- Pain is rated as moderate to severe.
- Pain gets worse with exertion. The pain may be so severe that it is difficult or almost impossible to continue with normal daily activities.
- Nausea, vomiting, and/or stomach pain commonly occur with the attacks.
- Light and/or sound sensitivity is also common.
- Pain may be relieved with rest or sleep.
- Other members of the family have had migraines or "sick headaches."
- Warnings called auras may start before the headache. These auras can include blurry vision, flashing lights, colored spots, strange tastes, or weird sensations, and usually precede the headache by 5 to 60 minutes.

Migraine Without Aura

- Much more common than classic migraine.
- 85% of children with migraine have common migraine.
- There is no aura.
- The headache is usually slower in onset then classic migraine, building over several minutes to hours. However, the time from onset to peak intensity may be as short as 15 to 30 minutes.
- These headaches are frequently bifrontal (forehead) in location but may be one sided.
- Many children will vomit within 30 minutes to 1 hour following onset of their headache.

- These headaches may be aggravated by exercise or movement.
- Child may have trouble concentrating when they have a headache.
- Other prominent symptoms may include
  - Nausea.
  - Vomiting.
  - Light sensitivity (photophobia).
  - Sensitivity to sound (phonophobia).
  - Sensitivity to strong odors (osmophobia).
- Children may seek a dark quiet room and attempt to sleep.
- Dizziness (an automatic feature) is seen, particularly in young females.
- Headaches last anywhere from 1 hour to 48 hours—sometimes longer.
- The child is normal between attacks.
- The children will frequently grab onto a nearby person or object.
- Episodes usually last less than 1 minute.
- Following the event, the child returns to normal.
- Though frightening to both child and parent, these are benign.
- If frequent, the attacks can be treated; however, treatment is usually not necessary.
- Typically this disorder resolves before age 5.
- A family history of migraine can usually be obtained.

Migraine With Aura

- Much less common than migraine without aura. (Common migraine.)
- Occurs in 10% to 15% of children with migraine.
- The aura may be visual, sensory, or somatic such as abdominal pain.
- An aura is an abrupt onset neurologic change and is fully reversible.
- The aura develops over minutes and lasts less than 1 hour.
- Visual auras are the most common and often frightening. They may consist of visual loss, flashing lights, or squiggly lines.
- The headache may begin during the aura or shortly after the aura clears.
- The headache should start within 60 minutes following the aura, although it may begin within the aura.
- The pain of a migraine headache is usually moderate to severe.
- In children it is frequently bifrontal (forehead) and throbbing.
- It may be unilateral (one sided) but is rarely in the back of the head.
- Other prominent symptoms may include:
  - Nausea.
  - Vomiting.

- Light sensitivity (photophobia).
  - Sensitivity to sound (phonophobia or sonophobia).
  - Sensitivity to strong odors (e.g., perfume) (osmophobia).
- The child will seek a dark room and attempt to sleep.
- Dizziness may occur especially in young females as an associated symptom.
- The headache may worsen by movement or exercise.
- Sleep generally alleviates the headache.
- The headache may last for 1 hour to 48 hours or more.

TENSION-TYPE HEADACHE

Tension-type headache has also been called tension headache, muscle contraction headache, stress-related headache, and "ordinary headache." These headaches can be either episodic or chronic and may include tightness in the muscles of the head or neck.

A tension-type headache can last from 30 minutes to several days. Chronic tension headaches may persist for many months. The pain usually occurs on both sides of the head, is steady and nonthrobbing. Some people say "it feels like a band tightening around my head." The pain is usually mild to moderate in severity. Most of the time the headache does not affect the person's activity level.

Tension-type headaches are usually not associated with other symptoms, such as nausea or vomiting. Some people may experience sensitivity to light or sound with the headache, but not both. Muscle tightness may be noticed by some patients but does not always have to occur.

CHRONIC DAILY HEADACHES

In adults, headaches that occur at least 15 days per month for at least 3 months have been called chronic daily headaches. In children there is not yet a clear definition.

Some chronic daily headaches may have started as migraine and build to a daily frequency. These are sometimes called transformed migraines. Tension-type headaches that increase to near-daily frequency are known as chronic tension-type headaches. Chronic headaches can result from taking some types of over-the-counter medication—for example, acetaminophen (Tylenol), ibuprofen (Motrin), caffeine—and some prescription medications almost every day. These are called drug rebound headaches. These headaches return either shortly after taking the medication or the medication stops working. The most effective way to make these headaches better is to stop taking pain medicines altogether for a few weeks. After that time, use of pain-relievers is limited to no more that 2 to 3 times per week.

Some people with chronic daily headaches are low in certain vitamins and minerals. It is important to eat balanced meals. Many children and adolescents may need to take a daily multivitamin.

CAUSES OF HEADACHES

There are different theories about the cause of migraine headaches. Often several family members are affected, suggesting genetic factors are partly responsible. Some individuals may become hypersensitive to triggers in their environment, such as flickering lights, changing weather patterns, or strong odors. The true cause may be a combination of factors. Some of the possible causes include blood vessel changes. Blood vessels in the head may first tighten and then expand during a migraine attack, changes that may explain the aura before and the throbbing pain during the migraine. Some migraine medication and other treatments may work by counteracting or blocking these changes in the blood vessels.

- *Brain and nervous system changes.* Imaging studies have identified an area in the brainstem at the back of the head that is activated during a migraine attack. A spreading wave of decreased activation occurs in the brain at the onset of an attack, which may account for the blurred vision or numbness that some people experience in the migraine aura.
- *Serotonin system abnormalities.* Serotonin is a natural chemical in the brain that has an important function in transmission of signals from one brain cell to another. Some migraine medication and other treatments affect serotonin action in the brain and can stop a migraine.

OTHER MIGRAINE-LIKE DISORDERS

Benign Paroxymal Vertigo

- Usually occurs in young children between 1 and 3 years of age.
- These are sudden attacks of dizziness experienced by young children.
- The child usually becomes pale, appears frightened, and staggers around as if he or she is drunk.

Cyclic Vomiting

- Usually beginning between 4 and 8 years of age.
- Children experience repetitive episodes.
- May be quite dramatic and lead to dehydration and hospitalization.

Hemiplegic Migraine

- A frightening attack of sudden onset of unilateral weakness (one-sided weakness).
- Weakness may involve the face, arm, or leg.
- If the right side of the body is the affected side, the individual may not be able to speak.
- May be triggered by mild head injury.
- There is a familial form, with a first-degree relative affected.
- The headache follows the onset of weakness.
- The weakness may last 1 hour to days, but usually resolves in 24 hours.
- The familial form has been identified on chromosome 19 in 50% to 60% of cases.
- Other causes of acute onset weakness must be considered before the diagnosis is made.

WHAT TO DO IF THE CHILD GETS A HEADACHE

Have the parent keep a record of the child's headaches. Have them write down everything that might relate to the child's headache (foods, odors, situations), how long it lasted, and how much pain the headache caused (Table 6-2).

Recommend that the child take pain medication for his or her headache as soon as pain is felt. He or she may be taking over-the-counter medication or prescription medication when getting a headache.

The child needs to be able to treat headaches at school. This means that the child's school nurse needs to know your treatment plan. It is important that permission is granted and all of the forms are completed for treating the child's headaches at school without having to go home. Suggest that the parent and you or your nurse educate the child's teachers about headaches and migraines.

Remember that using pain relievers (analgesics) every day can cause an increase in the child's headaches.

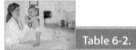

Table 6-2.

Worrisome Headache Symptoms

- Headaches that wake a child from sleep
- Early morning vomiting without nausea (upset stomach)
- Worsening or more frequent headaches
- Personality changes
- Complaints that "this is the worst headache I've ever had!"
- The headache is different from previous headaches
- Headaches with fever or a stiff neck
- Headaches that follow an injury

Drinking more fluids (especially sports drinks) during a headache may also be very important to help it to go away faster.

TREATMENT

The first step in treatment is to avoid known triggers, such as cheese or chocolate. The diagnosis of each headache type is dependent on a reliable history of the headache from the child or parent.

Many children have difficulty explaining their headaches, so to gain clues to the diagnosis you may want to include questions for the parents such as the following:

- Q. When did the headaches first begin?
- Q. How frequent are the headaches now?
- Q. How often did they occur when they first began?
- Q. Has there been a change in the severity of the headache?
- Q. What time of day do they occur?
- Q. Is there any warning that a headache is about to occur, such as changes in appetite, attitudes, or behavior?
- Q. Do the headaches appear sudden in onset?
- Q. Are there any outward physical changes? (pale, sweaty, color change)?
- Q. What does your child do when he or she complains of a headache?
- Q. Do they interfere with his or her ability to participate in activities?
- Q. Does he or she go lay down?
- Q. Does he or she seek a dark room?
- Q. Does he or she watch TV or listen to the stereo?
- Q. Does your child sleep to get rid of his or her headache?
- Q. How long does the headache appear to last?
- Q. When it is over, is there change in behavior and appetite?
- Q. Has there been any head trauma prior to the onset of the headache?
- Q. What have you used to treat the headache thus far?
- Q. Has the medication been effective?
- Q. Have you identified any triggers (food, weather, or stress)?
- Q. Is there a family history of headaches, migraine or otherwise?
- Q. Has there been any personality change in your child?
- Q. Has he or she missed any school because of the headache?
- Q. Has he or she missed any extracurricular activities because of the headache?

You may ask your patient many of the above questions *plus*:

Q. Where does your head hurt?

Q. What does it feel like?

Q. Do you know when you're going to get a headache?

Q. Do you see flashing lights or other changes in your vision before the headache starts?

Q. What do you do when you get a headache?

Q. When do you tell your parents?

Q. Does sleep help your headache?

Aside from the above, a complete medical history should be obtained in addition to inquiring about the family's significant medical history, especially history of headaches.

After a complete exam, a specific diagnosis such as common migraine or classic migraine may be given, and medication options for both acute and if needed preventive medications can be considered.

In cases of "worrisome" headache symptoms or an abnormal neurological examination, you may want to consider ordering a brain MRI, head CT, and blood tests (Figure 6-3).

Acute Treatment

■ Treatment of acute headaches can usually be accomplished at home with over-the-counter medication.

■ Dosages in children over 12 years of age are usually written on package labels for medication like Tylenol or ibuprofen.

■ However, dosages of over-the-counter pain medication for children under 12 vary with age and weight.

■ Triptans can be used in select circumstances.

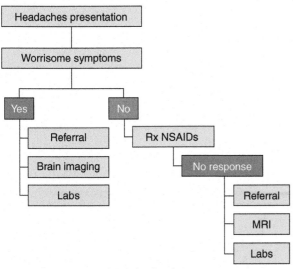

FIGURE 6-3 ■ Pediatric headache flowchart.

■ Aspirin is to be avoided in children because of its association with Reye syndrome.[2,3]

Preventive Medications

■ If headaches are frequent and disabling, medications to prevent headache occurrences may need to be considered.

■ These medications are given on a daily basis to prevent headaches from occurring.

■ Treatment with preventive medications needs to be individualized.

■ These medications can frequently be withdrawn after a period of good headache control.

■ There are several different medications that can be used in this regard.

■ After a complete medical evaluation, the child and parent can decide if preventive medication is needed and which one to choose.[2,3]

If you decide to prescribe daily medication to reduce headache frequency, remember to have the patient take it every day, whether having headaches or not.

Good sleep habits, going to bed at a consistent time and arising at about the same time each day, may alleviate some headaches.

PREVENTION

Taking good care of the child can decrease the frequency and severity of his or her headaches

1. Make sure the child drinks enough fluids. Children and adolescents need 4 to 8 glasses of fluid a day. Caffeine should be avoided. Sports drinks may help during a headache as well as during exercise by keeping sugar and sodium levels normal.

2. Make sure the child gets plenty of regular sleep at night (but do not let him or her oversleep). Fatigue and over-exertion are two factors that can trigger headaches. Most children and adolescents need to sleep 8 to 10 hours each night and keep a regular sleep schedule to help prevent headaches.

3. Be sure that the child eats balanced meals at regular hours. Do not let him or her skip meals.

4. Try to avoid foods that seem to trigger headaches. Remember that every child is different, so the child's triggers.

5. Plan and schedule the child's activities sensibly. Try to avoid overcrowded schedules or stressful and potentially upsetting situations.

SUMMARY

It is important to remember that the most headaches in children are benign, but when headaches begin, a thorough medical evaluation is important.

Treatment of headaches in children can be as simple as an over-the-counter medication in the correct dose. Some children need more aggressive treatment with both a preventive medication and possibly acute medication with subcutaneous injections of newer antimigraine headache agents such as sumatriptan.

The child need not suffer: appropriate treatment can significantly alter the course of headache frequency and severity.

REFERENCES

1. Bechtel KA. Migraine Headache: Pediatric Perspective. *Web MD.* May 2004;25(4):380-388. http://emedicine.medscape.com/article/802158-overview. Updated February 3, 2008.
2. American Academy of Neurology issues guidelines for pediatric migraine. *Neurology.* 2004;63:2215-2224.
3. New Guidelines for Treating Pediatric Migraine Released by American Academy of Neurology and Child Neurology Society, American Academy of Neurology, 2004.

CHAPTER 7

Ataxia

Farjam Farzam

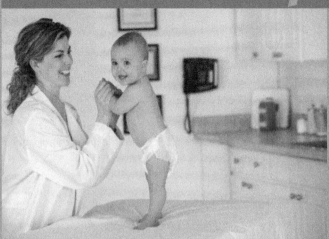

DEFINITION/EPIDEMIOLOGY

Ataxia is a term derived from Greek referring to impairment and lack of ability to coordinate or perform voluntary movements.[1] Ataxia can present and be noted in children of all age groups ranging from young infants to adolescents. Both genders, plus all racial and ethnic groups, may be affected. However, since there are many conditions and disorders that may cause ataxia in children, there is great variability in its underlying pathogenesis, risk factors, and presentation.

PATHOGENESIS

The cerebellum is the structure that, its dysfunction, is commonly attributed to the presentation of ataxia. On the other hand, disturbance to the structures or function of other sites such as the peripheral nerves, dorsal columns of the spinal cord, brainstem, or frontal cerebral cortex, which provide connections or pathways into and out of the cerebellum, may also play contributing roles in ataxia.[2,3]

CLINICAL PRESENTATION

Most children presenting with ataxia typically present with abnormal gait.[2] Some parents usually describe their children as clumsy, with poor coordination and balance, and unable to perform motor tasks smoothly[4,5]; whereas some are reported to walk as if under the influence of alcohol.[6] The gait is usually wide-based and staggering, with elevation of the feet and then slapping the soles on the ground.[2] The impaired balance and coordination may be worsened by closing both eyes (Romberg sign). Dysfunctions in the sensory and proprioceptive cerebellar inputs from the peripheral nerves and the posterior spinal columns may result in children looking at their feet during ambulation.[2,3] Frequent falls and fears of injury may urge parents to seek advice from health care professionals. Lesions affecting the cerebellar vermis may lead into ataxia affecting the trunk with difficulties in maintaining axial posture and balance in an upright position. In addition, titubation (bobbing of the head forward and backward)[4] may be noted with vermal lesions. The lesions affecting the cerebellar hemispheres may lead into hypotonia and ataxia affecting the limbs ipsilaterally.[4]

Associated findings in children presenting with ataxia may also include impaired speech, ocular movements, fine motor skills, and intentional tremors.[4] The speech may be described as slow, scanning, with uneven volume and separation of syllables.[2,4] Nystagmus and ocular dysmetria, overshooting and an inability to keep the moving eyes towards a targeted point, may be noted.[1,6] The smooth and accurate performance of rapid alternating movements (diadochokinesia) and complex motor activities may be impaired.[4] Tables 7-1 summarizes some of the common and rare presentations of signs and symptoms of ataxia in children.

HISTORY AND PHYSICAL EXAM

Obtaining an adequate history is the most essential part of evaluating children who present with ataxia. Some of the key elements in the history that can help with identifying the underlying causes include the child's age plus the course and pattern of onset at the time of presentation (acute versus chronic, intermittent, or progressive). Presence of fever, cough, congestion, rhinorrhea, rash, vomiting, or diarrhea at the time of or within few weeks

Table 7-1.

Signs and Symptoms Associated with Ataxia

Common Signs	Common Symptoms	Rare Signs	Rare Symptoms
Wide-based gait	Impaired walking	Opsoclonus	Headache
Slapping gait	Frequent falls	Myoclonus	Nausea
Abnormal speech	Poor balance	Papilledema	Vomiting
Hypotonia	Impaired motor coordination	Cranial nerve palsies	Visual impairment
Dysmetria		Titubation	Hearing impairment
Dysdiadochokinesia		Absent deep tendon reflexes	
Nystagmus		Tremors	
Mental status changes			
Seizures			

prior to presentation may identify an infectious or postinfectious source. Other features such as confusion, stiff neck, and seizures may be worrisome for more serious etiologies including meningitis, meningoencephalitis, or acute disseminating encephalomyelitis (ADEM). Experiencing head and neck trauma plus exposure to drugs and toxins should be determined. Headaches, emesis, and focal neurological findings are of concern for acute complications of mass lesions (tumors, abscess, arteriovenous malformations), strokes, or hemorrhage in the regions of the brainstem, cerebellum, or the posterior fossa. Intermittent and recurrent ataxia may be suggestive of migraines, epileptic seizures, postictal period, or disorders of inborn error of metabolism. Chronic or progressive ataxia may be caused by slowly developing tumors or congenital structural malformations, genetic, inherited disorders.

Additional information that may be beneficial in evaluating and diagnosing a child with ataxia include the presence of other medical or systemic illnesses, adequate assessment of the developmental milestones, plus the detailed family and social histories.

After gathering and obtaining a detailed history, a comprehensive general and neurological examination should be performed. The neurological examination should start with the evaluation of the child's mental status. The examiner should assess the alertness, social interaction, eye contact, and response to verbal and tactile stimuli. In older children, the speech, spelling, naming of objects, calculation, attention, recent or remote memory, and general fund of knowledge should be determined.

A detailed examination of the cranial nerve function and integrity with assessment of the vision, pupillary response to light and accommodation, extraocular movements, nystagmus, facial muscles strength and sensation, hearing, chewing, swallowing, gag reflex, neck and tongue sensation, plus movement should be

emphasized. A fundoscopic examination of the eyes should be performed to evaluate for papilledema.

The strength, sensation for light touch, pin prick, temperature, vibration, proprioception, muscle tone, and deep tendon reflexes can also be helpful in localizing other lesions within the nervous system that may be attributed to ataxia.

The cerebellar exam may reveal intentional tremor, dysmetria, abnormal diadochokinesia, and heel to shin or a positive Romberg sign. The gait exam focusing on heel, toe, and tandem walking are also essential in evaluating children with ataxia.

DIFFERENTIAL DIAGNOSIS

Acute presentation of ataxia may be caused by a variety of conditions including infections, postinfections, trauma, toxins, inflammatory, tumors, strokes, hemorrhage, and seizures (Table 7-2).[2,3,5] Among the infectious agents, viruses including varicella, Epstein–Barr virus, echovirus, coxsackievirus, measles, mumps, HIV, rubella, and polio are commonly associated with ataxia.[2,3,5] Bacterial agents such as *Streptococcus pneumoniae*, *Haemophilus influenzae*, *Listeria monocytogenes*,

Table 7-2.

Signs and Symptoms of Severe and Life-Threatening Conditions in Ataxic Children

Mental status changes
Severe headaches
Fever
Seizures
Vomiting
Papilledema
Cranial nerve dysfunction

and *Escherichia coli* are common pathogens.[2,3,5] Syphilis, Lyme disease, tuberculosis, and mycoplasma pneumoniae have also been associated with ataxia in children. Toxoplasmosis and cysticercosis are two parasitic agents commonly attributed to ataxia,[3] especially among individuals exposed to cat feces and the immigrant population from Latin America and Asia, respectively. Postinfectious conditions such as ADEM and inflammatory disorders such as multiple sclerosis can also lead to acute ataxia.

Head injuries sustained from falls or motor vehicle accidents to nonaccidental injuries due to child abuse can lead to acute ataxia. Exposure to toxins such as drugs (antiepileptics, benzodiazepines), alcohol, lead, mercury, and carbon monoxide must be excluded. Mass lesions such as tumors or vascular insults to the cerebellum or brainstem as the result of thrombosis, embolism, or hemorrhage may occur, along with cranial nerve deficits plus signs and symptoms worrisome for increased intracranial pressure.

Chronic, intermittent, and progressive ataxias may be caused by genetic, structural, or degenerative disorders. The hereditary causes are usually categorized into autosomal dominant and autosomal recessive disorders.[7] Some of the autosomal dominant conditions include the spinocerebellar ataxias (SCA types 1–28) and episodic ataxias (EA type 1 and 2). The autosomal recessive disorders include Friedreich ataxia (FRDA), ataxia-telangiectasia (A-T), and ataxia with vitamin E deficiency (AVED).[7] The urea cycle enzyme deficiencies, aminoacidurias, and impaired lactate and pyruvate metabolism are examples of inborn errors of metabolism that can lead to progressive ataxia in children.[2] Congenital structural malformations such as aplasia or dysplasia of the cerebellar hemisphere or vermis, plus Dandy-Walker and Chiari malformations, may also present with chronic ataxia.[2] Brain tumors such as ependymomas, medulloblastomas, and cerebellar astrocytomas should be excluded (Table 7-3).

SPECIFIC DISORDERS

There are several genetic disorders such as Friedreich and non-Friedreich ataxias that can present with ataxia among children.

Friedreich Ataxia

Epidemiology

Friedreich ataxia is an autosomal recessive triple repeat disease with a number of components. Symptoms are present by age 10 years in about half of those affected, and almost all have symptoms by the early 20s.

Table 7-3.

Causes of Ataxia in Children

Acute/Intermittent	Chronic/Progressive
Infectious	**Congenital/Structural**
Viral	Cerebellar vermis agenesis/ dysgenesis
Bacterial	Cerebellar hemisphere aplasia/ dysplasia
Parasitic	Chiari malformation
Fungal	Dandy-Walker syndrome
Trauma	**Mass Lesions**
Accidental	Medulloblastoma
Nonaccidental	Ependymoma
	Brainstem glioma
	Abcess, arteriovenous malformations
Toxic	**Genetic/Degenerative**
Antiepileptic drugs	Nutrition
Alcohol	Vitamin B_{12}
Benzodiazepines	Vitamin E
Carbon monoxide, lead	Thiamine
Vascular	**Endocrine**
Ischemia	Hypothyroidism
Hemorrhage	
Embolic	**Psychogenic**
	Major depressive disorder
Inflammatory/ Postinfectious	Anxiety disorder
	Conversion reaction
ADEM	Malingering
Multiple sclerosis	
Migraine	
Basilar	
Seizures	
Inborn error of metabolism	
Genetic	
Episodic ataxia[1,2]	
Psychogenic	
Hysteria	
Conversion reaction	
Malingering	

Etiology/pathogenesis

Friedreich ataxia occurs secondary to a mutation of the mitochondrial protein, frataxin, located on chromosome 9. Spinal cord degeneration occurs in three distinct regions: (1) posterior columns and dorsal root ganglia, (2) corticospinal tracts, and (3) spinocerebellar tracts. The sensory neuropathy associated with Friedreich ataxia occurs because of progressive degeneration of the dorsal ganglion and axon. There is some associated secondary demyelination.

Clinical features

The primary feature of Friedreich ataxia is gait ataxia. This ataxia is progressive and typically leads to the need for a wheelchair. There is associated peripheral neuropathy, dysarthria, and cardiomyopathy (in 50% of cases). Hearing loss and optic atrophy occur only rarely. Most patients are unable to walk by age 30 years.

Treatment

There is no specific treatment for Friedreich ataxia. The patient is at risk of falling, and appropriate safety measures should be taken. Furthermore, the patient's feet should be checked on a daily basis for cuts or blisters that might otherwise go unnoticed because of the sensory loss.

Non-Friedreich Ataxia

There are a number of distinct and unrelated diseases that have phenotypes similar to Friedreich ataxia.

Ataxia with vitamin E deficiency (AVED)

Ataxia with vitamin E deficiency arises secondary to abnormalities in vitamin E absorption or metabolism. AVED can result in a syndrome clinically indistinguishable from Friedreich ataxia. AVED is an autosomal recessive disease with a mutation in the gene encoding for alpha-tocopherol transfer protein (alpha-TTP), and results in low or undetectable levels of vitamin E without associated fat malabsorption.

Abetalipoproteinemia (Bassen-Kornzweig syndrome)

Abetalipoproteinemia is a rare autosomal recessive disorder of lipoprotein metabolism. There is malabsorption of vitamin E. There is an absence of apolipoprotein B-containing proteins (chylomicrons, LDL, VLDL), and diagnostic studies can help in distinguishing this disorder from Friedreich ataxia, including a low serum cholesterol level, acanthocytosis on peripheral blood smear, and an abnormal serum protein electrophoresis. Furthermore the presence of retinopathy distinguishes the disorder from Friedreich ataxia.

Acquired vitamin E deficiency

Acquired vitamin E deficiency can be associated with severe fat malabsorption in diseases such as cystic fibrosis, cholestatic liver disease, celiac disease, and short bowel syndrome. While there may be an ataxia clinically similar to Friedreich ataxia, there are typically symptoms associated with the primary disease that guide diagnosis.

Early-onset cerebellar ataxia with retained reflexes (EOCA)

The early-onset cerebellar ataxias are a heterogeneous group of disorders, most of which are autosomal recessive. The EOCA disorders have a childhood onset resembling Friedreich ataxia but with retained reflexes. There may be spasticity, but the diabetes, cardiac disease, and skeletal deformities are absent. The Friedreich ataxia triplet repeat test is negative and the prognosis is better than with Friedreich ataxia.

Progressive ataxia associated with biochemical abnormalities

Multiple inherited diseases can cause progressive ataxia, including ceroid lipofuscinosis, cholestanolosis, ataxia-telangiectasia, xeroderma pigmentosum, Cockayne syndrome, GM-2 gangliosidosis, adrenoleukodystrophy, metachromatic leukodystrophy, mitochondrial diseases (MERRF, KSS, NARP), sialidosis, and Niemann-Pick and sphingomyelin storage disorders.

Ataxia telangiectasia (Louis-Bar syndrome)

Ataxia telangiectasia is an autosomal recessive disease with a mutation in the ATM gene (leads to defect in DNA repair) on chromosome 11. Symptoms of ataxia telangiectasia typically begin during infancy. There is progressive truncal ataxia, usually resulting in the patient being wheelchair-bound by age 12 years. The hallmark oculocutaneous telangiectasias usually appear between ages 3 and 5 years, well after the onset of ataxia. Other symptoms include dysarthria, nystagmus, oculomotor dyspraxia, dystonia, athetosis, myoclonic jerks, polyneuropathy, and cognitive dysfunction.

Diagnostic studies reveal elevated AFP and CEA levels (alpha-fetoprotein and carcinoembryonic antigen), and decreased or absent IgA levels. Fibroblasts can be screened for increased x-ray sensitivity and radioresistant DNA synthesis. The associated immunodeficiency leads to recurrent respiratory infections. Ataxia telangiectasia is also associated with cancer, typically leukemias and lymphomas. The average age of death is 20 years and is usually from infection or neoplasm.

Progressive Myoclonic Ataxias

The progressive myoclonic ataxias are a heterogenous group of childhood disorders associated with progressive cerebellar ataxia and action myoclonus. Most of these disorders are due to mitochondrial disorders (MERRF, KSS, NARP). Rare cases of polyQ disease and dentatorubral-pallidoluysian atrophy (DRPLA) have juvenile onset.

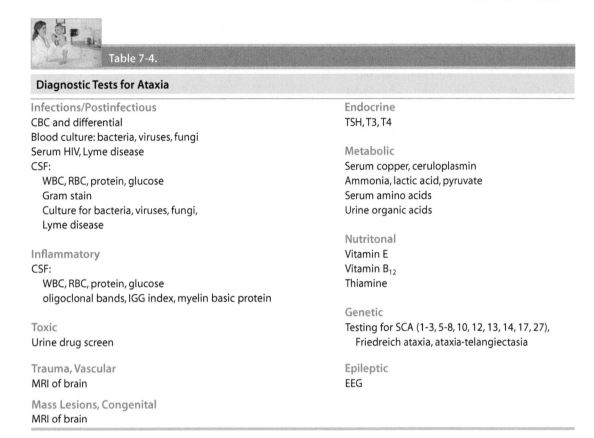

Table 7-4.

Diagnostic Tests for Ataxia

Infections/Postinfectious	Endocrine
CBC and differential	TSH, T3, T4
Blood culture: bacteria, viruses, fungi	
Serum HIV, Lyme disease	Metabolic
CSF:	Serum copper, ceruloplasmin
WBC, RBC, protein, glucose	Ammonia, lactic acid, pyruvate
Gram stain	Serum amino acids
Culture for bacteria, viruses, fungi,	Urine organic acids
Lyme disease	
	Nutritonal
Inflammatory	Vitamin E
CSF:	Vitamin B$_{12}$
WBC, RBC, protein, glucose	Thiamine
oligoclonal bands, IGG index, myelin basic protein	
	Genetic
Toxic	Testing for SCA (1-3, 5-8, 10, 12, 13, 14, 17, 27),
Urine drug screen	Friedreich ataxia, ataxia-telangiectasia
Trauma, Vascular	Epileptic
MRI of brain	EEG
Mass Lesions, Congenital	
MRI of brain	

DIAGNOSTIC TESTS

The information obtained from an adequate history and detailed exam can help the clinician select the appropriate diagnostic tests that can help identify the underlying causes of ataxia. Table 7-4 provides a list of some diagnostic tests commonly used in evaluating children who present with ataxia. Imaging techniques such as MRI and CT scans should be performed in children presenting with ataxia who are suspected of harboring mass lesions, stroke, or hemorrhage in the cerebellum and brainstem. In the case of suspected infectious etiologies, appropriate microbiological cultures and cerebrospinal fluid specimens should be obtained. A urine drug screen can be helpful in identifying any potential exposure to medications, drugs, or toxins. For those children with family histories of ataxia, specific genetic testing for either the autosomal dominant or recessive disorders is encouraged. Electroencephalograms (EEG) should be considered if the child presents with encephalopathy or suspected seizures. Testing the blood, urine, and CSF for metabolic disorders is emphasized in the progressive circumstances. Table 7-5 recommends appropriate specialists who may be helpful in evaluating and managing children presenting with ataxia.

TREATMENT

Antibiotics and antiviral agents may be used in the case of infectious sources of ataxia. Anti-inflammatory drugs such as corticosteroids and immunomodulating drugs can be helpful in postinfectious and autoimmune disorders such as ADEM and multiple sclerosis, respectively. Eliminating and discontinuing the use of toxins

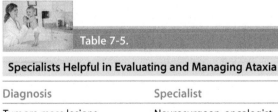

Table 7-5.

Specialists Helpful in Evaluating and Managing Ataxia

Diagnosis	Specialist
Tumors, mass lesions	Neurosurgeon, oncologist
Meningitis, encephalitis	Infectious disease
Stroke, hemorrhage	Neurologist, neurosurgeon
Trauma	Neurologist, neurosurgeon
Hereditary/genetic	Geneticist
Migraine	Neurologist
Epileptic	Neurologist
Psychogenic	Psychiatrist

or substances leading to ataxia should be emphasized. Surgical resection and radiation therapy of mass lesions may be appropriate. Providing the appropriate hormones such as thyroid and nutritional supplements such as vitamins E, B_{12} and thiamine may be helpful in preventing the progression of their corresponding disorders. Dietary restriction of proteins and glucose may be beneficial in children suffering from the inborn errors of metabolism. The anti-epileptic drugs can prevent ataxia related to epileptic seizures but in some cases can cause ataxia as a side effect. Acetazolamide may be beneficial in reducing the increased intracranial pressure in children with episodic ataxia. Referral of individuals with strong family histories of ataxia to a geneticist is highly recommended. Children presenting with conversion disorders (a rare cause) should be treated and managed by counselors and psychiatrists.

REFERENCES

1. Hensyl W. *Stedman's Pocket Medical Dictionary.* Baltimore, MD: Williams & Wilkins; 1987.
2. Fenichel GM. Ataxia. In: Pioli S. and Ryan J. eds. *Clinical Pediatric Neurology.* 5th ed. Philadelphia, PA: Elsevier Saunders; 2005:219-289.
3. Perlman SL. Ataxia. *Clin Geriatr Med.* 2006;22(4): 859-877.
4. Maricich SM, Zoghbi H. Cerebellum and the hereditary ataxias. In: Swaiman K., Ashwal S. and Ferriero D. Mosby eds. *Pediatric Neurology.* Philadelphia, PA: Elsevier; 2005: 1241-1262.
5. Agrawal D. Approach to the child with acute Ataxia. www.uptodate.com. September 2006.
6. Lynn DJ, Newton HB, Rae-Grant A. Ataxia. Philadelphia, PA: Lippincott Williams & Wilkins; 2004:4-6.
7. Bird TD. Hereditary ataxias: overview. *Gene Rev.* www.genetests.org. October 2006.

CHAPTER 8

Abnormalities of Head Size: Microcephaly and Macrocephaly

Paul R. Carney and James D. Geyer

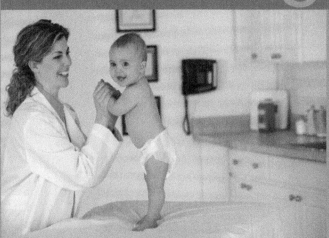

MICROCEPHALY

Definitions and Epidemiology

Head size is an easily measured clinical finding that can be followed over time. The head circumference is measured around the forehead and the occipital protuberance. Microcephaly is defined by a head circumference more than two standard deviations below the mean for a given demographic (age, gender, race). Small head size is an indication of the underlying brain size except in cases of craniosynostosis, or premature closure of the bony sutures.

The posterior fontanelle should close by age 3 months and anterior fontanelle by 20 months. Fibrous union of the suture lines occurs by about age 6 months. The craniobasal bones are ossified by age 8 years. The remaining sutures are visible on x-ray until approximately age 20 years but can resist elevated intracranial pressure by age 12 years.[1]

Pathogenesis

Primary microcephaly

Primary microcephaly occurs because of genetic or environmental factors that produce small brain size (micrencephaly). The genetic form of primary microcephaly can be inherited by either autosomal dominant or autosomal recessive mechanisms.[2] A variety of neuronal migrational disorders—lissencephaly, schizencephaly, agensesis of the corpus callosum, and polymicrogyria—can be associated with microcephaly. Incomplete neurogenesis can also cause microcephaly secondary to insufficient neuronal production. Disorders such as anencephaly can also result in microcephaly (Figure 8-1). While the inheritance for microcephaly has been linked to chromosomes 1, 9, and 19, linkages are likely to be found with genes mapping to a number of other chromosomes.[3-5] Chromosomal disorders including Down syndrome and other trisomy disorders can produce microcephaly.

Exposure to ionizing radiation during the first two trimesters can result in microcephaly.[6,7] It does not appear that exposure to low levels of radiation associated with diagnostic imaging (x-ray, CT, MRI) pose any significant increased risk for the development of microcephaly.

Prenatal infections do, however, increase the risk for microcephaly. Cytomegalovirus (CMV), rubella virus, and toxoplasmosis are the most well-known causes of microcephaly, but numerous infections in utero can increase this risk.[8]

Fetal exposure to certain chemicals during neuronal induction or cellular migration also increases the risk of microcephaly.

Secondary microcephaly

As opposed to disorders interrupting cerebral development associated with primary microcephaly, secondary microcephaly arises following neuronal injury. Prenatal cerebral infarction, meningitis, encephalitis, trauma, hypoxia, and metabolic disorders can result in this neuronal injury.

Craniosynostosis is premature closure of at least one of the cranial bony sutures.[9] Primary craniosynostosis is caused by abnormalities of the mesenchymal matrix. Secondary craniosynostosis can occur in association with a number of hematologic, metabolic, and in some cases mechanical disorders.

Craniosynostosis is associated with a number of genetic disorders including Aperts syndrome, Crouzon syndrome, Jackson-Weiss syndrome, Muenke syndrome,

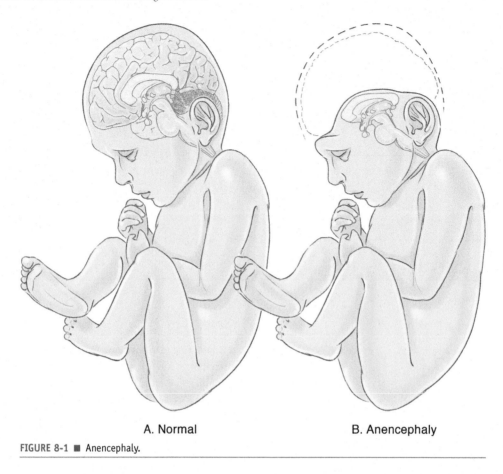

A. Normal   B. Anencephaly

FIGURE 8-1 ▪ Anencephaly.

Pfeiffer syndrome, Saethre-Chotzen syndrome, and Shprintzen-Goldberg syndrome.[10] Secondary craniosynostosis can occur in patients with hyperthyroidism, vitamin D deficiency, hypophosphatemia, inherited metabolic disorders such as Hurler disease, and hematologic disorders such as sickle cell anemia and thalassemia.

Clinical Presentation/Diagnosis

Microcephaly is defined by a head circumference more than two standard deviations below the mean for a given demographic (age, gender, race). Since small head size is usually an indication of the underlying brain size, it is associated with a variety of neurological disorders.

This physical finding does not guarantee abnormal development since approximately 2% of otherwise healthy school children will have a small head size with a head circumference more than two standard deviations below the mean size. The head circumference should be monitored along with the height and weight. Obviously a small child with a small head circumference would be less worrisome

than a small head circumference associated with average height and weight.

Craniosynostosis has numerous subtypes depending on which sutures are involved in the premature closure (Table 8-1). Oxycephaly is associated with the most severe neurological consequences, including increased intracranial pressure, anosmia, optic atrophy, weakness, and spasticity. Patients with Crouzon syndrome or craniofacial

Table 8-1.	
Craniosynostosis Subtypes	
Suture Prematurely Closed	Name of Subtype
Sagittal	Scaphocephaly or dolichocephaly
Sagittal and coronal	
Sagittal and lambdoid	
Bilateral coronal	Acrocephaly
Unilateral coronal	Plagiocephaly
Metopic	Trigonocephaly
All in vault	Oxycephaly

dysostosis have premature closure of multiple sutures, hypertelorism, high forehead, exophthalmos, choanal atresia, and relatively intact intelligence.

Diagnostic Tests

After the presence of microcephaly has been confirmed, additional neuroimaging is warranted. Routine radiography gives an excellent view of the bony sutures. CT provides information regarding calcifications associated with infectious and metabolic causes of microcephaly. Finally, MRI provides information regarding neuronal migration disorders, heterotopias, and schizencephaly.

Treatment

Primary microcephaly and secondary microcephaly associated with hypoxia, infarction, trauma, in utero infections, and metabolic disorders do not have any direct treatment other than supportive measures. Craniosynostosis secondary to hyperthyroidism or vitamin deficiencies is rarely as severe as the primary forms and should be treated via the management of these disorders.

Craniosynostosis involving multiple sutures is treated surgically to prevent increased intracranial pressure.[11] Surgery for craniosynostosis involving only one suture is much more controversial since this is typically a cosmetic procedure.

MACROCEPHALY

Definitions and Epidemiology

As with microcephaly, macrocephaly is easily identified by monitoring the head circumference. Macrocephaly is defined by a head circumference more than two standard deviations above the mean for a given demographic (age, gender, race). Unfortunately, the skull enlargement occurs after significant enlargement of the ventricles in cases of obstructive hydrocephalus.

Pathogenesis

Macrocephaly occurs because of one of two etiologies—increased brain size or hydrocephalus. Head size expands secondary to increased brain size, elevated intracranial pressure, or hydrocephalus if this occurs prior to fibrous closure of the sutures at approximately 12 years of age.

Brain Size

Megalencephaly arises secondary to brain overgrowth. This can occur because of cellular proliferation, insufficient apoptosis, or one of several storage diseases. Hemimegalencephaly is defined as a variably enlarged cerebral hemisphere, usually with neuronal migrational abnormalities such as lissencephaly, pachygyria, and abnormalities of the corpus callosum (Figure 8-2).[12] The occipital pole is usually shifted across the midline.

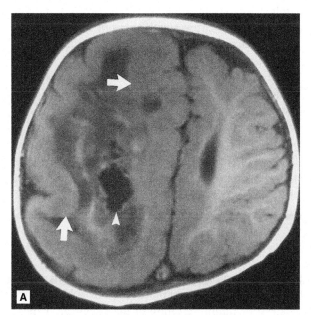
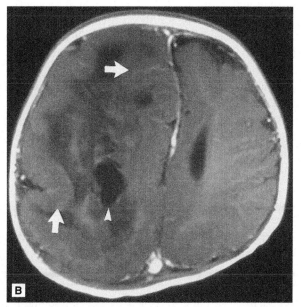

FIGURE 8-2 ■ Hemimegalencephaly. Axial unenhanced **(A)** and contrast material-enhanced **(B)** T1-weighted MR images show enlargement of the right cerebral hemisphere, cavitation in the region of the centrum semiovale (*arrowhead*), and diffuse gyral thickening (*arrows*) with diminished sulcation, a finding consistent with pachygyria. There are patchy, linear regions of increased signal intensity in the white matter of the right hemisphere. No pathologic enhancement is seen on the contrast-enhanced image **B.** (*Reproduced with permission from Broumandi DD, Hayward UM, Benzian JM, Gonzalez I, Nelson, MD. Best Cases from the AFIP: Hemimegalencephaly.* RadioGraphics. RSNA. *2004;24:843-848.*)

Hydrocephalus

In most cases, hydrocephalus occurs because of either decreased cerebrospinal fluid (CSF) absorption or blockage of the CSF pathways. The choroid plexus papilloma is a tumor that may result in increased CSF production. Obstruction of the foramen of Monro or of the foramina of Magendie or Lushka results in noncommunicating hydrocephalus. Such obstruction usually occurs because of a tumor, enlarged vein of Galen, or other posterior fossa lesion.

The aqueduct of Sylvius has a cross-sectional area of approximately 0.5 mm^2 in the normal. Aqueductal stenosis arises with a histologically normal but constricted aqueduct. The channel may, however, be branched or the stenosis can occur secondary to abnormalities of adjacent structures. Hydrocephalus secondary to aqueductal stenosis can occur from birth to middle age.

The aqueduct can also become blocked by a progressive gliotic process, usually following meningitis or intraventricular hemorrhage.[13] The onset of symptoms is insidious as the gliosis progresses.

Approximately half of the cases of hydrocephalus-related macrocephaly occur secondary to abnormalities involving the fourth ventricle. The most common of these is a Chiari malformation. Type I Arnold-Chiari malformation is an isolated displacement of the cerebellar tonsils into the cervical canal and a kinked cervical spinal cord. There is no obstruction of the fourth ventricle with type I malformation. Type II Arnold-Chiari malformation is a much more serious disorder with displacement of the cerebellum into cervical canal, displacement of the medulla and fourth ventricle into the cervical canal, and hydrocephalus due to fourth ventricle obstruction or aqueductal stenosis (Figure 8-3). All type II Chiari malformations are associated with myelomeningocele. Cortical malformations (heterotopias and polymicrogyria), brainstem malformations (hypoplasia of cranial nerves and pons), cerebellar dysplasia, thoracolumbar kyphoscoliosis, diastematomyelia (bifid cord), and syringomyelia frequently occur as well.[1] Type III Chiari malformation has the constituent part of the type II malformation plus an encephalocele, which is usually occipital.

The Dandy-Walker malformation is a less common cause of ventricular obstruction at the level of the fourth ventricle, occurring in approximately 1 in 30,000 births.[14] Agenesis of the cerebellar vermis, cystic dilation of the fourth ventricle, and an enlarged posterior fossa are the hallmark features of the Dandy-Walker malformation (Figure 8-4). The cystic changes in the fourth ventricle appear to block the CSF outflow pathways, resulting in hydrocephalus.

Communicating hydrocephalus or block CSF reabsorption accounts for 30% of cases of hydrocephalus. The reabsorption can be blocked by scarring following meningitis or hemorrhage.

Clinical Presentation/Diagnosis

Megalencephaly has been classically associated with cognitive dysfunction, seizures, hypotonia, and weakness but is often seen in patients with normal intellect. Megalencephaly is associated with a variety of syndromes with cutaneous findings, including hemagiomatosis, neurofibromatosis, angiomatosis and lipomatosis, Bannayan syndrome, Klippel-Trenaunay-Weber syndrome, and Beckwith-Wiedemann syndrome. Hemimegalencephaly is also associated with a number of neurological findings depending on the hemisphere involved and the degree of severity. Seizures are a common sequela.

The presentation of hydrocephalus is dictated by age at onset, duration of the elevated pressure, and the rate of development. Obviously, if the hydrocephalus develops secondary to other structural abnormalities, these findings may overshadow the hydrocephalus and dictate the overall clinical presentation. If the hydrocephalus occurs prior to 2 years of age, macrocephaly is an early indicator. The anterior fontanelle is usually tense and the skull is thin with wide suture lines. As the hydrocephalus progresses, divergent strabismus and a downward gaze often occur. Optic atrophy without papilledema is also common. Weakness and spasticity, worse in the legs than the arms, occurs because of stretching of the corticospinal fibers as they progress around the lateral ventricles. In severe cases, pseudobulbar palsy can occur, resulting in difficulty with sucking, feeding, and aspiration.

Hydrocephalus presenting in the older child, over age 2 years, has a different presentation. The increased intracranial pressure causes optic atrophy with papilledema, strabismus, headache that is worse on awakening but improves with vomiting and sitting up, and leg weakness with spasticity. Hypothalamic–pituitary dysfunction also commonly occurs.

In addition to the monitoring of the head circumference, transillumination of the skull can be very informative. In this age of technologically advanced imaging techniques, transillumination is becoming a lost art. Ultrasound can be used for monitoring ventricular size but is of limited utility for identifying the underlying etiology. MRI provides the most diagnostic information regarding the etiology of hydrocephalus and is the imaging modality of choice for this disorder.[15]

Treatment

Surgical intervention is the primary treatment for hydrocephalus. In cases of blockage of the CSF pathways by a cyst or tumor, resection of the lesion can be performed. This is rarely possible, and most cases of hydrocephalus must be managed by a shunting procedure. Extracranial shunts move the CSF through one-way valves to the peritoneum, atrium, or pleural space. The ventriculoperitoneal shunt is the most commonly used

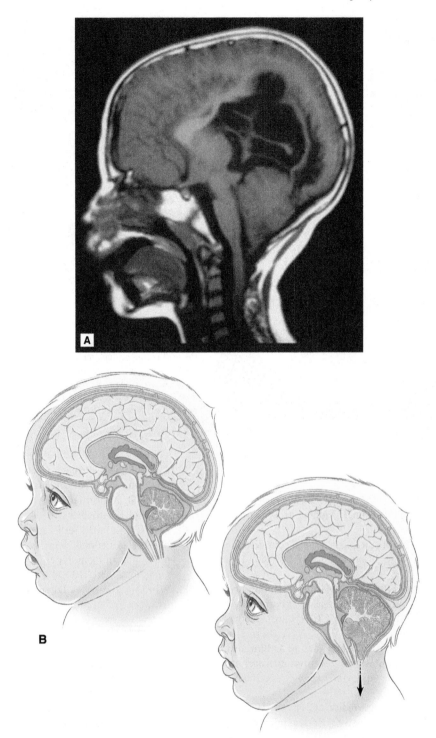

FIGURE 8-3 ■ **(A)** Chiari II malformation: Note herniation of the cerebellar vermis, fourth ventricle, and elongation of the brainstem into the vertebral canal. **(B)** Normal. **(C)** Chiari I malformation: Note elongation of the cerebellum and extension through the foramen magnum into the cervical spinal cord (arrow). (*Part A reproduced with permission from Photo Researchers, Inc.*)

shunt for obstructive hydrocephalus.[16] The lumboperitoneal shunt is restricted to treatment of communicating hydrocephalus, which is much less common in the pediatric population.

Shunt complications are common, with infection and failure being the two most common problems. Further complicating the situation is the possibility of intermittent failure. Suspected cases of shunt infection should be assessed by a shunt tap sent for cell counts, culture, and sensitivity. Treatment must be aggressive as delineated in the chapter on infectious diseases. The assessment of shunt patency is usually deferred to the neurosurgical team.

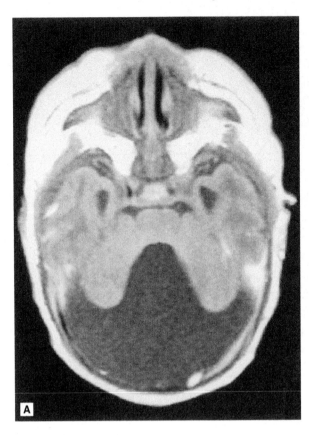

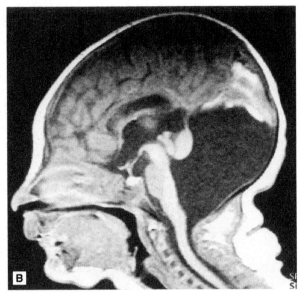

FIGURE 8-4 ▪ Dandy-Walker malformation. MRI showing agenesis of the midline cerebellum and large midline cyst, representing the greatly dilated fourth ventricle, which occupies almost the entire posterior fossa. **A.** Axial view. **B.** Sagittal view. (*Reproduced with permission from Ropper AH, Brown RH, eds. Adams and Victor's Principles of Neurology. 8th ed. New York: McGraw-Hill; 2005, Figure 38-2.*)

REFERENCES

1. Geyer J, Keating J, Potts D, Carney P, eds. *Neurology for the Boards*. 3rd ed. Philadelphia: Lippincott Williams & Wilkins; 2006.
2. Opitz JM, Holt MC. Microcephaly: general considerations and aids to nosology. *J Craniofac Genet Dev Biol*. 1990; 10:175-204.
3. Jamieson CR, Fryns JP, Jacobs J, Matthijs G, Abramowicz MJ. Primary autosomal recessive microcephaly: MCPH5 maps to 1q25-q32. *Am J Hum Genet*. 2000;67: 1575-1577.
4. Moynihan L, Jackson AP, Roberts E, et al. A third novel locus for primary autosomal recessive microcephaly maps to chromosome 9q34. *Am J Hum Genet*. 2000;66: 724-727.
5. Roberts E, Jackson AP, Carradice AC, et al. The second locus for autosomal recessive primary microcephaly (MCPH2) maps to chromosome 19q13.1-13.2. *Eur J Hum Genet*. 1999;7:815-820.
6. Greskovich JF Jr., Macklis RM. Radiation therapy in pregnancy: risk calculation and risk minimization. *Semin Oncol*. 2000;27:633-645.
7. Jensh RP, Eisenman LM, Brent RL. Postnatal neurophysiologic effects of prenatal X-irradiation. *Int J Radiat Biol*. 1995;67:217-227.
8. Bale JF, Miner L, Petheram SJ. Congenital cytomegalovirus infection. *Curr Treat Options Neurol*. 2002;4:225-230.
9. Blaser SI. Abnormal skull shape. *Pediatr Radiol*. 2008; 38(suppl 3):S488-S496.
10. Passos-Bueno MR, Serti Eacute AE, Jehee FS, Fanganiello R, Yeh E. Genetics of craniosynostosis: genes, syndromes, mutations and genotype-phenotype correlations. *Front Oral Biol*. 2008;12:107-143.
11. Wan DC, Kwan MD, Lorenz HP, Longaker MT. Current treatment of craniosynostosis and future therapeutic directions. *Front Oral Biol*. 2008;12:209-230.
12. Pang T, Atefy R, Sheen V. Malformations of cortical development. *Neurologist*. 2008;14:181-191.
13. Ment LR, Duncan CC, Scott DT, Ehrenkranz RA. Posthemorrhagic hydrocephalus. Low incidence in very low birth weight neonates with intraventricular hemorrhage. *J Neurosurg*. 1984;60:343-347.
14. Kalidasan V, Carroll T, Allcutt D, Fitzgerald RJ. The Dandy-Walker syndrome: a 10-year experience of its management and outcome. *Eur J Pediatr Surg*. 1995;5(suppl 1):16-18.
15. Shprecher D, Schwalb J, Kurlan R. Normal pressure hydrocephalus: diagnosis and treatment. *Curr Neurol Neurosci Rep*. 2008;8:371-376.
16. Drake JM. The surgical management of pediatric hydrocephalus. *Neurosurgery*. 2008;62(suppl 2):633-640; discussion 640-642.

CHAPTER 9

Attention-Deficit/ Hyperactivity Disorder

Eileen B. Fennell

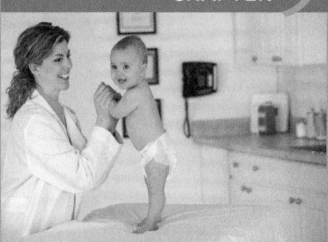

DEFINITION AND EPIDEMIOLOGY

Attention-deficit/hyperactivity disorder (ADHD) is one of the most frequently encountered disorders in pediatric and adolescent medical practice. ADHD is a complex developmental disorder of brain and behavior that makes its initial appearance in preschool ages, persists into adolescence, and, in some individuals, into adult life.[1] In 2007, the CDC summary of health statistics for U.S. children indicated that 4.5 million children (7%) between the ages of 3 and 17 years had been diagnosed with ADHD. The rate for boys (11%) was twice the rate for girls (4%).[2] While the degree of persistence of this disorder into adulthood is still unclear, estimates from longitudinal studies suggest between 1% and 6% of the adult population has symptoms of ADHD.[3]

Historically, symptoms of impulsivity, hyperactivity, and inattention were first attributed by Still (1902) to neurological disorder. Therefore, early clinical diagnosis were based upon presumptive "organic" etiological factors such as brain trauma, encephalitis, or other brain conditions that resulted in problems of attention, impulse control, emotional disregulation, and cognition. Gradually, however, the clinical diagnostic emphasis shifted to what Shelton[4] labeled "symptom-based" description of the disorder, which preceded current classification systems such as the American Psychiatric Association's *DSM-IV*. In 2000, the empirically updated *DSM-IV-TR*[5] was published and provides the current diagnostic criteria and ICD-9 codes for several subtypes of ADHD. These include (1) Attention-Deficit/Hyperactivity Disorder, Combined Type (314.01); (2) Attention-Deficit/ Hyperactivity Disorder, Predominantly Inattentive Type (314.00); (3) Attention-Deficit/Hyperactivity Disorder, Predominantly Hyperactive–Impulsive Type (314.01);

and (4) Attention-Deficit/Hyperactivity Disorder, Not Otherwise Specified (314.9). While the first three subtypes are differentiated from each other on the basis of predominant clinical presentation, the fourth subtype is reserved for those patients who, despite the presence of prominent symptoms of inattention or hyperactivity–impulsivity, do not meet full diagnostic criteria for a specific ADHD subtype. Similarly, for adolescents and/or adults who currently have symptoms but no longer meet full criteria, the label "In Partial Remission" would be added to the diagnostic code (eg, 314.01—In Partial Remission). Table 9-1 presents the common signs and symptoms described for diagnostic purposes under the three primary domains of inattention, hyperactivity, and impulsivity.

Current diagnostic criteria for any of the three ADHD subtypes noted above include

1. Six or more of the symptoms of inattention and six or more of the symptoms of hyperactivity–impulsivity must be present.
2. Symptoms must have been present for 6 or more months prior to diagnosis.
3. Some symptoms that have caused impairment must be present before age 7 years.
4. Symptoms causing some impairment must be present in two or more settings.
5. There must be clear evidence of clinically significant impairment in social, academic, or occupational functioning.
6. These symptoms do not occur exclusively during the course of another disorder, such as pervasive developmental disorder and are not better accounted for by another disorder.

There has been considerable controversy about the current diagnostic criteria,[6] primarily focused on the age

Table 9-1.

Common Signs and Symptoms of ADHD

Domain: Inattention

1. Poor attention to details or makes careless mistakes in academic or employment activities
2. Problems in sustained attention
3. Seems not to listen when spoken to
4. Poor follow-through on instructions, tasks, or duties in academic settings, work, or play
5. Difficulty organizing activities
6. Often avoids tasks requiring sustained concentration or effort
7. Often loses things that are needed
8. Often easily distracted by external stimuli
9. Often forgetful in daily activities

Domain: Hyperactivity

1. Often fidgets or squirms in seat
2. Often out-of-seat in classroom or other situations
3. Often runs about or climbs excessively in situations where it is inappropriate
4. Often has difficulty playing or engaging in leisure activities quickly
5. Is often "on the go" or often acts as if "driven by a motor"
6. Often talks excessively

Domain: Impulsivity

1. Often blurts out answers before questions have been completed
2. Often has difficulty awaiting turn
3. Often interrupts or intrudes on others

Diagnosis Requires:

1. Onset before age 7 years
2. Impairment from symptoms in two or more settings (eg, school, home, work)
3. Clinically significant impairment in social, academic, or occupational functioning
4. Symptoms do not occur exclusively in the course of other psychiatric, mental, or developmental disorder

Adapted with permission from American Psychiatric Association. Diagnostic Criteria from DSM-IV-TR. Washington, DC: American Psychiatric Association; 2000.

differences in presentation, gender differences in diagnosis, longitudinal course,[7,8] and impact of comorbid behavioral, emotional, and cognitive disorders accompanying ADHD.[9] What is not controversial is the need for careful, systematic diagnostic approaches to this very complex developmental disorder, and for continued refinement in our understanding of the disorder and its treatment.

PATHOGENESIS

A number of different causes of the brain dysfunctions that result in ADHD have been examined in the search for the etiology of this disorder. Among these are (1) differences in brain morphology and development, (2) differences in neurotransmitter activity, (3) differences in neuroelectrophysiology, (4) differences in genetics, and (5) interactions of genetic risk and environmental factors. Structural differences in the brains of children and adults with ADHD compared to normal control have included anterior and posterior regions of the corpus callosum, basal ganglia and related frontal-striatal structures, caudate nucleus, and prefrontal versus occipital volumes.[10,11] Whether smaller volumes in these anatomic sites for ADHD result in the symptoms assumes that smaller size equates to less functional capabilities. However, there appears to be some support for the importance of prefrontal-striatal systems in development of behavioral response inhibition. More recently, longitudinal imaging studies have also supported the role of delayed maturation of superior and dorsolateral prefrontal cortex and in the middle and superior temporal cortex in children diagnosed with ADHD.[12]

Studies have employed functional neuroimaging techniques in order to assess for differences in brain activity in selected structures of the brains of children and adults with ADHD. Studies of dorsolateral prefrontal cortex and ventrolateral prefrontal cortex, dorsal anterior cingulate cortex, and striatum predominate because these anatomic areas have been implicated in functions such as vigilance, selective and divided attention behavioral inhibition, and aspects of executive functioning including planning, response selection, and response initiation. Support for hypofunction in dorsal anterior and posterior cingulate cortex has been demonstrated in a number of recent FMRI studies.[13] Earlier PET and SPECT studies of ADHD subjects, although methodologically flawed due to lack of control groups, found increased regional cerebral blood flow in dorsolateral prefrontal cortex, caudate, and thalamus when methylphenidate was administered.[13]

Neuroelectrophysiological studies utilizing quantitative EEG (QEEG) and event-related potentials (ERPs), while problematic compared to MRI in terms of spatial resolution, have also been utilized to study brain functioning in ADHD subjects compared to controls. Results, however, have not yet enabled these two methodologies to explicitly address the specific anatomic substrates involved in the problems of inattention, impulsivity, and executive control functions in ADHD subjects. Genetic studies have focused upon the familial pedigree of individuals diagnosed with ADHD. Current views suggest that ADHD results from polygenetic rather than a single gene mode of inheritance with approximately 70% to 95% variance in symptoms. Concordance rates for identical twins are considerably higher compared to concordance rates in fraternal twins (70%-80% vs. 30%-40%). Specific dopamine receptor genes identified include *DRD2* and *DRD5*, the dopamine transport gene DAT1, and potentially defective alleles of the dopamine beta hydroxylase enzyme (DBH) that is important in the dopamine-to-norepinepherine conversion.[14] Recently, a large-scale assessment of 51 candidate genes in pathways related to dopamine, norepinepherine, and serotonin supported earlier reports of the role of DRD4 and DAT genes in the ADHD phenotype as well as 16 other potential genes, lending further support for the polygenetic model of ADHD.

A final group of studies have focused upon environmental factors, genetic profiles, and specific subtypes of ADHD. Previously, a number of acquired risk factors for the development of ADHD have been identified. These include pregnancy and birth complications, low birth weight, traumatic brain injury, prenatal substance exposure, and lead exposure. However, these factors likely carry less influence in the likelihood of developing ADHD, or at least are responsible for fewer cases, than genetic factors. Recently, Swanson and associates[15] presented a potential model that addresses gene–environment interactions that may affect fetal adaptations in development of dopamine neurons and contribute to development of different subtypes of ADHD. The authors critically review the research literature that provides support for the dopamine deficit theory underlying ADHD, and suggests future studies, in particular those needed to address the emergence of the ADHD phenotype over time.

CLINICAL PRESENTATION

The clinical presentation of ADHD varies by age. Children from age 3 years through the adolescent years and even adults can present with symptoms of overactivity, inattention, and impulsivity. Parents of children 7 years or younger may report the presence of overactivity, impulsivity leading to sometimes risky behavior, sleep disorders (eg, difficulty falling asleep, disruptive sleep, and early morning awakening), short attention spans, and inability to sustain focused attention. Some of these behavioral problems may have been noticed in the preschool years but emerged as clearly problematic upon entry to prekindergarten or kindergarten classes. Once in the school environment, teacher reports are also included in the presentation. Typical teacher reports focus on problems such as failure to follow classroom rules, frequent out-of-seat behavior, difficulty completing assigned work, interrupting others, easily distracted, distracting other students trying to do classroom activities, failure to turn in assignments, and less frequently, aggression towards other students or arguing with others.

During the primary grades, problems in academic functioning and achievement may lead to questions regarding a learning disability in reading, mathematics, or spelling/writing. While research has suggested that both boys and girls may exhibit some or all of these behavioral problems, a subset of children (more commonly girls than boys) present with parental and school complaints of failure to complete assigned school work, inattentive (sometimes "spacey") behaviors, slowness in initiating or completing assignments, and disorderly school papers and work habits.

In general, most research has reported that primary symptoms of hyperactivity may diminish during adolescence and into adult years. However, continuing problems in short attention span, difficulties with sustained attention and distractibility, inattention to detail, problems meeting deadlines, and excessive daydreaming have been reported. For some adolescents and adults, impulsivity remains a problem that can lead to poor decision making and risk-taking behaviors. Employment and/or educational/vocational underachievement may lead to depressive and anxiety complaints. Higher rates of alcohol and substance abuse, marital discord, and legal problems have been described in some longitudinal studies of childhood ADHD.[16,17]

DIAGNOSIS

History and Examination

In 2007, the American Academy of Child and Adolescent Psychiatry issued practice parameters for the assessment and treatment of children, adolescents, and adults with attention-deficit/hyperactivity disorder.[18] The report was an update of an earlier set of guidelines published in 1997 and complements the guideline issued by the American Academy of Pediatrics in 2000.[19] The following recommendations were made:

1. Screening for ADHD should be part of every patient's mental health assessment. Screening should specifically ask questions regarding presence of the major symptoms of ADHD (inattention, hyperactivity, and impulsivity) and whether these symptoms cause impairment. If the parent reports any symptoms or if the patient scores in the clinical range for ADHD symptoms, then a full evaluation is indicated.

2. Evaluation for ADHD should consist of clinical interview with patient and parent, obtaining information about the patient's school or day care functioning, review of patient's medical, social, and family history, and evaluation for comorbid psychiatric disorders.

3. Additional neuropsychological and neurological studies, including EEG, MRI, SPECT, or PET scanning, are not indicated for the diagnosis of ADHD in the presence of an unremarkable medical history.

4. Psychological and neuropsychological tests should be performed if the patient's history suggests low general cognitive ability or low achievement in language or mathematics relative to the patient's intellectual ability. Additional neuropsychological, speech and language assessments, and computerized testing of attention or inhibitory control may be indicated by the findings of standard psychological assessment.

5. The clinician must evaluate the patient with ADHD for the presence of comorbid psychiatric disorders. If the patient meets full DSM-IV criteria for a second disorder, then the clinician should develop a treatment plan to address each comorbid disorder in addition to ADHD.

6. A well thought-out and comprehensive treatment plan should be developed for the patient with ADHD.

7. The initial psychopharmacological treatment of ADHD should be a trial with an agent approved by the FDA for the treatment of ADHD (eg, dextroamphetamine, D- and DL-methyl-phenidate mixed salts amphetamine, and ato-moxetine).

8. If none of the above agents result in satisfactory treatment, the clinician should undertake a careful review of the diagnosis and then consider behavior therapy and/or the use of medications not approved by the FDA for treatment of ADHD.

9. During a psychopharmacological intervention for ADHD, the patient should be monitored for treatment-emergent side effects.

10. If a patient with ADHD has a robust response to psychopharmacological treatment and subsequently shows normative functioning in academic, family, and social functioning, then psychopharmacological treatment of ADHD alone is satisfactory.

11. If a patient with ADHD has a less than optimal response to medication, has a comorbid disorder, or experiences stressors in family life, then psychosocial treatment in conjunction with medication treatment is often beneficial.

12. Patients should be assessed periodically to determine whether there is continued need for treatment or if symptoms have remitted, treatment of ADHD should continue as long as symptoms remain present and cause impairment.

13. Patients treated with medication for ADHD should have their height and weight monitored throughout treatment.

Figure 9-1 presents a schematic of the diagnostic and intervention steps recommended by the AACAP.

Differential Diagnosis

As noted earlier, there are three subtypes of ADHD that have formal criteria for diagnoses in *DSM-IV-TR* (Attention-Deficit/Hyperactivity Disorder, Combined Type; Attention- Deficit/Hyperactivity Disorder, Predominantly Inattentive Type; and Attention-Deficit/hyperactivity Disorder, Predominantly Hyperactive–Impulsive Type). This listing of a total of 15 symptoms across the 3 domains of Inattention, Hyperactivity, and Impulsivity cannot occur exclusively during the course of a Pervasive Developmental Disorder, Schizophrenia, or other psychiatric disorders, and is not better accounted for by another mental disorder such as Mood Disorder, Anxiety Disorder, Dissociative Disorder, or Personality Disorder.

ADHD should also be distinguished from a number of medical disorders that can produce some of the symptoms, including sensory impairments (hearing and vision), brain injury, developmental language disorders, inborn errors of metabolism, renal insufficiency, endocrine deficiencies, lead toxicity, asthma, seizure disorders, progressive neurological disorders, and malnutrition.

Environmental factors that could lead to ADHD symptomatology include poor learning environment, curriculum not suited to the child, dysfunctional home environment, poor parenting, neglect or abuse, and parental psychopathology.

Comorbid psychiatric and developmental disorders that must also be identified and/or ruled out include specific learning disabilities, oppositional defiant disorder (ODD), conduct disorder (CD), developmental delay, anxiety disorder, obsessive-compulsive disorder (OCD), depressive disorders, and posttraumatic stress disorder. There is a fairly high incidence of four comorbid disorders in patients diagnosed with ADHD. These include Oppositional Defiant Disorder/Conduct Disorder (30%-50%), anxiety disorder (23%-30%), and depressive disorders (15%-38%). In addition, an estimated 20% to 25% of children with ADHD have a diagnosed learning disability as well. There is also an increased incidence of tic disorders among children diagnosed with ADHD (10%-15%). Table 9-2 presents the most frequent comorbid disorders among children and adolescents diagnosed with ADHD.

Diagnostic Tests

A recent review by Rapport and colleagues[20] supported the assertion that there is no one test that, used alone, can diagnose ADHD. However, a number of different behavioral interviews, checklists, and rating scales for the diagnosis have been developed to assist the clinician who is evaluating a patient for ADHD. These include diagnostic interviews such as the Diagnostic Interview

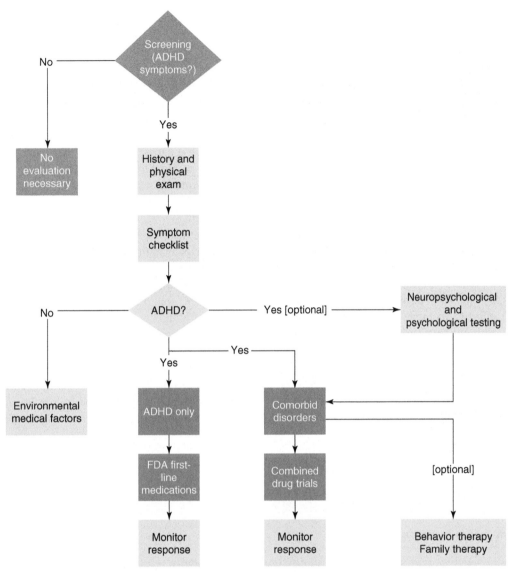

FIGURE 9-1 ■ Steps in assessment and treatment of ADHD in children, adolescents, and adults.

Schedule for Children–IV (DISC-IV) [21] and the Diagnostic Interview for Children and Adolescents–IV (DICA-IV), [22] which are based upon the DSM-IV diagnostic criteria. Behavioral checklists can be divided into

Table 9-2.

Common Comorbid Disorders in ADHD

- Oppositional Defiant Disorder (30%-50%)
- Conduct Disorder (30%-50%)
- Anxiety Disorders (23%-30%)
- Learning Disabilities (20%-25%)
- Depressive Disorders (15%-38%)
- Developmental Language Disorders (10%-15%)

two types: (1) broadband and (2) narrow band based upon the comprehensive sampling of problem behaviors. Broadband parent rating scales are often used in which parents rate a variety of problematic behaviors on Likert-type scales. Examples of these types of instruments include the Behavioral Assessment Rating System for Children–2 (BASC-2), [23] the Child Behavior Checklist (CBCL)–Parent Report Form, [24] and the Conners Rating Scales–3. [25] Narrow band rating scales and checklists include the Brown Attention-Deficit Disorder Scale (BADDS) [26] and the Swanson, Nolan, and Pelham Rating Scale (SNAP-IV). [27] Teacher rating scales are often available in parallel to both broadband and narrow band rating scales to allow for determination of problematic behaviors in school settings. These enable the clinician to evaluate for the requirement of symptoms in two or more settings. There are other psychological instruments available that assess for mood disorders, such as the Child Depression Inventory (CDI)[28] or the Revised Children's Manifest Anxiety Scale (RCMAS).[29] Finally, the clinician may obtain report cards from school and results from standardized achievement tests that allow for determination of problems in academic classroom performance and achievement, consistent with potential comorbid learning disabilities.

TREATMENT

Pharmacological treatment for the core symptoms of ADHD is typically the first-line intervention approach to this behavioral disorder.[18] As recommended by the American Academy of Child and Adolescent Psychiatry (AACAP), the patient's treatment plan, once developed, may consist of pharmacological and behavior therapy. If a drug therapy approach is taken, the physician must review both effective therapies and the family's preferences for treatment approaches. Medications to be employed can be broadly categorized into "first-line," "second-line," and other types according to their FDA approval guidelines and those of the AACAP. Second-line and other medications, such as antipsychotics, have been used by some physicians to treat comorbid disorders or severe behavioral problems arising in the course of treatment for ADHD.

Table 9-3 presents a listing of medications that have been utilized in treating ADHD. The physician should follow guidelines regarding any required tests prior to initiating drug therapy (eg, EKG). Once drug therapy is initiated, the physician should monitor response to the type and dosage of the medication as well as any apparent side effects. For many practitioners, this requires more frequent visits during the initiation of drug treatment. Once the efficacy of the drug therapy is established for the patient, less frequent follow-up visits are needed.

Despite the prevalence of pharmacological interventions, many of the social, family, and academic problems experienced by the patient may not be alleviated without additional interventions. A variety of therapies are available that address the problems attendant to a history of ADHD symptomatology. These include individual behavior therapy, social skills training, family therapies, and combinations of these treatments. The recent guidelines of the AACAP, however, suggest that research on these additional interventions suggests their results show only a relatively minor impact on the course of treatment. Equally important is the need for

Table 9-3.

Medications Used in Treatment of ADHD

First-Line Medications (Stimulants)			
	Short-Acting	Intermediate-Acting	Long-Acting
Methylphenidate (MPH)	Ritalin Methylin	Ritalin–SR Metadate–ER Methylin–ER	Ritalin–LA Metadate–CD Concerta Daytrana
Dextroamphetamine	Dexedrine Dextrostat	Dexedrine–ER spansule	
Dexmethylphenidate	Focalin	Focalin XR	Focalin XR
Amphetamine salts		Adderall XR	Adderall XR
Lisdexamfetamine			Vyvanase
Second-Line Medications			
Bupropion Clonidine (Catapres) Guanfacine (Tenex) Imipramine (Tofranil) Desipramine (Norpramine)	Wellbutrin	Wellbutrin SR	Wellbutrin XR
Other Medications			
Nonstimulants	Straterra		
Atypical antipsychotics	Risperdal, Seroquel, Abilify, Clozaril, Zyprexa, Geodon		
Antidepressants	Prozac, Paxil, Zoloft, Celexa, Luvox, Serzone, Lexa-pro, Effexor, Remeron		

psychoeducational interventions. For the child or adolescent with a diagnosed learning disability, an individualized educational plan (IEP) utilizing exceptional student education (ESE) resources is required by federal ADA legislation. For the child with academic deficiencies who does not meet criteria for the diagnosis of a learning disability, an IEP should still be developed under the 504 plan that may include modifications in classroom seating, weekly reports to parents, and academic support for identified areas of academic deficiencies. Most recently, school districts must also operationalize the specifics of any remediation plan and formally assess the child's response to the intervention (RTI).

A final concern to parents is the length of treatment. While clearly ADHD has been described as a chronic disorder with differing expression of symptoms (phenotype) with increasing age, the AACAP notes that the lack of large-scale longitudinal research in this disorder makes decisions regarding treatment "holidays" and duration difficult. For these, collaboration between physician and patient is critical to effective management of the child's care through his or her development. In particular, comorbid problems may emerge during adolescence, after high school matriculation, and extend into adult life.[9,30]

REFERENCES

1. Baron IS. Attention-deficit/hyperactivity disorder: new challenges for definition, diagnosis and treatment. *Neuropsychol Rev*. 2007;17:1-3.

2. Bloom B, Cohen RA. Summary health statistics for U.S. children: National Health Interview Survey, 2006. National Center for Health Statistics. *Vital Health Stat*. 2007;10:234.

3. Rowland AS, Lesesne CA, Abramowitz AJ. The epidemiology of attention-deficit/hyperactivity disorder (ADHD): a public heath view. *Ment Retard Dev Disabil Res Rev*. 2002;8:162-170.

4. Shelton T. Attention deficit/hyperactivity disorder. In: Roberts MC, ed. *Handbook of Pediatric Psychology*. New York: Guilford Press; 2003:617-635.

5. American Psychiatric Association. *Diagnostic Criteria from DSM-IV-TR*. Washington, DC: American Psychiatric Association; 2000.

6. Stefanatos GA, Baron IS. Attention deficit/hyperactivity disorder: a neuropsychological perspective towards DSM-V. *Neuropsychol Rev*. 2007;17:5-38.

7. Lahey BB, Pelham WE, Loney J, Lee SS, Willcutt E. Instability of the DSM-IV subtypes of ADHD from preschool through elementary school. *Arch Gen Psychiatry*. 2005; 62:896-902.

8. Wilens TE, Biederman J, Brown S, Monteaux M, Prince J, Spencer TJ. Patterns of psychopathology and dysfunction in clinically referred preschoolers. *J Dev Behav Pediatr*. 2002;23:531-536.

9. Spencer TJ, Biederman J, Mick E. Attention deficit/hyperactivity disorder: diagnosis, lifespan, comorbidities and neurobiology. *J Pediatr Psychol*. 2007;32:631-642.

10. Castellanos FX, Glaser PEA, Gerhardt GA. Towards a neuroscience of attention-deficit/hyperactivity disorder: fractionating the phenotype. *J Neurosi Methods*. 2006;151:1-4.

11. Seidman LJ, Valera EM, Makris N. Structural brain imaging of attention-deficit/hyperactivity disorder. *Biol Psychiatry*. 2005;57:1263-1272.

12. Shaw PE, Eckstrand K, Sharp W, et al. Attention-deficit/hyperactivity disorder is characterized by a delay in cortical maturation. *Proc Natl Acad Sci USA*. 2007;104:19649-19654.

13. Bush G, Valera EM, Seidman LJ. Functional neuroimaging of attention-deficit/hyperactivity disorder: a review and suggested future directions. *Biol Psychiatry*. 2005;57:1273-1284.

14. Faraone SV. Report from the third international meeting of the attention-deficit/hyperactivity disorder molecular genetics network. *Am J Med Genet*. 2002;114:272-276.

15. Swanson JM, Kinsbourne M, Nigg J, et al. Etiologic subtypes of attention-deficit/hyperactivity disorder: brain imaging, molecular genetics and environmental factors and the dopamine hypothesis. *Neuropsychol Rev*. 2007;17:39-60.

16. Lahey BB, Hartung CM, Loney J, Pelham WE, Chronis AM, Lee SS. Are there sex differences in the predictive validity of DSM-IV ADHD among younger children? *J Clin Child Adolesc Psychol*. 2007;36:113-126.

17. Biederman J, Monuteaux MC, Spencer T, et al. Young adult outcomes of attention deficit hyperactivity disorder: a controlled 10 year follow-up study. *Psychol Med*. 2006;36:167-179.

18. Pliska S. AACAP Work Group on Quality Issues. Practice parameters for the assessment and treatment of children and adolescents with attention deficit/hyperactivity disorder. *J Am Acad Child Adolesc Psychiatry*. 2007;46:894-921.

19. American Academy of Pediatrics. Clinical practice guideline: diagnosis and evaluation of the child with attention-deficit/hyperactivity disorder. *Pediatrics*. 2000;105:1158-1170.

20. Rapport MD, Timko TM Jr, Wolfe R. Attention-deficit/hyperactivity disorder. In: Hersen M, ed. *Clinician's Handbook of Child Behavioral Assessment*. Burlington, MA: Elsevier Academic Press; 2006:401-435.

21. Shaffer D, Fisher P, Lucas CP, Dulcan MK, Schwab-Stone ME. NIMH Diagnostic Interview Schedule for Children version IV (DISC-IV). *J Am Acad Child Adolesc Psychiatry*. 2000; 39:28-38.

22. Reich W, Weiner Z, Herjanic B. Diagnostic Interview for Children and Adolescents (DICA-IV) North Tonawanda, NY: Multi-Health Symptoms; 2000.

23. Reynolds CR, Kamphaus. *Behavioral Assessment System for Children*. 2nd ed. Bloomington, MN: Pearson Assessments; 2004.

24. Achenbach TM, Rescorea LA. *Child Behavior Checklist 6/18*. Lutz, FL: Psychological Assessment Resources; 2005.

25. Conners CK. *Conners Rating Scales–3*. Lutz, FL: Psychological Assessment Resources; 2008.

26. Brown TE. *Brown Attention Deficit Disorder Scales*. Lutz, FL: Psychological Assessment Resources; 2001.

27. Swanson JM. *The SNAP-IV Teacher and Parent Rating Form*. Irvine: University of California-Irvine; 1994.

28. Kovacs M. *Child Depression Inventory*. Lutz, FL: Psychological Assessment Resources; 1981.

29. Reynolds CR, Richmond BG. *Revised Children's Manifest Anxiety Scale*. 2nd ed. Lutz, FL: Psychological Assessment Resources; 2008.

30. Biederman J. Attention-deficit/hyperactivity disorder: a selective overview. *Biol Psychiatry*. 2005;57:1215-1220.

CHAPTER 10

Learning and Language Disorders

Anne-Marie Slinger-Constant and Maria Wojtalewicz

DEFINITIONS AND EPIDEMIOLOGY

Learning and language disorders are a heterogeneous group of neurobiological disorders involving impairments in the acquisition and/or use of spoken (oral) language, written language (reading/spelling/writing), and mathematical skills.[1-3] "Learning disability" (LD) is a broad term that encompasses language and learning disorders.

The definitions and diagnostic criteria outlined in the *Diagnostic and Statistical Manual of Mental Disorders, 4th Edition, Text Revision (DSM-IV-TR)*[1] provide a guide for the diagnosis of LDs in clinical settings. *DSM-IV-TR* uses a categorical approach to the classification of LDs and other disorders. Reading disorder (RD), disorders of written expression, mathematics disorder (MD), and learning disorder not otherwise specified fall into the learning disorders category (Table 10-1). As defined in *DSM-IV-TR*, learning disorders are "diagnosed when the individual's achievement on individually administered, standardized tests in reading, mathematics, or written expression is substantially below that expected for age, schooling, and level of intelligence."[1] The terms (developmental) dyslexia and (developmental) dyscalculia may be used synonymously with RD and MD, respectively.

Expressive and/or receptive language disorders are classified as communication disorders in *DSM-IV-TR* (Table 10-2). The defining features of these spoken language disorders are impairments in oral expression and/or listening comprehension associated with dysfunction in one or more subdomains of language, including morphology (word structure), semantics (word meaning), and syntax (sentence structure). By definition, these deficits significantly interfere with academic achievement and/or social communication.[1] As with learning disorders, *DSM-IV-TR* outlines specific inclusionary and exclusionary diagnostic criteria for language disorders, which are further defined as "developmental" or "acquired." Specific language impairment (SLI) and developmental dysphasia are terms that refer to developmental language disorders that are characterized by a delay in, or lack of, normal language acquisition at an appropriate age in the absence of pervasive cognitive impairments, sensorimotor abnormalities, and frank neurological deficits.[4,5] In contrast to developmental language disorders, acquired language disorders are, by definition, the "result of a neurological or other general medical condition (eg, encephalitis, head trauma, irradiation)."[1]

Table 10-1.

DSM-IV-TR Classification of Learning and Language Disorders

	Diagnostic Code[*]
Learning Disorders	
Reading disorder	315.00
Mathematics disorder	315.1
Disorder of written language	315.2
Learning disorder not otherwise specified	315.9
Communication Disorders[‡]	
Expressive language disorder	315.31
Mixed receptive-expressive language disorder	315.32

[*] *This is the numerical* International Classification of Diseases, 9th ed., *Clinical Modification (ICD-9-CM) code that appears with the disorder in DSM-IV-TR.*
[‡] *This category also includes phonological disorder (an articulation disorder involving disturbance of speech sound production), stuttering (a speech dysfluency disorder involving disruption of normal speech fluency and time patterning), and communication disorders not otherwise specified (a category that includes voice disorders).*[1]

While the clinical diagnosis of LDs is guided by *DSM-IV-TR*, identification and classification of LDs in public school systems, and thereby access to early intervention, exceptional student education (ESE), and related services, is governed by the federal definition of LD, as outlined in the Individuals with Disabilities Education Improvement Act of 2004 (commonly referred to as IDEA 2004). Clinicians should also be aware that consensus about the definition (both conceptual and operational) LD is lacking.[6] Furthermore, it is important to be familiar with differences in the use of terminology across disciplines and the potential implications thereof. For example, while the term "dyslexia" is often used synonymously with RD by clinicians, school districts generally do not recognize that term as referring to a "specific learning disability" in reading, as it is termed in educational settings. Thus, a child may be deemed ineligible for necessary educational supports and services if the clinical terminology used by physicians, neuropsychologists, and clinical psychologists is inadequately translated into terms that are more familiar to educators and other professionals who participate in educational planning teams in school settings. Two widely used definitions are included in Table 10-2.

Learning disabilities are common, and without effective intervention, children with these disorders are at high risk of school failure with far-reaching consequences on their economic and, thus, health outcomes. Data from the 2003 National Survey of Children's Health indicates that learning disabilities are the most common parent-reported diagnosis in children aged 6 to 17 years (11.5%).[7] A more recent U.S. Department of Education report indicates that approximately 5.6% of children aged 2 through 21 years served by federally supported programs (ie, 2.5 million prekindergarten through 12th grade students enrolled in public school) have a specific learning disability, and another 1.5 million (3.0%) are identified as speech or language impaired.[8] Moreover, data from the National Assessment of Education Progress (NAEP) suggest that a far greater percentage of students struggle to meet proficiency levels in reading, writing, and mathematics. According to 2007 NAEP results, only 31% of U.S. fourth graders, and 29% of eighth graders, read at or above proficiency levels, while 70% of eighth graders are below proficiency in writing.[9,10] Mathematics proficiency levels were similar, with only 38% of fourth graders and 31% of eighth graders at or above proficiency levels.[11]

Reading disorder (dyslexia) affects 80% of individuals with learning disabilities, comprising the most common type of LD.[6,12] Prevalence rates for reading disorder range from 5% to 17.5%,[13] depending on what definitions are applied and the method of ascertainment. In contrast, disorders of written expression are rare in the absence of comorbid learning and/or attention problems, thus, prevalence estimates are difficult to determine.[1] Population-based estimates of the prevalence of mathematics disorder (developmental dyscalculia) in school-age children are in the range of 3% to 6%.[14] Reported prevalence rates for language disorders vary with age.[1] As noted in the *DSM-IV-TR*, expressive language delays occur in 10% to 15% of children under the age of 3 years with a subsequent drop in prevalence estimates to between 3% and 7% by school age. Prevalence estimates for mixed receptive/expressive language disorder of approximately 5% in preschoolers and 3% in school-age children are reported.[1]

Table 10-2.

Definitions of Learning Disability

Federal Statutory Definition
The Individuals with Disabilities Education Improvement Act of 2004 (Public Law 108-446) defines a "specific learning disability" as "a disorder in 1 or more of the basic psychological processes involved in understanding or in using language, spoken or written, that may manifest itself in the imperfect ability to listen, think, speak, read, write, spell, or to do mathematical calculations," including "such conditions as perceptual disabilities, brain injury, minimal brain dysfunction, dyslexia, and developmental aphasia" and excluding "a learning problem that is primarily the result of visual, hearing, or motor disabilities, of mental retardation, of emotional disturbance, or of environmental, cultural, or economic disadvantage."[3]

National Joint Committee on Learning Disabilities (NJCD) Definition
Learning disabilities "is a general term that refers to a heterogeneous group of disorders manifested by significant difficulties in the acquisition and use of listening, speaking, reading, writing, reasoning, or mathematical skills. These disorders are intrinsic to the individual, presumed to be due to central nervous system dysfunction, and may occur across the life span. Problems in self-regulatory behaviors, social perception, and social interaction may exist with learning disabilities but do not, by themselves, constitute a learning disability. Although learning disabilities may occur concomitantly with other disabilities (eg, sensory impairment, mental retardation, serious emotional disturbance), or with extrinsic influences (such as cultural differences, insufficient or inappropriate instruction), they are not the result of those conditions or influences."[2]

PATHOGENESIS

Learning disabilities have complex etiologies involving multiple genetic and environmental influences.[15-17] Reading disorder (dyslexia), the most common type of LD, has been studied most extensively. Among investigators there is broad consensus that the underlying cognitive basis is a phonological deficit associated with poor awareness of the sound-structure of spoken language and limited appreciation of the relationship between phonemes (the discrete, elemental sound units of spoken language—for example, the words "you" and "see" each consist of two phonemes) and graphemes (letters, eg, the words "you" and "see" each consist of three graphemes), resulting in impaired word reading (decoding) and spelling (encoding) abilities.[12,16] Research has revealed a significant genetic influence on both word reading and spelling abilities.[18,19] While the mode(s) of transmission of this genetically and phenotypically heterogeneous disorder remains unclear, there is strong evidence that reading disorder (dyslexia) is both highly familial and heritable.[20-23] Family studies indicate that first-degree relatives are four to ten times as likely as controls to be affected.[24] Heritability estimates from twin studies indicate that between 44% and 65%, and 62% and 75%, of the variance in reading and spelling abilities, respectively, is explained by genetic factors.[18,19,24,25] Susceptibility loci have been identified on several chromosomal regions including 2p, 3p, 6p, 15q, and 18p.[24,26] Cytoarchitectonic studies of dyslexic brains have found cortical anomalies in areas important for language, and more recently molecular genetic studies have linked (four) genes involved in neuronal migration and cortical development to dyslexia.[27-30] Imaging studies comparing the brains of individuals with dyslexia to those of controls have found a number of structural differences, including normal or increased planum temporale asymmetry.[31-33] Functional neuroimaging studies examining brain activation patterns during phonological and reading tasks provide additional insight into the neural basis of dyslexia, with converging evidence implicating aberrant functional connectivity in the left hemispheric regions subserving language functions, including the inferior frontal gyrus, middle and superior temporal gyrus, and the angular gyrus.[22,34-37]

Written expression disorders usually occur in association with other disorders, notably reading disorder, and there is little evidence to support a specific learning disability in written expression when not associated with other learning disabilities.[38] Thus, difficulty with written expression warrants assessment for underlying deficits including language and executive dysfunction.

Unlike RD, mathematics disorder (developmental dyscalculia) has not been studied extensively, and so the underlying cognitive deficits and neurobiological factors that may play a role in mathematical difficulties are less well understood. Current evidence implicates deficits in the mental representation of numerical quantities ("number sense")[39-41] or impaired links between numerical magnitude representations and learned numerical symbols[42] as the neuropsychological basis of mathematics disorder. Neuroimaging studies indicate that intraparietal brain regions play a key role in numerical cognition,[43] and functional abnormalities in this area appear to underlie impairment in numerical processing.[44] As with RD, twin and family studies provide strong evidence of a genetic component to mathematical disorder. The prevalence rate in twins is approximately ten times that of the general population (58% of monozygotic and 39% of dizygotic twins of a child with MD meet the criteria).[45,46] Furthermore, among first-degree relatives of individuals with mathematical disorder, more than half have mathematical difficulties.[47] There appear to be different subgroups of children with mathematical difficulties, including those with isolated MD and those with MD in association with other LDs or comorbid conditions.[48,49] The latter constitutes two-thirds of children with MD.[50] Numeracy deficits are common among children with ADHD, epilepsy, and genetic disorders, including Turner, fragile X, Down, Williams, and velocardiofacial syndromes.[51,52] Whether the mathematical difficulties experienced by these subgroups are related to general cognitive deficits or a specific deficit in numerical cognition is uncertain.[49]

Language disorders comprise a wide range of phenotypes with diverse etiologies. In the case of developmental language disorders, as with other types of LDs, evidence implicates a complex interplay of environmental, neurobiological, and genetic influences.[53-56] In addition to decreased cerebral volumes, neuroimaging findings in developmental dysphasia have most consistently involved a loss of normal left-right asymmetry in perisylvian and planum temporale regions (which are known to subserve language).[32,57] Known causes of language impairments include hearing loss, global cognitive impairment, specific genetic and chromosomal disorders (Down, fragile X, and Klinefelter syndromes), neurobehavioral disorders (autism), and neurological disorders (Landau-Kleffner syndrome).[58,59] A period of typical development before the occurrence of language impairments suggests an acquired etiology and the need for prompt medical investigation.

CLINICAL PRESENTATION

The clinical presentation of learning disabilities is diverse and reflects the underlying deficits, the severity of the disorder, and the age of the child.[1] Children with developmental language disorders typically present prior to school entrance with a delay in emergence of spoken language, while learning disorders are often not recognized until after a child enters school and is identified as lagging behind peers in the acquisition of foundational academic skills. Signs and symptoms that can serve to alert the clinician to a language or learning problem are listed in Table 10-3.

Expressive and/or receptive language disorders are characterized by deficits in vocabulary (lexical development), acquisition and use of appropriate word conjugations and derivations, knowledge and understanding of word meanings, and/or aberrations in sentence structure.[60] Caregivers may characterize children with expressive language impairments as "quiet" due to sparse speech output, trouble putting thoughts into words, and short, simplified, agrammatical utterances.[1] Children with receptive language impairments often have trouble following directions and may respond tangentially or inappropriately to questions.[1] As a result of their limited understanding of oral instructions and narratives, they may be described as confused and/or be perceived as inattentive.

Prior to school entrance, when compared to peers, children at risk for reading problems exhibit relative deficits in syntax (grammar) and difficulty pronouncing words correctly; but by school entrance, deficits in phonological awareness are predominant.[61] School-aged children with RD exhibit difficulty decoding ("sounding out") unfamiliar words, trouble recognizing sight words, and difficulty spelling (encoding) new or unfamiliar words. Their oral reading is dysfluent or "choppy," and they often have trouble understanding what they have read. Thus, notwithstanding a comorbid attention or core language problem, children with RD usually find it easier to understand a passage that is read aloud to them (ie, their listening comprehension is better than their reading comprehension).

Clinical features of mathematical disorder are included in Table 10-3. Early manifestations include difficulty grasping basic numerical concepts and trouble learning to count.[62] As they progress through school, children with MD have trouble learning and recalling basic mathematical facts as well as difficulty performing arithmetic computations and learning mathematical procedures, and struggle to solve complex mathematical problems.[63]

It is important to note that rather than language or learning difficulties, behavioral disturbance and/or social/emotional problems may be the presenting concern for a child with LD, and some children with LD may be simply be (mis)labeled "lazy" or "unmotivated."

History and Physical

A primary focus of the history and physical examination is identification of medical, psychiatric, or psychosocial problems that may underlie or be contributing to the child's language or learning difficulties.[64] Table 10-4 outlines important elements of the history and physical examination.

Table 10-3.

Signs and Symptoms of Learning Disability[64–67]

Preschool-Aged Child	School-Aged Child
Delayed emergence of spoken language	Trouble learning letter sounds[a]
Poor vocabulary growth	Difficulty "sounding out" words
Poor comprehension of words and sentences	Difficulty segmenting words into syllables
Difficulty understanding and following directions	Problems spelling unfamiliar words
Trouble rhyming words and learning nursery rhymes	Difficulty acquiring arithmetical facts
Trouble learning to recognize the letters of the alphabet [a]	Trouble understanding the complementarity of addition and subtraction
Difficulty learning color and object names	Difficulty learning names and/or slow recall of names
Trouble learning to recite the alphabet	Difficulty finding words (slow word retrieval)
Difficulty learning to count	Slow, dysfluent reading (reading is laborious)[b]
Struggle to grasp basic numerical concepts	Reluctance to reading aloud (resists reading)
Difficulty learning to pronounce words correctly	Trouble applying mathematical concepts
Confusing similar-sounding words	Poor listening and/or reading comprehension[c]
Sentence structure lacks age-typical complexity	Difficulty with written composition (organization and flow, idea development, sentence structure)

[a,b] Evidence indicates that letter-name knowledge in preschool and early kindergarten and letter-sound knowledge in later kindergarten are strong predictors of later reading abilities.[68-72] Along with text reading fluency, difficulty quickly and accurately sounding out unfamiliar/nonsense words (ie, weak phonemic decoding efficiency) is the strongest indicator of dyslexia when children start to read (typically by the end of first grade).[69]
[c] Children with RD typically exhibit better listening than reading comprehension, while children with receptive language impairments often have difficulty understanding both written and spoken language (a finding that is not surprising given that spoken language lays the foundation for written language[73]).

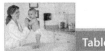

| Table 10-4. | | |

History and Physical Examination[82,87,88]

Important Elements of the History

Medical history	Exposure to teratogens (including alcohol) Low birth weight Prematurity Risk factors for hearing loss and neurocognitive impairments Symptoms of an underlying neurological disorder, other medical conditions, psychiatric disturbance
Developmental history	Delays in speech, language, personal/social, cognitive, and/or motor development Loss of previously acquired skills; any other signs or symptoms of psychomotor regression
Family history	Parents and/or siblings with LD Relatives with genetic, psychiatric, neurological, or medical conditions associated with LD
Psychosocial history	Limited or poor linguistic and/or early literacy experiences Psychosocial deprivation, neglect/abuse, family dysfunction, emotional disturbance, bullying Substance abuse (parent, child)
Scholastic/ academic history	Limited learning opportunities Inadequate academic instruction Lack of response to evidence-based interventions

Important Elements of the Physical Examination

General examination	Vision and hearing Head circumference (microcephaly, macrocephaly) Dysmorphic features (genetic disorders) Macroorchidism (fragile X syndrome) Stigmata of phakomatoses Hepatosplenomegaly (metabolic disorders)
Neurological	Atypical behaviors Abnormal speech (prosody, articulation) Abnormal neurological findings

Thorough medical and family histories are key components of the clinical evaluation of a child with language impairments or learning problems. Risk factors for language delays and learning difficulties include complications during the prenatal and perinatal periods (in-utero infections, exposure to teratogens, prematurity, hyperbilirubinemia), infections of the central nervous system, traumatic brain injury, epilepsy, psychiatric disorder, and chronic or debilitating health conditions. A positive family history of speech and/or language delay, difficulty learning to read or spell, grade retention, behavior problems or trouble in school, and/or school failure (or "drop out") is also a risk factor.

A detailed review of the development history is important in identifying aberrations in fine-motor, gross-motor, language, personal-social, cognitive, and adaptive skill acquisition. Language delay is often the presenting feature of a pervasive developmental disorder or general cognitive impairment, and delay in more than one domain is indicative of global neurocognitive dysfunction. A history suggesting loss of previously acquired skills or functions or other evidence of psychomotor regression should shift the focus of the examination to a medical investigation targeted at pinpointing the underlying cause.

The review of systems should include a thorough sleep history. Sleep problems affect one in three school-aged children and can adversely impact attention, memory, and learning.[74] A history of snoring, snorting or gasping during sleep, and daytime sleepiness (symptoms that have been found to predict poor academic performance[75]) should prompt consideration of polysomnographic evaluation.

A detailed psychosocial history is necessary to identify socioemotional problems, environmental factors (economic disadvantage, impoverished linguistic environment, chaotic family life), and other psychosocial and emotional disturbances that can impact language acquisition, learning, and exposure to appropriate academic instruction. Compared to unaffected peers, children with LD more commonly exhibit poor self-concept, social adjustment problems, frustration, loneliness, withdrawal behavior, anxiety, mood, and emotional problems.[76-81] Thus, it is important to assess the child's relationships with peers and teachers, emotional state, adaptive functioning, family situation, and the extent of peer, community, and family support. Information about the child's self-concept and experiences as a learner, as well as his or her interests and parental attitudes, should also be sought.

Physical examination findings in children with isolated, primary LDs are usually minimal;[82] however, subtle ("soft") neurological signs (eg, obligatory synkinesis) may be present.[57, 83-86] Hearing and vision screening is essential, particularly if records indicate a lack of prior vision and audiometric testing. If the child fails screening tests or results are equivocal, referral for full ophthalmologic and/or audiologic evaluation is indicated. A detailed physical examination targeted at identifying dysmorphic features, neurological deficits, and other abnormal findings indicative of an underlying congenital or acquired disorder should be completed.

DIFFERENTIAL DIAGNOSIS AND COMMON COMORBID CONDITIONS

Communication difficulties, academic underachievement, and school performance problems may arise from a range of conditions, examples of which are included in Table 10-5. The differential diagnosis of LD includes

Table 10-5.

Differential Diagnosis¹

Prolonged or repeated school absences
Psychosocial deprivation/neglect
Vision/hearing impairment
Attention-deficit hyperactivity disorder
Sleep disorder
Mood and/or anxiety disorder
Tourette syndrome
Epilepsy
Other neurological and neurodevelopmental disorders
Mental retardation
Genetic disorders (eg, Down, fragile X, Williams, and Turner syndromes)
Teratogentic exposure (eg, fetal alcohol syndrome or fetal alcohol effects)
Other medical conditions (eg, lead poisoning, anemia, thyroid disease, metabolic disorders)

vision and hearing impairments; genetic, neurological, and psychiatric disorders; psychosocial deprivation or neglect; sociocultural disadvantage; excessive school absenteeism; and inadequate academic instruction.¹

Attention-deficit hyperactivity disorder (ADHD) may result in academic underachievement independent of a learning disability; however, the coexistence of ADHD and LD is common and diagnosis of either disorder warrants assessment for the other. Of children with ADHD, an estimated 25% to 40% have a comorbid language or learning disorder,[89] and approximately 20% to 50% of children with a reading disorder have co-occurring ADHD.[90,91] High rates of ADHD and other behavioral disorders are also found in children with language impairments.[92] Overall, some 50% of children with language and learning disorders have a co-occurring psychiatric disorder,[93] and receptive language impairment appears to place a child at particularly high risk.[94]

Mood and anxiety disorders are associated with an increased risk of low academic achievement.[95,96] Distinguishing a primary emotional or behavioral disorder from emotional problems generated by LD-related difficulties—including frustration, performance anxiety, poor self-efficacy, and low self-esteem as a result of recurrent or chronic failure—requires a careful history to determine the chronology of symptom onset and identify risk factors, such as a positive family history of anxiety or depression.

Numerous neurological disorders are associated with language and learning difficulties. For example, the rate of comorbid LD is high in children with Tourette syndrome (1 in 3 have LD and 50% to 60% have co-occurring ADHD).[97] Children with epilepsy are also known to be vulnerable to attention, learning, memory,

and behavior problems.[59,98-100] Approximately half meet criteria for LD,[101,102] and learning impairments may occur even when seizures are well controlled.[103] Children with neurocutaneous disorders (eg, 20%-61% of children with neurofibromatosis-1 have LD[97,104]), neuromuscular disorders (eg, Duchenne and Becker muscular dystrophies[105-108]), and central nervous system lesions may also exhibit impairments in language and learning.

Marked impairment in communication is a characteristic feature of disorders within the autism spectrum. While children with LDs exhibit higher levels of withdrawn behavior and poorer social competence than peers without LDs,[6,109-111] they lack the pronounced deficits in pragmatic language (language *use*), abnormal prosody of speech, atypical eye gaze, poor or absent joint attention, profound limitations in perspective taking, marked impairments in social reciprocity, and stereotypical behaviors that define autism spectrum disorders. Children who are deaf and hard of hearing may also exhibit marked impairments in language and literacy development, particularly in cases where identification and appropriate interventions occur after 6 months of age.[112]

Mild mental retardation (MR) may not be identified until school entry when the child's generalized cognitive impairments and learning problems become apparent. Unlike LD, mild MR is associated with globally depressed critical thinking, problem-solving, reasoning abilities, and deficits in adaptive functioning.[1] Moderate to profound MR is associated with marked global developmental delays and is usually identified prior to school entrance.

General medical conditions impacting a child's general health and well-being, school attendance, and cognitive functioning should also be considered. The prevalence of sleep-disordered breathing is remarkably higher among low-performing students. While it affects 1% to 2% of children as a whole,[113] in a prospective study of low-performing elementary school students who were screened for obstructive sleep apnea (OSA), 18% were found to have sleep-associated gas exchange abnormalities.[114] As one might predict, the severity of neurocognitive (attention, memory, learning, and language) deficits associated with OSA appears to be inversely related to the frequency of apneic/hypopneic events.[115-117] Importantly, therapeutic intervention can result in significant improvements in school grades.[114] Physical examination findings such as obesity, tonsillar hypertrophy, and other risk factors for OSA, warrant further investigation including polysomnography.

Environmental factors, such as the amount and type of parental input, and psychosocial disadvantage and neglect, may either underlie or contribute to deficits in language development and academic achievement.

Lastly, it should be noted that one type of LD commonly coexists with another; thus, as is the case with ADHD, identification of one should prompt evaluation for another (Table 10-5).[6,16,118]

DIAGNOSIS

Definitive diagnosis of a learning or communication disorder requires a multidisciplinary approach. A comprehensive history and physical examination by the physician is the first step in the diagnostic process, as outlined in Table 10-6 and Figure 10-1. Subsequent steps include evaluation of oral language, cognitive function, academic achievement, socioemotional function, and adaptive skills using standardized, norm-referenced measures. Such assessment requires the involvement of a qualified speech/language pathologist, school psychologist, clinical psychologist, or neuropsychologist, as indicated by the presenting concern and findings of the clinical examination. Referrals to other clinicians and specialists may also be warranted. For example, if dysgraphia (or handwriting) is a concern, the child may be referred to a pediatric occupational therapist for evaluation of graphomotor and related skills.

The clinical evaluation process is typically informed by the diagnostic criteria delineated in *DSM-IV-TR*. Thus the psychological evaluation involves determination of whether the child's performance on individually administered, standardized tests of academic achievement is substantially below that anticipated for chronological age, measured intellectual abilities, and exposure to

Table 10-6.

Diagnostic Steps for Evaluation of Suspected Language or Learning Disorder

Steps in the Diagnostic Process	Tests/Procedures
Step 1: Detailed history and physical examination	▪ Parent and child interviews ▪ Teacher interviews (when applicable) ▪ Review of medical records, including the developmental surveillance data from pediatric records if available ▪ Review of scholastic records ▪ General physical and extended neurological/neurodevelopmental examinations
Step 2: Consider specific diagnostic studies as in dicated by the medical history and physical examination findings	▪ MRI ▪ EEG ▪ Polysomnogram ▪ Cytogenetic and metabolic studies
Step 3: Detect vision or hearing impairments	▪ Vision and hearing screens ▪ Formal vision/audiologic evaluation
Step 4: Identify attention deficits & psychiatric disorders	▪ Parent and teacher (norm-referenced) behavior rating scales and interviews ▪ Child interview ▪ Neuropsychological testing to assess attention and executive function

Step 5: Identify language impairment	▪ Systematic evaluation of language subsystems and global language function
	  ▪ Phonology
	  ▪ Morphosyntax
	  ▪ Semantics
	  ▪ Pragmatics
	  ▪ Receptive and expressive language

Step 6: Assess cognitive function	▪ Standardized assessment of
	  ▪ Thinking and reasoning ability (verbal and nonverbal)
	  ▪ Memory (including visual and verbal; short-term, long-term, and working memory)
	  ▪ Cognitive efficiency/processing speed

Step 7: Identify learning disorder	▪ Review of scholastic records
	▪ Standardized assessment of academic skills and proficiency including
	  ▪ Written language
	    ▪ Reading (phonemic decoding, sight-word recognition, fluency, passage comprehension)
	    ▪ Spelling (encoding of real and nonsense words)
	    ▪ Written expression (sentence/paragraph construction)
	  ▪ Mathematical skills
	    ▪ Calculation, conceptual understanding, reasoning, fluency

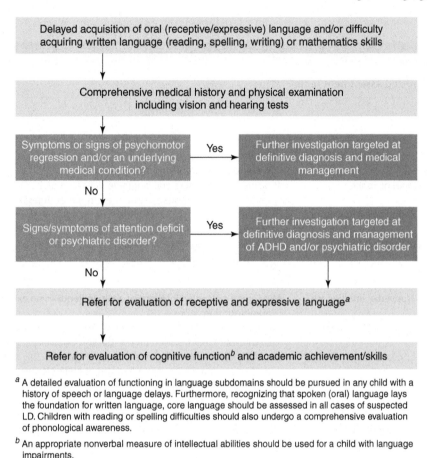

Delayed acquisition of oral (receptive/expressive) language and/or difficulty acquiring written language (reading, spelling, writing) or mathematics skills

Comprehensive medical history and physical examination including vision and hearing tests

Symptoms or signs of psychomotor regression and/or an underlying medical condition? — Yes → Further investigation targeted at definitive diagnosis and medical management

No

Signs/symptoms of attention deficit or psychiatric disorder? — Yes → Further investigation targeted at definitive diagnosis and management of ADHD and/or psychiatric disorder

No

Refer for evaluation of receptive and expressive language[a]

Refer for evaluation of cognitive function[b] and academic achievement/skills

[a] A detailed evaluation of functioning in language subdomains should be pursued in any child with a history of speech or language delays. Furthermore, recognizing that spoken (oral) language lays the foundation for written language, core language should be assessed in all cases of suspected LD. Children with reading or spelling difficulties should also undergo a comprehensive evaluation of phonological awareness.

[b] An appropriate nonverbal measure of intellectual abilities should be used for a child with language impairments.

FIGURE 10-1 ■ Algorithm for diagnosis of LD.

age-appropriate education; and whether the child's difficulty "significantly interferes with academic achievement or activities of daily living" that require the particular skill (eg, reading).[1] "Substantially below" is variably defined as a discrepancy of 1 to 2 standard deviations between aptitude and achievement.[1] Similarly, diagnosis of an expressive or mixed receptive-expressive disorder involves demonstration that "scores obtained from a battery of standardized individually administered measures [expressive language development or both receptive and expressive language development, respectively] are substantially below those obtained from standardized measures of nonverbal intellectual capacity."[1] As noted in *DSM-IV-TR*, a detailed functional assessment of language ability may serve as the basis for diagnosis "when standardized instruments are not available or appropriate." A list of commonly used measures of language, intellectual abilities, and academic skills is included in Table 10-7. Test selection and result interpretation should both be guided by, and take into consideration, variables that may impact test performance such as language proficiency, attention regulation, the sociocultural background of the individual, and any motor or sensory deficiencies.

A large number of children undergo evaluations for LD within school systems. The assessment procedures employed by local education agencies (LEAs) are shaped by the guidelines for determination of LD specified by federal and state statutes.

While both *DSM-IV-TR* and special education laws include aptitude-achievement discrepancy criteria, this discrepancy-based approach for identification of LD has long been criticized by researchers and leaders in the field. Such criticism has highlighted the poor reliability and discriminant validity of the discrepancy model, as well as concerns about the limited instructional relevance of the type of assessments that are typically conducted when determination of intellectual quotient (IQ)-achievement discrepancy is the focus, and the frequently long gap between identification of a struggling learner and determination of eligibility and initiation of appropriate interventions.[16,119-124] The latter is of particular concern because remediation becomes an increasingly challenging undertaking as time elapses, and the prognosis for achieving typical skills declines.[6,125]

In part spurred by these concerns, the 2004 reauthorization of IDEA by Congress brought new guidelines and directions for LD determination. Of particular interest is the option that local education agencies (LEAs) may employ a "process that determines if [a] child responds to scientific, research-supported intervention as part of the

Table 10-7.

Examples of Standardized Assessment Tools[149, 150]

Area Assessed	Brief Description (Age range)
Language	
Clinical Evaluation of Language Fundamentals, Fourth Edition (CELF-4)[151]	Measure used to diagnose language disorders and assess strengths and weaknesses in specific domains. (Ages 5-21)
Comprehensive Assessment of Spoken Language (CASL)[152]	Measure used to assess oral language skills (comprehension, expression, and retrieval) in four language structure categories (Ages 3-21)
Comprehensive Test of Phonological Processing (CTOPP)[153]	Measure of phonological awareness, phonological memory, and rapid naming. (Ages 5-24)
Lindamood Auditory Conceptualization Test, Third Edition (LAC 3)[154]	Measures the ability to perceive and conceptualize speech sounds using visual stimuli. (Ages 5-18)
Intelligence	
Comprehensive Test of Nonverbal Intelligence (CTONI)[155]	Measure of nonverbal intellectual abilities. Requires no expressive language for administration. (Ages 6-18)
Das-Naglieri Cognitive Assessment System (CAS)[156]	Measure of cognitive processing ability. Authors report this test is appropriate to use with students from diverse backgrounds. (Ages 5-17)
Differential Ability Scales, Second Edition (DAS-II)[157]	General measure of intelligence and cognitive skills. This test is divided into three main composites, including Verbal Ability, Nonverbal Reasoning Ability, and Spatial Ability that yield an overall General Cognitive Ability (GCA) score. In addition, it includes additional clusters measuring Working Memory and Processing Speed. (Ages 2:6-17:11)
Kaufman Assessment Battery for Children, Second Edition (KABC-II)[158]	Measure of cognitive abilities. This test provides two pathways for administration and scoring. One yields an overall Mental Processing Index (MPI). The other yields an overall Fluid-Crystallized Index (FCI). Additionally, this test also provides a Nonverbal Composite. (Ages 3-18)
Reynolds Intellectual Assessment Scales (RIAS)[159]	Short measure of verbal and nonverbal intelligence and memory. (Ages 3-94 years)
Stanford-Binet Intelligence Scale, Fifth Edition (SB-V)[160]	Measures verbal and nonverbal domains of five factors including Fluid Reasoning, Knowledge, Quantitative Reasoning, Visual-Spatial Processing, and Working Memory. (Ages 2-85+ years)
Universal Nonverbal Intelligence Test (UNIT)[161]	Measure of nonverbal intelligence and memory useful for children who are linguistically diverse or exhibit language impairments. This test minimizes verbal output and does not require the individual to provide a verbal response. (Ages 5:0-17:11)
Wechsler Adult Intelligence Scale, Third Edition (WAIS-3)[162]	General measure of intellectual and cognitive abilities. This test is based on a six factor model including Verbal Comprehension, Perceptual Reasoning, Working Memory, Processing Speed, Verbal Memory and Visual Memory. (Ages 16-89)
Wechsler Intelligence Scales for Children, Fourth Edition (WISC-4)[163]	A widely used measure of intellectual and cognitive abilities. This test is divided into four main composites (Verbal Comprehension, Perceptual Reasoning, Working Memory, and Processing Speed) that yield a Full IQ score. When statistically significant differences are noted among the four composites an alternative score (General Ability Index, GAI) can be derived to estimate overall cognitive ability. (Ages 6-16)
Wechsler Nonverbal Test of Ability (WNV)[164]	Measure of nonverbal ability for individuals who are not English language proficient or have other language considerations. (Ages 4-21)
Woodcock-Johnson III Cognitive Battery (WJ III Cog)[165]	Measure of general intellectual ability and specific cognitive skills. (Ages 2-90+ years)

(Continued)

Table 10-7. (Continued)

Examples of Standardized Assessment Tools[149, 150]

Area Assessed	Brief Description (Age range)
Memory and Learning	
Children's Memory Scale[166]	Comprehensive assessment of learning and memory. Provides information regarding children's visual and verbal memory, attention/concentration, learning, and delayed recognition. (Ages 5-16)
Test of Memory and Learning, Second Edition (TOMAL)[167]	Measure of general and specific memory functions. (Ages 5-19)
Wechsler Memory Scale, Third Edition (WMS-III)[162]	Measure of general memory, visual and auditory immediate, visual and auditory delayed, and working memory. (Ages 16-89)
Wide Range Assessment of Memory and Learning, Second Edition (WRAML-2)[168]	Measures memory functioning (visual, verbal, and working memory) and verbal learning. (Ages 5-90)
Academic Skills	
Gray Oral Reading Tests, Fourth Edition (GORT-4)[169]	Measure of oral reading ability. (Ages 6-18)
KeyMath-Revised/NU[170]	Measure of understanding and application of mathematics concepts and skills for grades kindergarten through 8.
Kaufman Test of Educational Achievement, Second Edition (KTEA-II)[171]	Measure used to assess reading, mathematical, written language skills and oral language. (Ages 4:0 through 25)
Stanford Diagnostic Mathematics Test, Fourth Edition (SDMT 4)[172]	Measure of basic academic concepts and skills. Can be group administered for grades 1.5 through beginning college level.
Stanford Diagnostic Reading Test, Fourth Edition (SDRT 4)[173]	Measure of essential reading components for grades kindergarten through beginning college level.
Test of Early Mathematics Ability, Third Edition (TEMA-3)[174]	Measure of early mathematics performance. (Ages 3-8)
Test of Early Reading Ability, Third Edition (TERA-3)[175]	Measure of early reading skills. (Ages 3-8)
Test of Early Written Language, Third Edition (TEWL-3)[176]	Measure of basic and contextual writing. (Ages 4-10)
Test of Reading Comprehension, Third Edition (TORC-3)[177]	Measure of silent reading comprehension. (Ages 7:0-17:11)
Test of Word Reading Efficiency (TOWRE)[178]	Measure of word reading accuracy and fluency. (Ages 6:0-24:11)
Test of Written Expression (TOWE) (McGhee et al., 1995)[179]	Comprehensive assessment of writing achievement. (Ages 6-14)
Test of Written Language, Third Edition (TOWL-3)[180]	Measure of written language skills. (Ages 7:6-17:11)
Wechsler Individual Achievement Test, Second Edition (WIAT-II)[181]	Comprehensive assessment of academic achievement. (Ages 4-85)
Wide Range Achievement Test 4 (WRAT4)[182]	Measures the basic academic skills of reading, spelling, and mathematical computation. (Ages 5-94)
Woodcock-Johnson III Tests of Achievement (WJ III Ach)[165]	Comprehensive measure of academic skills in reading, mathematics, written language, and oral language. (Ages 5-90+)
Woodcock-Johnson III Diagnostic Reading Battery (WJ III DRB)[183]	Measure of phonological awareness, phonics knowledge, reading achievement, and related oral language abilities. (Ages 2-90+)

evaluation procedures." Importantly, LEAs are no longer required to "take into consideration whether a child has a severe [IQ-achievement] discrepancy."[3] This response-to-intervention (RTI) approach to LD determination is a multi-tiered process that targets early intervention and prevention.[16,126-128] In general, the first tier involves universal screening at the beginning of the school year to identify children who may be at risk for LD, along with the provision of empirically supported classroom instruction to all students in the general education setting. At-risk children who demonstrate poor responsiveness to tier 1 interventions as determined by serial (curriculum-based) assessments receive further interventions at the tier 2 and 3 levels, which include small-group tutoring and more intensive, individualized instruction. Progress monitoring occurs throughout, and those at-risk children who continue to struggle (ie, "nonresponders") are considered for multidisciplinary evaluation for possible LD or other disability classification (eg, intellectual disability) and special education and related services (eg, language therapy).[126–129] The LD designation is reserved for those students who demonstrate "unexpected underachievement" (a core LD construct) in spite of evidence-based interventions that are validated as effective for most students.[16,122,130] The dynamic, formative assessment methods employed in RTI models differ from the singular, summative assessment approach that characterizes the evaluation procedures used in the discrepancy model.[124,131]

In addition to providing options for LD determination, IDEA 2004 further delineated guidelines regarding required components of the evaluation and information-gathering process. As a result, in addition to a multidisciplinary evaluation, LEAs must include procedures for gathering information from the student's parents, as well as conducting classroom observations of the student in the areas being targeted (eg, academic achievement domains). Once this information is collected, the child study team or educational planning team, including the parent(s), meets to develop treatment recommendations for the child.

As may be gleaned from the foregoing, in order to provide informed guidance to families, awareness is necessary of the federal and state statutes that govern LD determination in local school districts, and thus access to remedial intervention services. Links to useful online resources for information about IDEA 2004 and RTI are included in Table 10-8 (Figure 10-1).

Table 10-8.

Resources for Information on IDEA 2004, RTI, and Section 504

▪ The U.S. Department of Education, Office of Special Education Programs (OSEP) IDEA Web site
http://idea.ed.gov/
▪ The U.S. Department of Education, Office of Civil Rights Web site containing answers to "Frequently Asked Questions About Section 504 and the Education of Children with Disabilities"
http://www.ed.gov/about/offices/list/ocr/504faq.html
▪ The National Dissemination Center for Children with Disabilities (NICHCY) Web site provides information on IDEA, Individualized Education Programs (IEPs), and related topics
http://www.nichcy.org/
▪ The National Research Center on Learning Disabilities Web site includes extensive information on RTI
http://www.nrcld.org/free/

TREATMENT

Subsequent to the clinical evaluation and diagnosis of an LD, the physician's role in the management of learning and language disorders is primarily one of providing appropriate treatment for underlying and/or co-occurring medical or psychiatric conditions, initiating and facilitating referrals for appropriate treatment interventions as indicated by the child's specific needs; educating, supporting, and providing anticipatory guidance to the child and family; monitoring the child's progress and evolving needs; and advocating on their behalf wherever possible.

Parent education helps caregivers to understand their child's learning differences and strengths and to provide appropriate assistance to their child. By educating and supporting parents, clinicians can play a crucial role in building parent/school collaboration and developing effective intervention plans in both the home and school setting.

While pharmacotherapy is not a recommended treatment modality for isolated LD, it is important to recognize and treat comorbid attention deficits, which can otherwise hinder response to appropriate interventions and impede a child's progress.[6,132-134] Pharmacologic management may also be indicated for other co-occurring conditions.

For children with LDs, treatment is centered around the implementation of educational interventions and/or language therapy through an early intervention program or the school system. Through the passage of the Education of All Handicapped Children Act in 1975, LD was established as a category of disability under federal law. Reauthorized and renamed by Congress since then, IDEA 2004 mandates the provision of early intervention and special education services for children with disabilities. Infants and toddlers (birth through 3 years) with disabilities and their families receive early intervention services under IDEA part C, while children and youth (ages 3 to 21 years) with disabilities are entitled to receive special education and related services under IDEA part B. Thus, state and local education agencies are required to provide appropriate interventions for children (birth through 21 years) with language and learning disabilities. Children with disabilities who do not qualify for special education services under IDEA's narrower definition of disability, may otherwise be eligible for accommodations, modifications, and support services in their public preschool, elementary, and secondary education programs under Section 504 of the Rehabilitation Act of 1973, a civil rights statute that protects the rights of children with disabilities in schools that receive federal funds.[135]

Both IDEA and Section 504 require all states receiving federal special education funds to provide a

Table 10-9.

Learning Disability Interventions*

- ▪ Early intervention services
- ▪ Special education and related services (IEP)
- ▪ Academic accommodations (504 Plan)
- ▪ Language therapy
- ▪ Academic tutoring using effective instructional approaches to build requisite skills and develop proficiency (ie, intensive, systematic, explicit instruction that includes mastery-orientated progression through targeted skills, frequent opportunities for guided practice, and appropriate scaffolding to facilitate application of skills in meaningful contexts). The importance of a highly skilled teacher should be underscored.
- ▪ General supportive measures
  - ▪ Parent–child book-sharing activities (daily)
  - ▪ Use of audio books and textbooks
  - ▪ Limit television viewing in favor of board games and other interactive activities that build language and mathematical skills

*Parent education is an important part of caring for children with LD. For example, misinformation about RD (dyslexia) may lead a parent to pursue costly and unproven therapies, which can delay initiation of evidence-based interventions. As such, parents should be advised that dyslexia is not a "problem seeing words backwards" and be cautioned against pursuing therapies for reading problems that evidence does not support (eg, vision therapy[139-141] and motor coordination training[142-145]).

"free and appropriate public education" (FAPE) in the "least restrictive environment" (LRE) (ie, with their peers who are not disabled to the greatest degree that is appropriate given their needs) for all students with disabilities.[136] IDEA requires the development in writing of an individualized education plan (IEP) for a school-aged child or an individualized family support plan (IFSP) for a child aged 3 and under, which in essence outlines a plan to address the identified needs of the child.[3] In contrast, while Section 504 provides for accommodations and supports to enable a student with disabilities equal access to education programs and activities, it neither requires the development of an IEP that sets out *measurable* annual goals nor provides the extensive legal safeguards afforded by IDEA.[136] Further information about these federal laws and issues related to determination of eligibility for special programs and services can be assessed via the links included in Table 10-8.

For infants and toddlers with language disorders, treatment typically involves home-based individual therapy through an early intervention program. Optimally, parents serve as "treatment partners," providing daily reinforcement of the concepts and skills targeted by the language therapist. This is particularly important, when therapy is provided infrequently (eg, once or twice a week) and for school-aged children with moderate to

Table 10-10.

Findings of the National Research Council's National Reading Panel and Mathematics Learning Study Committee*‡

National Reading Panel
- ▪ Key components of effective reading instruction[146]
  - ▪ Phonological awareness
    - ▪ Students should learn to identify and manipulate the sounds (phonemes) in spoken syllables and words
  - ▪ Phonics
    - ▪ Students should be explicitly taught letter-sound relationships
  - ▪ Vocabulary
    - ▪ Students should learn word meanings/build their vocabularies (eg, through repeated exposure to vocabulary words embedded in rich contexts).
  - ▪ Fluency
    - ▪ Providing systematic and explicit guidance and feedback to students during repeated oral reading helps to build reading fluency (provided the reader has the requisite decoding skills)
  - ▪ Comprehension
    - ▪ Students should be taught a combination of comprehension techniques (eg, how to monitor their understanding of text, how to use graphic and semantic organizers)

Mathematics Learning Study Committee
- ▪ Five components of mathematics proficiency (successful mathematics learning)[147,148]
  - ▪ Conceptual understanding ("understanding mathematics")
  - ▪ Procedural fluency ("computing fluently")
  - ▪ Strategic competence ("applying concepts to solve problems")
  - ▪ Adaptive reasoning ("reasoning logically")
  - ▪ Productive disposition ("engaging with mathematics, seeing it as sensible, useful, and doable")

*While the National Research Council's findings do not specifically address the learning needs of students with LD, they are included because of their relevance to all students, including those with learning difficulties.
‡The National Research Council has incorporated these findings into practical guides for parents (and teachers). References are included in Table 10-11.

severe language impairments who receive therapy in group settings that afford limited opportunity to target an individual child's needs. For all children with LD regardless of severity, the importance of implementing effective treatment interventions as early as possible, and of careful monitoring of treatment efficacy, should be emphasized. For example, the rate of reading failure in children with a history of language impairments is six times that of nonimpaired controls/peers, with 50% developing a reading disability,[137] and those with persistence language impairments have particularly poor reading outcomes. In addition, children with LDs who do not receive effective, early intervention often exhibit persistent deficits into adolescence and adulthood.[6,16,138] Tables 10-9 to 10-11 include an outline of LD interventions that may be considered as well as suggested parent resources.

In addition to the implementation of empirically supported language and learning interventions, supportive counseling aimed at improving the child's self-concept and renewing his or her interest and enthusiasm in learning may be helpful. For children who have experienced repeated academic failure, the process of undoing the accumulated effects of chronic "failure" on their self-concept involves showing them that they *can* learn by providing appropriate educational instruction, related interventions, and supports.

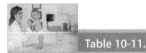

Table 10-11.

Parent Resources

Books Providing Practical Advice and Information on LD Topics
- *Starting Out Right: A Guide to Promoting Children's Reading Success* by the National Research Council
- *Overcoming Dyslexia: A New and Complete Science-Based Program for Reading Problems at Any Level* by Sally Shaywitz, M.D. Published by Alfred A. Knopf, New York, 2004
- *Unlocking Literacy: Effective Decoding & Spelling Instruction* by Marcia Henry, Ph.D.
- *Helping Children Learn Mathematics* by the National Research Council
- *How Students Learn: Mathematics in the Classroom* by the National Research Council
- *A Mind At a Time* by Mel Levine, M.D. Published by Simon & Schuster, New York, 2002
- *The Myth of Laziness* by Mel Levine, M.D. Published by Simon & Schuster, New York, 2003

Online Resources
- What Works Clearinghouse (www.whatworks.gov)
  - U.S. Department of Education's Institute of Education Sciences site is a "source of scientific evidence for what works in education" for educators, researchers, policymakers, and the public
- Florida Center For Reading Research (www.fcrr.org)
  - Source of information about evidence-based literacy instruction and assessment practices for parents, teachers, and researchers
- LD OnLine (www.ldonline.org)
  - LD OnLine provides information on a broad range of LD-related topics, and includes reports from the National Joint Committee on Learning Disabilities (NJCLD) and information about IDEA 2004, IEPs, and 504 Plans

REFERENCES

1. *Diagnostic and Statistical Manual of Mental Disorders*, 4th ed., text revision: DSM-IV-TR. Washington, DC: American Psychiatric Association; 2000.
2. National Joint Committee on Learning Disabilities. Learning disabilities: issues on definition. *ASHA*. 1991;33(5):18-20.
3. Individuals with Disabilities Education Improvement Act of 2004, 20 USC §1400 et seq. Available at: http://www.copyright.gov/legislation/pl108-446.pdf.
4. Campbell WN, Skarakis-Doyle E. School-aged children with SLI: the ICF as a framework for collaborative service delivery. *J Commun Disord*. 2007;40:513-535.
5. Gauger LM, Lombardino LJ, Leonard CM. Brain morphology in children with specific language impairment. *J Speech Lang Hear Res*. 1997;40:1272–1284.
6. Lyon GR. Learning disabilities. *Future Child*, 1996;6:54-76
7. Blanchard LT, Gurka MJ, Blackman JA. Emotional, developmental, and behavioral health of American children and their families: a report from the 2003 National Survey of Children's Health. *Pediatrics*. 2006;117:e1202-e1212.
8. Digest of Education Statistics: 2007. U.S. Department of Education National Center for Education Statistics, 2007. Available at: http://nces.ed.gov/programs/digest/d07/tables/dt07_047.asp?referrer=list. Accessed July, 2008.
9. Lee J, Grigg WS, Donahue P. *The Nation's Report Card: Reading 2007* (NCES 2007-496). Washington, DC: National Center for Education Statistics, Institute of Education Sciences, U.S. Department of Education; 2007.
10. Salahu-Din D, Persky H, Miller J. *The Nation's Report Card: Writing 2007* (NCES 2008-468). Washington, DC: National Center for Education Statistics, Institute of Education Sciences, U.S. Department of Education; 2008.
11. Lee J, Grigg WS, Dion GS. *The Nation's Report Card: Mathematics 2007* (NCES 2007-494). Washington, DC: National Center for Education Statistics, Institute of Education Sciences, U.S. Department of Education; 2007.
12. Lyon G, Shaywitz S, Shaywitz B. A definition of dyslexia. *Ann Dyslexia*. 2003;53:1-14.
13. Shaywitz SE, Gruen JR, Shaywitz BA. Management of dyslexia, its rationale, and underlying neurobiology. *Pediatr Clin North Am*. 2007;54:609-623, viii.
14. Shalev RS, Auerbach J, Manor O, Gross-Tsur V. Developmental dyscalculia: prevalence and prognosis. *Eur Child Adolesc Psychiatry*. 2000;9(suppl 2):II58-II64.

15. Grigorenko EL. Developmental dyslexia: an update on genes, brains, and environments. *J Child Psychol Psychiatry.* 2001;42:91-125.

16. Fletcher JM, Lyon GR, Fuchs LS, Barnes MA. *Learning Disabilities: From Identification to Intervention.* New York, NY: Guilford Press; 2007.

17. Olson RK. Genes, environment, and dyslexia: The 2005 Norman Geshwind Memorial Lecture. *Ann Dyslexia.* 2006;56(2): 205-238.

18. Friend A, DeFries J, Wadsworth S, Olson R. Genetic and environmental influences on word recognition and spelling deficits as a function of age. *Behav Genet.* 2007;37:477-486.

19. Wadsworth S, DeFries J, Olson R, Willcutt E. Colorado longitudinal twin study of reading disability. *Ann Dyslexia.* 2007;57:139-160.

20. Hawke JL, Wadsworth SJ, DeFries JC. Genetic influences on reading difficulties in boys and girls: the Colorado twin study. *Dyslexia.* 2006;12:21-29.

21. Voeller KK. Dyslexia. *J Child Neurol.* 2004;19:740-744.

22. Richards TL, Aylward EH, Field KM, et al. Converging evidence for triple word form theory in children with dyslexia. *Dev Neuropsychol.* 2006;30:547-589.

23. Snowling MJ, Muter V, Carroll J. Children at family risk of dyslexia: a follow-up in early adolescence. *J Child Psychol Psychiatry.* 2007;48:609-618.

24. Williams J, O'Donovan MC. The genetics of developmental dyslexia. *Eur J Hum Genet.* 2006;14:681-689.

25. Harlaar N, Dale PS, Plomin R. From learning to read to reading to learn: substantial and stable genetic influence. *Child Dev.* 2007;78:116-131.

26. Bates TC, Luciano M, Castles A, Coltheart M, Wright MJ, Martin NG. Replication of reported linkages for dyslexia and spelling and suggestive evidence for novel regions on chromosomes 4 and 17. *Eur J Hum Genet.* 2006;15:194-203.

27. Galaburda AM, LoTurco J, Ramus F, Fitch RH, Rosen GD. From genes to behavior in developmental dyslexia. *Nat Neurosci.* 2006;9:1213-1217.

28. McGrath LM, Smith SD, Pennington BF. Breakthroughs in the search for dyslexia candidate genes. *Trends Mol Med.* 2006;12:333-341.

29. Paracchini S, Scerri T, Monaco AP. The genetic lexicon of dyslexia. *Annu Rev Genomics Hum Genet.* 2007;8:57-79.

30. Ramus F. Neurobiology of dyslexia: a reinterpretation of the data. *Trends Neurosci.* 2004;27:720-726.

31. Peterson RL, McGrath LM, Smith SD, Pennington BF. Neuropsychology and genetics of speech, language, and literacy disorders. *Pediatr Clin North Am.* 2007;54:543-561.

32. Leonard C, Eckert M, Given B, Virginia B, Eden G. Individual differences in anatomy predict reading and oral language impairments in children. *Brain.* 2006;129:3329-3342.

33. Eckert MA, Leonard CM, Richards TL, Aylward EH, Thomson J, Berninger VW. Anatomical correlates of dyslexia: frontal and cerebellar findings. *Brain.* 2003; 126:482-494.

34. Shaywitz BA, Lyon GR, Shaywitz SE. The role of functional magnetic resonance imaging in understanding reading and dyslexia. *Dev Neuropsychol.* 2006;30:613-632.

35. Hoeft F, Meyler A, Hernandez A, et al. Functional and morphometric brain dissociation between dyslexia and reading ability. *Proc Natl Acad Sci.* 2007;104:4234-4239.

36. Vellutino FR, Fletcher JM, Snowling MJ, Scanlon DM. Specific reading disability (dyslexia): what have we learned in the past four decades? *J Child Psychol Psychiatry.* 2004;45:2-40.

37. Eden GF, Jones KM, Cappell K, et al. Neural changes following remediation in adult developmental dyslexia. *Neuron.* 2004;44:411-422.

38. Barnes MA, Fuchs LS. Learning disabilities. In: Wolraich ML, Drotar DD, Dworkin PH, Perrin EC, eds. *Developmental-Behavioral Pediatrics: Evidence and Practice.* Philiadelphia, PA: Mosby; 2008:445-466.

39. Gersten R, Jordan NC, Flojo JR. Early identification and interventions for students with mathematics difficulties. *J Learn Disabil.* 2005;38:293-304.

40. Wilson A, Dehaene S, Pinel P, Revkin S, Cohen L, Cohen D. Principles underlying the design of "the Number Race," an adaptive computer game for remediation of dyscalculia. *Behav Brain Func.* 2006;2:19.

41. Dehaene S. *The Number Sense: How the Mind Creates Mathematics.* New York, NY: Oxford University Press; 1997.

42. Rousselle L, Noël M-P. Basic numerical skills in children with mathematics learning disabilities: a comparison of symbolic vs non-symbolic number magnitude processing. *Cognition.* 2007;102:361-395.

43. Dehaene S, Molko N, Cohen L, Wilson AJ. Arithmetic and the brain. *Curr Opin Neurobiol.* 2004;14:218-224.

44. Price GR, Holloway I, Rasanen P, Vesterinen M, Ansari D. Impaired parietal magnitude processing in developmental dyscalculia. *Curr Biol.* 2007;17:R1042-R1043.

45. Alarcon M, DeFries JC, Light JG, Pennington BF. A twin study of mathematics disability. *J Learn Disabil.* 1997;30:617-623.

46. Shalev RS, Gross-Tsur V. Developmental dyscalculia. *Pediatr Neurol.* 2001;24:337-342.

47. Shalev RS, Manor O, Kerem B, et al. Developmental dyscalculia is a familial learning disability. *J Learn Disabil.* 2001;34:59-65.

48. Geary DC. Learning disabilities in arithematic: problem-solving differences and cognitive deficits. In: Swanson HL, Harris KR, Graham S, eds. *Handbook of Learning Disabilities.* New York, NY: Guilford Press; 2003:199-212.

49. Ansari D, Karmiloff-Smith A. Atypical trajectories of number development: a neuroconstructivist perspective. *Trends Cogn Sci.* 2002;6:511-516.

50. Von Aster MG, Shalev RS. Number development and developmental dyscalculia. *Dev Med Child Neurol.* 2007;49:868-873.

51. Kadosh RC, Walsh V. Dyscalculia. *Curr Biol.* 2007;17:R946-R947.

52. Murphy MM, Mazzocco MMM. Mathematics learning disabilities in girls with fragile X or Turner syndrome during late elementary school. *J Learn Disabil.* 2008; 41:29-46-R947.

53. Bishop DVM, Hayiou-Thomas ME. Heritability of specific language impairment depends on diagnostic criteria. *Genes Brain Behav.* 2008;7:365-372.

54. Hayiou-Thomas ME. Genetic and environmental influences on early speech, language and literacy development. *J Commun Disord.* 2008;41:397-408.

55. McMahon A, McMahon R. Genetics and language. In: Keith B, ed. *Encyclopedia of Language & Linguistics.* Oxford, England: Elsevier; 2006:21-24.

56. Fisher SE. On genes, speech, and language. *N Engl J Med.* 2005;353:1655-1657.

57. Webster RI, Erdos C, Evans K, et al. The clinical spectrum of developmental language impairment in school-aged children: language, cognitive, and motor findings. *Pediatrics.* 2006;118:e1541-e1549.

58. Feldman HM. Evaluation and management of language and speech disorders in preschool children. *Pediatr Rev.* 2005;26:131-142.

59. Kramer U. Atypical presentations of benign childhood epilepsy with centrotemporal spikes: a review. *J Child Neurol.* 2008;23:785-790.

60. Nelson HD, Nygren P, Walker M, Panoscha R. Screening for speech and language delay in preschool children: systematic evidence review for the U.S. Preventive Services Task Force. *Pediatrics.* 2006;117:e298-e319.

61. Grizzle KL, Simms MD. Early language development and language learning disabilities. *Pediatr Rev.* 2005;26:274-283.

62. Butterworth B. The development of arithmetical abilities. *J Child Psychol Psychiatry.* 2005;46:3-18.

63. Shalev RS. Developmental dyscalculia. *J Child Neurol.* 2004;19:765-771.

64. Kelly DP, Aylward GP. Identifying school performance problems in the pediatric office. *Pediatr Ann.* 2005;34:288-298.

65. Snowling MJ, Maughan B. Reading and other learning disorders. In: Gillberg C, Harrington R, Steinhausen HC, eds. *A Clinician's Handbook of Child and Adolescent Psychiatry.* New York, NY: Cambridge University Press; 2006:417-446.

66. Fletcher JM, Barnes MA, Francis DJ, Shaywitz SE, Shaywitz BA. Classification of learning disabilities: an evidence-based evaluation. In: Bradley R, Danielson L, Hallahan DP, eds. *Identification of Learning Disabilities: Research to Practice.* Mahwah, NJ: Erlbaum; 2002:185-250.

67. Grizzle KL, Simms MD. Early language development and language learning disabilities. *Pediatr Rev.* 2005;26:274-283.

68. Puolakanaho A, Ahonen T, Aro M, et al. Developmental links of very early phonological and language skills to second grade reading outcomes: strong to accuracy but only minor to fluency. *J Learn Disabil.* 2008;41:353-370.

69. Schatschneider C, Torgesen JK. Using our current understanding of dyslexia to support early identification and intervention. *J Child Neurol.* 2004;19:759-765.

70. Schatschneider C, Fletcher JM, Francis DJ, Carlson CD, Foorman BR. Kindergarten prediction of reading skills: a longitudinal comparative analysis. *J Edu Psychol.* 2004;96:265-282.

71. De Jong PF, Olson RK. Early predictors of letter knowledge. *J Exp Child Psychol.* 2004;88:254-273.

72. Lonigan C, Burgess SR, Anthony JL. Development of emergent literacy and early reading skills in preschool children: evidence from a latent-variable longitudinal study. *Dev Psychol.* 2000;36:596-613.

73. Storch SA, Whitehurst GJ. Oral language and code-related precursors to reading: evidence from a longitudinal structural model. *Dev Psychol.* 2002;38:934-947.

74. Meltzer LJ, Mindell JA. Sleep and sleep disorders in children and adolescents. *Psychiatr Clin North Am.* 2006;29:1059-1076.

75. Perez-Chada D, Perez-Lloret S, Videla AJ, et al. Sleep disordered breathing and daytime sleepiness are associated with poor academic performance in teenagers. A study using the pediatric daytime sleepiness scale (PDSS). *Sleep.* 2007;30:1698-1703.

76. Maag JW, Reid R. Depression among students with learning disabilities: assessing the risk. *J Learn Disabil.* 2006;39:3-10.

77. Elbaum B, Vaughn S. Self-concept and students with learning disabilities. In: Swanson HL, Harris KR, Graham S, eds. *Handbook of Learning Disabilities.* New York, NY Guilford Press; 2003:229.

78. Sideridis GD. Why are students with LD depressed? A goal orientation model of depression vulnerability. *J Learn Disabil.* 2007;40:526-539.

79. Martinez RS, Semrud-Clikeman M. Emotional adjustment and school functioning of young adolescents with multiple versus single learning disabilities. *J Learn Disabil.* 2004;37:411-420.

80. Lackaye T, Margalit M, Ziv O, Ziman T. Comparisons of self-efficacy, mood, effort, and hope between students with learning disabilities and their non-LD-matched peers. *Learn Disabil Res Pract.* 2006;21:111-121.

81. Sundheim ST, Voeller KK. Psychiatric implications of language disorders and learning disabilities: risks and management. *J Child Neurol.* 2004;19:814-826.

82. Capin DM. Developmental learning disorders: clues to their diagnosis and management. *Pediatr Rev.* 1996;17:284-290.

83. Jäncke L, Siegenthaler T, Preis S, Steinmetz H. Decreased white-matter density in a left-sided fronto-temporal network in children with developmental language disorder: evidence for anatomical anomalies in a motor-language network. *Brain Lang.* 2007;102:91-98.

84. Manor O, Shalev RS, Joseph A, Gross-Tsur V. Arithmetic skills in kindergarten children with developmental language disorders. *Eur J Paediatr Neurol.* 2001;5:71-77.

85. Webster RI, Erdos C, Evans K, et al. Neurological and magnetic resonance imaging findings in children with developmental language impairment. *J Child Neurol.* 2008;23:870-877.

86. Trauner D, Wulfeck B, Tallal P, Hesselink J. Neurological and MRI profiles of children with developmental language impairment. *Dev Med Child Neurol.* 2000;42:470-475.

87. Coplan J. Language delays. In: Parker S, Zuckerman BS, Augustyn M, eds. *Developmental and Behavioral Pediatrics: A Handbook for Primary Care.* 2nd ed. Philadelphia, PA: Lippincott Williams & Wilkins; 2005:222-226.

88. Dworkin PH. School failure. In: Parker S, Zuckerman BS, Augustyn M, eds. *Developmental and Behavioral Pediatrics: A Handbook for Primary Care.* 2nd ed. Philadelphia, PA: Lippincott Williams & Wilkins; 2005:280-284.

89. Semrud-Clikeman M. Neuropsychological aspects for evaluating learning disabilities. *J Learn Disabil.* 2005; 38:563-568.

90. Pliszka S. Practice parameter for the assessment and treatment of children and adolescents with attention-deficit/hyperactivity disorder. *J Am Acad Child Adolesc Psychiatry.* 2007;46:894-921.

91. Del'Homme M, Kim TS, Loo SK, Yang MH, Smalley SL. Familial association and frequency of learning disabilities in ADHD sibling pair families. *J Abnorm Child Psychol.* 2007;35:55-62.

92. Tomblin JB, Zhang X. The association of reading disability, behavioral disorders, and language Impairment among second-grade children. *J Child Psychol Psychiatry.* 2000;41: 473-482.

93. American Academy of Child and Adolescent Psychiatry. Practice parameters for the assessment and treatment of children and adolescents with language and learning disorders. *J Am Acad Child Adolesc Psychiatry* 1998; 37(suppl):46S-62S.

94. Toppelberg C, Shapiro T. Language disorders: a 10-year research update review. *J Am Acad Child Adolesc Psychiatry.* 2000;39:143-152.

95. Fergusson DM, Woodward LJ. Mental health, educational, and social role outcomes of adolescents with depression. *Arch Gen Psychiatry.* 2002;59:225-231.

96. Grover R GG, Ialongo N. Psychosocial outcomes of anxious first graders: a seven-year follow-up. *Depress Anxiety.* 2007;24:410-420.

97. Cutting L, Denckla M. Attention: relationship between attention-deficit hyperactivity disorder and learning disabilities. In: Swanson H, Harris K, Graham S, eds. *Handbook of Learning Disabilities.* New York: Guilford Press; 2003:125-139.

98. Oostrom KJ, van Teeseling H, Smeets-Schouten A, Peters ACB, Jennekens-Schinkel A, Dutch Study of Epilepsy in Childhood (DuSECh). Three to four years after diagnosis: cognition and behaviour in children with "epilepsy only." A prospective, controlled study. *Brain.* 2005;128:1546-1555.

99. Selassie GR-H, Viggedal G, Olsson I, Jennische M. Speech, language, and cognition in preschool children with epilepsy. *Dev Med Child Neurol.* 2008;50:432-438.

100. Nolan MA, Redoblado MA, Lah S, et al. Memory function in childhood epilepsy syndromes. *J Paediatr Child Health.* 2004;40:20-27.

101. Fastenau PS, Jianzhao S, Dunn DW, Austin JK. Academic underachievement among children with epilepsy: proportion exceeding psychometric criteria for disability and associated risk factors. *J Learn Disabil.* 2008;41:195-207.

102. Piccinelli P, Borgatti R, Aldini A, et al. Academic performance in children with rolandic epilepsy. *Dev Med Child Neurol.* 2008;50:353-356.

103. Henkin Y, Sadeh M, Kivity S, Shabtai E, Kishon-Rabin L, Gadoth N. Cognitive function in idiopathic generalized epilepsy of childhood. *Dev Med Child Neurol.* 2005;47: 126-132.

104. Hyman SL, Arthur Shores E, North KN. Learning disabilities in children with neurofibromatosis type 1: subtypes, cognitive profile, and attention-deficit- hyperactivity disorder. *Dev Med Child Neurol.* 2006;48:973-977.

105. Cyrulnik SE, Hinton VJ. Duchenne muscular dystrophy: a cerebellar disorder? *Neurosci Biobehav Rev.* 2008;32:486.

106. Hendriksen JG, Vles JS. Are males with Duchenne muscular dystrophy at risk for reading disabilities? *Pediatric Neurol.* 2006;34:296-300.

107. Marini A, Lorusso ML, D'Angelo MG, et al. Evaluation of narrative abilities in patients suffering from Duchenne muscular dystrophy. *Brain Lang.* 2007;102:1-12.

108. Young HK, Barton BA, Waisbren S, et al. Cognitive and psychological profile of males with Becker muscular dystrophy. *J Child Neurol.* 2008;23:155-162.

109. Hart KI, Fujiki M, Brinton B, Hart CH. The relationship between social behavior and severity of language impairment. *J Speech Lang Hear Res.* 2004;47:647-662.

110. Fujiki M, Spackman MP, Brinton B, Hall A. The relationship of language and emotion regulation skills to reticence in children with specific language impairment. *J Speech Lang Hear Res.* 2004;47:637-646.

111. Marton K, Abramoff B, Rosenzweig S. Social cognition and language in children with specific language impairment (SLI). *J Communication Disord.* 2005;38:143-162.

112. Yoshinaga-Itano C. Sensitive periods in the development of language of children who are deaf or hard of hearing. In: Accardo P, Rogers B, Capute AJ, eds. *Disorders of Language Development.* Timonium, MD: York Press; 2002: 57-81.

113. Caspari SS, Strand EA, Kotagal S, Bergqvist C. Obstructive sleep apnea, seizures, and childhood apraxia of speech. *Pediatr Neurol.* 2008;38:422-425.

114. Gozal D. Sleep-disordered breathing and school performance in children. *Pediatrics.* 1998;102:616-620.

115. Rhodes SK, Shimoda KC, Waid LR, et al. Neurocognitive deficits in morbidly obese children with obstructive sleep apnea. *J Pediatr.* 1995;127:741-744.

116. Suratt PM, Peruggia M, D'Andrea L, et al. Cognitive function and behavior of children with adenotonsillar hypertrophy suspected of having obstructive sleep-disordered breathing. *Pediatrics.* 2006;118:e771-e781.

117. Kurnatowski P, Putynski L, Lapienis M, Kowalska B. Neurocognitive abilities in children with adenotonsillar hypertrophy. *Int J Pediatr Otorhinolaryngol.* 2006;70: 419-424.

118. Schuele CM. The impact of developmental speech and language impairments on the acquisition of literacy skills. *Mental Retard Dev Disabil.* 2004;10:176-183.

119. Fletcher JM, Francis DJ, Morris RD, Lyon GR. Evidence-based assessment of learning disabilities in children and adolescents. *J Clin Child Adolesc Psychol.* 2005; 34:506-522.

120. Lyon GR, Fletcher JM, Shaywitz SE, Shaywitz BA, Torgesen JK. Rethinking learning disabilities. In: Finn C, Rotherham A, Hokanson C, eds. *Rethinking Special Education for a New Century.* Washington, DC: Thomas B. Fordham Foundation and the Progressive Policy Institute; 2001:259-287.

121. Fletcher JM, Denton C, Francis DJ. Validity of alternative approaches for the identification of learning disabilities: operationalizing unexpected underachievement. *J Learn Disabil.* 2005;38:545-552.

122. National Research Center on Learning Disabilities. SLD Identification Overview. Winter 2007. Available at: http:// www.nrcld.org/resource_kit/tools/SLDO verview2007.pdf. Accessed May 18, 2008.

123. Francis DJ, Fletcher JM, Stuebing KK, Lyon GR, Shaywitz BA, Shaywitz SE. Psychometric approaches to the identification of LD: IQ and achievement scores are not sufficient. *J Learn Disabil.* 2005;38:98-108.

124. Fletcher JM, Coulter WA, Reschly DJ, Vaughn S. Alternative approaches to the definition and identification of learning disabilities: some questions and answers. *Ann Dyslexia.* 2004;54:304-331.

125. Shaywitz SE, Morris R, Shaywitz BA. The education of dyslexic children from childhood to young adulthood. *Annu Rev Psychol.* 2008;59:451-475.

126. Fuchs D, Deshler DD. What we need to know about responsiveness to intervention (and shouldn't be afraid to ask). *Learn Disabil Res Pract.* 2007;22:129-136.

127. Reschly DJ. Learning disabilities identification: primary intervention, secondary intervention, and then what? *J Learn Disabil.* 2005;38:510-515.

128. Bradley R, Danielson L, Doolittle J. Response to intervention. *J Learn Disabil.* 2005;38:485-486.

129. Vaughn S, Fuchs LS. Redefining learning disabilities as inadequate response to instruction: the promise and potential problems. *Learn Disabil Res Pract.* 2003;18:137-146.

130. Gresham F. Responsiveness to intervention: an alternative approach to the identification of learning disabilities. In: Bradley R, Danielson L, Hallahan DP, eds. *Identification of Learning Disabilities: Research to Practice.* Mahwah, NJ: Erlbaum; 2002:467-519.

131. Fuchs D, Fuchs LS. Introduction to response to intervention: what, why, and how valid is it? *Reading Res Q.* 2006;41:93-99.

132. Torgesen JK, Alexander AW, Wagner RK, Rashotte CA, Voeller KKS, Conway T. Intensive remedial instruction for children with severe reading disabilities: immediate and long-term outcomes from two instructional approaches. *J Learn Disabil.* 2001;34:33-58.

133. Bental B, Tirosh E. The effects of methylphenidate on word decoding accuracy in boys with attention-deficit/hyperactivity disorder. *J Clin Psychopharmacol.* 2008;28:89-92.

134. Keulers EH, Hendriksen JG, Feron FJ, et al. Methylphenidate improves reading performance in children with attention deficit hyperactivity disorder and comorbid dyslexia: An unblinded clinical trial. *Eur J Paediatr Neurol.* 2007; 11:21-28.

135. U.S. Department of Education, Office for Civil Rights. Free Appropriate Public Education for Students with Disabilites: Requirements Under Section 504 of the Rehabilitation Act of 1973. Washington, DC: 2007. Available at: http://www.ed.gov/about/ offices/list/ocr/ docs/FAPE504.pdf. Accessed June 1, 2008.

136. Wright PW, Wright P. Wrights law: special education law. 2nd ed. Hartfield, VA: Harbor House Law Press; 2008.

137. Catts HW, Fey ME, Tomblin JB, Zhang X. A longitudinal investigation of reading outcomes in children with language impairments. *J Speech Lang Hear Res.* 2002;45:1142-1157.

138. Shaywitz SE, Fletcher JM, Holahan JM, et al. Persistence of dyslexia: the Connecticut longitudinal study at adolescence. *Pediatrics.* 1999;104:1351-1359.

139. American Academy of Pediatrics Committee on Children with Disabilities: American Association for Pediatric Ophthalmology and Strabismus, and American Academy of Ophthalmology: Learning disabilities, dyslexia, and vision. *Pediatrics.* 1992;90:124-126.

140. Committee on Children with Learning Disabilities. Dyslexia, and Vision: a subject review. *Pediatrics.* 1998;102:1217-1219.

141. Wright C. Learning disorders, dyslexia, and vision. *Aust Fam Physician.* 2007;36:843-845.

142. Bishop DVM. Curing dyslexia and attention-deficit hyperactivity disorder by training motor co-ordination: miracle or myth? *J Paediatr Child Health.* 2007;43:653-655.

143. McArthur G. Test-retest effects in treatment studies of reading disability: the devil is in the detail. *Dyslexia.* 2007;13:240-252.

144. Snowling MJ, Hulme C. A critique of claims from Reynolds, Nicolson & Hambly (2003) that DDAT is an effective treatment for children with reading difficulties—"lies, damned lies and (inappropriate) statistics?" *Dyslexia.* 2003;9:127-133.

145. Singleton C, Stuart M. Measurement mischief: a critique of Reynolds, Nicolson and Hambly (2003). *Dyslexia.* 2003;9:151–160.

146. National Reading Panel. *Teaching Children to Read: An Evidence-Based Assessment of the Scientific Research Literature on Reading and Its Implications for Reading Instruction.* Rocksville, MD: NICHD Clearinghouse; 2000.

147. National Research Council. *Adding It Up: Helping Children Learn Mathematics.* Kilpatrick J, Swafford J, and Findell B, eds. Mathematics Learning Study Committee, Center for Education, Division of Behavioral and Social Sciences and Education. Washington, DC: National Academy Press; 2001.

148. National Research Council. *Helping Children Learn Mathematics.* Mathematics Learning Study Committee. Kilpatrick J, and Swafford J, eds. Center for Education, Division of Behavioral and Social Sciences and Education. Washington, DC: National Academy Press; 2002.

149. Sattler JM. *Assessment of Children: Cognitive Applications.* 4th ed. La Mesa, CA: Jerome M. Sattler; 2001.

150. Baron IS. *Neuropsychological Evaluation of the Child.* New York, NY: Oxford University Press; 2004.

151. Semel E, Wiig E, Secord WA. *Clinical Evaluation of Language Fundamentals.* 4th ed. San Antonio, TX: PsychCorp; 2003.

152. Carrow-Woolfolk E. *Comprehensive Assessment of Spoken Language.* Circle Pines, MN: American Guidance Service, Inc.1999.

153. Wagner RK, Torgesen JK, Rashotte CA. *Comprehensive Test of Phonological Processing.* Austin: PRO-ED; 1999.

154. Lindamood PC, Lindamood P. *Lindamood Auditory Conceptualization Test.* 3rd ed. Austin, TX: PRO-ED; 2004.

155. Hammill DD, Pearson NA, Wiederholt JL. *Comprehensive Test of Nonverbal Intelligence.* Austin, TX: PRO-ED; 1996.

156. Naglieri JA, Das JP. *Das-Naglieri Cognitive Assessment System.* Itasca, IL: Riverside Publishing; 1997.

157. Elliott CD. *Differential Ability Scales.* 2nd ed. San Antonio, TX: The Psychological Corporation; 2007.

158. Kaufman AS, Kaufman NL. Kaufman-Assessment Battery for Children. Circle Pines, MN: AGS Publishing; 2004.

159. Reynolds CR, Kamphaus RW. *Reynolds Intellectual Assessment Scales and the Reynolds Intellectual Screening Test.* Lutz, FL: Psychological Assessment Resources, Inc.; 2003.

160. Roid GH. *Stanford-Binet Intelligence Scales.* 5th ed. Itasca, IL: Riverside Publishing; 2003.

161. Bracken BA, McCallum RS. *Universal Nonverbal Intelligence Test.* Itasca, IL: Riverside Publishing; 1998.

162. Wechsler D. *Wechsler Adult Intelligence Scale.* 3rd ed. San Antonio, TX: The Psychological Corporation; 1997.

163. Wechsler D. *Wechsler Intelligence Scale for Children.* 4th ed. San Antonio, TX: The Psychological Corporation; 2003.

164. Wechsler D, Naglieri J. *Wechsler Nonverbal Scale of Ability.* San Antoni, TX: The Psychological Corporation; 2006.

165. Woodcock RW, McGrew KS, Mather N, Schrank FA. *Woodcock-Johnson(r) III.* Itasca, IL: Riverside Publishing; 2001.

166. Cohen MJ. *Children's Memory Scale*. San Antonio,TX: The Psychological Corporation; 1997.

167. Reynolds CR, Bigler ED. *Test of Memory and Learning*. Austin, TX: PRO-ED; 1994.

168. Sheslow D, Adams W. *Wide Range Assessment of Memory and Learning*. 2nd ed. Lutz, FL: Psychological Assessment Resources, Inc.; 2003.

169. Wiederholt JL, Bryant BR. *Gray Oral Reading Tests*. 4th ed. Austin, TX: PRO-ED; 2001.

170. Connolly AJ. *KeyMath Revised: A Diagnostic Inventory of Essential Mathematics [1998 Normative Update]*. Circle Pines, MN: American Guidance Service; 1998.

171. Kaufman, A., Kaufman N. Kaufman Test of Educational Achievement-Second Edition, Comprehensive Form. Circle Pines, MN: AGS Publishing; 2004.

172. Harcourt Brace Educational Measurement *Stanford Diagnostic Mathematics Test*. 4th ed. San Antonio, TX: Harcourt Brace Educational Measurement; 1996.

173. Karlsen B, Gardner EF. *Stanford Diagnostic Reading Test*. 4th ed. San Antonio, TX: Harcourt Brace Educational Measurement; 1996.

174. Ginsburg HP, Baroody AJ. *Test of Early Mathematics Ability*. 3rd ed. Austin, TX: PRO-ED; 2003.

175. Reid DK, Hresko WP, Hamill DD. *Test of Early Reading Ability*. 3rd ed. Austin, TX: PRO-ED; 1981.

176. Hresko WP, Herron SR, Peak PK. *Test of Early Written Language*. 2nd ed. Austin, TX: PRO-ED; 1996.

177. Brown VL, Hammill DD, Wiederholt JL. *Test of Reading Comprehension*. 3rd ed. Austin, TX: PRO-ED; 1995.

178. Torgesen JK, Wagner RK, Rashotte CA. *Test of Word Reading Efficiency*. Austin, TX: PRO-ED, 1999.

179. McGhee R, Bryant BR, Larsen SC, Rivera DM. *Test of Written Expression*. Austin, TX: PRO-ED; 1995.

180. Hammill DD, Larsen SC. *Test of Written Language*. 3rd ed. Austin, TX: PRO-ED; 1993.

181. The Psychological Corporation, *Wechsler Individual Achievement Test,* 2nd ed. San Antonio, TX: The Psychological Corporation; 2001

182. Wilkinson, G., *Wide Range Achievement Test,* 4th ed. Los Angeles, CA: Western Psychological Services; 2004

183. Schrank FA, Mather N, Woodcock RW. *Woodcock-Johnson III(r) Diagnostic Reading Battery*. Rolling Meadows, IL: Riverside Publishing; 2004.

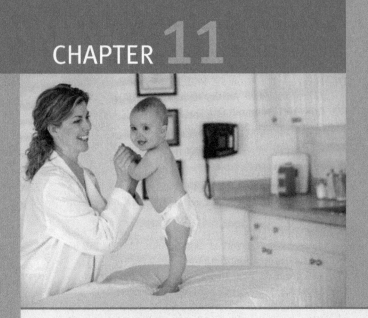

CHAPTER 11

Cerebral Palsy

Deborah Ringdahl, Carolyn Carter, Paul R. Carney, and James D. Geyer

DEFINITION AND EPIDEMIOLOGY

Cerebral palsy (CP) is a general term used for a group of nonprogressive disorders of movement and posture caused by abnormal development of, or damage to, parts of the brain that control muscle movements.[1] The term does not imply severity, cause, treatment, or prognosis. The overall prevalence of the condition ranges from 1.9 to 2.6 of every 1000 live-born children in the Western world.[2] The rate of CP is much higher in preterm versus term infants and increases with decreasing birth weight and gestational age. It increases at the extremes of birth weight across gestational ages.[3] CP is newly diagnosed in approximately 6000 infants and young children every year in the United States. This overall amount has not changed in the last 20 to 30 years, although recent studies suggest that there may be a decreasing trend.[2,4,5]

PATHOGENESIS

CP is caused by events occurring before, during, or after birth up to age 3 years.[6] The etiology is multifactorial. Birth injuries such as hypoxic ischemic encephalopathy, or head injuries after delivery such as those from car accidents, child abuse, falls, or intracranial hemorrhages, can lead to CP. Illnesses such as meningitis in the first few weeks or months of life, or strokes that occur in the newborn period, may result in cerebral palsy. CP is often, but not always, diagnosed in children with congenital cerebral malformations of microcephaly or hydrocephalus. Perinatal asphyxia, intrapartum hypoxia, prematurity, intrauterine growth retardation, intrauterine infection, antepartum hemorrhage, severe placental abnormalities, and multiple pregnancies can all be associated pathologies.[7] Unfortunately, the cause is not always clear.[8]

CLINICAL PRESENTATION

CP is characterized by abnormalities of movement and posture. Young children are often identified with signs of CP when motor milestones are not met. Children may also have increased (stiffness) and/or decreased tone on the motor exam or asymmetries may be found.

These children may show a lack of muscle coordination when performing voluntary movements. A young child may appear *ataxic* when ambulating. *Spasticity* may be noted as the child has stiff or tight muscles in his or her arms and/or legs, exaggerated reflexes, walking with one foot or leg dragging, toe walking, a crouched, or a "scissored" gait, and muscle tone that is either too stiff or too floppy.[9] Common terms used to describe the clinical presentation of CP include static encelphalopathy, spasticity, or developmental delay.[10]

The classification of CP is based on the number of limbs involved and the associated resting tone, or movement abnormalities (Figure 11-1).

Types of Cerebral Palsy

- **Spastic CP**—Most common type accounting for approximately 80%, is due to pyramidal tract lesions with subsequent rate-dependent increase in tone, hyperreflexia, clonus, and an abnormal Babinski reflex.[11] Muscles are stiff, body position may be abnormal, and fine motor control is affected.

- **Dyskinetic CP** (Athetoid CP, dystonic CP, and choreoathetoid CP)—Extrapyramidal signs characterized by involuntary movements such as twisting, jerking, rigid

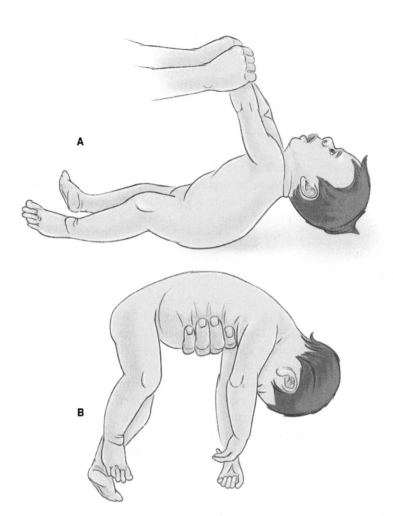

FIGURE 11-1 ■ Delay in motor milestones or abnormal tone may be associated with CP. **(A)** Development of Head Control: At 1 month of age, the head lags after the shoulders, but by 5 to 6 months of age, the child raises the head before the shoulders in the pull-to-sit maneuver. **(B)** Ventral suspension: This drawing shows a normal posture for a 1 to 3 month old held in ventral suspension. The head, hips, and knees are flexed. For an infant 4 months of age or older, this posture would be abnormal as the head, hips, and knees may be extended when held in this manner.

posturing or other movements; increased tone is often present.[11]

- **Ataxic CP**—Abnormal movements involving tremors, unsteady gain, and loss of coordination.
- **Mixed CP**—May have both hyper and hypotonia and there is often a mixture of spastic and dyskinetic components.[6]
- **Hypotonic CP**—Hypotonia in both trunk and extremities with increased reflexes and persistent primitive reflexes; occurs infrequently.[6]

The location usually of impairment falls into one of three broad categories[11]:

- **Hemiplegia**—CP predominantly affecting one side of the body, with the arm usually more impaired than the leg.
- **Diplegia**—CP affecting bilateral lower extremities; arms may be partially involved.
- **Quadriplegia**—CP affecting all 4 extremities (full body).

CP may also be termed mild, moderate, or severe, although there are no firm boundaries.

DIAGNOSIS

Children with CP usually present with a delay in reaching early developmental milestones. The diagnosis of CP depends upon a combination of findings including motor delay, tone abnormalities, weakness, persistence or asymmetry of primitive reflexes, and abnormal postural reactions. A detailed history and thorough physical and neurological examinations are necessary to rule out other potential causes such as progressive neurodegenerative disorders or other inherited or metabolic diseases. It is important to note that these children are not losing motor skills.

Infants with an abnormal obstetric or perinatal history should be monitored closely as they may be at increased risk to develop CP. Potential findings include abnormal behavior such as excessive passivity or irritability, poor feeding and/or sleeping, and poor visual attention. The baby may be hypotonic or hypertonic, have increased tendon reflexes, and clonus. Primitive reflexes such as fisting may be asymmetric or persistent, and postural reflexes may be exaggerated or their disappearance may be delayed. Oromotor skills may be abnormal with tongue retraction and thrust, tonic bite, oral hypersensitivity, and grimacing. Furthermore, achievement of motor milestones should be evaluated. Serial examination of motor milestones can be an effective screening tool for CP.[12,13] It should also be noted that although the damage in CP is nonprogressive, clinical signs develop as the nervous system matures. An absolute diagnosis usually requires repeated examinations and often is not possible until later infancy or early childhood.

Laboratory Tests

No specific studies confirm the diagnosis of CP. Children with unusual components in the history or other abnormalities on physical or neurological examination should be thoroughly evaluated and a metabolic disorder excluded.

Neuroimaging

Imaging studies are useful to identify specific lesions such as periventricular leukomalacia, hydrocephalus, or porencephaly; or developmental abnormalities such as migrational defects or agenesis of the corpus callosum. Magnetic resonance imaging (MRI) of the brain can identify a lesion in the majority of cases of CP and can help determine whether the injury was prenatal, perinatal, or postnatal in occurrence.[14-16] However, a normal MRI does not rule out CP.

Metabolic and Genetic Testing

The American Academy of Neurology and the Child Neurology Society recommend in their practice parameter that metabolic and genetic testing be considered if the clinical history or findings on neuroimaging do not determine a specific structural abnormality, or if there are suggestive or atypical features in the history or clinical examination.[16]

Recommendations

The practice parameter from the American Academy of Neurology and the Child Neurology Society recommends the following approach to the evaluation of the child with CP (Figure 11-2)[16]:

- The diagnosis of CP is based on a comprehensive history and physical examination. It is important to confirm that there is not a progressive or degenerative condition. It is also important to classify the type of CP.
- Screening for developmental delay/mental retardation, ophthalmologic disturbances, hearing impairment,

speech and language problems, and oral-motor dysfunction are advised as part of the initial assessment because these problems are commonly found with CP.
- An EEG is recommended when there are signs or symptoms suggestive of seizures.
- Neuroimaging is advised to establish an etiology and for aiding with prognosis. MRI is preferred to CT scan.
- Metabolic and genetic testing should be considered if evidence of regression or episodes of metabolic decompensation. It should also be considered if an etiology has not been found by the medical work up.

DIFFERENTIAL DIAGNOSIS

CP is a diagnosis of exclusion. It is important that children with signs or symptoms of CP be evaluated for a possible cause. Muscle weakness may be confused for hypotonia diplegia or quadriplegia; may result from inborn errors of metabolism or degenerative disorders dystonia and choreoathetosis from metabolic disorders; and ataxia may arise from genetic abnormalities. Another diagnosis should especially be considered if there is a positive family history of a neurodegenerative disease or inborn error of metabolism, loss of developmental milestones, worsening during times of illness, sensory loss, or hypotonia with muscle weakness.[17] See Table 11-1.

TREATMENT

Every child with CP is different in that no two patients have the exact same impairment so treatment must be individualized as well. All treatment should be targeted at improving function and reducing disability. A multidisciplinary team is necessary to address the many needs including social and emotional development, communication, education, nutrition, and mobility as well as achieving maximal independence in activities of daily living. It is also important to keep appearance as nearly normal as possible.[18]

Treatment of CP may be intervention and preventive based. For example, therapy and the use of adaptive equipment may prevent the patient's spasticity from worsening and evolving to contractures. The goal of most adaptive equipment is focused on preventing tightening of heel cord tendons, preventing scoliosis issues, and preventing bone issues in the non–weight-bearing patient.

Adaptive equipment has the goal of minimizing long-term complications of CP. For example, a footstool at the dining table or in the car can help prevent the "dangling" of feet and helps prevent shortening of the

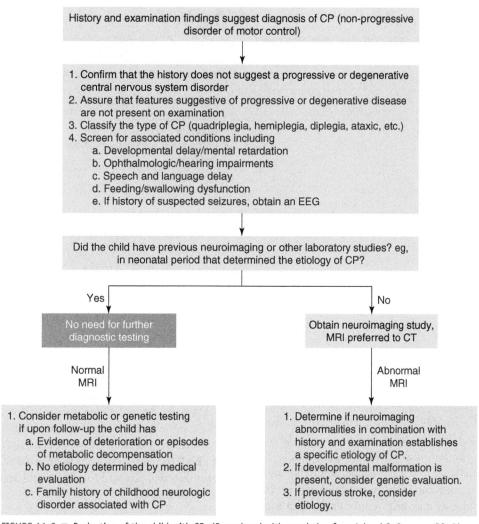

FIGURE 11-2 ■ Evaluation of the child with CP. *(Reproduced with permission from Ashwal S, Russman BS, Blasco PA, et al. Practice parameter:diagnostic assessment of the child with cerebral palsy. Report of the quality standards subcommittee of the American Academy of Neurology and the Practice Committee of the Child Neurology Society. Neurology. 2004;62:851.)[16]*

heel cord tendon. High-top shoes may also keep the foot at a 90-degree angle. The therapist may suggest seating support for feeding or various orthotics. Standers help the non–weight-bearing child to have daily periods of weight bearing. Wheelchairs must be fitted and adapted as the child grows to meet the physical and changing needs. For the child with mild CP, the use of a bicycle is also an excellent source of therapy. Trials of hippo therapy have shown beneficial effects on body structures and functioning.[19]

Many children with CP receive therapy services (Table 11-2) during the school year at school. When summer approaches, many are without therapy. It is important that therapy be maintained throughout the calendar year. In some situations, schools can help the child to have the necessary standers at home during summers and holidays.

Several medications are useful in managing CP (Table 11-3). The most common use of botulinum toxin A (Table 11-4) is for equinous foot deformity.[20] Other uses for BtA include crouched gait, pelvic flexion contractures, cervical spasticity, seating difficulties, and UE deformity. Casting after BtA may be done to assist with maximum stretching of injected tendons.

Table 11-1.

Differential Diagnosis

Neurodegenerative diseases
Inherited metabolic disorders
Developmental lesions of the brain or spinal cord
Traumatic lesions of the brain or spinal cord
Neuromuscular or movement disorders
Neoplasm
Rett syndrome
Hyperkinetic movement disorders

Table 11-2.

Types of Therapy

Physical
Occupational
Speech
Voice box
Dance
Hippo
Swimming
Conductive education
Hyperbaric chamber

Table 11-4.

Four Uses for Botulinum Toxin A[20]

- Balance muscle forces and improve motor function
- Decrease spasticity
- Decrease pain
- Improve self-esteem by diminishing inappropriate motor responses

SURGICAL INTERVENTIONS

Selective Dorsal Rhizotomy

SSDR is the permanent severing of selective dorsal rootlets in the lumbosacral regions (L1-S2). It is thought that cutting these rootlets decreases spasticity or muscle stiffness by inhibiting the muscle stretch reflex. The role of SDR in spastic quadriparesis is to improve hip stability by preventing progressive lateral migration of the femoral head. (If hip instability is untreated, there is up to a 60% risk of painful hip subluxation and dislocation.) SDR in the child with severe spastic quadriparesis may help reduce tone which may also improve the physical care of the child. The role of SDR in spastic diplegia requires thorough investigation. These patients are less affected by their CP and may do well without SDR. The principle impairment of CP is the inability of the patient to effectively be in command of their muscles and this disability persists even after spasticity is removed.[21]

Other issues of treatment include time and money for appointments and therapy. The home requires modification. Schools require modification to meet the needs of the child with a disability. The cost of lost wages and the loss of independence may be devastating for some. The estimated yearly cost to care for children with cerebral palsy is $11.5 billion.[22]

CLOSING COMMENT

The terms neuromotor dysfunction, developmental delay, motor disability, static encephalopathy, and central nervous system dysfunction are less emotional terms in labeling the condition until certain of diagnosis. However, once the diagnosis of CP is made, much can be done to help the individual reach his or her potential. We, as healthcare providers, need to work with the child and family to help them overcome the challenges they will face and to achieve and maintain a rich and rewarding life.

REFERENCES

1. Nelson KB, Ellenberg JH. Epidemiology of cerebral palsy. *Adv Neurol.* 1978;19:421-435.
2. Robertson CMT, Watt MJ, Yasui Y. Changes in the prevalence of cerebral palsy for children born very prematurely within a population-based program over 30 years. *JAMA.* 2007;297:2733-2740.
3. Jarvis S, Glinianaia S, Torrioli MG, et al. Cerebral palsy and intrauterine growth in single births. European collaborative study. *Lancet.* 2003;362:1106-1111.
4. Answers.com. Cerebral Palsy. Available at: http://www.answers.com/ cerebral+palsy&r=67. 2007.
5. Platt MJ, Cans C, Johnson A, et al. Trends in Cerebral palsy among infants of very low birthweight (<1500 g) or born prematurely (<32 weeks) in 16 European centres: a database study. *Lancet.* 2007;369:43-50.
6. eMedicine from WebMD. Cerebral Palsy. Available at: http://www. emedicine.com/NEURO/topic533.htm. 2007.
7. Hankins GD, Speer M. Defining the pathogenesis and pathophysiology of neonatal encephalopathy and cerebral palsy. *Obstet Gynecol.* 2003;102:628.
8. Garne E, Dolk H, Krageloh-Mann I, Ravn SH, Cans C, and SCPE Collaborative Group. Cerebral palsy and congenital malformations. *Eur J Paediatr Neurol.* 2008;12:82-88.

Table 11-3.

Types of Medication

Baclofen—oral versus pump infusion
Valium
Tizanidine
Clonzepam
Botulinum toxin type A (BtA)

9. National Institute of Neurological Disorders and Stroke. Cerebral Palsy Information Page. Available at: http://www.ninds.nih.gov/ disorders/cerebral_palsy.htm. 2007.

10. Rosenblaum P. Cerebral palsy: what parents and doctors want to know. *BMJ.* 2003;326:970-974.

11. Stanley F, Blair E, and Alberman E. Cerebral palsies: epidemiology and causal pathways, in clinics in developmental medicine. London: Cambridge University Press: 2000 p. 14-15.

12. Allen MC, Alexander GR. Using motor milestones as a multistep progress to screen preterm infants for cerebral palsy. *Dev Med Child Neurol.* 1997;39:12.

13. Capute AJ. Identifying cerebral palsy in infancy through study of primitive-reflex profiles. *Pediatr Ann.* 1979;8:589.

14. Truwit CL, Barkovich AJ, Koch TK, Ferriero DM. Cerebral palsy: MR findings in 40 patients. *AJNR.* 1992;13:67.

15. Yin R, Reddihough D, Ditchfield M, Collins K. Magnetic resonance imaging findings in cerebral palsy. *J Paediatr Child Health.* 2000;36:139.

16. Ashwal S, Russman BS, Blasco PA, et al. Practice parameter: diagnostic assessment of the child with cerebral palsy: report of the quality standards subcommittee of the American Academy of Neurology and the Practice Committee of the Child Neurology Society. *Neurology.* 2004;62:851.

17. Miller G. Clinical features and diagnosis of cerebral palsy. http://www.utdol.com/content/cerebralpalsy 2007.

18. Miller G. Management and prognosis of cerebral palsy. http://www.utdol.com/content/cerebralpalsy 2007.

19. Liptak G. Complementary and alternative therapies for cerebral palsy. *Ment Retard Dev Disabil Res Rev.* 2005;11:156-163.

20. Koman A, Smith BP, Balkrishnan R. Spasticity associated with cerebral palsy in children. Guidelines for the use of botulinum A toxin. *Pediatr Drugs.* 2003;5:11-23.

21. Brunstrom JE. Cerebral palsy. Curr Manag Child Neurol. 1999;35:163-168.

22. Centers for disease control: Cerebral Palsy. http://www.cdc.gov/ncbddd/dd/cp3.htm Atlanta, GA 2007.

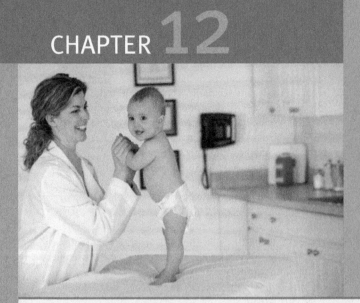

CHAPTER 12

Pediatric Sleep Medicine

Paul R. Carney, James D. Geyer, and Stephenie C. Dillard

DEFINITIONS AND EPIDEMIOLOGY

Pediatric and adolescent sleep disorders are common and often disturbing to either the patient or the family. Sleep disorders can adversely impact physical and mental health. Nonrestorative sleep can hamper a child's ability to concentrate and control emotions and behavior. Sleep disorders vary among age groups, but most can occur with varying frequency at any age. Several disorders are typically seen only during the first 3 years of life, including colic, excessive nighttime feedings, and sleep-onset association disorder. A number of conditions are common during childhood but begin to improve as the child ages. The non-REM sleep parasomnias—including sleepwalking, confusional arousals, and night terrors—are the most common in this category. Nightmares are also common in childhood but can occur at any age.

The sleep-related breathing disorders include obstructive sleep apnea, central sleep apnea, central alveolar hypoventilation syndrome, and Cheyne-Stokes respirations. These disorders can occur at any age, although the treatment options vary by age (Table 12-1).

DISORDERS DURING THE FIRST 3 YEARS OF LIFE

The most frequent sleep-related problem for children between ages 6 months and 3 years is difficulty going to sleep or staying asleep throughout the night.[1] Multiple factors have been implicated in the occurrence of repetitive night waking and inability to fall asleep: infant temperament, nutrition, physical discomfort, mild allergy, and parental marital conflict.[2,3]

Table 12-1.

Pediatric Sleep Disorders

Disorders Occurring During the First 3 Years of Life	Parasomnias	Other Pediatric Sleep Disorders
Sleep-onset association disorder	Restless legs syndrome	Narcolepsy
Difficulties learning to sleep alone	Periodic limb movement disorder	Circadian rhythm sleep disorders
Excessive nighttime feedings	Rhythmic movement disorder	Delayed sleep phase syndrome
Limit setting	REM sleep behavior disorder	Pediatric obstructive sleep apnea
Fear	Sleep terrors	
Colic	Confusional arousals	
	Nocturnal epilepsy	

Sleep-Onset Association Disorder

Clinical features

Complaints of sleep problems in the infant and young child usually come from the parents, not the child. Nighttime awakenings sometimes become worrisome to parents. However, most often the problems reflect certain established patterns of interaction between the parent and the child at time of sleep transition. Nighttime arousals are very common in all ages; however, older children and adults are usually unaware of these disruptions.

Causes/pathogenesis

A parent may incorrectly conclude that nocturnal awakenings are abnormal, becoming involved in the sleep transition process. The child may become accustomed to parental intervention and become unable to make the transition back to sleep alone, creating a sleep problem or sleep-onset association disorder. The child becomes reliant on the parent to help complete the sleep transition regardless of the time of night.

Diagnosis and treatment

Diagnosis is usually made with a careful history. Children with this disorder often rapidly respond to simple gradual behavioral interventions, which helps the child learn a new set of sleep-associated habits.[4]

Difficulties Learning to Sleep Alone

Clinical features

Sleeping alone throughout the night without parental intervention is a learned process. All children wake up 5 to 8 times per night, at the end of each sleep cycle, but some children are able to put themselves back to sleep without parental awareness. Most infants are capable of learning this process from about 5 to 7 months of age.[1]

Diagnosis and treatment

The key is to gradually withdraw the amount of parental involvement at sleep onset. The same parental behavior response is required for middle-of-the-night awakenings. Consistency is also of critical importance if a treatment plan is going to work, especially in conditioning the child to sleep throughout the night. If fear is affecting the progression of this process, it is important to effectively deal with child and/or parental anxiety. Fear can prevent sleep, and fear of safety for one's child can alter a planned behavioral intervention. In certain cases, it will be important to have parents problem solve about their child's fear and how to best accommodate the behavioral treatment plan.

Excessive Nighttime Feedings

Clinical features

Studies have shown that an increase in nighttime awakenings among infants and toddlers may be related to nighttime feedings. Infants fed large quantities at night (8-32 oz) have been shown to have continued and frequent awakenings, ranging up to eight per night.[4-7] Repeated awakenings for ingestion of fluid directly disrupt the functioning of circadian-modulated systems, which may cause further deleterious effects on sleep–wake stabilization.[4,8,9]

Diagnosis and treatment

Diagnosis can be made from a characteristic history: multiple nighttime awakenings, return to sleep only with feeding, significant fluid intake during the night, and extremely wet diapers. Treatment consists of a gradual decrease in the frequency of feedings during the night.[4] Frequent awakenings, three or more per night in a child over 6 months of age, may cause sleep fragmentation that is harmful to the child. As feedings are decreased and associated habits are eliminated over a couple of weeks, sleep consolidation usually promptly occurs.[7]

Limit Setting

Inability to set limits at bedtime can also lead to sleep deterioration. Typical bedtime struggles may consist of requests for water, stories, use of the bathroom, and adjustment of lights.[4,7] A diagnosis of this sort can be made from the history. Through history-taking it may become clear that the parents are unable to enforce nighttime rules with enough consistency to keep the child in bed and quiet so that he or she falls asleep. Parents may have to learn to be firm in their limit setting, enforcing a regular bedtime ritual with an end-point. The child should also be kept in his or her bedroom with the use of a gate of some sort or closure of the door if necessary. Positive behavior modification, such as a sticker, star chart, or other prizes for staying in bed, may elicit a positive response.[4]

Fear

Fear and nightmares are also commonly seen in early childhood, as part of normal development. A truly anxious child at night should be handled in the same manner whether the child's fears were initially expressed during waking or sleep. Mild fears often respond to supportive firmness and a stable social setting. Positive reinforcement, with rewards for staying in bed, may help motivate the child. Treatment may also consist of sleep schedule correction, progressive relaxation,[10] and progressive desensitization.[11]

Colic

Clinical features

Colic is the most common medical condition that affects the sleep of young infants. It causes inconsolable fussiness and crying, typically in the late afternoon and evening. Although symptoms usually remit by 3 to 4 months of age, continuing sleep disturbances are common, secondary to altered sleep schedules and habitual patterns of parental responsiveness.[7]

Diagnosis and treatment

Colic is diagnosed when there are unexplained spells of crying in healthy infants. Treatment mainly focuses around education and management strategies for helping parents cope with the stresses of caring for the infant.[12]

PARASOMNIAS: NOCTURNAL EVENTS

In the course of clinical practice many unusual nocturnal phenomena may be described by patients or parents. The correct diagnosis can usually be ascertained from the clinical history alone, but in some cases polysomnography may be necessary. Additional EEG leads should be used if a seizure disorder is suspected. Additional EMG leads can be useful in patients with movement disorders.

Nocturnal movement disorders are extremely common in the pediatric population. In some cases, these events are so common that they may be considered a normal component of childhood and are usually "outgrown."

Restless Legs Syndrome

Clinical features

Restless legs syndrome (RLS) is a disorder composed of four principal diagnostic criteria:

1. Intense, irresistible desire to move limbs, usually with uncomfortable feeling in the limbs
2. Symptoms worsen with decreased activity
3. Symptoms improve with activity
4. Symptoms are typically worse at night[13]

Patients, especially young children may have difficulty describing the symptoms. Children may get into trouble at school or at home because they have difficulty sitting still. RLS is underdiagnosed or misdiagnosed because of these factors.

RLS may cause significant sleep disturbance, especially with sleep onset. Patients may describe the subjective symptoms of RLS in a number of ways including creepy, crawly, tingly, like worms or bugs crawling under the skin, painful, burning, aching, and electrical. They may have difficulty describing the symptoms. In children, these symptoms can easily be mistaken for "growing pains."

Restless legs syndrome may coexist with periodic limb movements disorder (PLMD, described below) but are not always seen together. A comparison of the two syndromes appears in Table 12-2.

Epidemiology

RLS has an age-adjusted prevalence of up to 10% of adults. It is less common in children and increases with increasing age. The symptom severity also typically worsens with increasing age. Primary RLS is a genetic disorder with an autosomal dominant pattern. Secondary RLS associated with a precipitating factor, is less common. Renal failure, iron deficiency, and diabetes may contribute to the restlessness. In children, growing pains may mimic or cause restless legs.

Evaluation

The laboratory evaluation of RLS includes serum ferritin, screening for uremia, and screening for diabetes. Low normal ferritin levels (20-60) may be associated with RLS and frequently respond to treatment with iron.[14] Polysomnography is not indicated in the evaluation of RLS, unless there is suspicion of a concomitant sleep disorder.

Treatment

Dopamine agonist therapy is the mainstay of RLS treatment in adults. No agents have been FDA approved for treatment of RLS in children. Use of simple nonpharmacological therapies may be of some benefit, including teaching the child to visualize an activity or simply allowing the child to move the legs. Teachers should be informed of the condition and the fact that it is not a form of attention-deficit disorder should be reinforced. Symptoms may be caused by an underlying iron or vitamin deficiency, and supplementing with iron, vitamin B_{12}, or folate (as indicated) may be sufficient to relieve symptoms in these specific cases. A potential treatment algorithm is outlined in Figure 12-1.

Table 12-2.

Comparison Between RLS and PLMD

RLS	PLMD
RLS is a symptom	PLMD are an electromyographic finding
RLS is diagnosed in the physician's office	PLMD are diagnosed in the sleep laboratory
80% of people who have RLS will have PLMs	30% of individuals who have PLMD have RLS symptoms

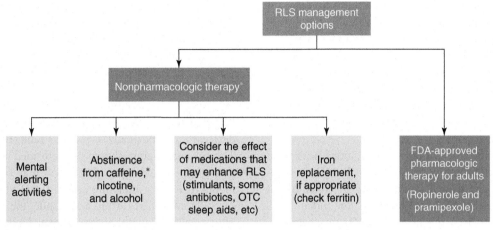

*Extremely important in the control of symptoms in children

FIGURE 12-1 ■ Restless legs syndrome treatment algorithm. Dopamine agonist therapy is FDA approved only for adults and should be considered with caution.

Periodic Limb Movement Disorder

Clinical features

Periodic limb movement disorder (PLMD) is "characterized by periodic episodes of repetitive and highly stereotyped limb movements that occur during sleep."[15] While these movements usually occur in the legs, they can also occur in the arms. There is usually extension of the toe and flexion of the ankle, knee, and hip. Most patients are not aware of the movements. The sleep disruption associated with the movements can lead to insomnia or daytime somnolence. There is a repetitive increase in EMG activity (most often measured over the anterior tibialis muscle) lasting 0.5 to 5 seconds. The movement can be synchronous or asynchronous with the other leg or only involve one extremity. Both legs (and even the arms) should be monitored if PLMD is suspected. The movements are between 5 and 90 seconds apart. Most of the time, the movements occur every 20 to 40 seconds. Four or more consecutive movements are needed to count them as periodic limb movements (PLMs). The PLM index is the total number of PLMs divided by the total hours of sleep. A PLM index over 5 is considered abnormal. Often, PLMs are associated with arousals. A PLM-arousal index may also be noted on the sleep study interpretation. While many assume that the higher the PLM-arousal index, the more likely one is to suffer from daytime sleepiness, this has not been proven.[16]

Individuals with RLS, narcolepsy, and obstructive sleep apnea often have PLMs on a polysomnogram. While all patients with PLMD and most patients with RLS have periodic limb movements on a sleep study, only the RLS patients have the daytime annoying sensations in their limbs that improve with movement. Use of caffeine, neuroleptics, alcohol, monoamine oxidase inhibitors, or tricyclic antidepressants can cause periodic limb movements.

Withdrawal of benzodiazepines, barbiturates, and certain hypnotics can cause or aggravate PLMS. PLMs are reportedly rare in children but increase in prevalence with age. PLMs may be seen in patients who are asymptomatic from them. Inadequate sleep habits, psychophysiologic insomnia, and other causes of daytime tiredness need to be considered and treated before placing a patient on medication for PLMs.

There are a few conditions that mimic PLMs. Sleep starts or hypnic jerks are frequently mentioned by patients. These occur in drowsiness, may be associated with a feeling of falling, and do not recur repetitively throughout sleep. Seizures can cause nighttime kicking movements but may also cause nocturnal enuresis, morning musculoskeletal soreness, or bleeding from oral laceration. An expanded additional 16-lead EEG on the polysomnogram is invaluable in identifying these individuals. Many people with sleep apnea have PLMs that disappear with initiation of effective treatment of the obstructive sleep apnea including surgery or continuous positive airway pressure (CPAP).

Rhythmic Movement Disorder

Clinical features

Rhythmic movement disorder (RMD) "comprises a group of stereotyped, repetitive movements involving large muscles, usually of the head and neck; the movements typically occur immediately prior to sleep onset and are sustained into light sleep" (ICSD (15)). This can manifest as repetitive head banging, leg banging or body rolling. The movements typically start during drowsiness. Movements typically occur at a frequency of 0.5 to 2 times per second. While very common in normal infants, it is sometimes associated with a static encephalopathy, autism, or psychopathology in older children and adults. It is thought to have a self-soothing effect for some individuals. It appears to be more common in males. The noise from the movements can be disturbing to family members. While injuries, even serious injury such as subdural hematoma, are is possible, they are not common. It is very important to have the technologist accurately document what was seen at the time this occurs in the sleep laboratory. Continuous video monitoring usually easily confirms the diagnosis.

The differential diagnoses includes nocturnal seizures, masturbation, bruxism, and PLMD. Nocturnal seizures can usually be diagnosed by concomitant extra 16 channel EEG and review of the video. Masturbation has been mistaken for RMD. Bruxism and PLMD are usually easily distinguished on the sleep study. Gasping respirations from sleep apnea can cause rhythmic movements.

Nocturnal Bruxism

Clinical features

Nocturnal bruxism is "a stereotypical movement disorder characterized by grinding or clenching of the teeth during sleep."[15] This often leads to abnormal destruction of the surface of teeth, which may first be noticed by a dentist. It often causes headaches or jaw and facial pain. Its prevalence has been estimated at 5% to 20% or even higher.[17] It is not uncommon in patients with a static encephalopathy.[18] It occurs equally among males and females. Most people with bruxism are of normal intelligence. While a link has been questioned with anxiety and psychosocial stress, psychological problems are not more common in patients with bruxism. There is a familial tendency toward bruxism. Temporal mandibular joint dysfunction and malocclusion are sometimes accredited as being underlying causes or results of bruxism. There is no guarantee that correction of these abnormalities will cure bruxism in an individual. It can occur in all stages of sleep and is often disturbing to family members. Rhythmic muscle artifact is usually noted on most electrodes placed on the head.

The only significant differential diagnosis is a seizure disorder. Seizure disorders can cause masticatory movements in some individuals. Usually, there is additional history to lead to this diagnosis.

REM Sleep Behavior Disorder

Clinical features

REM sleep behavior disorder (RBD) is characterized "by the intermittent loss of REM sleep electromyographic atonia and by the appearance of elaborate motor activity associated with dream mentation."[15] The patient physically acts out a dream, leading to a variety of movements and actions. Episodes can be violent. It is more common in males. Although it can be seen at any age, it is most prevalent in the sixth and seventh decades, occurring more frequently in patients with Parkinson disease. REM sleep behavior disorder is uncommon in childhood but may be seen in young patients with narcolepsy. The polysomnogram shows episodes of sustained increased muscle tone in REM sleep instead of the decreased tone normally seen at this time (Figure 12-2). The polysomnogram should be preformed with continuous time-locked video. The video may show movements including punching and guttural utterances. If carefully awakened during an episode, the patient can often recall the content of the dream and a reason for the movements can sometimes be ascertained. There is often an increase in NREM periodic limb movements and REM density.

A careful general medical and neurological history is necessary. Tricyclic antidepressants and other anticholinergic medications may lead to RBD symptoms. There are also reports of transient RBD symptoms following hypnotic or alcohol withdrawal. The differential includes nocturnal seizures. Concomitant 16 channel-EEG can be useful in this situation. Another REM-related parasomnia, the nightmare, is sometimes confused with RBD. A nightmare is a frightening dream that often awakens the sleeper. Rarely, striking out can be part of a nightmare. RBD patients tend to be more explosive and usually do not awaken with the frightening aspect so common in a true nightmare. The differential also includes other NREM parasomnias including sleepwalking, confusional arousals, and sleep terrors (Table 12-3).

Sleep Terrors

Clinical features

Sleep terrors are "characterized by a sudden arousal from slow-wave sleep with a piercing scream or cry, accompanied by autonomic and behavioral manifestations of intense fear."[15] There are various autonomic phenomena present including tachycardia, mydriasis, diaphoresis, and flushing. Patients often sit up in bed and scream inconsolably. The facial expression is one of fear. The patient is very difficult to awaken. Once awakened, the person often seems confused. While a dream may be recalled, it is often fragmented and usually makes no sense. The patient is amnestic for the event. It is usually seen between ages 4 and 12 years of age, occurring in approximately 3% of children, but in rare cases may persist into adulthood. Like most NREM parasomnias, it usually disappears in adolescence. It is seen more commonly in males. Other family members may have NREM parasomnias.[19] Sleep terrors begin in slow-wave sleep, usually in the first third of the night, but can happen anytime during the night.

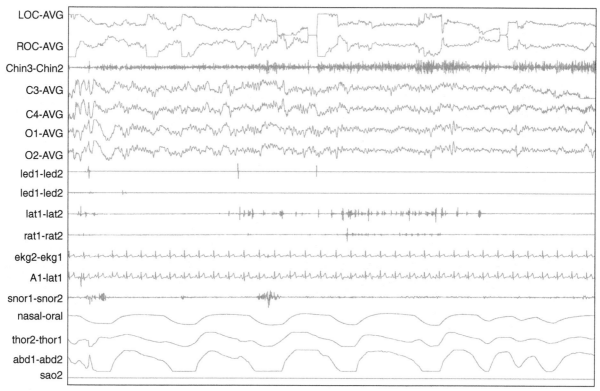

FIGURE 12-2 ■ Sample of a polysomnogram with elevated muscle tone during REM sleep in a patient with REM sleep behavior disorder. *(Reproduced with permission from Geyer JD, Payne TA, Carney PR, Aldrich MS. Atlas of Digital Polysomnography. Philadelphia: Lippincott Williams & Wilkins; 2000:190.)*

Table 12-3.

Parasomnias

	Sleep Terror	Nightmare	Confusional Arousals	Sleepwalking	REM Sleep Behavior Disorder
Prevalence	Uncommon	Common	Uncommon	Common	0.5%; more common in Parkinson, MSA
Sleep stage	SWS	REM	SWS	SWS	REM
Onset	First 90 minutes of sleep	Second half of night	First 1/3 of the night	First 1/3 of the night	Last 1/3 of the night
Features	Intense; vocalization, fear, motor activity	Less intense; vocalization, fear, motor activity	Complex behavior; slow, confused speech	Complex behaviors not limited to walking	Acting out dreams; may be violent; increased EMG tone
Mental content	Sparse	Elaborate	N/A	N/A	
Violent behavior	Common	None	Occasional	Rare	Frequent
Injury	More likely	Unlikely	Rare	Rare	Occasional
Amnesia	Often	Rare	N/A	N/A	N/A
Ability to arouse	Difficult	Easy	N/A	N/A	N/A
On awakening	Confused	Oriented	N/A	N/A	N/A
Treatment	N/A	N/A	Benzodiazepines	Benzodiazepines, TCAs	Clonazepam, carbamazepine

The differential includes nightmares, confusional arousals, and epileptic seizures. When people awaken from nightmares, they are usually clear of mind and often can remember a dream with some detail. While some children can remember an image when awakened from a sleep terror, there is no frightening story such as with a nightmare. Nightmares are more common in the last third of the night, where REM sleep is more concentrated. There are usually fewer autonomic phenomena in a nightmare. If there is a partial arousal during slow-wave sleep, the person often seems stuck in a confused state without the fear seen in sleep terrors. This is called a confusional arousal. These people do not have the autonomic phenomena represented in sleep terrors. Epileptic seizures can present with a cry and the patient can be confused afterward. Ictal fear can be seen in certain epileptic syndromes. Most epileptics do not have seizures solely in sleep. Focal dystonic posturing or tonic–clonic activity points to a seizure as the likely diagnosis. Sometimes, continuous video-EEG monitoring is needed to distinguish a night terror from a nocturnal seizure.

Confusional Arousals

Clinical features

Confusional arousals "consist of confusion during and following arousals from sleep, usually from deep sleep in the first part of the night."[15] Patients may not respond, or may respond inappropriately, and are usually amnestic for the event. Confusional arousals usually arise in the first third of the night from slow-wave sleep. They are sometimes associated with incontinence. Typical of many NREM parasomnias, it is common in young children and it usually disappears with adolescence. While usually seen in children, it can be seen in adults when there is interference with awakening. Examples include sleep deprivation, metabolic encephalopathies, and use of medications that suppress the central nervous system. It is seen equally in both sexes. There is a familial predisposition to NREM parasomnias.

The differential includes sleep terrors, sleepwalking, and nocturnal seizures. Sleep terrors are associated with a frightful scream and more autonomic phenomena such as tachycardia, tachypnea, diaphoresis, and flushing. Sleepwalking is very similar to confusional arousals, except that people do get up and walk with sleepwalking. Most epileptics with nocturnal seizures also have diurnal seizures. Sometimes video-EEG monitoring is needed to distinguish nocturnal seizures from parasomnias.

Treatment

Reassurance for the patient and the patient's family is the most important component of care. In rare cases pharmacotherapy may be necessary. It is recommended that children with confusional arousals and sleepwalking may be safer not using a bunk bed.

Nocturnal Epilepsy

Clinical features

Epilepsy is "a disorder characterized by an intermittent, sudden discharge of cerebral neuronal activity."[15] There has been a growing interest in the relationship between sleep and epilepsy.[20] Almost any seizure type can occur during sleep. In some epileptic syndromes seizures occur primarily during sleep (eg, benign epilepsy with central-temporal spikes or Rolandic epilepsy). The manifestation of the seizure depends on its anatomic origin. Generalized tonic–clonic seizures are associated with loss of awareness, tonic flexion and then extension, a forced expiratory "cry," and then clonic rhythmic jerking of the extremities. Focal (partial) seizures may or may not be associated with alteration of consciousness but are associated with unilateral sensory or motor phenomena. Automatisms consisting of repetitive picking movements or lip smacking may be seen. Seizures may start focally and then secondarily generalize (Figure 12-3). Sleep deprivation, noncompliance with antiepileptic medication, fever, and alcohol can contribute to breakthrough seizures. Epilepsy can be idiopathic or symptomatic of an underlying discernable brain lesion. The lesions could be a tumor, stroke, brain dysgenesis, hippocampal sclerosis, or due to posttraumatic changes. The EEG may show generalized, bilateral, synchronous spike-and-wave activity or generalized polyspike activity in patients with generalized seizures. The EEG often shows focal, regional epileptiform activity including spikes or sharp waves and focal slowing of background activity in patients with focal (partial) seizures. Focal epileptiform activity is more common in NREM sleep and suppressed in REM sleep. Epileptiform activity is much more common in sleep than wakefulness in children with Rolandic epilepsy. A diurnal EEG may be all that is needed to confirm the diagnosis. An EEG after sleep deprivation or overnight continuous video-EEG may be needed in more complicated cases. Sleep deprivation from other sleep disorders such as sleep apnea has been shown to worsen seizures in some patients.

The differential includes nocturnal paroxysmal dystonia, sleepwalking, rhythmic movement disorder,

---

Box 12-1. Common Signs and Symptoms of Nocturnal Epilepsy

Life-threatening
　Falls or injuries
Severe
　Falls or injuries
　Sleepiness
　Effect on family (sleep disruption for others)
Mild
　Effect on school performance
Benign
　The movements or events themselves are often troubling
　　only to the parent

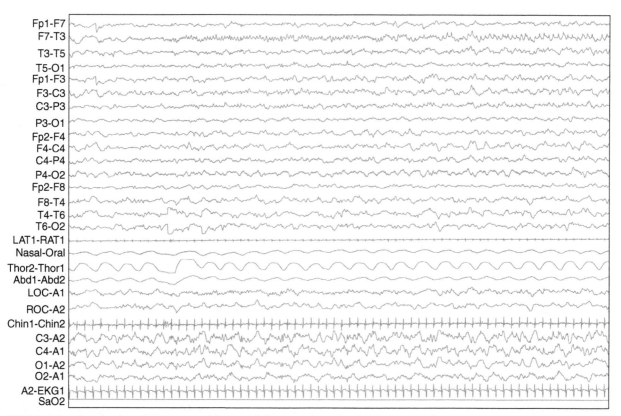

FIGURE 12-3 ▪ Sample of a polysomnogram with a recorded seizure. *(Reproduced with permission from Geyer JD, Payne TA, Carney PR, Aldrich MS.* Atlas of Digital Polysomnography. *Philadelphia: Lippincott Williams & Wilkins; 2000:204.)*

and REM behavior disorder. Nocturnal paroxysmal dystonia occurs in a short form (15-60 seconds) and a longer form (up to 60 minutes). It is characterized by repeated stereotypical dyskinetic episodes of ballismus or choreoathetosis often associated with vocalizations in NREM sleep.[21] Sleepwalking, rhythmic movement disorder, and REM behavior disorder are not associated with epileptiform activity.

Narcolepsy

Clinical features

Narcolepsy is a disorder of excessive sleepiness with a loss of control of the boundaries between sleep and wakefulness. The classic tetrad of symptoms (see Table 12-4) defining narcolepsy includes (1) excessive daytime sleepiness, (2) cataplexy, (3) sleep paralysis, and (4) hypnapompic or hypnagogic hallucinations.[15] A minority of patients, between 10% and 15%, will actually have the entire tetrad of symptoms. Excessive sleepiness is the most common symptom. Sleep attacks, sudden and unpredictable episodes of severe sleepiness or sleep, are less common but can result in serious accidents and injury.

Cataplexy is a loss of muscular tone elicited by emotion, including laughing, excitement, anger, fear, and so forth. Cataplexy occurs in 76% to 80% of narcoleptic patients. The degree of weakness is variable, but weakness at the knees is the most common complaint.

Extraocular muscles are typically spared, though blurred vision may occur. The episodes of weakness typically last a few seconds to greater than 30 minutes.

Sleep paralysis is the sudden onset of paralysis at sleep onset or at awakening. Patients are awake and conscious during the event. These episodes are of variable duration but typically last between several seconds and 10 minutes. Patients are able to move following any tactile stimuli. Sleep paralysis occurs in approximately 50% to 80% of narcoleptics.

Hypnogogic (sleep onset) and/or hypnopompic (awakening) hallucinations are typically bizarre or frightening dreams. The dreams consist primarily of visual hallucinations but in rare cases may include vestibular

---

Box 12-2. Common Signs and Symptoms of Narcolepsy

Life-threatening
    Falls or injuries
Severe
    Falls or injuries
    Sleepiness
    Effect on family
    Effect on school performance
    Cataplexy
Mild
    Sleep paralysis
    Hypnagogic/hypnapompic hallucinations

Table 12-4.

Features of the Classic Narcolepsy Tetrad

Feature	Duration	Age at Onset	Occur (%)
Excessive daytime sleepiness (EDS)	Continuously, with exacerbations	Typically teens–30s but may occur earlier	100
Cataplexy	Seconds–minutes	Typically after EDS	60-70
Hypnagogic/hypnapompic hallucinations	Minutes	Teens	30-60
Sleep paralysis	Minutes	Teens	25-50

symptoms, auditory hallucinations, and a sense of levitation. These hallucinations occur in approximately 67% of narcoleptic patients (Table 12-4).

Nocturnal sleep disruption is common with repeated awakenings and frightening dreams. Patients are typically light sleepers despite being very sleepy during the day. REM behavior disorder is more common in narcoleptics than the general population.

Epidemiology

Narcolepsy occurs in approximately 1 in 2000 persons and peaks in the second decade of life. Subtle symptoms may be present much earlier. Parents often refer the child with narcolepsy as having been a "sleepyhead" as a young child. There is no significant gender difference for narcolepsy but there is a significant ethnic difference, with the disorder occurring more frequently in Japan. Monozygotic twins are discordant for narcolepsy. Eighty-six percent of narcoleptics with definite cataplexy have HLA DQB1-0602 on chromosome 6, but greater than 99% of patients with these haplotypes are normal. Orexin or hypocretin may also be involved in narcolepsy.[22]

Treatment

Several treatment options are available—see Table 12-5. Treatment of the excessive sleepiness is vital to improve daytime function and school performance. Modafinil (Provigil) is a pro-alerting drug that is FDA approved for the treatment of narcolepsy in adults and can dramatically improve daytime sleepiness. If modafinil proves ineffective, traditional stimulants such as methylphenidate and dextroamphetamine may also be of benefit. Xyrem is also FDA approved for cataplexy and narcolepsy in adults. In an off-label use, tricyclic antidepressants are also quite effective for cataplexy.

Circadian Rhythm Sleep Disorders

For optimal sleep and alertness, desired sleep time and wake times should be synchronized with the timing of the endogenous alertness promoting circadian rhythm. Misalignment between the circadian timing system and the 24-hour physical environment or work and social schedules can result in symptoms of insomnia and excessive daytime sleepiness. Circadian rhythm sleep disorders arise when the physical environment is altered relative to the internal circadian timing system, such as in jet lag and shift work, or when the timing of endogenous circadian rhythms is altered, such as in circadian rhythm sleep phase disorders. The latter is thought to occur predominantly because of chronic alterations in the circadian clock or its entrainment mechanisms (Figure 12-4). This chapter focuses on this second group of disorders.

Delayed Sleep Phase Syndrome

Clinical features

Delayed sleep phase syndrome (DSPS) is characterized by bedtimes and wake times that are usually delayed 3 to 6 hours relative to desired or socially acceptable sleep/wake times. The patient typically cannot fall asleep before 2 to 6 AM and has difficulty waking up earlier than 10 to 1 PM.[23,24] Attempts to advance the sleep times are frequently unsuccessful. Patients with DSPS often report feeling most alert in the evening and most sleepy in the early morning.[25] In general, individuals with DSPS seek treatment or are brought in for treatment because enforced socially acceptable bedtimes and wake-up times result in insomnia, excessive sleepiness, and functional impairments, particularly during the morning hours.[23]

Clinical epidemiology

DSPS is probably the most common of the primary circadian rhythm sleep disorders.[26] The prevalence of DSPS among adolescents and young adults is 7% to 16%.[23,27] It is a relatively common cause of the presenting symptom of insomnia in this age group.[24]

Table 12-5.

Medications Used to Treat Excessive Daytime Sleepiness of Narcolepsy (not FDA-Approved for Children)

Drug	Typical Initial Dose	Half-Life (hr)	Selected Side Effects
Pemoline (Cylert)	18.75-37.5 mg qd	12 (adults)	Hepatitis, liver failure
Methylphenidate* (Ritalin)	10-30 mg bid or tid	2-4	Nervousness, tremulousness, headache, palpitations
Methylphenidate SR† (Concerta)	18 mg SR qam	8-12	Same
Medidate ER	20 mg		
Dextroamphetamine* (Dexedrine, Dextrostat, and others)	5-30 mg qd to bid	10-30	Nervousness, tremulousness, headache, palpitations
Dextroamphetamine* (SR preparation)	10 mg		Palpitations
Methamphetamine* (Desoxyn)	5-20 mg qd to bid	12-34	Nervousness, tremulousness, headache, palpitations
Selegiline (Eldepryl)	20-40 mg	9-14	Nausea, dizziness, confusion, dry mouth‡
Modafinil* (Provigil)	200-400 mg qd	10-12	Headache, drug interactions, nervousness

*Schedule II medication.
†SR, slow release.
‡FDA-approved for treatment of narcolepsy in adults.

Alcohol and excessive caffeine may be used to self-treat in order to cope with symptoms of insomnia and excessive sleepiness, which in turn, may exacerbate the underlying circadian rhythm sleep disorder.

There is a family history present in approximately 40% of individuals with DSPS. The DSPS phenotype occurs as an autosomal dominant trait.[28]

Diagnostic evaluation

The diagnosis of DSPS relies largely on the clinical history. However, diagnostic studies such as actigraphy and sleep diaries can be very useful to confirm the delayed sleep phase pattern. Recordings of sleep diaries and actigraphy over a period of at least 2 weeks demonstrate delayed sleep onset and sleep offset, with sleep onsets typically delayed until 2 to 6 AM and wake-up times in the late morning or early afternoon. Daily work or school schedules may result in earlier than desired wake time during weekdays, but a delay in bedtime and wake-up time is almost always seen during weekends and while on vacation. Polysomnographic (PSG) parameters of sleep architecture, when performed at the natural

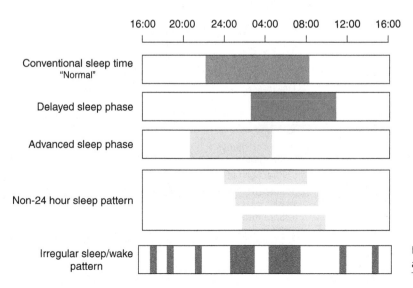

FIGURE 12-4 ■ Depiction of the phase shifts associated with various circadian rhythm disorders.

delayed sleep times, are essentially normal for age. However, if a conventional bedtime and wake-up time is scheduled, PSG recording will show prolonged sleep latency and decreased total sleep time.

Clinical management

Approaches aimed at resetting circadian rhythms include chronotherapy and timed bright light therapy. Chronotherapy is a treatment in which sleep times are progressively delayed by approximately 3 hours per day until the desired earlier bedtime schedule is achieved.[29] Although effective, the length and repeated nature of treatment and need for adherence to restrictive social and professional schedules limit practicality in the clinical setting. However, in adolescents, in whom behavioral factors often contribute to the delayed sleep phase, chronotherapy in conjunction with enforcement of regular sleep and wake times are important components of the clinical management.

Exposure to bright light for 1 to 2 hours in the morning results in an advance of the phase of circadian rhythms, whereas evening light exposure causes phase delays. Therefore, bright light exposure during the early morning hours and avoidance of bright light in the evening have been shown to be effective treatments for DSPS.[30] Following 2 weeks of exposure to 2 hours of bright light of 2500 lux each morning and restricted evening light, individuals with DSPS showed earlier sleep times and reported improved morning alertness level. However, many patients, particularly those who are severely delayed, find it difficult to awaken earlier for the 1 to 2 hours of bright light therapy. Despite the potential utility of bright light therapy, the necessary timing, intensity, and duration of treatment are not known. Exposure to broad spectrum light of 2000 to 10,000 lux for approximately 1 to 2 hours is generally recommended for use in clinical practice.

Pediatric Obstructive Sleep Apnea

Epidemiology

The prevalence of pediatric obstructive sleep apnea (OSA) is estimated at 2% to 4% for children between the ages of 2 and 18.[35,36] Obstructive apnea is very uncommon in normal children. In the past, obstructive sleep apnea was primarily seen in patients with significant adenotonsillar hypertrophy or neurological impairment.[37] More recently, pediatric sleep apnea has been associated with the obesity epidemic in children.

The symptoms of obstructive sleep apnea in children differ from those seen in adults. Although daytime sleepiness and fatigue are reported in children, behavioral problems, hyperactivity, and neurocognitive deficits are much more common in children with sleep apnea compared to normal controls.[38]

Diagnosis

Pediatric OSA can be confirmed with polysomnography. The severity of OSA has been defined by use of AHI criteria alone. There are inherent problems with such an approach, most notably that there are substantial differences in how different sleep laboratories define respiratory events. This problem becomes more pronounced in the pediatric population. The criteria are different than adults, with an apnea index of > 1/hr considered abnormal.

In children, a cessation of airflow of any duration (usually 2 or more respiratory cycles) is considered an apnea when the event is obstructive.[35-39] Of note, the respiratory rate in children (20-30/min) is greater than in adults (12-15/min). The obstructive apnea hypopnea index (AHI) > 1 is considered abnormal in children as opposed to 5 in adults (Figure 12-5). There is usually a mild decrease in the arterial oxygen desaturation.

The significance of central apnea in older children is less certain than in infants. Most do not consider central apneas following sighs (big breaths) to be abnormal. Some central apnea is probably normal in children, especially during REM sleep. In one study, up to 30% of normal children had central apneas. Central apneas longer than 20 seconds or those of any length associated with arterial oxygen desaturation below 90% are often considered abnormal, although a few such events have been noted in normal children.[38] Therefore, most would recommend observation unless the events are frequent and the arterial oxygen desaturations severe.

There is a shortage of sleep laboratories that can accommodate children. Other potential screening techniques have not proved successful thus far. Therefore, in a child with behavioral problems, hyperactivity, or daytime sleepiness, a polysomnogram should be considered,

Box 12-3. Common Signs and Symptoms of Pediatric Obstructive Sleep Apnea
Life-threatening
Falls or injuries
Cardiac rhythm changes
Severe
Falls or injuries
Sleepiness
Effect on family (sleep disruption for others)
Effect on school performance
Mild
Sore throat
Dry mouth
Benign

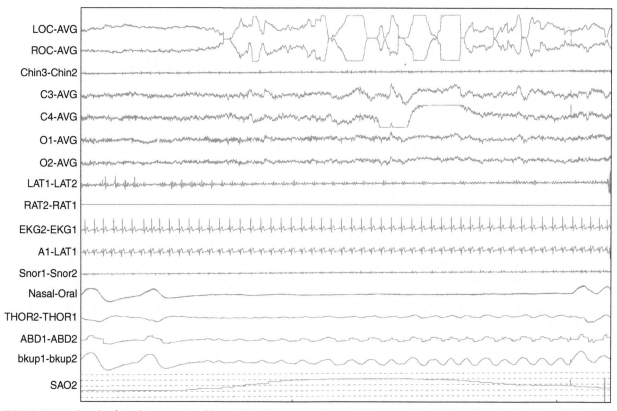

FIGURE 12-5 ▪ Sample of a polysomnogram with an obstructive apnea and associated oxygen desaturation. *(Reproduced with permission from Geyer JD, Payne TA, Carney PR, Aldrich MS. Atlas of Digital Polysomnography. Philadelphia: Lippincott Williams & Wilkins; 2000:102.)*

especially if obesity, tonsillar and/or adenoidal hypertrophy, or other upper airway anatomic abnormalities are present.

Treatment

In contrast to adults, the treatment of choice for the majority of pediatric OSA cases is adenotonsillectomy. There are some specific groups who are at increased risk for postoperative morbidity: children < 3 years of age; severe OSA; and those with underlying medical disorders. Weight loss and nasal CPAP are also used in pediatric OSA for those cases who do not improve after adenotonsillectomy or are not surgical candidates. Craniofacial surgeries are also an option in selected children with anatomic abnormalities.

Box 12-4. When to Refer to a Sleep Specialist

Evaluation of possible OSA
Evaluation of possible narcolepsy
Refractory parasomnias (after initial management by
 primary care)
Refractory insomnia or DSPS (after initial management by
 primary care)

REFERENCES

1. Anders TF, Halpern LF, Hua J. Sleeping through the night: a developmental perspective. *Pediatrics.* 1992; 90:554-560.
2. Beltramini AU, Hertzig ME. Sleep and bedtime behavior in preschool-aged children. *Pediatrics.* 1983;71:153-158.
3. Dahl DE. The development and disorders of sleep. *Advan Pediatr.* 1998;45:73-90.
4. Anders TF, Eiben LA. Pediatric sleep disorders: a review of the past 10 years. *J Am Acad Child Adolesc Psychiatry.* 1997;36:9-20.
5. Carskadon MA. Patterns of sleep and sleepiness in adolescents. *Pediatrician.* 1990;17:5-12.
6. Ferber R. Introduction: pediatric sleep disorders medicine. In: Ferber R, Kryger M, eds. *Principles and Practice of Sleep Medicine in the Child.* Philadelphia: Saunders; 1995:1-5.
7. Ferber R. Assessment of sleep disorders in the child. In: Ferber R, Kryger M, eds. *Principles and Practice of Sleep Medicine in the Child.* Philadelphia: Saunders; 1995:45-53.
8. Beal VA. Termination of night feeding in infancy. *J Pediatr.* 1969;75:690-692.
9. Zuckerman B, Stevenson J, Bailey V. Sleep problems in early childhood: continuities, predictive factors, and behavioral correlates. *Pediatrics.* 1987;80:664-671.
10. Ferber R. Sleeplessness in children. In: Ferber R, Kryger M, eds. *Principles and Practice of Sleep Medicine in the Child.* Philadelphia: Saunders; 1995:79-89.

11. Van Tassel EB. The relative influence of child and environmental characteristics on sleep disturbances in the first and second years of life. *J Develop Behav Pediatr.* 1985;6:81-86.

12. Richman N. A community survey of characteristics of one- to two-year-olds with sleep disruptions. *J Am Acad Child Adolesc Psychiatry.* 1981;20:281-291.

13. Ferber RA. *Solve your Child's Sleep Problems.* New York: Simon & Schuster; 1985.

14. Ferber RA. Sleeplessness, night awakening, and night crying in the infant and toddler. *Pediatr Rev.* 1987;9:69-82.

15. *The International Classification of Sleep Disorders, Revised.* Rochester, MN: Davies; 1997.

16. Mendelson WB. Are periodic leg movements associated with clinical sleep disturbance? *Sleep.* 1996;19:219-223.

17. Glaros AG. Incidence of diurnal and nocturnal bruxism. *J Prosthet Dentistry.* 1981;45:545-549.

18. Richmond G, Rugh JD, Dolfi R, Wasilewsky JW. Survey of bruxism in an institutionalized mentally retarded population. *Am J Ment Deficiency.* 1984;88:418-421.

19. Kales A, Soldatos CR, Bixler EO, et al. Heriditary factors in sleepwalking and night terrors. *Br J Psychiatry.* 1980; 37:111-118.

20. Bazil CW, Malow BA, Sammaritano MR. *Sleep and Epilepsy: The Clinical Spectrum.* Amsterdam: Elsevier Science; 2002.

21. Provini F, Plazzi G, Lugaresi E. From nocturnal paroxysmal dystonia to nocturnal frontal lobe epilepsy. *Clin Neurophysiol.* 2000;111(suppl 2):S2-S8.

22. Oka Y, Inoue Y, Kanbayashi T, et al. Narcolepsy without cataplexy: 2 subtypes based on CSF hypocretin-1/orexin-A findings. *Sleep.* 2006;29:1439-1443.

23. Regestein QR, Monk TH. Delayed sleep phase syndrome: a review of its clinical aspects. *Am J Psychiatry.* 1995; 152:602-608.

24. Czeisler CA, Richardson GS, Zimmerman JC, et al. Entrainment of human circadian rhythms by light-dark cycles: a reassessment. *Photochem Photobiol.* 1981;34:239-247.

25. Horne JA, Ostberg O. A self-assessment questionnaire to determine morningness-eveningness in human circadian rhythms. *Int J Chronobiol.* 1976;4:97-110.

26. Yamadera H, Takahashi K, Okawa M. A multicenter study of sleep-wake rhythm disorders: clinical features of sleep–wake rhythm disorders. *Psychiatry Clin Neurosci.* 1996;50:195-201.

27. Pelayo R, Thorpy MJ, Govinski P. Prevalence of delayed sleep phase syndrome among adolescents. *Sleep Res.* 1988;17:392.

28. Ancoli-Israel S, Schnierow B, Kelsoe J, et al. A pedigree of one family with delayed sleep phase syndrome. *Chronobiol Int.* 2001;18:831-840.

29. Weitzman ED, Czeisler CA, Coleman RM, et al. Delayed sleep phase syndrome. A chronobiological disorder with sleep-onset insomnia. *Arch Gen Psychiatry.* 1981;38:737-746.

30. Chesson AL Jr., Littner M, Davila D, et al. Practice parameters for the use of light therapy in the treatment of sleep disorders. Standards of Practice Committee, American Academy of Sleep Medicine. *Sleep.* 1999;22:641-660.

31. James SP, Sack DA, Rosenthal NE, et al. Melatonin administration in insomnia. *Neuropsychopharmacology.* 1990; 3:19-23.

32. Moldofsky H, Musisi S, Phillipson EA. Treatment of a case of advanced sleep phase syndrome by phase advance chronotherapy. *Sleep.* 1986;9:61-65.

33. Schrader H, Bovim G, Sand T. The prevalence of delayed and advanced sleep phase syndromes. *J Sleep Res.* 1993; 2:51-55.

34. Reid KJ, Chang AM, Dubocovich ML, et al. Familial advanced sleep phase syndrome. *Arch Neurol.* 2001; 58:1089-1094.

35. Redline S, Tishler P, Schluchter M, et al. Risk factors for sleep-disordered breathing in children: associations with obesity, race and respiratory problems. *Am J Respir Crit Care Med.* 1999;159:1527-1532.

36. Guilleminault C, Korobkin R, Winkle R. A review of 50 children with obstructive sleep apnea syndrome. *Lung.* 1981;159:275-287.

37. Ali N, Pitson D, Stradling J. Sleep disordered breathing: effect of adenotonsillectomy on behaviour and psychological functioning. *Eur J Pediatr.* 1996;155:56-62.

38. Rosen C. Clinical features of obstructive sleep apnea hypoventilation syndrome in otherwise healthy children. *Pediatr Pulmonol.* 1999;27:403-409.

39. Geyer JD, Payne TA, Carney PR, Aldrich MS. *Atlas of Digital Polysomnography.* Philadelphia: Lippincott Williams & Wilkins; 2000.

General Neurologic Disorders

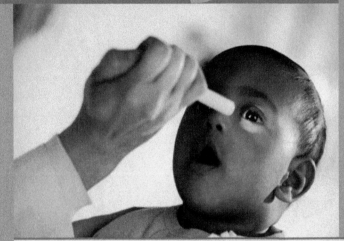

CHAPTER 13

Movement and Balance Disorders

Harrison C. Walker, Leon S. Dure IV, and Ray L. Watts

Although large-scale epidemiologic studies are lacking, pediatric movement disorders are relatively common. Many movements that are brought to clinical attention are transient and may be associated with normal development. Additionally, the natural history of specific disorders varies and must be interpreted in the context of a child's developmental stage. A careful history, physical examination, and direct observation of the movements in question are critical for diagnosis and management of pediatric movement disorders (Table 13-1). Factors that should prompt consideration of more significant underlying neurological disorder include the progression of symptoms, a family history of a heritable neurological disease, complications during childbirth, a failure of the child to reach developmental milestones, and significant functional impairment. Serological tests, electroencephalography, and imaging studies may contribute in unusual cases, but in the majority of cases it is the clinical impression of the treating physician that drives both diagnosis and treatment of pediatric movement disorders.

Movement disorders can be broadly classified based upon whether they are hyperkinetic or hypokinetic. Hyperkinetic disorders involve excessive involuntary movements, including tics, chorea, myoclonus, dystonia, and tremor. Hypokinetic disorders manifest with bradykinesia (paucity or slowness of movement) and rigidity (abnormal muscle stiffness), as can be seen in parkinsonism. In contrast to adults, the overwhelming majority of movement disorders in children are hyperkinetic. In a tertiary pediatric neurology movement disorders practice, Fernandez-Alvarez and Aicardi reported tics (39%), dystonia (24%), tremor (19%), chorea (5%), myoclonus (3%), akinetic-rigid syndromes (2%), and mixed disorders (8%) out of a sample of 684 children.[1]

This chapter will focus on the most common types of movement disorders encountered in pediatric neurology practice, emphasizing correct identification and appropriate initial management.

Table 13-1.

History and Physical Exam

History
Birth history
Developmental history
Location of symptoms
Rate of onset of symptoms (acute, subacute, chronic?)
Frequency of symptoms (normal function between paroxysms?)
Change in symptoms over time
Perceived disability level
Functional deficits (writing, dressing, gait)
Family history of neurological symptoms
Effects of physical activity on symptoms
Perception of illness/symptoms
Associated neurological symptoms
Associated psychiatric comorbidities

Physical Exam
Spontaneous activity
Cranial nerve exam
Deep tendon reflexes
Strength in all extremities
Sensory exam
Muscle tone
Dexterity
Rest, postural, and action tremor
Gait

DEFINITIONS AND EPIDEMIOLOGY

Tics are sudden, rapid, nonrhythmic repetitive movements or vocalizations, usually in the presence of an otherwise normal neurological exam. Most experts regard tic disorders along a spectrum of disease from transient tic disorders, characterized by the presence of simple tics that spontaneously resolve, to Tourette syndrome (TS), a chronic disorder featuring both motor and vocal tics. Since the overall incidence of tics may be as high as 20% in the school-age population,[2] the development and resolution of a simple tic in a child could almost be considered a part of normal development. Tic disorders are five times more common in boys than in girls, and the median age of onset is 5 to 6 years.[3] Recent epidemiologic studies suggest that approximately 3% of school-age children meet the diagnostic criteria for Tourette syndrome.[4-7]

Virtually any voluntary movement can manifest as a tic. Simple tics may include eye-blinking or squinting, facial grimacing, licking the lips, head jerking, shoulder shrugging, spasms of the abdominal wall, or rapid arm movements. Complex tics involve more formed or stereotyped movements, such as touching, smelling, shaking, hair combing, or jumping. Vocalizations often include grunting, coughing, throat-clearing, and in a minority of cases, repetition of words (echolalia), screaming, or outbursts of profanities (coprolalia).[8] In contrast to other paroxysmal movement disorders, such as stereotypy and myoclonus, tics characteristically migrate from one area of the body to another over time (Table 13-2). Tics have been described as being "suppressible yet irresistible," illustrating how patients may disguise the abnormal movements in public settings, only later to relieve the accumulated urge to perform tics at a higher frequency in private. However, this phenomenon of a "rebound" has come into question with

work specifically examining tics after a period of suppression.[9]

Patients who have either motor or vocal tics satisfy the diagnostic criteria for chronic tic disorder or transient tic disorder, depending upon whether or not the symptoms resolve within 12 months of onset. The DSM-IV criteria for Tourette syndrome require both motor and vocal tics, which do not have to occur simultaneously; a duration of greater than 3 months; onset before age 18; and resultant disability. Additionally, the symptoms must not be explained by drug exposure, or another medical condition such as Huntington disease, cerebral palsy, pervasive developmental disorder, or encephalitis.

Importantly, Tourette syndrome is associated with various behavorial syndromes, including attention deficit–hyperactivity disorder (approximately 50% of TS patients), oppositional-defiant disorder, conduct disorder, rage, obsessive-compulsive symptoms, and depression.[10-13] These potential comorbidities can cause disability, which in many cases is more important to address than the tics themselves. Patients with TS are said to have obsessive compulsive behaviors (OCBs) rather than obsessive compulsive disorder (OCD) per se, because patients with TS seldom meet the DSM IV criteria for that diagnosis.[14]

Stereotypy is in the differential diagnosis of a suspected tic disorder. Motor stereotypies are relatively complex, seemingly purposeful, stereotyped movements, generally of the arms, head, face, or neck. Examples of stereotypy may include recurrent raising or lowering of the arms, flapping of the hands, thumb-sucking, body-rocking, and head-banging. Although stereotypies can be severely disabling if they are sufficiently intrusive or violent, they usually do not interfere with daily function. Characteristically, stereotypies are triggered by

Table 13-2.

Paroxyms of Movement

Paroxysm	Duration	Suppressible	Migratory	Evolution
Tic	Brief	Yes	Yes	Tics may change and migrate within an individual patient
Stereotypy	Brief	Yes	No	None
Tremor	Often intermittent, but repetitive and sustained when present	Sometimes, when mild	No	May progress to other limbs or become more constant; should not completely change in character
Myoclonus	Very brief	No	Yes	Variable
Chorea	Brief	No	Usually	None

excitement, fatigue, or anxiety. The majority of the literature on stereotypy describes such movements in the context of developmental disorders such as autism and Rett syndrome or cases of congenital blindness, although they can occur in developmentally normal children.[15-18] Unlike tics, stereotypies do not migrate among different locations nor do the movements themselves evolve significantly over time; and in a study by Mahone and associates, the age of onset of stereotypies in 90% of patients was younger than 3 years.[19] Despite this, it may be difficult in some situations to distinguish among complex tics, obsessive compulsive behaviors, and stereotypies, and differentiating these entities may be important, as the pharmacotherapies for tic disorders and obsessive compulsive disorders are different, and there have been no well-designed treatment studies of stereotypies.

Tremor is a rhythmic, repetitive movement oscillation of one or more limbs or of the head. Tremor typically involves alternating contractions of agonist and antagonist muscle groups. Tremor may occur at rest or during posture and action. Rest tremor is very uncommon in children. It is assessed with the patient seated with the arms and legs at rest. Having the patient close his or her eyes or introducing a distraction such as a cognitive task can reveal latent subclinical rest tremor or exacerbate baseline rest tremor. Postural tremor is assessed with the arms extended in front of the patient or with the patient holding a cup of water in the hand. Action tremor may be demonstrated by finger to nose testing or by mimicking drinking or using a spoon or fork.

Both action and postural tremor are common manifestations of essential or familial tremor, which is likely the most common type of tremor in children. As the name implies, familial tremor is often genetic and transmitted in an autosomal dominant manner, although penetrance is variable, and typical essential tremor (ET) can occur sporadically. Despite intense investigations, the identification of a gene associated with familial tremor has remained elusive, supporting a role for multiple gene interactions contributing to the phenotype. Although often characterized as a disease of senescence, reports by Lou and Jankovic and Louis and associates underscore that essential tremor can have childhood onset.[20,21] Hornabrook and Nagurney reported adults with essential tremor had a childhood onset in 4.6% of cases.[22] Childhood-onset essential tremor is phenomenologically similar to essential tremor in adults, although there is evidence that childhood-onset ET may be more common in boys than in girls.[23] ET only rarely causes significant disability in the pediatric population, and many of the children with more severe tremor likely gravitate toward hobbies or professions with which the tremor does not interfere.

Another type of tremor that may be noted in children is enhanced physiologic tremor. A recognizable example of enhanced physiologic tremor can be appreciated upon attempting to write immediately after intense physical activity. The emergent tremor is an exaggeration of typically minimal oscillatory motor activities.[24,25] Physiologic tremor may be enhanced by hypoglycemia, pheochromocytoma, thyrotoxicosis, alcohol withdrawal, valproate, lithium, theophylline, corticosteroids, adrenergic agonists, and other medications, and it can also result from intense emotional or physical stress. The disability associated with enhanced physiologic tremor primarily involves very fine hand movements such as writing or repairing a watch. The elimination of exacerbating factors can be very helpful, although some patients may have persistent difficulties and benefit from propranolol prior to such activities.

Some additional tremor syndromes should be mentioned. Jitteriness of infancy is relatively common and usually resolves within the first few hours of life. More prolonged jitteriness may result from drug withdrawal or hypoxic-ischemic encephalopathy, and the tremulousness in these cases almost always resolves within one year.[26,27] Geniospasm (hereditary chin trembling) refers to a rapid, repetitive chin tremor and is regarded as an ET variant, as it tends to cluster in families.[28,29] Shuddering attacks are benign, brief episodes that occur in infants or young children. These spells have the appearance of shivering with no accompanying loss of consciousness, and they typically last no more than 5 to 7 seconds. The attacks may occur multiple times per day, and shuddering spells may be difficult to diagnose by history and clinical examination alone, because they are seldom observed during a clinic visit. A home videotape recording or video EEG will usually facilitate the diagnosis.[30,31] Like geniospasm, shuddering attacks have been considered an early manifestation of ET, as some patients with the attacks have primary relatives with ET.

Although debilitating tremor in children is rare, it usually is associated with other neurological abnormalities such as traumatic brain injury, cerebral palsy, or an underlying degenerative, genetic, or metabolic syndrome. These causes of tremor in children are far less common than essential tremor or enhanced physiologic tremor, and they are often much more difficult to manage medically than more common forms of tremor. A large-amplitude, proximal "wing-beating" tremor may suggest the diagnosis of Wilson disease, particularly if it is accompanied by hepatic dysfunction, dystonia, parkinsonism, and/or psychiatric abnormalities. The so-called Holmes tremor (or rubral tremor) is caused by an interruption of the dentatorubrothalamic tract, usually by trauma or by a demyelinating disease in the midbrain in or around the red nucleus. This tremor arises from interruption of the dentatothalamic outflow tract from the cerebellum to the thalamus and then to motor areas of the cerebral cortex. Rubral tremor is a debilitating, large-amplitude, proximal, low-frequency tremor (2-3 Hz) that characteristically is present both at rest and with posture and action.

Cerebellar tremor can range greatly in severity, but it characteristically presents as an action tremor that increases in amplitude as the target is approached during finger-to-nose testing. Other associated cerebellar findings may include dysarthria, a wide-based, unstable gait; and in severe cases, dysfunction of the cerebellar vermis may result in truncal ataxia, which renders the patient unable to sit up without assistance. Cerebellar tremor may be seen as a result of postinfectious cerebellitis, such as is seen in association with varicella zoster infection.[32] Most cases of postviral cerebellitis improve significantly over time; however, a minority of patients are left with persistent disability. Lesions in the posterior fossa from trauma or a neoplasm should be considered in children with the new onset of cerebellar dysfunction, particularly considering that posterior fossa tumors are the most common type of solid tumor in childhood.[33] The most common genetic form of cerebellar ataxia is Freidreich ataxia. The genetic basis of the disease is a triplet expansion of the nucleotide sequence of cytosine, adenine, and guanine (CAG) in the protein *frataxin*; in addition to ataxia, patients also develop peripheral neuropathy, corticospinal tract signs, and dysarthria.[34] The mutation is carried in one out of 30,000 to one out of 50,000 persons, and it is inherited in an autosomal recessive fashion. Other genetic causes of ataxia are more rare and beyond the scope of this text, but have been described more extensively elsewhere.[35,36]

Dystonia is a hyperkinetic involuntary movement disorder in which twisting, writhing movements that produce abnormal postures occur at rest and/or with action, often associated with co-contraction of agonist and antagonist muscle groups. These involuntary movements are slower, with the muscle contractions typically lasting a second or more. The definition of dystonia is complicated by the fact that it refers to a group of symptoms rather than a specific disease, and aspects of dystonia may be present in the context of other neurological abnormalities. Any patient who develops the acute onset of dystonia with no prior history should raise the suspicion of an acute dystonic reaction from antiemetics such as metoclopramide or from a neuroleptic medication. Another cause of acute dystonic movements in early childhood is Sandifer syndrome, in which dystonic postures occur after the intake of food, usually in association with a hiatal hernia or gastroesophageal reflux.[37,38]

Dystonic movements are usually stereotyped within and across patients. Characteristic dystonic postures in children may include arching of the back or neck with or without kyphosis or scoliosis, a flexed or "spooned" appearance of the hand, or curling or pointing of the toes during walking. In general, dystonia is worsened by voluntary movements and lessened by a lack of movement or by distraction, and although the dystonic postures may appear uncomfortable, pain may not be a prominent complaint.[39-43] During the execution of motor tasks, patients with dystonia may exhibit "overflow," in which additional muscle groups are involuntarily recruited, often interfering with the performance of the task. An important characteristic of dystonia that can often aid in its identification is the "sensory trick," which patients use to temporarily alleviate their dystonic movements. A sensory trick involves initiating somatosensory contact in the region of the body affected by dystonia, such as placing a finger on the chin in a patient with spasmodic torticollis or touching the lateral aspect of the orbit in a case of blepharospasm, the result of which is the temporary alleviation of the dystonic movement or posture. In children, the sensory trick may actually be performed by the parent.

Dystonia may be subclassified by the distribution of the body regions affected or by the age of onset of symptoms (eg, juvenile vs. adolescent). By definition, children have childhood-onset dystonia, and they tend to develop generalized dystonia, which typically begins in a lower extremity and spreads to other parts of the body. This underscores that the symptoms of children with idiopathic torsion dystonia are often driven by genetic or metabolic factors, such as the mutation of the protein *torsin A* in cases of DYT-1 dystonia.[42] Focal dystonias, in contrast, affect a single part of the body. Unlike children, adults with the new onset of dystonia are more likely to develop a focal dystonia of the face or neck, and the symptoms are not likely to generalize to other parts of the body over time. Focal dystonias seldom occur in isolation in children; however, it is useful to identify focal dystonia syndromes, as they individually can form the constituents of a segmental or generalized dystonia phenotype. Some focal dystonias commonly seen in adults, such as blepharospasm (repetitive eye-blinking) and task-specific dystonias (writer's cramp or musician's cramp), are rarely seen in children; but other focal dystonias, such as cervical dystonia (torticollis) and opisthotonus, are seen in pediatric populations. Cervical dystonia involves twisting, turning movements of the muscles of the neck (eg, torticollis or retrocollis), and opisthotonus refers to a particularly severe abnormal extension posture of the neck and cervicothoracic spine.

Dystonia is often associated with other neurological symptoms and/or disorders. Secondary dystonias in children may occur in association with cerebral palsy or other causes of spasticity, lesions of the basal ganglia, and with the effects of medications. It is estimated that dystonia is the primary abnormality in as many as 15% of patients with cerebral palsy.[39] Although cerebral palsy is regarded as a static condition present since birth, secondary dystonia associated with spasticity can progress as the nervous system matures,[40] and a similar evolution of dystonia secondary to upper motor lesion can be observed in adults following stroke and traumatic brain injury.[44] Some have referred to dystonic or choreoathetoid cerebral palsy as being nonprogressive but everchanging, to emphasize how the dystonia phenotype may evolve over time. Wilson disease is a rare but treatable autosomal recessive cause of dystonia and parkinsonism secondary to abnormal copper metabolism, and it usually begins in childhood or early adulthood.

Dystonic tremor refers to the irregular tremor that sometimes accompanies dystonic movements. It has a lower frequency and a more irregular quality than essential tremor or parkinsonian tremor, and it is often exacerbated by certain postures, such that it can appear to be an attempt to return the affected body part to a more normal position. In addition to its association with spasticity and tremor, generalized dystonia may be associated with myoclonus. Some cases of myoclonus-dystonia have been associated with mutations in the protein *epsilon sarcoglycan* (DYT-11).[45] Hemidystonia refers to dystonia present only on one side of the body. Hemidystonia, particularly when it is progressive, is suggestive of secondary dystonia related to a structural lesion (often in the contralateral striatum), and should prompt consideration of neuroimaging.[46]

Chorea ("to dance") is a hyperkinetic movement disorder in which the involuntary movements are irregular, brief, migratory, purposeless, and unsuppressible. Chorea often involves the proximal limbs, the neck, or the trunk. The superimposition of chorea upon voluntary movements has been described as being "dance-like." Analogous to benign tics, chorea has been described as a manifestation of normal development in some children, and a piano-playing movement with the arms outstretched ("chorea minima"), is present in many children in a general pediatric clinic.[47] The most common cause of pathologic chorea in children is Sydenham chorea (SC). It constitutes one of the major criteria in the clinical definition postinfectious rheumatic fever and is associated with prior group A beta-hemolytic *Streptococcus* infection. The choreatic movements observed in this disorder classically form part of the triad of chorea, emotional lability, and hypotonia.[48] Presumably, the hyperkinetic movements in SC are driven by molecular mimicry between antigens on the *Streptococcus* and the basal ganglia, which are both targeted by antineuronal antibodies.[49] Most commonly, Sydenham chorea remits spontaneously within a year, although there are reports of chronic SC and reemergence of chorea during pregnancy (chorea gravidarum).[50]

Other potential causes of chorea include so-called choreoathetoid cerebral palsy, medication side effects (secondary to digoxin, valproate, or pemoline),[51-53]

metabolic derangements such as hypoparathyroidism, and electrolyte imbalances. Benign hereditary chorea is rare, but it is usually inherited in an autosomal dominant fashion. The specifics of the family history are very important in such cases, as chorea may be associated rarely with the development of juvenile Huntington disease, although that disease usually presents with dystonia and parkinsonism in children, as described below.

Spasticity is associated with upper motor neuron lesions. An upper motor neuron lesion results from damage to neurons or tracts anywhere rostral to the alpha motor neuron in the ventral spinal cord. On examination, there is characteristically "clasp-knife" or velocity-dependent hypertonia, in which the examiner can detect a change in muscle tone comparing slow and fast rates of passive extremity movement. In spasticity, increased muscle tone is detected at fast rates of passive movements relative to slow rates of passive movement. In children, spasticity is most commonly caused by cerebral palsy, although any upper motor neuron lesion (eg, from brain trauma or stroke) can result in spasticity. Associated examination findings in spastic hypertonia include brisk reflexes, a Babinski sign (an extensor response), ankle clonus, upper extremity extensor weakness, and lower extremity plantar ankle and dorsiflexion weakness (Table 13-3). Ankle clonus is demonstrated by briskly dorsiflexing the ankle, which evokes a rhythmic, continuous oscillating flexion–extension movement, analogous in some ways to tremor. Weakness, in addition to the hypertonicity associated with the spasticity itself, is often the most important cause of disability in these patients, in contrast to patients with a primary dystonia syndrome. In some cases of spasticity, it is the preservation of lower extremity extensor strength that permits a spastic gait ("scissor gait"). As mentioned above, dystonia and spasticity may coexist in a patient, complicating the evaluation, and there is an increasing appreciation of overlapping features between pyramidal (upper motor neuron) and extrapyramidal (basal ganglia) disorders of movement.[43,54]

Myoclonus is a very rapid, jerking, hyperkinetic movement disorder of the limbs, which is often bilateral. Myoclonus is stereotyped, repetitive, and unsuppressible. Myoclonus may originate from the cerebral cortex, brainstem, or spinal cord, and its differential diagnosis is extensive.[55] Myoclonus in isolation in a child is not necessarily an ominous sign. The occurrence of myoclonus immediately after birth or in the neonate is benign and almost always resolves spontaneously.[56,57] Nocturnal myoclonus is a normal variant that is very common in the general population. Additionally, myoclonus may be noted with metabolic derangements or in association with medications. Opsoclonus-myoclonus syndrome is characterized by rapid, involuntary, chaotic conjugate movements of the eyes, accompanied by myoclonus. The eye movements can be horizontal, vertical, or rotatory, and they are

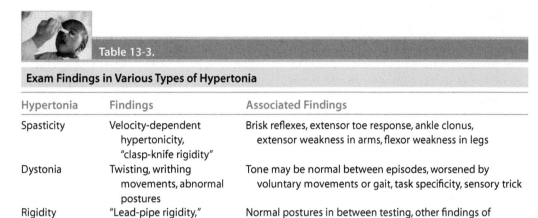

Table 13-3.

Exam Findings in Various Types of Hypertonia

Hypertonia	Findings	Associated Findings
Spasticity	Velocity-dependent hypertonicity, "clasp-knife rigidity"	Brisk reflexes, extensor toe response, ankle clonus, extensor weakness in arms, flexor weakness in legs
Dystonia	Twisting, writhing movements, abnormal postures	Tone may be normal between episodes, worsened by voluntary movements or gait, task specificity, sensory trick
Rigidity	"Lead-pipe rigidity," malleability	Normal postures in between testing, other findings of parkinsonism, "cogwheeling" if rest tremor is present

often accompanied by oscillopsia, or the sensation the world is moving. Like Sydenham chorea, opsoclonus-myoclonus is thought to be autoimmune in origin, and more than half of the pediatric patients with opso-clonus-myoclonus syndrome have underlying neuro-blastoma.[58] Other potential associations with opsoclonus may include parainfectious encephalitis, systemic diseases such as celiac disease or AIDS, side effects of medications, or toxins. Myoclonus can also be an associated finding in a variety of neurological syndromes including myoclonus dystonia (DYT-11) and certain forms of epilepsy (juvenile myoclonic epilepsy, Lennox-Gastaut syndrome); therefore, the occurrence of other neurological abnormalities in addition to myoclonus should prompt consideration of such an underlying diagnosis.

Akinetic-rigid syndromes from primary neurological disorders are very rare in children with movement disorders. Parkinsonian syndromes are characterized by muscle rigidity, bradykinesia (slow movements), rest tremor, postural instability, and decreased facial expression. Movements typically are slower and become more difficult with repetition. In all cases, a thorough history and review of the medication records should be undertaken to rule out neuroleptic use, metoclopramide use, or possible ingestion of medications taken by other family members. Although rare, there are juvenile-onset parkinsonian syndromes usually associated with a predominance of dystonia, and these syndromes are generally driven by genetic or metabolic abnormalities, some of which may involve the interruption of normal dopamine synthesis. Examples include dopa-responsive dystonia/parkinsonism (DYT-5), also known as Segawa disease or dystonia with diurnal variations. Juvenile Parkinson disease and Juvenile Huntington disease (HD) both cause early onset of dystonia and parkinsonism as well. A large proportion of cases of levodopa-responsive juvenile parkinsonism are attributed to alterations in both copies of the gene *parkin* (ie, autosomal recessive).[59] In contrast to adult-onset Huntington disease, juvenile HD usually presents initially with dystonia and

bradykinetic-rigid parkinsonism rather than isolated chorea.[60]

CLINICAL PRESENTATION

A detailed history and neurological examination are the most important components of the evaluation of a patient with a movement disorder. Many movement disorders wax and wane over time or consist of paroxysms, but specific questioning almost always reveals that their onset and evolution are gradual. Acute or subacute onset of a movement disorder in a child suggests that a potentially reversible medication reaction, a metabolic abnormality, or structural lesion may underlie the symptoms.

Movement disorders must be distinguished historically from other causes of neurological dysfunction, such as seizures, neuromuscular disease, or normal variants. Seizures, in contrast to movement disorders, are commonly preceded by an aura, and are usually associated with alteration of consciousness and postictal confusion. Most movement disorders worsen during situations of anxiety or emotional stress, and primary movement disorders only rarely occur during sleep. Relevant details about the delivery of the child and the attainment of developmental milestones must be obtained, and the family history can be very useful in diagnosing both common and rare pediatric movement disorders. In particular, tic disorders along with their behavioral comorbidities and essential tremor are commonly familial, so history and even a brief physical examination of available family members can often be helpful.

Distinguishing pathologic movements from transient, benign abnormalities of movement in children can sometimes be challenging, and the history alone may be insufficient in such cases. Patients with abnormal movements are occasionally evaluated with video electroencephalography; however, families now commonly have portable video cameras, and viewing the activity recorded in the home situation usually is sufficient to make a diagnosis. In particular, video recordings can be invaluable in children who are able to suppress the movements in question while in the clinical setting.

Assessing the movements of a child often requires a great deal of patience on the part of the clinician. The examination of any movement disorder should begin with passive observation while the patient and family are providing the details of the history. The child's level of spontaneous activity should be noted, as well as any hyperkinetic involuntary movements. Vocal tics, in particular, may appear as throat clearing or other easily disguised sounds, and prior to diagnosis, these manifestions of a tic disorder may be misconstrued by the family as upper respiratory symptoms or reflux. The examination of sensory function, complex motor tasks, and higher cognitive function can be unreliable in children, particularly considering their age and developmental history, further underscoring the need for a history of attainment of various developmental milestones.

In many patients, the evaluation of gait is the most important part of the neurological examination, because walking is an important functional measure requiring the integration of multiple neurological subsystems. Specific gait patterns can suggest whether the underlying disorder is hypo- or hyperkinetic, or whether dystonia or spasticity are present. Patients with parkinsonism characteristically take small, shuffling steps with stooped posture and freezing of gait, whereas patients with cerebellar disorders or severe peripheral proprioceptive loss may walk with a wide-based ataxic gait. Dystonic movements and postures are frequently exacerbated or exposed during walking and other voluntary movements.

Despite the importance of classifying movement disorders into one of the categories described previously (tremor, tics, myoclonus, and so forth), such categorization can occasionally be difficult, and in some cases, even experienced movement-disorder clinicians may not agree on the classification of the movement. Comments and some suggested guidelines for the neurological examination of movement disorders are included in Table 13-4.

Table 13-4.

Potential Manifestations of Movement Disorders in the Neurological Examination

Exam Section	Comments
Spontaneous activity	Note the overall level of activity and any spontaneous movements. Observation often provides as much information as any other modality, as cooperation with some aspects of the exam may be limited.
Cranial nerve exam	Transient end-gaze nystagmus is a normal variant. Persistent end-gaze nystagmus or nystagmus in primary gaze may suggest inner ear dysfunction, or less commonly a brainstem or cerebellar lesion. Note the velocity of saccadic eye movements and whether or not there are saccadic pauses or overshoot. Opsoclonus consists of random, chaotic, conjugate eye movements.
Deep tendon reflexes	Elevated in spasticity from upper motor neuron lesions, diminished in peripheral nerve lesions. Normal in basal ganglia and cerebellar disorders.
Muscle tone	Muscle tone must be assessed independent of limitations caused by resistance at the joint, such as from contractures or other orthopedic issues. The patient is instructed to relax. The examiner observes muscle tone at baseline and then with passive flexion and extension of the elbow, wrist, knees, and ankles. Tone is classified as being hypotonic (abnormally loose), normal, or hypertonic (abnormally stiff). Decreased muscle tone or hypotonia is most commonly a manifestation of peripheral nervous system or cerebellar dysfunction. Increased muscle tone or hypertonia may result from spasticity, rigidity, dystonia, or in some cases, a combination of factors.
Rest tremor	Observe tremor of the arms, legs, or head at rest. Subclinical rest tremor or very mild rest tremor can be elicited by distraction or by having the patient perform a mentally stressful task with the eyes closed. Predominant rest tremor is very uncommon in children.
Postural tremor	Assessed with the upper limbs extended and outstretched for a period of time in front of the patient. Postural tremor can also be assessed holding an object like a glass of water in a stationary position.
Action tremor	Assessed by finger-to-nose testing or by imitating the use of an eating utensil. Having the patient write his or her name, write some sentences, and draw an Archimedes spiral provide useful objective information that can be stored in medical record for later reference.
Dexterity	Repetitive tapping of the index finger to the thumb, hand opening and closing, rapid alternating movements of the forearms, and foot/leg tapping on the floor are tests of dexterity. Complex motor tasks may be difficult to assess in very young or less cooperative children.
Gait	Observe for toe walking or worsening of postures seen at rest in dystonia. Shuffling gait may be observed in parkinsonian conditions. Postural instability is specifically associated with parkinsonism, but gait dysfunction can result with dysfunction of multiple neurological systems, and warrants evaluation by a specialist.

DIFFERENTIAL DIAGNOSIS

Table 13-5 contains different classifications of movement disorders in children and potential differential diagnoses within each category. The list is not meant to be exhaustive, but rather to point out the most common diagnostic entities, and to highlight other rare, specific entities that should be considered.

Table 13-5.

Differential Diagnosis of Pediatric Movement Disorders

Tics
    Transient tic disorder
    Chronic tic disorder
    Tourette syndrome
    Medication-induced tics
Stereotypy
Dystonia
    Primary
        Idiopathic torsion dystonia
        DYT-1 dystonia (Oppenheim dystonia, autosomal dominant)
        DYT-3 dystonia (X-linked Filipino dystonia)
        DYT-5 dystonia (Segawa disease, dopa-responsive dystonia)
        DYT-11 dystonia (myoclonus dystonia)
    Secondary
        Wilson disease
        Pantothenate kinase-associated neurodegeneration
        Juvenile Huntington disease
        Juvenile parkinsonism
        Mitochondrial disease
        Machado–Joseph disease
        Ataxia telangiectasia
    Acquired/Other
        Hypoxic encephalopathy
        Stroke
        Encephalitis
        Trauma
        Tumor
        Neuroleptic drugs
        Conversion disorder/psychogenic
Tremor
    Enhanced physiologic tremor
        Lithium
        Valproate
        Theophylline/caffeine
        Glucocorticoids
        Adrenergic agonists
        Stress/physical exertion
        Hyperthyroidism
        Drug withdrawal
    Benign tremor variants
        Geniospasm
        Shuddering spells
        Jitteriness of infancy
    Essential tremor
    Cerebellar tremor
        Postinfectious
        Structural lesions
        Friedreich ataxia/genetic diseases
        Vitamin E deficiency
        Celiac disease
    Dystonic tremor
    Psychogenic tremor
Chorea
    Primary
        Benign hereditary chorea (autosomal dominant)
        Juvenile Huntington disease
    Secondary
        Cerebral palsy
        Sydenham chorea
        Hyperthyroidism
        Hypoparathyroidism
        Hypocalcemia
        Hyper- or hyponatremia
        Medications
Spasticity
    Cerebral palsy
    Demyelinating disease
    Other conditions affecting upper motor neurons
Myoclonus
    Benign infantile myoclonus
    Nocturnal myoclonus
    Epilepsy syndrome (JME, LGS)
    Post-anoxic myoclonus
    Metabolic abnormalities
    Medications and drug withdrawal
Akinetic-rigid syndromes
    Dopa-responsive dystonia/parkinsonism
    Juvenile parkinsonism
    Juvenile Huntington disease
    Neuroleptic medications and antiemetics (metoclopramide)
    Carbon monoxide toxicity
    Manganese toxicity
    Anticonvulsants

DIAGNOSIS

Diagnostic Testing

The neurological history and examination leading to classification of the movements in question may indicate that specific laboratory or radiographic studies are necessary to narrow the differential diagnosis. This being said, the results of extensive laboratory or imaging studies often do not add to the clinical evaluation, as such studies are often normal in patients with movement disorders. In particular, patients with both Tourette syndrome and straightforward cases of essential tremor do not necessarily require further blood tests or imaging studies. As mentioned previously, home video footage of the patient's abnormal movements can be invaluable in making the diagnosis. Video EEG may be helpful in some cases, as an abnormal EEG is not expected in patients with movement disorders; however, a normal EEG does not necessarily rule out seizures. Unexplained focal neurological signs elicited by the history and neurological exam should prompt consideration of imaging studies. The new onset of idiopathic dystonia requires imaging of the brain and cervical spinal cord to rule out mass lesions, although studies in patients with dystonia as an isolated feature are unlikely to be revealing.

All patients with young-onset dystonia or parkinsonism should undergo 24-hour urine collection for copper, serum ceruloplasmin measurement, and an ophthalmologic slit-lamp examination for Kayser–Fleischer rings in the cornea to rule out Wilson disease, as it is a very rare but treatable cause of these symptoms.[61] Older patients with Wilson disease may present with neurological manifestions only, with subclinical hepatic disease to progress later. Pediatric-onset cases, in contrast to adults, more often present with hepatic dysfunction alone, which may make the diagnosis more challenging. Only 2% of patients who have neurological symptoms of Wilson disease will not have Kayser–Fleischer rings on slit lamp examination.

Despite the myriad genetic causes of generalized dystonia, routine genetic testing may not be recommended unless the diagnosis of dystonia is in question, particularly if the result of the test will not impact clinical management. In appropriate cases, DYT-1 testing is recommended as an initial screening test, since the well-characterized DTY-1 mutation is the most common genetic cause of generalized limb-onset dystonia ("Oppenheim dystonia"). DYT-1 mutations have variable penetrance, so the absence of family history of dystonia does not necessarily exclude it as a diagnostic possibility.

MRI should be considered for de novo movement disorders, particularly when there are concomitant focal abnormalities on the neurological exam such as spasticity, focal weakness, or other abnormalities not explained historically or with prior investigations. Acute or subacute onset of symptoms, in particular, suggests a potentially reversible etiology such as an electrolyte disturbance or adverse effects of medications. Routine screening for electrolyte abnormalities, thyroid dysfunction, vasculitides, the anti-phospholipid syndrome, and vitamin B_{12} or vitamin E deficiencies are recommended in appropriate cases.

INITIAL MANAGEMENT

Once the movements in question have been classified and a diagnosis made, initial management must focus on the objective level of disability, the family's perception of the patient's illness, and the family's expectations from therapy. Many patients with mild tics, tremor, or chorea do not develop significant functional disability from the abnormal movements themselves. In these cases, an appreciation of the natural history of the disease in question, that a partial response to pharmacotherapy should be expected, and caveats about common adverse effects from the specific medications are important. With this knowledge, families may be less inclined initially towards pharmacological interventions. Although the abnormal movements are frequently a source of embarrassment or irritation, establishing a diagnosis and counseling the patient on the nature of the disease are critical. Simply having the patient respond to peers who mention the symptoms, saying "I have tics" or "I have tremor," may in many cases begin the process of education. Encouraging the family to develop a supportive, understanding environment for the child at home and among peers is invaluable. Subsequent education of school teachers and peers by the family can also be extremely helpful, since acceptance by others contributes greatly to a child's sense of wellness. In patients who have persistent, disabling symptoms requiring pharmacotherapy, it should be mentioned that no drugs have been formally approved by the FDA for the treatment of pediatric movement disorders. Common practice is to initiate therapy at the lowest dose possible and slowly increase the dose over time while assessing the response to treatment. The maintenance dose should be the lowest dose that provides adequate clinical efficacy.

For more severe **tic disorders**, if patients choose medical therapy, the natural history of tics is to wax and wane over time, and this can complicate the evaluation of response to therapy.[64] Patients frequently improve spontaneously after they reach the state of symptomatic worsening that prompted their initial medical evaluation, simply as a manifestation of the natural ebb and flow of the disease rather than some specific response to a medication. Target symptoms should be identified prior to the initiation of treatment, and patients should not leave the clinic with the expectation that their tics will be eliminated completely. No single pharmacological therapy has been shown to be universally effective for tic disorders; however, a number of agents have been investigated in randomized clinical trials.[65] Initial management is often attempted with a presynaptic alpha-2 antagonist, such as clonidine or guanfacine. Adverse effects from treatment may include somnolence, depression, hypotension, and dry mouth. Other potential choices for therapy include haloperidol or atypical neuroleptics. These latter medications are not generally chosen as first-line agents, because of potential adverse effects including sedation, weight gain, acute dystonic reaction, parkinsonism, and, rarely, tardive dyskinesia. Numerous other medications have been advocated for the medical treatment of tic disorders including calcium channel blockers, buspirone, and antidepressants. Dopamine-depleting medications such as tetrabenazine have been reported to be effective for tics in Europe, but use of this agent has been limited in the United States.[66] It should be emphasized again that concomitant obsessive-compulsive behaviors, ADHD symptoms, and depression may actually cause more disability than the tics in Tourette syndrome; therefore addressing these comorbidities with a multidisciplinary approach and serotonin reuptake inhibitors may be extremely helpful in such cases. Stimulants such as dextroamphetamine should be used judiciously in patients with ADHD symptoms, since stimulant medications have been reported to exacerbate tic disorders; however, more recent studies suggest this may not be the case.[67]

Similar to tic disorders, pharmacotherapy for children with **tremor** may not be necessary after careful consideration of the patient's level of disability. Various medical therapies can be attempted for tremor disorders. Propranolol and primidone are traditional first-line agents for essential treatment, but like tic disorders, complete resolution of the tremor is an unrealistic expectation, and a balance between therapeutic effects of medications and possible side effects such as somnolence and depression must be achieved. Evidence is now available for the use of topiramate for moderate to severe essential tremor in adults.[68]

Chorea must be assessed carefully clinically prior to treatment since the hyperkinetic movements may not be a cause of significant disability. Symptomatic treatment with neuroleptics, anticonvulsants, or with dopamine-depleting agents such as reserpine or tetrabenazine are often effective, but potential benefits of therapy must be weighed against potential adverse effects such as somnolence, depression, parkinsonism, and in the case of neuroleptics, tardive dyskinesia. In cases of chorea associated with autoimmune disease, corticosteroids, intravenous immunoglobulin, or plasmapheresis may be considered, but again considering the natural history of the chorea in SC, many patients with mild symptoms may not require treatment.[69]

All patients with young-onset dystonia or parkinsonism should be treated initially with levodopa, as the symptoms of some patients with Segawa disease (dopa-responsive dystonia) normalize completely with modest doses of levodopa supplementation. Other syndromes may be caused by dysfunction in the enzymes responsible for the metabolic conversion of precursor amino acids into catecholamines in the substantia nigra pars compacta, and guidelines are available for performing lumbar puncture to diagnose neurotransmitter deficiencies including Segawa disease, tyrosine hydroxylase

deficiency, and aromatic acid decarboxylase deficiency, if clinical suspicion of such a disorder is present.[63] Another diagnostic test that may be considered in addition to a therapeutic levodopa trial is the phenylalanine loading test.[63] This assay nonspecifically measures the function of the enzymatic pathway that converts phenylalanine to tyrosine, and it may be useful in cases of dopa-responsive dystonia in which clinical or genetic tests are unrevealing or ambiguous. An abnormal phenylalanine loading test shows prolonged elevation phenylalanine and little or no rise in tyrosine following loading. Interestingly, patients with confirmed dopa-responsive dystonia do not develop the motor complications of levodopa therapy seen in idiopathic Parkinson disease in adults, such as peak-dose dyskinesias and the "wearing off" phenomenon.

The pharmacological treatment of **dystonia** depends on the etiology of the symptoms. Acute onset of dystonia from neuroleptic medications or antiemetics requires cessation of the offending medication and intravenous treatment with an anticholinergic such as benztropine or diphenhydramine and a subsequent benzodiazepine, if needed. Every child with **idiopathic dystonia** or **parkinsonism** should undergo a trial of levodopa to rule out dopa-responsive dystonia. Even children with dystonic cerebral palsy may have a dopamine-responsive element to their symptoms, and the response to therapy may not be immediate.[70] Excessive doses of levodopa, however, are generally not necessary to provide symptomatic benefit. Generally, the first-line agent for **focal, segmental,** or **generalized dystonia** following a levodopa trial is an anticholinergic. Children may be able to tolerate remarkably high doses of anticholinergics, in particular, and response rates in open label studies have been reported to be as high as 60% with trihexyphenidyl.[71] Additional agents may be tried including baclofen, benzodiazepines, and amantadine, and some patients may respond to combinations of therapies based upon trial and error. Paroxysmal dystonias and dyskinesias may respond preferentially to anticonvulsant medications such as carbamazepine.[72–74]

Deep brain stimulation (DBS) has not been rigorously studied in large populations of pediatric patients; therefore, DBS in children should only be considered for severe, refractory disease in experienced tertiary centers. Appropriate young adults with severely debilitating, medically refractory dystonia or essential tremor should be considered for DBS,[75,76] and neurostimulation of the internal segment of globus pallidus, in particular, is very effective for symptoms of severe idiopathic torsion dystonia. More recently DBS has been promoted for refractory Tourette syndrome in adults; however, such an invasive therapy will not be indicated in the vast majority of children with tics, as their symptoms are expected to resolve or improve significantly over time.[77,78] Any invasive procedure in the central nervous system carries with it initial risk, but once successfully implanted, deep brain stimulation for dystonia or tremor in many severe cases is superior to medical therapy and can greatly improve quality of life.

INDICATIONS FOR CONSULTATION OR REFERRAL

Most pediatric patients with movement disorders would be well-served by at least an initial screening visit with a pediatric neurologist or pediatric movement disorders specialist to confirm the diagnosis and suggest options for therapy. However, in the initial stages of a mild tic or tremor disorder, immediate referral to a pediatric movement specialist may not be necessary. Indications for referral include complex cases associated with significant disability, patients where the diagnosis is unclear, and cases in which therapy has been unsuccessful or patients want a thorough discussion of therapeutic options. Occasionally the diagnosis of movement disorders requires longitudinal follow-up. Following the evaluation, a therapeutic strategy can be agreed upon by the clinician and family, and depending upon a variety of factors including disease severity, response to initial attempts at therapy, and practical issues such as distance from the consulting physician's practice, the patient could follow-up with either the referring physician or with the movement disorders specialist.

REFERENCES

1. Fernandez Alvarez E, Aicardi J. *Movement Disorders in Children.* London: MacKeith Press; 2001.
2. Scahill L, Tanner C, Dure L. The epidemiology of tics and Tourette syndrome in children and adolescents. *Adv Neurol.* 2001;85:261-271.
3. Dooley JM. Tic disorders in childhood. *Semin Pediatr Neurol.* 2006;13:231-242.
4. Mason A, Banerjee S, Eapen V, Zeitlin H, Robertson MM. The prevalence of Tourette syndrome in a mainstream school population. *Dev Med Child Neurol.* 1998; 40: 292-296.
5. Kurlan R, Whitmore D, Irvine C, McDermott MP, Como PG. Tourette's syndrome in a special education population: a pilot study involving a single school district. *Neurology.* 1994;44:699-702.
6. Mason A, Banerjee S, Eapen V, et al. The prevalence of Gilles de la Tourette syndrome in a mainstream school population: a pilot study. *Dev Med Child Neurol.* 1998; 40: 292-296.
7. Hornsey H, Banerjee S, Zeitlin H, et al. The prevalence of Tourette syndrome in 13-14 year-olds in mainstream schools. *J Child Psychol Psychiatry.* 2001;42:1035-1039.
8. Goldenberg JN, Brown SB, Weiner WJ. Coprolalia in younger patients with Gilles de la Tourette syndrome. *Mov Disord.* 1994;9:622-625.
9. Himle MB, Woods DW. An experimental evaluation of tic suppression and the tic rebound effect. *Behav Res Ther.* 2005;43:1443-1451.
10. Kurlan R, Como PG, Miller B, et al. The behavioral spectrum of tic disorders: a community-based study. *Neurology.* 2002;59:414-420.
11. Scahill L, Williams S, Schwab-Stone M, et al. Disruptive behavior problems in a community sample of children with tic disorders. *Adv Neurol.* 2006;99:184-190.
12. Robertson MM. Attention deficit hyperactivity disorder, tics and Tourette syndrome: the relationship and treatment implications. A commentary. *Eur Child Adolesc Psychiatry.* 2006;15:1-11.
13. Robertson MM, Orth M. Behavioral and affective disorders in Tourette syndrome. *Adv Neurol.* 2006;99:39-60.
14. Singer HS. Tourette's syndrome. From behavior to biology. *Lancet Neurol.* 2005;4:149-159.
15. Rojahn J. Self-injurious and stereotypic behavior of noninstitutionalized mentally retarded people: prevalence and classification. *Am J Ment Defic.* 1986;91:268-276.
16. Aichner F, Gerstenbrand F, Poewe W. Primitive motor patterns and stereotyped movements. A comparison of findings in early childhood and in the apallic syndrome. *Int J Neurol.* 1982-1983;16–17:21-29.
17. MacLean WE Jr, Ellis DN, Galbreath HN, Halpern LF, Baumeister AA. Rhythmic motor behavior of preambulatory motor impaired, Down syndrome and nondisabled children: a comparative analysis. *J Abnorm Child Psychol.* 1991;19:319-330.
18. FitzGerald PM, Jankovic J, Percy AK. Rett syndrome and associated movement disorders. *Mov Disord.* 1990;5:195-202.
19. Mahone EM, Bridges D, Prahme C, Singer HS. Repetitive arm and hand movements (complex motor stereotypies) in children. *J Pediatr.* 2004;145:391-395.
20. Louis ED, Dure LS, Pullman S. Essential tremor in childhood: a series of nineteen cases. *Mov Disord.* 2001;16: 921-923.
21. Lou JS, Jankovic J. Essential tremor: clinical correlates in 350 patients. *Neurology.* 1991;41:234-238.
22. Hornabrook RW, Nagurney JT. Essential tremor in Papua New Guinea. *Brain.* 1976;99:659-672.
23. Louis ED, Fernandez-Alvarez E, Dure LS 4th, Frucht S, Ford B. Association between male gender and pediatric essential tremor. *Mov Disord.* 2005;20:904-906.
24. Elble RJ, Randall JE. Motor-unit activity responsible for 8- to 12-Hz component of human physiological finger tremor. *J Neurophysiol.* 1976;39:370-383.
25. Elble RJ, Randall JE. Mechanistic components of normal hand tremor. *Electroencephalogr Clin Neurophysiol.* 1978;44: 72-82.
26. Kramer U, Nevo Y, Harel S. Jittery babies: a short-term follow-up. *Brain Dev.* 1994;16:112-114.
27. Shuper A, Zalzberg J, Weitz R, Mimouni M. Jitteriness beyond the neonatal period: a benign pattern of movement in infancy. *J Child Neurol.* 1991;6:243-245.
28. Danek A. Geniospasm: hereditary chin trembling. *Mov Disord.* 1993;8:335-338.

29. Soland VL, Bhatia KP, Sheean GL, Marsden CD. Hereditary geniospasm: two new families. *Mov Disord*. 1996;11:744-746.

30. Holmes GL, Russman BS. Shuddering attacks. Evaluation using electroencephalographic frequency modulation radiotelemetry and videotape monitoring. *Am J Dis Child*. 1986;140:72-73.

31. Vanasse M, Bedard P, Andermann F. Shuddering attacks in children: an early clinical manifestation of essential tremor. *Neurology*. 1976;26:1027-1030.

32. Ziebold C, von Kries R, Lang R, Weigl J, Schmitt HJ. Severe complications of varicella in previously healthy children in Germany: a 1-year survey. *Pediatrics*. 2001;108:E79. Erratum in *Pediatrics*. 2004;113:1470.

33. Packer RJ. Brain tumors in children. *Arch Neurol*. 1999;56:421-425.

34. Thyagarajan D. Genetics of movement disorders: an abbreviated overview. *Stereotact Funct Neurosurg*. 2001;77:48-60.

35. Fogel BL, Perlman S. Clinical features and molecular genetics of autosomal recessive cerebellar ataxias. *Lancet Neurol*. 2007;6:245-257.

36. Mariotti C, Di Donato S. Cerebellar/spinocerebellar syndromes. *Neurol Sci*. 2001;22(suppl 2):S88-S92.

37. Kinsbourne M. Hiatus hernia with contractions of the neck. *Lancet*. 1964;1:1058-1061.

38. Webb HE, Sutcliffe J. Neurological basis for the abnormal movements in Sandifer's syndrome. *Lancet*. 1971;2:818.

39. Kyllerman M, Bager B, Bensch J, et al. Dyskinetic cerebral palsy. I. Clinical categories, associated neurological abnormalities and incidences. *Acta Paediatr Scand*. 1982;71:543-550.

40. Sanger TD, Delgado MR, Gaebler-Spira D, et al. Classification and definition of disorders causing hypertonia in childhood. *Pediatrics*. 2003;111:e89-e97.

41. Fahn S, Marsden CD, Calne DB. Classification and investigation of dystonia. In: Marsden CD, Fahn S, eds. *Movement Disorders*. London: Butterworths; 332-358.

42. Ozelius L, Kramer PL, Moskowitz CB, et al. Human gene for torsion dystonia located on chromosome 9q32-q34. *Neuron*. 1989;2:1427-1434.

43. Sanger TD. Toward a definition of childhood dystonia. *Curr Opin Pediatr*. 2004;16:623-627.

44. Jankovic J. Delayed-onset progressive movement disorders after static brain lesions. *Neurology*. 1996;46:68-74.

45. Zimprich A, Grabowski M, Asmus F, et al. Mutations in the gene encoding epsilon-sarcoglycan cause myoclonus-dystonia syndrome. *Nat Genet*. 2001;29:66-69.

46. Pettigrew LC, Jankovic J. Hemidystonia: a report of 22 patients and a review of the literature. *J Neurol Neurosurg Psychiatry*. 1985;48:650-657.

47. Swaiman KF. Movement disorders. In: Swaiman KF, ed. *Pediatric Neurology Principles and Practice*. Vol 1. St. Louis:Mosby; 1898:205-218.

48. Swedo SE, Leonard HL, Schapiro MB, et al. Sydenham's chorea: physical and psychological symptoms of St Vitus dance. *Pediatrics*. 1993;91:706-713.

49. Church AJ, Cardoso F, Dale RC, Lees AJ, Thompson EJ, Giovannoni G. Anti-basal ganglia antibodies in acute and persistent Sydenham's chorea. *Neurology*. 2002;59:227-231.

50. Cardoso F, Vargas AP, Oliveira LD, Guerra AA, Amaral SV. Persistent Sydenham's chorea. *Mov Disord*. 1999;14:805-807.

51. Sekul EA, Kaminer S, Sethi KD. Digoxin-induced chorea in a child. *Mov Disord*. 1999;14:877-879.

52. Lancman ME, Asconape JJ, Penry JK. Choreiform movements associated with the use of valproate. *Arch Neurol*.1994;51:702-704.

53. Nausieda PA, Koller WC, Weiner WJ, Klawans HL. Pemoline-induced chorea. *Neurology*. 1981;31:356-360.

54. Delgado MR, Albright AL. Movement disorders in children: definitions, classifications, and grading systems. *J Child Neurol*. 2003;18(suppl 1):S1-S8.

55. Vercueil L. Myoclonus and movement disorders. *Neurophysiol Clin*. 2006;36:327-331.

56. Lombroso CT, Fejerman N. Benign myoclonus of early infancy. *Ann Neurol*. 1977;1:138-143.

57. Resnick TJ, Moshe SL, Perotta L, Chambers HJ. Benign neonatal sleep myoclonus. Relationship to sleep states. *Arch Neurol*. 1986;43:266-268.

58. Wong A. An update on opsoclonus. *Curr Opin Neurol*. 2007;20:25-31.

59. Lucking C, Durr A, Bonifati V, Vaughan J, et al. Association between early-onset Parkinson's disease and mutations in the parkin gene. French Parkinson's Disease Genetics Study Group. *N Engl J Med*. 2000;342:1560-1567.

60. Gonzalez-Alegre P, Afifi AK. Clinical characteristics of childhood-onset (juvenile) Huntington disease: report of 12 patients and review of the literature. *J Child Neurol*. 2006;21:223-229.

61. Harris S, Naina HV, Siddique S. Wilson's disease. *Lancet*. 2007;369:397-408.

62. Hyland K. The lumbar puncture for diagnosis of pediatric neurotransmitter diseases. *Ann Neurol*. 2003;54(suppl 6):S13-S17.

63. Hyland K, Fryburg JS, Wilson WG, et al. Oral phenylalanine loading in dopa-responsive dystonia: a possible diagnostic test. *Neurology*. 1997;48:1290-1297.

64. Leckman JF, Bloch MH, King RA, et al. Phenomenology of tics and natural history of tic disorders. *Adv Neurol*. 2006;99:1-16.

65. Swain JE, Scahill L, Lombroso PJ, King RA, Leckman JF. Tourette syndrome and tic disorders: a decade of progress. *J Am Acad Child Adolesc Psychiatry*. 2007;46:947-968.

66. Jankovic J, Beech J. Long-term effects of tetrabenazine in hyperkinetic movement disorders. *Neurology*. 1997;48:358-362.

67. Kurlan R. Tourette's syndrome: are stimulants safe? *Curr Neurol Neurosci Rep*. 2003;3:285-288.

68. Ondo WG, Jankovic J, Connor GS, et al. Topiramate Essential Tremor Study Investigators. Topiramate in essential tremor: a double-blind, placebo-controlled trial. *Neurology*. 2006;66:672-677.

69. Garvey MA, Swedo SE. Sydenham's chorea. Clinical and therapeutic update. *Adv Exp Med Biol*. 1997;418:115-120.

70. Edgar TS. Oral pharmacotherapy of childhood movement disorders. *J Child Neurol*. 2003;18(suppl 1):S40-S49.

71. Marsden CD, Marion MH, Quinn N. The treatment of severe dystonia in children and adults. *J Neurol Neurosurg Psychiatry*. 1984;47:1166-1173.

72. Marsden CD. Paroxysmal choreoathetosis. *Adv Neurol.* 1996;70:467-470.

73. Hirsch E, Sella F, Maton B, et al. Nocturnal paroxysmal dystonia: a clinical form of focal epilepsy. *Neurophysiol Clin.* 1994;24:207-217.

74. Biary N, Singh B, Bahou Y, et al. Posttraumatic paroxysmal nocturnal hemidystonia. *Mov Disord.* 1994;9:98-99.

75. Vidailhet M, Vercueil L, Houeto JL, French SPIDY. Bilateral, pallidal, deep-brain stimulation in primary generalised dystonia: a prospective 3 year follow-up study. *Lancet Neurol.* 2007;6:223-229.

76. Kupsch A, Benecke R, Muller J, et al., Deep-Brain Stimulation for Dystonia Study Group. Pallidal deep-brain stimulation in primary generalized or segmental dystonia. *N Engl J Med.* 2006;355:1978-1990.

77. Temel Y, Visser-Vandewalle V. Surgery in Tourette syndrome. *Mov Disord.* 2004;19:3-14.

78. Mink JW, Walkup J, Frey KA, Tourette Syndrome Association. Patient selection and assessment recommendations for deep brain stimulation in Tourette syndrome. *Mov Disord.* 2006;21:1831-1838.

CHAPTER 14

Neuropathy

Paul R. Carney, James D. Geyer, and Juan Idiaquez

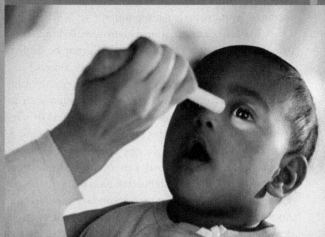

GENERAL APPROACH TO PERIPHERAL NEUROPATHIES

History

A thorough history is vital in the evaluation of neuromuscular diseases. The presentation of a peripheral neuropathy in the pediatric population may be different from that of an adult. The nature of the chief complaint helps define the type of neuropathic process. Patients may present with weakness, sensory disturbances, pain, autonomic disturbance, atrophy, ataxia, or a combination thereof. The time course of the symptoms is an important diagnostic clue, whether it is acute, subacute, or chronic (relapsing, recurrent, progressive, and so forth). Neuropathies can present with a number of different anatomic patterns. Symmetric or asymmetric, focal or diffuse, helps differentiate between a mononeuropathy, mononeuropathy multiplex, polyneuropathy, radiculopathy, polyradiculopathy, or plexopathy.[1]

In the history of a neuromuscular disorder, the examiner should always ask specifically about trauma, toxic exposures (including recreational drugs and alcohol), infections or vaccinations, dietary deficiencies, medications (both past and present), and concomitant medical conditions (Table 14-1).[1] Constitutional symptoms such as weight loss or unexplained fever may direct the evaluation toward an underlying etiology. Family history may be extremely important in the neuropathies seen during childhood since many of these disorders have a genetic basis.

Physical Examination

A thorough physical examination is very important in the evaluation of neuromuscular disorders. The cranial nerves are rarely involved in a typical peripheral neuropathy but are commonly involved in Guillain–Barré syndrome (GBS), sarcoid, carcinomatosis, and diphtheria.[1] Atrophy and its distribution can assist with certain diagnoses such as Charcot-Marie-Tooth disease with the classic champagne bottle legs. As with atrophy, the distribution of weakness guides diagnosis. Most polyneuropathies affect distal muscles of lower extremities first. Most demyelinating and certain acute motor and toxic neuropathies affect all muscles of limbs, trunk, neck, and some facial muscles. With the help of the history, try to narrow weakness into a pattern of mononeuropathy, mononeuropathy multiplex, polyneuropathy, radiculopathy, polyradiculopathy, or plexopathy.

While the sensory examination is very important in the assessment of a patient with a neuropathy, it may be very difficult to formally assess in children, especially the very young. Most peripheral neuropathies have

Table 14-1.

Medical Conditions Related to Neuropathy

Diabetes
Thyroid disease
Vascular disease
Liver disease
GI disease
Sarcoidosis
Renal disease
Connective tissue disease
Lupus erythematosis
Cancer

distal, symmetric, sensory loss in lower extremities first (stocking-glove distribution). Sensory loss exceeds weakness in most toxic neuropathies.

The reflex examination usually reveals diminished or completely lost reflexes. The reflexes may be diminished out of proportion to the degree of weakness.[1]

A general skin and musculoskeletal examination is also of great importance. Pes cavus is often seen in hereditary neuropathies secondary to weakness of peroneal and pretibial muscles more than calf muscles. A "claw" hand may arise in the upper extremity for similar reasons. Kyphoscoliosis can occur secondary to weakness of paravertebral muscles. Skin ulcers, pressure sores, and burns are often seen secondary to analgesia. Analgesic joints become traumatized resulting in a deformity known as Charcot arthropathy. Hypertrophied nerves are seen in a number of neuropathies including chronic inflammatory demyelinating polyneuropathy (CIDP), Refsum disease, leprosy, hereditary sensory motor neuropathy (HMSN; III > II > I), acromegaly, neurofibromatosis, and amyloidosis.

Diagnostic Testing

Electrophysiologic studies (nerve conduction studies) can further categorize neuropathies as primarily demyelinating or axonal, sensory or motor, or both. This information helps to differentiate between mononeuropathy, polyneuropathy, mononeuropathy multiplex, plexopathy and radiculopathy.[1]

Most peripheral neuropathies are axonal and usually have symmetrical distal sensory loss with weakness, atrophy, and lost ankle jerks. The nerve conduction study shows significantly decreased amplitudes of compound motor action potential (CMAP) and sensory nerve action potential (SNAP) (often no obtainable potential), but only mild slowing without conduction block or temporal dispersion. Needle EMG shows evidence of distal denervation (frequently not performed in children).[1]

Demyelinating neuropathy is a less common category of peripheral neuropathy. Early generalized reflex loss, mild atrophy, proximal and distal muscle weakness, sensory loss of large fiber; small fiber modalities, motor usually; sensory involvement, tremor, and hypertrophied nerves are common physical findings in a patient with a demyelinating neuropathy. Nerve conduction studies reveal marked nerve conduction velocity slowing, conduction block, temporal dispersion, and prolonged F-wave and distal latencies. The needle EMG may show denervation, based on the chronicity of the neuropathy. GBS, CIDP, and some hereditary neuropathies are demyelinating. Many neuropathies are mixed axonal and demyelinating and mixed sensory and motor.

Laboratory studies are very important in the evaluation of neuropathy. A wide array of laboratory tests may be ordered but the exact panel depends on the history and the physical examination. Suggested laboratory studies are listed in the following sections.

Lumbar puncture is especially helpful in the diagnosis of a demyelinating neuropathy such as GBS or CIDP. In these patients, the CSF protein is elevated.

Treatment

Specific treatment modalities aimed at the underlying etiology are not possible in most neuropathies (especially chronic sensory motor polyneuropathies); nevertheless, the search for a specific, treatable cause should be undertaken. In approximately 25% of all chronic polyneuropathies, an etiology cannot be determined. Treatments for specific neuropathies, such as GBS and CIDP, are discussed later in this chapter.

ACUTE INFLAMMATORY DEMYELINATING POLYNEUROPATHY OR GUILLAIN-BARRÉ SYNDROME

Epidemiology

Acute inflammatory demyelinating polyneuropathy (AIDP) or GBS is the most frequent cause of acute generalized weakness. The incidence is 1 to 2 per 100,000 per year. It occurs in a nonseasonal, nonepidemic pattern affecting both genders, all ages, and in all parts of the world. While incidence increases with increasing age (highest ages 50-74 years), childhood cases are not unheard of.[1]

Two-thirds of patients have a preceding event 1 week to 1 month prior to onset (URI, 60%; GI syndrome, 20%; surgery, 5%; vaccinations, 5%).[1] Antecedent infections associated with GBS are listed in Table 14-2. Lymphoma, particularly Hodgkin disease, has been associated with GBS. Surgery and spinal/epidural anesthesia may also precipitate GBS.

Table 14-2.

Infections Associated with the Development of GBS

Cytomegalovirus (CMV)
Epstein-Barr virus (EBV)
HIV
Hepatitis B
Herpes simplex virus (HSV)
Mycoplasma pneumoniae
Campylobacter jejuni—associated with poor outcome and Miller-Fisher variant
Borrelia burgdorferi—Lyme disease
Influenza

Etiology/Pathogenesis

Immune-mediated segmental demyelination is initiated by an undetermined antigenic reaction (possibly viral). There is a cell-mediated component in which T-cell lines are sensitized to P2, a basic protein found in peripheral nerve myelin. A clinically and pathologically indistinguishable disease called experimental allergic neuritis (EAN) develops in animals 2 weeks after immunization with a peripheral nerve homogenate containing P2.

An antibody-mediated component also occurs with immunoglobulins and complement found on myelinated fibers, and anti-peripheral nerve myelin antibodies found in some patients' serum (titers correlate with clinical course). An antibody to the GD1a ganglioside has been associated with a worsened clinical course.

Pathology specimens show perivascular mononuclear cell infiltrates early, associated with perivenular demyelination. Later, segmental demyelination and secondary Wallerian degeneration occur, affecting entire peripheral nerves, cranial nerves, dorsal and ventral roots, and dorsal root ganglia.

Clinical Presentation

Most patients present with rapidly progressive symmetrical weakness with areflexia.[2] The weakness is usually ascending (distal to proximal) with the lower extremities affected first, then trunk, arms, and cranial muscles.[3] In rare cases, proximal muscles can be affected first. Cranial nerves are rarely affected first, but more than 50% of patients have cranial nerve involvement, with facial diplegia being the most common deficit.

The maximum deficit typically occurs within days of onset up to maximum of 4 weeks after onset and then plateaus.[3] Total motor paralysis with respiratory failure and death may occur in a few days in severe cases. Weakness is so rapid that atrophy is rarely seen. The weakness is associated with hypotonia. An acute cord lesion should be considered in patients with low back pain, areflexia, and leg paralysis. The reflexes are initially decreased and then absent in GBS.

While GBS is a motor neuropathy, sensory complaints are common.[2,3] Low-back pain and myalgias occur in many patients, often involving the hips and thighs. Severe myalgias are rare and increased CPK levels should suggest other disorders. Paresthesias are a common early symptom but resolve rapidly. Objective sensory loss is usually mild and usually affects large fiber modalities (vibration and position sense).

Autonomic instability is fairly common but highly variable in expression.[1-3] Patients may experience one or more dysfunctions of the autonomic system, occasionally with rapid fluctuations. Sinus tachycardia, bradycardia, other tachyarrhythmias, orthostatic hypotension, hypertension, anhidrosis, diaphoresis, sphincter dysfunction, pupil changes, gut atony, and flushing can occur. The autonomic dysfunction usually lasts less than 1 to 2 weeks. Urinary retention occurs in 15% of cases.

Clinical variants are even less common than GBS. Miller-Fisher syndrome consists of gait ataxia, ophthalmoparesis, and areflexia, with normal limbs (some patients have mild proximal limb weakness). It is associated with IgG antibody to ganglioside GQ1b and prior *Campylobacter jejuni* infection.[4,5]

Pharyngeal–cervical–brachial GBS consists of blurred vision or diplopia, ptosis, marked oropharyngeal, neck and shoulder weakness, respiratory failure, areflexia in arms only, and normal sensation (occasionally leg areflexia present). This disorder simulates botulism and diphtheria clinically. There is no dry mouth, dizziness, or GI symptoms that are typical of botulism.

Differential Diagnosis

Acute demyelinating inflammatory polyneuropathy is relatively uncommon in children and may mimic a variety of disorders making diagnosis a challenge. Rapid diagnosis is important as treatments are available that may help avoid complications. Table 14-3 outlines the differential diagnosis with differentiating factors.

Diagnostic Testing

Electrodiagnostic studies

Nerve conduction studies reveal focal nerve conduction velocity (NCV) slowing, motor conduction block, temporal dispersion, and prolongation of F-wave and terminal latencies. All parameters may be normal for the first few days. The initial abnormality is prolonged (or absent) F-waves. Nerve conduction studies can remain normal in up to 10% of cases.[9]

Laboratory studies

CSF studies typically exhibit an elevated protein with normal cell count (albuminocytologic dissociation). In rare cases, patients will have 10 to 50 cells/mm^3 (mostly lymphs). Protein may remain normal for the first few days, rising to peak in 4 to 6 weeks. Unfortunately, CSF protein remains normal in 10% of patients, making diagnosis even more challenging. The opening pressure and CSF glucose are usually normal.

Blood should be sent for complete blood count, metabolic profile with Ca, Mg, Phos, hepatic studies, HIV, ESR, and Lyme disease. If suggested by history, heavy metal studies should be obtained.

Table 14-3.

Differential Diagnosis of GBS/AIDP with Factors that Can Help Distinguish the Disorders

Spinal cord lesion
Diphtheria—impaired visual accommodation, EOM, and oropharyngeal paresis
Poliomyelitis—epidemic, meningismus, fever
Porphyria—abdominal crisis and psychological symptoms
Acute myelopathy—sensory level, sphincter dysfunction
Basilar artery thrombosis—positive Babinski sign, brisk reflexes
Acute myasthenia gravis—no sensory symptoms, reflexes retained, weak mandibular muscles
Botulism—pupillary reflexes lost, bradycardia present
Tick paralysis—can exactly mimic GBS, except no sensory loss and CSF protein normal
Hypophosphatemia and hypokalemia
Hexane inhalation
Thallium, arsenic, or lead poisoning
Lyme disease[6]
HIV seroconversion
Complication of IV methylprednisolone
Saxitoxin from contaminated shellfish, tetrodotoxin from puffer fish, and ciquatera toxin
Conversion disorder (rare in children)
Rare disorders misdiagnosed as GBS
Polyarteritis nodosa
Vasculitis
Severe musculoskeletal pain
Polymyositis
Critical illness polyneuropathy
Encephalomyeloneuritis
Sarcoid
Mycoplasma pneumoniae

Treatment

Supportive therapy is vital with respiratory assistance and careful nursing. Frequent forced vital capacity (FVC) measurements should be obtained. Intubation should be considered if the FVC falls below 12 to 15 mL/kg, regardless of arterial blood gas testing. If there is significant bulbar weakness even with a good FVC, the patient may need intubation for airway protection. Respiratory therapy should be consulted for aggressive pulmonary toilet. Tracheostomy may be necessary if the patient requires prolonged intubation.

Cardiac monitoring and frequent vital signs are important given the risk of autonomic dysfunction. As with all pediatric patients, special attention must be given to the fluid status.

Physical therapy should be consulted early in the hospital stay for range of motion, but the patient should not be pushed aggressively during therapy sessions, given the risk of respiratory insufficiency.

The patient must be monitored for the development of decubitus ulcers. The patient should be turned frequently to avoid the prolonged pressure leading to skin breakdown.

Artificial tears during the day, and lubricating gel with eye patches at night, should be used if there is significant facial weakness.

Immune modulating therapy

In mild cases, careful observation and supportive care may be all that is needed. Patients who are progressing, are ambulatory only with assistance or recently have become nonambulatory, or those with respiratory compromise or autonomic instability, should be considered for immune modulating therapy. Two treatment options exist for GBS: therapeutic plasma exchange and intravenous immunoglobulin.[10-12]

Therapeutic plasma exchange (TPE) is a common treatment in adults but has significant limitations in children.[12] It is most effective if given within 7 days of disease onset and for patients who require intubation. Use of TPE results in decreased hospitalization time, mechanical ventilation time, and time until the patient walks again. The side effects include hypotension, bleeding, arrhythmias, and infection. The volume exchanged limits this treatment option in children.

Intravenous immunoglobulin (IVIg) was proven effective in one multicenter trial at dosage of 400 mg/kg/d × 5 days. There appears to be a reduced complication rate over TPE, and less need for mechanical ventilation. The side effects include allergic reactions, renal failure, aseptic meningitis, increased serum viscosity with vasoocclusive phenomena, and headache. Always check an IgA level prior to IVIg initiation, given the increased risk of anaphylaxis in IgA-deficient patients when administered IVIg.[10,11]

Glucocorticoids are ineffective.

CHRONIC INFLAMMATORY DEMYELINATING POLYNEUROPATHY

Epidemiology

Chronic inflammatory demyelinating polyneuropathy (CIDP) is also known as chronic inflammatory demyelinating polyradiculoneuropathy, chronic relapsing GBS, chronic relapsing polyneuritis, and relapsing corticosteroid-dependent polyneuritis. The peak incidence occurs between 40 and 60 years of age, but can occur from infancy to late adulthood.[1] Less than 10% have preceding viral infections. The age of onset can influence disease course, with younger patients tending to have a relapsing course, and older patients a more chronic progressive course.[13]

Etiology/Pathogenesis

There is immune-mediated segmental demyelination with a cell-mediated component based on mononuclear cell infiltration of spinal roots, ganglia, and proximal nerve trunks.[13] The evidence for a humoral component is based on detection of IgM (less often IgG) and complement fragment C3d on myelin sheaths of sural nerve biopsies and also the fact that CIDP patients tend to respond to plasmapheresis. Pathology specimens, usually from sural nerve biopsy, show interstitial and perivascular inflammatory cell infiltrates, loss of many myelinated fibers and degeneration of others with segmental demyelination–remyelination (onion-bulb formations). Large fibers are more severely involved. In predominantly motor disease, changes in the sensory nerves may not be fully representative of the pathologic process.

Clinical Features

The onset of CIDP is typically insidious with a steady or stepwise progression of symmetric proximal and distal muscle weakness of both upper and lower extremities. Asymmetric signs are much less common. The formal diagnostic criteria for CIDP are shown in Table 14-4.[1,13,14]

Weakness must be present for at least 2 months. The weakness can vary from mild to severe, requiring assisted ambulation, but rarely assisted ventilation. Proximal muscle weakness may be equal to or greater than distal weakness. This sets CIDP apart from most other neuropathies. Arms and legs are usually affected, but the legs are usually more severely involved. Neck flexor weakness may also occur, which is also a distinguishing feature of CIDP. Facial muscles are rarely involved. Reflexes are diminished or absent.[1,16]

Sensory findings are usually mild but sensory involvement is more prominent than in GBS. Touch, vibration, and proprioception are more commonly involved than pain/temperature. Numbness, paresthesias, and dysesthesias of the hands may be initial symptoms. Painful paresthesias are uncommon. Some patients may have severe proprioceptive loss, with ataxia, wide-based gait, and positive Romberg sign.[1,16]

Diagnostic Evaluation

Electrodiagnostic testing

Nerve conduction studies usually reveal a non-uniform reduction in NCV in the demyelinating range in at least 2 motor nerves. Conduction block or abnormal temporal dispersion should be present in at least 1 motor nerve. Distal latencies should be prolonged in at least 2 nerves. F-waves are usually prolonged or absent.[16]

Laboratory studies

Cerebrospinal fluid (CSF) evaluation reveals albuminocytologic disassociation. The CSF protein is elevated in most cases, with CSF protein greater than 55 mg/dL in 95% of patients. The CSF white blood cell count is usually less than 10/mm³.

Nerve biopsy results are described under "Etiology/Pathogenesis" above.

Laboratory testing for patients with suspected or confirmed CIDP includes a wide array of tests, as outlined in Table 14-5.

Treatment

The mainstays of treatment in the adult population are prednisone and TPE. Prednisone is dosed at 1.5 mg/kg/d

Table 14-4.

Diagnostic Criteria for CIDP

Definite CIDP—all mandatory clinical features and major laboratory features must be present (50% of patients). Mandatory clinical features include

1. Progression of proximal and distal upper and lower extremity weakness for at least 2 months
2. Areflexia or hyporeflexia

Probable CIDP—all mandatory clinical features and 2 of 3 major laboratory features.

Possible CIDP—all mandatory clinical features and one of three major laboratory features.

Mandatory exclusion criteria must be met in all groups. (For an extensive list, see reference 15.)

Table 14-5.

Laboratory Studies in Patients with CIDP

ESR
ANA
RF
Vitamin B$_{12}$
Folate
TSH, free T4
Serum immunofixation electrophoresis
Hepatic panel
HIV

Consider the following if clinically indicated:
RBC protoporphyrin
Urine porphobilinogen
Serum lead level
24-hour urine for heavy metals

in children.[17,18] The prednisone should be continued until significant improvement in weakness is apparent. The mean time to initial response is approximately 2 months. Following improvement, the prednisone should be changed to an alternating day, single-dose regimen and continued until the patient reaches maximum therapeutic response. The prednisone should then be tapered slowly. Patients should be carefully monitored for side effects related to steroid use including increased blood pressure, hyperglycemia, and weight gain.

IVIg is administered as described earlier in the GBS treatment section. Following the initial treatment, patients may need additional treatments every 3 to 6 months depending on the clinical course.

Other treatment options include azathioprine (Imuran), cyclosporine A, or cyclophosphamide.[19,20]

TICK PARALYSIS

Tick paralysis is an uncommon disorder that occurs with a tick bite. The neuropathy has a rapid onset and symptoms resolve quickly when the tick is removed. Any patient presenting with symptoms of a rapid-onset motor neuropathy (generalized paralysis) should have a thorough skin examination for ticks.

CRITICAL ILLNESS POLYNEUROPATHY

Critical illness polyneuropathy (CIP) is uncommon in children but is likely under-recognized. Critical illness polyneuropathy occurs in approximately 50% of adults in the ICU with sepsis and in approximately 70% of adults with sepsis and multiorgan system failure.[21] Usually patients have been in the ICU for at least 1 week when the earliest signs develop (eg, difficulty weaning from the ventilator). Later signs include distal weakness, decreased deep tendon reflexes, and, if severe, complete quadriplegia and respiratory paralysis. CIP may occur outside the ICU in patients who develop sepsis in the course of severe renal failure. Physical signs occur in 50% of patients and the other 50% are diagnosed by NCS/EMG.

Nerve conduction studies are compatible with primary axonal degeneration, and EMG shows signs of denervation. Decreased diaphragmatic CMAPs and signs of chest wall denervation establish CIP as the cause of difficulty of weaning from the ventilator.[1]

SYNDROMES OF HEREDITARY CHRONIC POLYNEUROPATHY

There are a number of hereditary chronic polyneuropathies that tend to be more chronic than acquired, progressive, symmetrical, and degenerative. One major category

Table 14-6.

Hereditary Neuropathy with Autonomic Features

Type	Inheritance	Onset
HSAN I	AD	Second decade
HSAN II	AR	Infancy
HSAN III	AR	Birth
HSAN IV	AR	Birth
Friedreich's ataxia	AR	Before age 20 years
Ataxia telangiectasia	AR	Before age 5 years

HSAN, hereditary sensory autonomic neuropathy.
From Chance PF. Molecular basis of hereditary neuropathies. Phys Med Rehabil Clin North Am. *2001;12:277.*[23]

presents with autonomic features (Table 14-6). These disorders are inheritable and usually appear early in life.

Friedreich Ataxia

Epidemiology

Friedreich ataxia is an autosomal recessive, triple repeat disease with a number of components.[22] The disorder is described in more detail in Chapter 13.

Etiology/pathogenesis

The sensory neuropathy associated with Friedreich ataxia occurs because of progressive degeneration of the dorsal ganglion and axon. There is some associated secondary demyelination.[22] The characteristics of the hereditary neuropathies with autonomic features are outlined in Table 14-6.

Clinical features

The primary feature of Friedreich ataxia is the gait ataxia. This ataxia is progressive and typically leads to the need for a wheelchair. The sensory neuropathy is not usually the most important component of the disorder but does add to the effect of the ataxia.

Treatment

There is no specific treatment for Friedreich ataxia. The patient is on a fall risk and appropriate safety measures should be taken. Furthermore, the patient's feet should be checked on a daily basis for cuts or blisters that might otherwise go unnoticed because of the sensory loss.

CHARCOT-MARIE-TOOTH DISEASE

Epidemiology

The hereditary motor and sensory neuropathies also typically appear early in life, as described in Table 14-7.[23]

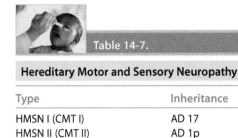

Table 14-7.

Hereditary Motor and Sensory Neuropathy

Type	Inheritance	Onset	Neuropathy
HMSN I (CMT I)	AD 17	Childhood	D
HMSN II (CMT II)	AD 1p	Second decade	A
HMSN III (Dejerine-Sottas)	AR 1q or 17p	Infancy	D
Rousy–Levy syndrome	AD	Infancy	D
HMSNIV (Refsum)	AR	Childhood	D

A, axonal; D, demyelinating; HMSN, hereditary motor sensory neuropathy.
From Geyer J, Keating J, Potts D, Carney P, eds. Neurology for the Boards. 3rd ed. Philadelphia: Lippincott Williams & Wilkins; 2006:163-189; Birouk N, Gouider R, Le Guern E, et al. Charcot-Marie-Tooth disease type Ia with 17p11.2 duplication. Clinical and electrophysiological phenotype study and factors influencing disease severity in 119 cases. Brain. 1997;120:813; and Loprest LJ, Pericek-Vance MA, Stajich J, et al. Linkage studies in Charcot-Marie-Tooth disease type 2: evidence that CMT types 1 and 2 are distinct genetic entities. Neurology. 1992;42:597.[1,24,25]

Charcot-Marie-Tooth (CMT) disease occurs in several subtypes. Type I CMT is an autosomal dominant disorder and is localized to chromosome 17 for type Ia and to chromosome 1 for type Ib (Table 14-7).[24]

Etiology/Pathogenesis

In Type I CMT, peripheral nerves hypertrophy and are occasionally palpable. Onion bulb formations occur in the nerve sheaths because of excessive collagen. Type II CMT, however, has no nerve hypertrophy and the onion bulb formations are rarely seen.[25]

Clinical Features

Type I CMT is characterized by distal muscle atrophy beginning in the lower extremities with progressive weakness of the anterior tibialis and peroneus muscles. This atrophy results in the classic "champagne bottle" legs. Similar changes in the upper extremities result in a clawed hand deformity. Distal sensory loss, paresthesias, and diminished or absent deep tendon reflexes also occur. Patients often develop skeletal changes as well, including an equinovarus deformity and kyphoscoliosis. The muscle atrophy and weakness are much less pronounced in type II CMT.

Diagnostic Testing

Nerve conduction studies reveal demyelinating range slowing even in infants. Over time, the amplitude seems to decrease with increasing age. Nerve biopsies reveal the demyelination, nerve hypertrophy and onion bulb formations in Type I CMT.

Treatment

Treatment is supportive. Aggressive splinting can help avoid the clawed hand deformity. Patients may also benefit from orthotics for the feet because of the equinovarus deformities.

Other Considerations

There exist a group of inherited neuropathies that in addition to neuropathy present with non neural tissue involvement.[26,27] Some of them are related with a specific inherited metabolic disorder, Table 14-8 outlined main neuropathies. Diagnostic testing include metabolic, genetic and nerve biopsy. There exist treatment for some disorders. Hereditary and acquired peripheral neuropathies show a wide range of sympathetic and parasympathetic nerve fiber lesions.[28,29] Table 14-9 described principal clinical autonomic dysfunction.

PLEXOPATHIES

Brachial Plexus Neuritis/Parsonage-Turner Syndrome/Neuralgic Amyotrophy

Epidemiology

Brachial plexus neuritis is relatively uncommon in the pediatric population. There is a seasonal variation in the incidence since the disorder is often related to viral infections. There are also sporadic cases related to surgery or trauma.

Etiology/pathogenesis

Most cases of brachial plexus neuritis are felt to be related to post-infectious inflammation.[1] The disorder has not been linked to a single virus but, on the contrary, has been associated with a wide variety of infections. There have also been reports of brachial plexus neuritis occurring after anesthesia, injection of serum,

Table 14-8.

Hereditary Neuropathies in Children with Systemic Features

Neuropathy	Inheritance	Onset	Disorder level
Axonal			
Giant axonal protein	AR	Birth	Gigaxonin
Fabry peroxisomal	XR	Child	
Acute intermitent pathway porphyria	AD	Before 20 years	Porphyrin
Ataxia telangectasia	AR	Child	ATM protein
NARP mitochondrial	X	Before 20 years	
MELAS mitochondrial	X	Before 20 years	
Demyelinating			
Metachromatic leukodystrophy	AR	Child	
Krabbe leukodystrophy	AR	Infant	
MERRF mitochondrial	X	Before 20 years	
Karnes Sayre mitochondrial	Varied	Before 20 years	
Myelin and Axon			
Tangier	XR	Child	Lipoprotein
MNGIE	X	Before 20 years	Mitochondrial

Table 14-9.

Autonomic Dysfunction Associated to Peripheral Neuropathies in Children

Type	Autonomic Dysfunction		
	Blood Pressure	Gastrointestinal	Bladder
Sweating			
Hereditary			
HSAN (Type III) Riley Day	Lability, OH	Dysmotility	Normal
Fabry anhidrosis	Normal	Dysmotility	Normal
Acute intermittent porphyria lability	Lability, OH	Constipation	Retention
Acquired			
Diabetes mellitus anhidrosis	OH	Gastroparesia, constipation, diarrhea	Retention
Guillain-Barré anhidrosis	Lability, OH	Constipation	Retention
Autoimmune neuropathy anhidrosis	OH	Dysmotility	Retention
Infections			
HIV anhidrosis	OH	Dysmotility	Retention
Leprosy anhidrosis	Normal	Normal	Normal
Toxic			
Thallium anhidrosis	Lability	Dysmotility	Retention
Acute			
Organophosphate hyperhidrosis	Lability	Dysmotility	Urination
Vincristine anhidrosis	OH	Constipation, ileus	Retention

OH, orthostatic hypotension.

vaccination, antibiotic administration, IV heroin injection, unaccustomed vigorous exercise, trauma, asthmatic attack in children (Hopkins syndrome), or Lyme disease.

Clinical presentation

The distribution of the symptoms depends on the portion of the brachial plexus involved. There is usually local pain at the shoulder described as a boring or toothache-like pain. Weakness then develops in the affected muscles 3 to 10 days after the onset of pain. Some muscles may become completely paralyzed which is uncommon in radiculopathies. Over time, atrophy develops in the weakened muscles. Sensory changes are also possible occurring most commonly in the axillary region.

Differential diagnosis

Diagnostic testing. Cerebrospinal spinal fluid testing is unremarkable. Blood testing may reveal antibodies against the causative agent (viral etiologies, Lyme disease, and so on).

Electrodiagnostic testing (NCV/EMG) is helpful in the diagnosis but may be normal if tested too early in the course of the syndrome. The two most useful NCVs are the latency from the Erb point to shoulder girdle muscles and sensory NCV from Erb point through brachial plexus. Needle EMG is best means of confirming diagnosis with fibrillation potentials/positive sharp waves and MUP changes indicative of denervation in affected limb muscles, with paraspinous muscles usually normal (as distinguished from radiculopathies).

Treatment

Approximately 80% of patients completely recover within 2 years. Treatment with steroids may help the pain. Treatment is primarily supportive.

TRAUMATIC BRACHIAL PLEXOPATHIES

Erb-Duchenne syndrome or upper radicular syndrome involves injury to the C4, C5, and C6 nerve roots, or the upper trunk of the brachial plexus.[1] This syndrome typically occurs following a hard blow to the neck or a birth injury. The signs consist of loss of arm abduction, elbow flexion, supination, and lateral arm rotation. The patient's arm assumes a "waiter's tip" arm position.

The middle radicular syndrome occurs following an injury of the C7 nerve root or the middle trunk of the brachial plexus. There is typically loss of radially innervated muscles except brachioradialis and part of the triceps. This syndrome can occur with the inappropriate use of crutches (crutch paralysis).

Klumpke syndrome or lower radicular syndrome occurs with an injury of the C8 and T1 nerve roots or the lower trunk of the brachial plexus.[1,30] It appears clinically as a combined median and ulnar palsy. There is paralysis of the thenar muscles and flexors resulting in a flattened simian hand. The syndrome usually occurs after a sudden pull of the arm or during delivery.

Thoracic Outlet Syndrome

Thoracic outlet syndrome (TOS) occurs secondary to compression of the neurovascular bundle between the neck and axilla, causing variable hand and arm muscle weakness and wasting, pain, and vascular symptoms.

Etiology/pathogenesis

Thoracic outlet syndrome can occur because of a number of disorders. An incomplete cervical rib with fibrous band passing from its tip to first rib is the most common cause. An elongated transverse process of C7 with fibrous bands passing to the first rib, a complete cervical rib that articulates with the first rib, and anomalies of position/insertion of the anterior and medial scalene muscles (neurovascular bundle passes between these), are other anatomic causes of TOS. Fractures of the clavicle and first rib, pseudoarthrosis of the clavicle, and traumatic injury to upper thorax can also result in TOS.

Clinical presentation

Non-Neurogenic TOS. Non-neurogenic TOS is usually seen in slender, "droop-shouldered" females with long necks, large breasts, and often poor muscle tone. This syndrome is usually accompanied by an ill-defined pain complex, with aching discomfort in shoulder, lower neck, pectoral region, upper arm, and sometimes hands, exacerbated by pulling down on and relieved by elevating the shoulder. In more severe cases, the patient may have signs of vascular compromise: subclavian vein compression—dusky color of the arm, venous distension, edema and thrombosis of vein after exercise (effort—thrombotic syndrome of Paget and Schroetter); or subclavian artery compression—digital gangrene, Raynaud phenomenon, brittle nails, or fingertip ulceration with or without supraclavicular bruit.

Tests for vascular compression are not very sensitive or specific but may be of some diagnostic help. For the test to be considered positive, the patient's symptoms should be reproduced during the maneuver. The Adson test is performed with the patient seated with hands on the thighs; both radial pulses are palpated simultaneously, the breath is held after full and rapid inspiration, the neck is hyperextended, and the head is turned to the side. The test is positive if the radial pulse on the affected side is diminished or obliterated, with the unaffected side remaining normal.

The shoulder hyperabduction test (Wright maneuver) is performed with the arm hyperabducted and externally rotated while the radial pulse is palpated; the pulse in normal subjects diminishes. The test is positive if the pulse diminishes asymmetrically in the presence of symptoms.

In the shoulder bracing test, the shoulders are braced backwards in an "exaggerated military position." The pulse on the affected side decreases more markedly than normal in the presence of symptoms.

Nerve conduction studies and EMG in non-neurogenic TOS are usually normal.

Neurogenic TOS. Neurogenic TOS is extremely rare. The syndrome typically consists of weakness and wasting of hypothenar and thenar muscles (in severe cases, of other hand intrinsics as well as flexors of fourth and fifth digits). There is usually an aching pain and sensory loss in the C8/T1 dermatomes (lower trunk involvement). Sensory symptoms may be reproduced by applying firm supraclavicular pressure or downward traction on the arm. Reflexes are usually preserved.

Nerve conduction studies and EMG show reduced amplitude of ulnar CNAP distally and across the thoracic outlet, prolonged ulnar F-wave latency, low CMAP in the median > ulnar nerve, and signs of chronic denervation in ulnar and median hand muscles.

Evaluation for both types of TOS should include C-spine films (may show cervical rib, elongated C7 spinous process, or T2 vertebral body visible above shoulder), nerve conduction studies, EMG, and possibly somatosensory evoked potentials.

SPINOMUSCULAR ATROPHY

The spinomuscular atrophy (SMA) syndromes are discussed in Chapter 30.

REFERENCES

1. Geyer J, Keating J, Potts D, Carney P, eds. *Neurology for the Boards.* 3rd ed. Philadelphia: Lippincott Williams & Wilkins; 2006:163-189.
2. Albers JW, Kelly JJ Jr. Acquired inflammatory demyelinating polyneuropathies: clinical and electrodiagnostic features. *Muscle Nerve.* 1989;12:435.
3. Rantala H, Uhari M, Niemala M. Occurrence, clinical manifestations, and prognosis of Guillain-Barré syndrome. *Arch Dis Child.* 1991;66:706; discussion,708.
4. Willison HJ, O'Hanlon GM. The immunopathogenesis of Miller Fisher syndrome. *J Neuroimmunol.* 1999;100:3.
5. Ang CW, De Klerk MA, Endtz HP, et al. Guillain-Barré syndrome-and Miller Fisher syndrome-associated *Campylobacter jejuni* lipoplysaccharides induce anti-GM1 and anti-GQ1b antibodies in rabbits. *Infect Immun.* 2001;69:2462.
6. Beiman AL, Iyer M. Coyle PK, et al. Neurologic manifestations in children with North American Lyme disease. *Neurology.* 1993;43:2609.
7. Hughes R. Campylobacter jejuni in Guillain-Barré syndrome. *Lancet Neurol.* 2004;3:644.

8. Grose C, Feorino PM. Epstein–Barr virus and Guillain-Barré syndrome. *Lancet.* 1972;2:1285.
9. Alma TA, Chaudhry V, Cornblath DR. Electrophysiological studies in the Guillain-Barré syndrome: distinguishing subtypes by published criteria. *Muscle Nerve.* 1998;21:1275.
10. al-Qudah AA. Immunoglobulins in the treatment of Guillain-Barré syndrome in early childhood. *J Child Neurol.* 1994;9:178.
11. Abd-Allah SA, Jansen PW, Ashwal S, et al. Intravenous immunoglobulin as therapy for pediatric Guillain-Barré syndrome. *J Child Neurol.* 1997;12:376.
12. Epstein MA, Sladky JT. The role of plasmapheresis in childhood Guillain-Barré syndrome. *Ann Neurol.* 1990;28:65.
13. Baba M, Takada H, Tomiyama M, et al. Chronic inflammatory demyelinating polyneuropathy in childhood. *No To Shinkei.* 1993;45:233.
14. Berger AR, Bradley WG, Brannagan TH, et al. Guidelines for the diagnosis and treatment of chronic inflammatory demyelinating polyneuropathy. *J Peripher Nerv Syst.* 2003;8:282.
15. Mendell JR. Chronic inflammatory demyelinating polyradiculoneuropathy. *Annu Rev Med.* 1993;44:211-219.
16. Connolly AM. Chronic inflammatory demyelinationg polyneuropathy in childhood. *Pediatr Neurol.* 2001;24:177.
17. Baba M, Ogawa M, Matsunaga M. Treatment of chronic inflammatory demyelinating polyneuropathy (CIDP). *Rinsho Shinkeigaku.* 1996;36:1336.
18. Dyck PJ, O'Brien PC, Oviatt KF, et al. Prednisone improves chronic inflammatory demyelinating polyradiculoneuropathy more than no treatment. *Ann Neurol.* 1982;11:136.
19. Dyck PJ, O'Brien P, Swanson C, et al. Combined azathioprine and predisone in chronic inflammatory-demyelinating polyneuropathy. *Neurology.* 1985;35:1173.
20. Brannagan TH 3rd, Pradhan A, Heiman-Patterson T, et al. High-dose cyclophosphamide with stem-cell rescue for refractory CIDP. *Neurology.* 2002;58:1856.
21. Bolton Cf, Laverty DA, Brown JD, et al. Critically ill polyneuropathy: Electrophysiological studies and differentiation from Guillain-Barré syndrome. *J Neurol Neurosurg Psychiatry.* 1986;49:563.
22. Dunn HG. Nerve conduction studies in children with Feiedreich's ataxia and ataxia-telangiectasia. *Dev Med Child Neurol.* 1973;15:324.
23. Chance PF. Molecular basis of hereditary neuropathies. *Phys Med Rehabil Clin North Am.* 2001;12:277.
24. Birouk N, Gouider R, Le Guern E, et al. Charcot-Marie-Tooth disease type Ia with 17p11.2 duplication. Clinical and electrophysiological phenotype study and factors influencing disease severity in 119 cases. *Brain.* 1997;120:813.
25. Loprest LJ, Pericek-Vance MA, Stajich J, et al. Linkage studies in Charcot-Marie-Tooth disease type 2: evidence that CMT types 1 and 2 are distinct genetic entities. *Neurology.* 1992;42:597.
26. Klein CJ. The inherited neuropathies. *Neurol Clin.* 2007; 25:173-207.
27. Stickler DE, Valenstein E, Neiberger RE, et al. Peripheral neuropathy in genetic mitochondrial disease. *Pediatr Neurol.* 2006;34:127-131.
28. Axelrod FB, Gold-von Simson G. Hereditary sensory and autonomic neuropathies: types II, III and IV. *Orphanet J Rare Dis.* 2007;2:39.
29. Freeman R. Autonomic peripheral neuropathy. *Neurol Clin.* 2007;25:277-301.
30. al-Qattan MM, Clarke HM, Curtis CG. Klumpke's birth palsy. Does it really exist? *J Hand Surg.* 1995;20:19.

CHAPTER 15

Disorders of Muscle and Motor Function

Juan Idiaquez, Paul R. Carney, and James D. Geyer

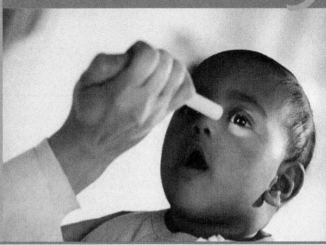

MUSCLE DISEASES

The myopathies are neuromuscular disorders in which the primary symptom is muscle weakness due to dysfunction of muscle fiber. In pediatric patients, myopathies can be inherited (such as the muscular dystrophies) or acquired. The distribution of muscle weakness is proximal but it could be generalized or distal. Patients may also complain of muscle pain and cramps. Presentation of weakness may be acute or insidious (Figure 15-1). Acute weakness can occur in neuromuscular junction disorders. Some diseases are present since childbirth, and in this group the differential diagnosis is important to distinguish the disorders from other causes of hypotonic infants. Figure 15-2 shows a diagnostic algorithm in infants with suspected neuromuscular hypotonia. Evidence of reduced fetal movement and polyhidroamnios could be found early. Also respiratory and feeding difficulties can occur. Other physical signs such as joint contractures (severe arthrogryposis), foot deformities, and facial, palatal, and pharyngeal abnormalities are also useful in detecting an inherited myopathy.

This chapter includes the principal inherited myopathies: congenital and acquired neuromuscular junction disorders, congenital myopathies, congenital muscular dystrophies, muscular dystrophies, inherited metabolic myopathies, mitochondrial myopathies, inflammatory myopathies, muscle channelopathies, and endocrine and toxic myopathies.

MYASTHENIC SYNDROMES

Myasthenia Gravis

Definitions and epidemiology

Myasthenia gravis (MG) is a disorder involving the neuromuscular junction that results in fatigable weakness as its primary symptom. The onset can be insidious, and it is often difficult to make the diagnosis initially (Table 15-1).[1]

Myasthenia gravis is a relatively common disorder, affecting approximately 2 to 10 per 100,000 people in the United States. Before age 40 years, MG is three times more common in women than men. It may begin at any age but is rare before age 10 years or after age 60 to 70 years. There are bimodal age-related peaks, with the earlier peak involving more women between ages 10 and 40 years and slightly more men between ages 50 and 70 years. The older patients more often have associated thymomas.

The male-to-female ratio is essentially equal in prepubertal patients of Northern European decent. Myasthenia gravis is usually a less severe disease in this group, with more spontaneous remissions and shorter disease duration. More patients in this group are seronegative (50%). The disease becomes more common in females during and after puberty, taking on more of the characteristics associated with myasthenia in the adult. The female-to-male ratio is 4.5:1 in the postpubertal group. Females in this group tend to have more severe disease than males. Thirty-two percent of prepubertal

Muscle weakness with normal peripheral nerve function

Acute or episodic → Check for:
Myoglobinuria
Hyper or hypokalemia
Myasthenic syndrome

Chronic → Check for:
Muscular dystrophy
Inflammatory myopathy
Myasthenic syndrome
Metabolic myopathy
Endocrine myopathy

FIGURE 15-1 ■ Algorithm for diagnosis of muscle weakness in children.

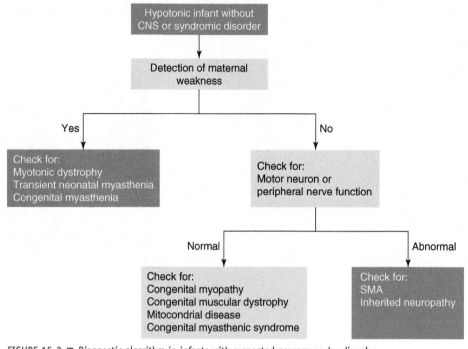

FIGURE 15-2 ▪ Diagnostic algorithm in infants with suspected neuromuscular disorder.

Table 15-1.

Acquired Neuromuscular Junction Diseases in Infants and Children

		Diagnostic tools		
	Synaptic Site	Repetitive Nerve Stimulation	ACH Esterase Inhibitors	Antibodies to
Autoimmune				
Transient neonatal myastenia gravis	Post	Decrement	Recovery	Nicotin AChR
Recurrent congenital arthrogryposis	Post	Decrement	N/A	Nicotin AChR
Childhood myastenia gravis	Post	Decrement	Recovery	Nicotin AChR
Anti MuSK	N/A	Decrement	None	MuSK protein
Eaton-Lambert syndrome	Pre	Increment High rate	None N/A	VG Ca^{++} channel N/A
Thymoma	Post	Decrement	Recovery	Nicotin AChR
Others				
Botulism	Pre	Increment High rate	N/A N/A	Absent N/A
Snake venom toxin	Post	N/A	N/A	Absent
Drug-induced myasthenia gravis	Post	Decrement	N/A	Nicotin AChR

children are seronegative, and 9% of postpubertal children are antibody negative. The disease appears more common in female African Americans of all ages than in males (2:1). The percentage of African-American children negative for AChR antibodies is the same as for whites.[1,2]

Patients and their first-degree relatives have an increased incidence of other autoimmune disorders (eg, systemis lupus erythematosus [SLE], rheumatoid arthritis [RA], thyroiditis, Grave disease) and hyperthyroidism (3-8%). Therefore, these disorders should be screened for on the initial evaluation.[1,2]

Children with MG are at an increased risk for a seizure disorder, with seizures occurring in 3% to 12% of patients. Neoplasms are rare but have also been associated with juvenile myasthenia.

Pathogenesis

Myasthenia arises as the result of the abnormal production of autoantibodies to nicotinic acetylcholine receptors (AChR). Overall, 80% to 90% of patients with MG are positive for AChR antibodies. Children less often have detectable AChR antibodies. Only 40% of children with ocular myasthenia are Ab+ as compared to 50% in adults. Only 58% of children with generalized MG are Ab+, as compared to 80% to 90% in adults. It is thought that the 10% to 20% of patients who have "antibody-negative" MG do have autoantibodies that may be directed at epitopes not present in the AChR extract used in testing, or they may have too low an affinity for detection in the assay system.[2]

The AChR antibodies are synthesized by B-cells in the thymus gland. The thymus gland of MG patients is almost always abnormal. Most of the pateints (>75%) have lymphoid hyperplasia of the thymus. Thymomas occur in approximately 15% of myasthenia patients (slightly more common in older patients).

Clinical presentation/diagnosis

The three cardinal features of MG are (1) fluctuating weakness, (2) weakness varies from day to day or during the course of a single day, and (3) excessive fatigability with exercise. There are several areas that are commonly affected by the weakness. Ocular muscle weakness is common, with ocular muscles affected at presentation in 40% of patients and are eventually affected in 85%. This produces the characteristic symptoms of diplopia and ptosis. Purely ocular myasthenia is relatively uncommon and differs from generalized myasthenia. Only 50% of these patients have AChR antibodies (as opposed to 80% to 90% with generalized MG). If myasthenia remains restricted to the eye muscles for more than 3 years, it is likely to remain restricted.

Bulbar muscle weakness is also a common finding. This results in complaints of dysphagia, dysarthria, and facial weakness. Speech may be "mushy" or nasal. Limb and neck weakness is common. Limb weakness is usually more prominent in the proximal muscles than the distal ones. Limbs are almost never affected alone.

Diagnostic tests

The history must be compatible and supported by physical examination findings. The sensory, cerebellar, and reflex examinations should be unremarkable.

The Tensilon test is performed with the administration of the short-acting acetylcholinesterase inhibitor edrophonium. The onset of action is approximately 30 seconds and the duration is about 5 minutes. The adult form of the test is described below.

1. Decide on a readily observable sign of weakness that you can measure (eg, ptosis, FVC [forced vital capacity]).
2. Make sure that the patient has a functioning IV line.
3. Keep 10-mg Tensilon and 1-mg atropine at bedside.
4. Inject 2-mg Tensilon and watch for side effects (bradycardia, hypotension, arrhythmias).
5. If patient tolerates the test dose well, inject the remaining 8-mg Tensilon.
6. Observe the patient for improvement and continue watching for side effects.
7. If at any point during the test the patient has serious side effects or becomes unstable, abort the test and give atropine 0.5- to 1-mg IV.

Placebo injections with NS are sometimes used in evaluation of limb weakness, but are not usually necessary when evaluating cranial muscle weakness, as this is difficult for most patients to simulate.

An alternate test is the ice-pack test. Cooling the eyelids can improve ptosis.

The repetitive nerve stimulation (Jolly test) is the most commonly used electrodiagnostic test for MG. Trains for electrical stimuli are applied for stimulation of the orbicularis oculi or the ADQ muscle in the hand. A decremental response to low rates of stimulation (2-5 Hz) suggests a defect in neuromuscular transmission (MG).

The most important laboratory test for MG is the acetylcholine receptor antibody (AChRAb) assay. It is positive in 80% to 90% of patients with generalized MG and in 50% with pure ocular MG. Antibody titers do *not* correlate with severity of disease.

Additional antibody testing may also be helpful for diagnosis in some cases. Muscle-specific tyrosine kinase antibodies (MuSK) are positive in 71% of AChR antibody-negative patients.[3] Antistriated muscle antibodies are positive in 85% of patients with a thymoma.

Chest x-ray and chest CT scan are important studies during the initial evaluation of MG. These studies help screen for infection and thymoma. The chest CT should be performed without contrast, since the contrast agent can exacerbate MG and potentially result in a myasthenic crisis.

The single-fiber EMG may be helpful in difficult cases. On this needle EMG study, increased "jitter" and blocking is seen. It is positive in about 90% of patients but is very nonspecific.

Additional evaluation of the newly diagnosed myasthenia patient should include ANA, RF, and ESR, ± anti–double stranded DNA (screen for SLE, RA, etc.). Thyroid studies should also be obtained, since hyperthyroidism is a common comorbid disorder. The CBC with differential and a urinalysis should be obtained since infection can exacerbate MG. Blood sugar and electrolytes must be studied.

Treatment

After the diagnosis of MG has been made, the patient's medication list should be reviewed to eliminate or avoid medications that may exacerbate MG. Box 15-1 gives an overview of medications that can worsen MG.

Acetylcholinesterase inhibitors (anticholines-terases) are the mainstay of therapy. Pyridostigmine (Mestinon) is the most commonly used agent. It has an onset of 30 minutes, a peak dose of 2 hours, and a duration of approximately 3 to 6 hours. The dosage is usually 30 to 90 mg every 3 to 4 hours. The IV dose is 1/30 of the oral dose. Potential side effects include diarrhea, nausea/ vomiting, sweating, increased salivation, miosis, bradycardia, and hypotension. The oral agent glycopyrrolate (Robinul), which is an anticholinergic, can be used for the GI side effects caused by pyridostigmine. The dosage is typically 1 to 2 mg orally three times daily.[4,5]

Immunosuppressive agents are used when symptoms are not adequately controlled by anticholinesterases alone.[4,5] Prednisone can help suppress the autoimmune activity. Patients should be hospitalized when high-dose steroids are initiated because they can precipitate weakness. After the initially high dosing, the dose should be tapered to the lowest dose needed to maintain the patient's functional status. As with any patient being treated with steroids, the patient should be monitored for side effects including hyperglycemia, sodium abnormalities and water retention (hypertension, edema, heart failure), psychosis, ulcers, osteoporosis, aseptic necrosis, and so forth.

A number of other immunosuppressive agents can be used when steroids prove ineffective.

> ### Box 15-1. Medications That Can Exacerbate Myasthenia Gravis
>
> - ᴅ-penicillamine
> - Aminoglycoside and polymyxin antibiotics (eg, gentamicin)
> - Antiarrhythmics (quinidine, procainamide)
> - Beta blockers (propranolol)
> - Thyroid hormones
> - Lithium, chlorpromazine
> - Intravenous CT contrast, IVP dye

Thymectomy is recommended for virtually all patients with thymoma.[6] The exceptions include those with poor surgical risk, the elderly, and those with limited life expectancy, because it may take years before a benefit is noted. It may also be beneficial for patients with severe generalized myasthenia without thymoma and for selected patients with severe, disabling ocular myasthenia requiring immunosuppressants.

Myasthenic Crisis

A myasthenic crisis occurs when respiratory weakness becomes severe enough to require mechanical ventilation. This can also result from severe dysphagia with airway compromise secondary to inability to clear secretions. The myasthenic crisis may be provoked by an infection (particularly respiratory), surgical procedures, drugs, IV contrast dye, emotional stress, or systemic illness.

There are two types of crisis: myasthenic crisis due to underlying disease, and cholinergic crisis due to overmedication. Symptoms include miosis, increased salivation and secretions, diarrhea, cramps, and fasciculations. Cholinergic crisis is treated by withdrawal of medications.

If unsure which type the patient has, you can challenge with edrophonium. If the patient improves, this is myasthenic crisis, and the patient needs more medication. If the patient worsens, this is cholinergic crisis, and the patient needs less medication. (Be prepared for marked worsening with this approach!)

In addition to aggressive management with acetylcholinesterase inhibitors such as pyridostigmine, there are several approaches to the patient in myasthenic crisis. The choice of the treatment depends in part on what therapies are available at that particular hospital. Total plasma exchange (TPE)/plasmapheresis and intravenous immunoglobulin (IVIg) therapy can both provide significant and fairly rapid improvement in the degree of weakness.[4,5] At present, IVIg given every 4 to 8 weeks until remission is the preferred treatment. TPE is usually reserved for cases in which IVIg fails or "tuning-up" is required prior to an intervention, surgery, or when the child is ventilator dependent and requires immediate attention.

Myasthenic Exacerbation

For myasthenic exacerbation, but not yet in crisis, close monitoring and aggressive management are warranted.[2,4,5] Since respiratory compromise can occur, the patient should be monitored with forced vital capacity (FVC) every 4 to 6 hours. Intubatation should be considered for those with FCV less than 12 to 15 mL/kg. FVC is the best indicator of respiratory weakness, and *not* arterial blood gas or pulse oximetry! Blood gases can remain unremarkable until just prior to respiratory failure, but the FVC will show a decline as the weakness worsens. Patients can decompensate quickly and must be monitored very closely. In addition to the respiratory status, the patient's bulbar function must be monitored closely.

Botulism

Pathogenesis

Botulism is caused by the exotoxin of *Clostridium botulinum*. The toxin interferes with the presynaptic release of AChR from the nerve terminal. There are three types of botulism: foodborne, wound-related, and infant.[7,8]

Foodborne botulism is most often due to ingestion of *C botulinum* in home-preserved foods. It is much less commonly caused by improperly canned commercial products. Public health authorities must be notified. Wound-related botulism is secondary to a penetrating injury or IV drug abuse. *C botulinum* from the soil colonizes the wound. Gas production in the wound can often be seen on x-ray. Infant-related botulism has a peak incidence 2 to 7 months of age and arises secondary to colonization of the GI tract by *C botulinum* after ingestion of spores or during periods of constipation. It may be a cause of sudden infant death syndrome (SIDS).

Clinical presentation/diagnosis

Symptoms usually appear within 12 to 36 hours after ingestion of contaminated food and evolve rapidly over 2 to 4 days. The characteristic progression of symptoms begins with ophthalmoparesis, progresses to loss of pupillary reactions, bulbar weakness (dysphagia, dysarthria), and finally results in generalized weakness and respiratory compromise. Pupils are often unreactive. Severe constipation and paralytic ileus frequently occur, which would be unusual in MG. The infantile form also has a similar progression of symptoms.

Diagnostic tests

C. botulinum toxin assays are available for stool and serum.[9] Furthermore, stool can be sent for *C. botulinum* culture. Repetitive nerve stimulation testing reveals an incremental response to high rates of stimulation. As with MG, single-fiber needle EMG reveals increased jitter and blocking.

Treatment

Trivalent antiserum (antitoxin) can be obtained from the Centers for Disease Control and Prevention. This is a horse serum product and can cause serum sickness or anaphylaxis. Guanidine can help with the weakness. Penicillin may help in both the wound and infant forms. Supportive care is vital regardless of the subtype of botulism. Improvement, in those who recover, begins within a few weeks, but complete recovery may take many months. Recovery mirrors symptom onset, with ocular movement typically improving first followed by other cranial nerves and finally limb/trunk and respiratory muscles.

Neonatal Myasthenia

Pathogenesis

Neonatal myasthenia is a transient disorder seen in 15% of infants born to mothers with MG. It is caused by placental transfer of AChR antibodies.[10,11] Symptomatic infants are thought to synthesize the antibodies de novo as well.

Clinical presentation/diagnosis

Symptoms may appear prenatally with intrauterine hypotonia, and affected infants can be born with arthrogryposis. Symptoms usually become evident within the first 24 hours of life and always by day of life 3. The mean duration of symptoms is 18 days. The most common symptoms include weakness of bulbar muscles with a weak cry, weak suck, and difficulty feeding. Approximately half of patients have generalized hypotonia. Respiratory insufficiency is uncommon.

Diagnostic testing

The mother should have a diagnosis of MG; however, it would be possible for the mother to be previously undiagnosed. Patients are usually AChR-antibody positive. The Tensilon test is positive.

Treatment

For those with severe generalized weakness and respiratory distress, exchange transfusion may be of benefit. For others, administer Neostigmine IM 0.01 to 0.04 mg/Kg/dose (or oral dose of 0.2 mg, 20 minutes before feeding). Recall that this is a self-limited disease.[10,11]

CONGENITAL MYASTHENIA

Pathogenesis

Congenital myasthenia is a heterogeneous disorder due to genetic defects in the presynaptic or postsynaptic neuromuscular junction.[11] It is *not* associated with antibodies to the AChR (Tables 15-2 and 15-3).

Clinical Presentation/Diagnosis

Symptoms usually begin in the neonatal period. Ocular, bulbar, and respiratory weakness, worse with crying or activity, are common symptoms. Congenital myasthenia is a heterogeneous set of disorders, however, and some disorders may not cause symptoms until the second or third decade of life (eg, slow channel syndrome).

Diagnostic Testing

There is a positive family history in some, but this is not required. The AChRAb tests must be negative.[11] Most forms are also Tensilon-test negative. The repetitive

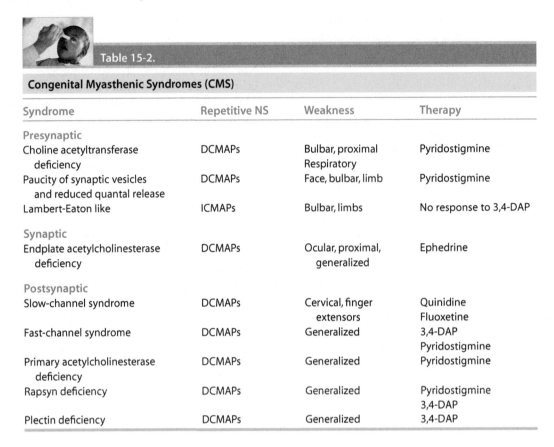

Table 15-2.

Congenital Myasthenic Syndromes (CMS)

Syndrome	Repetitive NS	Weakness	Therapy
Presynaptic			
Choline acetyltransferase deficiency	DCMAPs	Bulbar, proximal Respiratory	Pyridostigmine
Paucity of synaptic vesicles and reduced quantal release	DCMAPs	Face, bulbar, limb	Pyridostigmine
Lambert-Eaton like	ICMAPs	Bulbar, limbs	No response to 3,4-DAP
Synaptic			
Endplate acetylcholinesterase deficiency	DCMAPs	Ocular, proximal, generalized	Ephedrine
Postsynaptic			
Slow-channel syndrome	DCMAPs	Cervical, finger extensors	Quinidine Fluoxetine
Fast-channel syndrome	DCMAPs	Generalized	3,4-DAP Pyridostigmine
Primary acetylcholinesterase deficiency	DCMAPs	Generalized	Pyridostigmine
Rapsyn deficiency	DCMAPs	Generalized	Pyridostigmine 3,4-DAP
Plectin deficiency	DCMAPs	Generalized	3,4-DAP

Table 15-3.

Differential Diagnosis of Congenital Myasthenic Syndromes in Infants and Children

Syndrome	Useful Tests
Infancy	
Central nervous system hypotonia	Brain MRI
Werning-Hoffmann (SMA1)	EMG, genetic testing
Transient neonatal myasthenia	Anti-AChR antibodies
Congenital myopathies	Mucle MRI, muscle biopsy, genetic testing
Congenital muscular dystrophies	CK, muscle MRI, genetic testing
Children	
Muscular dystrophies	CK, muscle MRI, genetic testing
Spinal muscular atrophies	EMG, genetic testing
Myasthenia gravis	Edrophonium test, anti-AChR antibodies
Inherited peripheral neuropathies	Conduction velocity, EMG, genetic testing

nerve stimulation test shows a decremental response, and the single-fiber needle EMG has increased jitter.

Treatment

The course is usually protracted, with mild to moderate symptoms refractory to both medical and surgical treatments.[11]

INHERITED MUSCLE DISEASES

There exists a flourishing knowledge about inherited muscle diseases derived from myopathology including immunofluorescence and Western blotting analysis, and from identification of errors in many genes involved in structural protein complexes of muscle cells. Due to this increasing molecular and clinical understanding, the array of inherited myopathies is continuously increasing, so that any attempt to classify them is difficult. But classifications that combine in different degrees the clinical features with pathologic, genetic, and molecular findings are useful to study a child with suspected myopathy. The clinical features are discussed in more detail in Chapter 30.

CONGENITAL MYOPATHIES

Congenital myopathies show distinctive and specific morphologic abnormalities in skeletal muscles (within the myofibril) as the main pathologic feature. They are grouped into subtypes depending on the predominant pathologic finding in light and/or electronic microscopic biopsy study. Although weakness and hyptonia occur at birth or in the first year of life, there exists a wide clinical variation within each subtype including adult onset. Genetic diagnosis is available for the majority of these conditions, but they are genetically heterogeneous; one gene can result in multiple pathologies or multiple genes can result in only one myopathic phenotype. Therefore clinical study and muscle biopsy are very important in directing genetic testing. A morphologic classification of the main congenital myopathies is outlined in Table 15-4.

Myopathies with Cores: Central Core Myopathy

Central core myopathy is probably the most common congenital myopathy.[12-14] It arises because of a mutation in the skeletal muscle ryanodine receptor (*RYR1*) gene at chromosome 19 q13.1, which is also implicated in the malignant hyperthermia susceptibility trait. *RYR1* mutations associated with myopathies can occur as either dominant or recessive traits.[15] Genotype-phenotype correlations associated with the *RYR1* gene are complex, with some dominant mutations being related to malignant hyperthermia and others to congenital myopathy.

Clinical description

Onset of symptoms occurs in infancy with hypotonia or in early childhood with motor delay (begin walking at 4-5 years); however, marked clinical variation can occur within the same family. The slowly progressive weakness is more proximal, with prominent involvement of the hip girdle and axial muscles. Orthopedic complications are common, including scoliosis, dislocation of hips, and foot deformities.

Diagnostic methods

The diagnosis depends on the presence of muscle fibers with typical central cores without oxidative and glycolytic enzymatic activity (histochemical staining). On electron microscopy, there is reduction of mitochondria with myofibrillar disorganization and accumulation of abnormal Z-band material within the core area. Muscle MR imaging may complement clinical evaluation. CK and EMG are not useful.

Myopathies with Protein Accumulation: Nemaline (Rod) Myopathy

Inheritance could be dominant, recessive, or sporadic. It is genetically heterogeneous.[12,13] At present, there are seven known genetic loci and there are cases without link to any of the identified loci. All the known genes encode components of the sarcomeric thin filaments or proteins that regulate depolymeratization of the actin filament. The possible mechanism for rod formation could be an accumulation of sarcomeric components.

Clinical description

Onset varies from congenital weakness (90%) to adult presentation.

1. The congenital form includes severe hypotonia, joint contractures (severe arthrogryposis), foot deformities, and sucking and swallowing dysfunction. Respiratory and cardiac failure is the most common cause of death during infancy.
2. There is a mild form, with onset at birth or in childhood, that produces mild proximal weakness. Facial, palatal, and pharyngeal involvement also occurs. Usually the patient remains ambulatory. Patients may show dysmorphic features like a narrow face, micrognathia, prognathism, high arched palate, and chest deformities.
3. The adult form results in a progressive proximal and distal weakness. In some patients, there is a mild proximal weakness that slowly progresses to adult life.[12,13]

Diagnostic method

Diagnosis is based on morphologic identification of rods in myofibrils (frozen section stained with the modified trichrome technique). Electron microscopy shows that rods are elongated osmophilic structures. Immunohistochemical studies of rods shows presence of α-actinin.

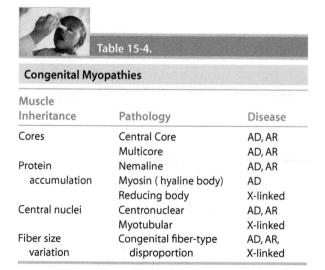

Table 15-4.

Congenital Myopathies

Muscle Inheritance	Pathology	Disease
Cores	Central Core	AD, AR
	Multicore	AD, AR
Protein accumulation	Nemaline	AD, AR
	Myosin (hyaline body)	AD
	Reducing body	X-linked
Central nuclei	Centronuclear	AD, AR
	Myotubular	X-linked
Fiber size variation	Congenital fiber-type disproportion	AD, AR, X-linked

Myopathies with Central Nuclei: Centronuclear Myopathy

There are autosomal dominant and recessive forms and an X-linked recessive form (myotubular myopathy).[12,13,16,17] The autosomal recessive form usually has an onset in infancy or childhood but there is a less common form with later onset. The X-linked recessive form (myotubular) progresses with severe myopathy and systemic features. The gene responsible for the autosomal dominant form is dynamin 2, for the autosomal recessive form is amphiphysin 2, and for the X-linked form is myotubularin.[12,13,16,17]

Clinical description

The early-onset cases represent the commonest presentation. Myotubular myopathy with onset in infancy shows severe hypotonia, proximal weakness, ophthalmoplegia with ptosis, and respiratory insufficiency. Polyhydramnios occurs in 50% of cases. Dysmorphic features include a large head, thin face, and long digits. Most infants have an early death. Survivors show systemic features like pyloric stenosis, gall and renal stones, hepatic dysfunction, spherocytosis, and a bleeding diathesis.[12,13,16,17]

Diagnostic method

Morphologic studies show numerous fibers with central nuclei (with NADH dehydrogenase reaction).

Fiber Size Variation Myopathies: Congenital Fiber-Type Disproportion

Fiber size variation myopathies are a condition characterized by type 1 fibers being smaller than type 2 fibers. There are dominant and recessive inheritances.[12,13]

Clinical presentation

The presentation is nonspecific and includes hypotonic infants with diffuse or proximal weakness and with facial and bulbar involvement. Other nonspecific features are arthrogryposis, scoliosis, and a high-arched palate. The course is variable, with slow progression or static.[12,13,16,17]

Diagnostic method

Type 1 fibers are at least 12% smaller than Type 2 fibers. Serum CK is normal or slightly elevated. EMG may show myopathic or some neuropathic features.

CONGENITAL MUSCULAR DYSTROPHIES

Congenital muscular dystrophy is a group of genetic diseases due to an error in one or more genes responsible for making structures of connective tissue molecules. The common clinical features are early diffuse weakness with some degree of contracture. The clinical features are discussed in more detail in Chapter 30. Also a central nervous system lesion related with myelin or neural migration occurs in severe forms. They manifest at birth. Inheritance is mainly autosomal recessive. Table 15-5 outlines the principal clinical features.

Primary Merosin Deficiency

The mutation in laminin α2 (chromosome 6q22) is inherited in a recessive pattern.[18] There is usually normal intelligence, but seizures can occur. MRI shows diffuse white matter abnormalities. There are mild and severe progressive forms.

Diagnostic method

Serum CK is moderately high. Immunohytochemistry with laminin α2 staining shows absence or partial loss of laminin.

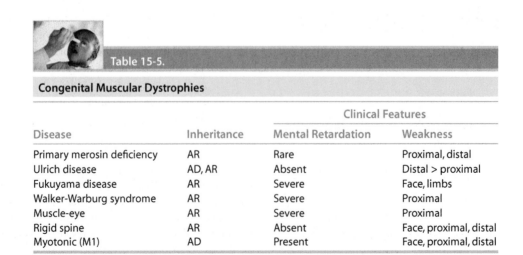

Table 15-5.

Congenital Muscular Dystrophies

Disease	Inheritance	Clinical Features	
		Mental Retardation	Weakness
Primary merosin deficiency	AR	Rare	Proximal, distal
Ulrich disease	AD, AR	Absent	Distal > proximal
Fukuyama disease	AR	Severe	Face, limbs
Walker-Warburg syndrome	AR	Severe	Proximal
Muscle-eye	AR	Severe	Proximal
Rigid spine	AR	Absent	Face, proximal, distal
Myotonic (M1)	AD	Present	Face, proximal, distal

Ulrich Disease

Ulrich disease is caused by collagen IV protein deficiency. It is inherited in either a recessive or a dominant pattern (chromosomes 21q22.3 and 2q37). While there is usually normal intelligence, skeletal abnormalities (joint contracture, scoliosis, foot deformities) and skin lesions like keratosis and atrophic scars can occur.

Diagnostic method

Serum CK is normal or elevated. Needle EMG may show myopathic features. Muscle biopsy reveals collagen IV absent from skeletal muscle.

Fukuyama Disease

Fukuyama disease is caused by a mutation of the Fukutin gene (Chromosome 9q31-q33) which occurs in an autosomal recessive pattern.[19-22] It is common in Japan. There is prominent central nervous system involvement with severe mental retardation, seizures, and progressive hydrocephalus. Pathology shows lissencephaly type II, pachygyria, and cerebellar lesions. There are also ocular lesions like myopia, retinal detachment, microphthalmos, and optic nerve atrophy.

Diagnostic method

Serum CK has moderate elevation. Needle EMG may show a myopathic pattern. Immunohistochemical staining shows a reduced α-dystroglycan pattern. There is greatly reduced surface membrane α-dystroglycan and reduced laminin α2.[19-22]

Walker-Warburg Syndrome

The Walker-Warburg syndrome is caused by a mutation of O-mannosyltransferase 1 (chromosome 9q34.1).[19-23] This is inherited as a recessive trait. It is lethal within the first years of life. There are severe central nervous system lesions with mental retardation and seizures. Pathology shows lissenchephaly type II, pachygiria, hydrocephalus, occipital encephalocele, and brainstem and cerebellar lesions. Ocular lesions like cataracts and microphthalmos are common.

Diagnostic method

Serum CK may be normal. Immunohistochemistry shows reduced β-dystroglycan and normal merosin staining patterns.[19-23]

Muscle-Eye-Brain Disease

Muscle-eye-brain disease is a result of a mutation of O-linked mannose β1,2-N-acetylglucosaminyltransferase (chromosome 1p32-p34).[19-23] This is inherited in an autosomal recessive pattern. There is severe mental retardation. Pathology shows disorganization of the cerebral cortex without horizontal lamination (cobblestone), hydrocephalus, and cerebellar hypoplasia with an absent inferior vermis. Eye malformations include severe myopia, glaucoma, cataracts, and retinal dysplasia.

Diagnostic method

Immunohistochemical staining shows α-dystroglycan and laminin β2 increased.[19-22]

Rigid Spine

Rigid spine disease occurs secondary to a mutation of selenoprotein N,1 (chromosome 1p35-p36), which is transmitted in an autosomal recessive pattern. Intelligence remains normal. There are skeletal abnormalities with a rigid spine, limited flexion, progressive scoliosis, and joint contractures.

Diagnostic method

Serum CK is normal. Insulin resistance can occur in some cases. MRI of muscle is useful to detect selective involvement of muscles (vastus lateralis, biceps femoris) and it is useful to choose the muscle for biopsy. Pathology shows minicores. Immunohistochemical studies reveal normal laminin α2 and normal merosin.

Myotonic Dystrophy (DM1 with Congenital Onset)

Myotonic dystrophy DM1 is a CTG triple repeat disease and has a congenital onset in 10% to 15% of patients. Myotonic dystrophy is inherited in an autosomal dominant pattern. There is a prenatal onset and during pregnancy it is possible to find decreased fetal movements and polyhydramnios. At delivery, a breech presentation with preterm labor is common. Neonatal respiratory distress is a common complication. Hypotonia, including facial and jaw weakness, is relevant, but there is not clinical myotonia. Mental retardation and autistic behavior frequently occur. Skeletal malformation such as arthrogryposis, high-arched palate, prominent brow, and tapered chin are present.

Diagnostic method

Serum CK is normal. EMG is nonspecific, without myotonia. MRI shows global cerebral atrophy and ventricular dilatation at birth. Muscle biopsy could be normal. Measurement of CTG triplet repeat sequences in the mother and fetus can assist in prenatal diagnosis.

MUSCULAR DYSTROPHIES

The muscular dystrophies are a group of genetic diseases in which the primary pathology affects the stability of the sarcolemma membrane. In congenital myopathies, there is a different process that affect primary the myofibrils. Presently, there are more than 30 different kinds of muscular dystrophies, but Duchenne muscular dystrophy is the most common and one of the most severe types. Table 15-6 outlines principal muscular dystrophies.

Duchenne Muscular Dystrophy

Duchenne muscular dystrophy is due to the complete lack of dystrophin (chromosome Xp21).[24] It is inherited in an X-linked recessive pattern.

Clinical description

Duchenne muscular dystrophy affects approximately 1 in 3500 boys.[25] Although serum CK is high beginning in the neonatal period, the onset of weakness is between 3 and 5 years of age. The gait becomes lordotic and waddling. Proximal weakness is symmetric and there is a Gowers sign (standing up with the aid of hands pushing on knees). Calf muscle hypertrophy due to muscle fibrosis is also seen. There is a progressive decline in strength, so boys are unable to walk about the age of 9 to 13 years. There is mild mental retardation, and night blindness (abnormal response to flashes of light in the dark) can occur. After loss of ambulation occurs, scoliosis and joint contractures can arise. Dilated cardiomyopathy and respiratory failure associated with infections contribute to death most commonly between 15 and 25 years of age.[25]

Diagnostic method

Serum CK is very high. Muscle biopsy shows endomysial fibrosis, muscle fiber degeneration and regeneration. Immunohistochemical staining for dystrophin protein is absent. Genetic testing shows deletion, duplication, and mutations.

Treatment

Prednisone prolongs the ability to walk by 2 to 5 years. Doses should be in the 5 to 10 mg/kg/wk range.[26,27] Deflazacort dosed at 0.9 to 1.2 mg/kg/d could be better in preserving cardiac function and for nonsurgical management of scoliosis, in countries where available.[28] For joint contractures, passive stretching exercises and night splints on the ankles are useful. Surgical contracture release of the ankles, knees, or hips may be necessary.[29] For scoliosis, surgical insertion of a spinal rod may be necessary.[29]

Becker Muscular Dystrophy

Becker muscular dystrophy is similar to the Duchenne type, but it is milder because boys with Becker have some dystrophin. Becker muscular dystrophy starts later in life and survival is much longer than in Duchenne muscular dystrophy.

Table 15-6.

Muscular Dystrophies

Disease	Inheritance	Protein	Weakness
Duchenne	X-linked, AR	Dystrophin	Proximal > distal
Becker	X-linked	Dystrophin	Proximal > distal
Myotonic			
DM 1	AD	DMPK	Face, proximal, distal
DM 2	AD	ZNF9	Face, proximal, distal
Facial-scapulo-humeral	AD, sporadic	Sarcoglycan	Face, scapular, asymmetric
Emery-Dreifuss			
Type 1	X-recessive	Emerin	Humeroperoneal
Type 2	AD, AR	Laminin	Limb-girdle
Type 3	AD	SYNE1	Girdle
Type 4	AD	SYNE2	Limb-girdle
Limb-girdle			
LG2A	AR	Calpain	Limb-girdle
LG2B	AR	Dyferlin	Legs
LG2C	AR	Sarcoglycan	Proximal > distal
LG2D	AR	Sarcoglycan	Proximal
LGE	AR	Sarcoglycan	Proximal
Miyoshi	AR, sporadic	Dysferlin	Distal
Bethlem	AD	Collagen VI	Proximal > distal

SYNE, synaptic nuclear envelope protein; MPK, myotonin protein kinase; ZNF9, zinc finger protein 9.

Clinical description

Mean age onset is about 12 years (range, 1-70 years) for the Becker type. There is a proximal and symmetric slow progressive weakness, with calf muscle hypertrophy and calf pain on exercise. The mean age at loss of ambulation is in the fourth decade. Other features include cardiomyopathy, joint contractures, and mild mental retardation.[25]

Diagnostic method

Serum CK is very high. Muscle biopsy shows muscle fibers degeneration and regeneration. Immunohistochemical studies reveal reduced dystrophin staining.

Myotonic Dystrophy

There are two genetic foci. Type DM 1 myotonin protein kinase (DMPK) is inherited via chromosome 19q13.3, as an autosomal dominant pattern, and the DM 2 type PROMM, via the zinc finger protein 9 (ZNF9) on chromosome 3q21, which is also autosomal dominant.

Clinical description

Type DM 1. Myotonic dystrophy is the most prevalent inherited neuromuscular disease in adults (13.5 per 100,000 live births). Onset could be from the neonatal period to late adulthood. In childhood, there is motor delay and mental retardation. Physical examination shows a hatchet face with frontal balding, temporal wasting, and ptosis. Weakness and myotonia occur during muscle contraction (grip) or are evoked by percussion.[30,31] Other features are cataracts, hypogonadism, insulin resistance, hypoventilation, cardiac dysfunction (conduction defects, arrhythmias, cardiomyopathy), megacolon, constipation, and intestinal pseudo-obstruction.

Diagnostic method. Serum CK is normal or mildly elevated. EMG shows myotonic discharges. Endocrine tests show low testosterone and insulin insensitivity. Serum IgG is low. Muscle MRI usually reveals significant compromise of the medial head of the gastrocnemius and soleus muscles. Genetic testing shows a mutated gene DMPK ZNF9. CTG repeats have a size of 100 to 4000.

Type DM 2. Type 2 has onset of weakness and myotonia from 8 years to 60 years. There is variable cardiac, gonadal, and ocular compromise in this subtype. Genetic testing shows mutated gene ZNF9. CTG repeats occur with more than 5000 repeats.

Treatment

For myotonia there are different drugs like quinine, phenytoin, and procainamide.

Facial-Scapulo-Humeral Myopathy

Facial-scapulo-humeral myopathy is caused by a double homeobox protein 4 (DUX4) (D4Z4 repeat DNA deletion), located on chromosome 4q35. This is an autosomal dominant disorder.[32] The prevalence is 1 to 5 per 100,000, and it is the third most common dystrophy after Duchenne and myotonic dystrophy.

Clinical description

There is a variable onset between the first and fifth decades. Infantile onset is uncommon and it is associated with severe facial weakness. Actually the disease has usually been present for many years before the parents seek medical attention. Weakness is often asymmetric and involves face (there is an unusual asymmetric expression) and scapular muscles. There can also be compromise of the distal posterior leg. There is a slowly descending pattern of weakness, from face to arms and then to legs.[32] Although progression is very slow, periods of acceleration may be observed. The disease has a broad clinical spectrum, mainly due to detection of atypical and sporadic cases by DNA testing. Prognosis is worse with younger onset, and about 20% of patients present with wheelchair confinement. Other systemic features include sensorineural hearing loss, Coats disease (retinal vasculopathy), cardiac arrhythmia, and conduction block.

Diagnostic method

Serum CK is normal or moderately elevated. EMG may show a myopathic pattern. Muscle biopsy shows hypertrophic muscle fibers with some necrotic fibers. There is inflammation located at the endomysial and perivascular spaces. DNA Eco RI fragment restriction analysis can help with diagnosis.

Treatment

Albuterol treatment produces increased muscle mass with no significant change in strength.

Emery-Dreifuss Myopathy

There are four types of Emery-Dreifuss myopathy depending on protein gene mutation. (Table 15-6).[33] The first recognized was the X-linked form (type 1) that presents as a dystrophy more benign than Duchenne.

Clinical description

Type 1. Onset could be at birth with neonatal hypotonia. Muscle contractures of the elbow and flexion of the neck and paraspinal muscles develop before the slowly progressive weakness. Upper limb weakness and scapular winging occur first with a later involvement of the legs.[34] Cardiac dysfunction is prominent and includes rhythm disturbances, AV conduction defects, and left ventricular myocardial fibrosis. Most patients need a pacemaker and the severity of cardiopathy increases with age.[35]

Diagnostic method. Serum CK is mildly elevated to <10 times normal. EMG shows a myopathic pattern with some fibrillations. MRI shows selective soleus muscle involvement. Muscle immunohistochemistry reveals absent emerin.

Type 2. There are contractures and cardiac dysfunction.

Diagnostic method. Serum CK is normal or mildly elevated. EMG shows myopathic pattern. MRI shows involvement of the medial head of gastrocnemius with the lateral head spared. Immunohistochemistry staining shows absent laminin.

Types 3 and 4. Type 3 and 4 are very rare conditions, onset of both conditions is during childhood. Type 4 may present cardiopathy.

Limb-Girdle Muscular Dystrophy

Limb-girdle muscular dystrophy occurs because of a mutation in the gene that controls the production of the sarcoglycan components of the dystrophin. It gets its name because there is a primary weakness of the shoulder, chest, hip, and thigh. The weakness is characterized by wide genetic and clinical heterogeneity.[36]

Clinical description

Onset could be in childhood, adolescence, or adulthood. Patients show a slow progression and weakness becomes severe after 20 to 30 years. Intelligence is normal. The clinical assessment must consider geographical and ethnic origin of patients, because locally the frequency of the different forms of the disease varies considerably.

Diagnostic method

Serum CK is elevated. MRI shows changes in specific muscles according to the subtype. EMG shows a myopathic pattern. Muscle biopsy shows nonspecific changes with hypertrophic and atrophic fibers. Regeneration and inflammation can also be seen. In most patients, a definite diagnosis can be obtained only by genetic analysis.

Miyoshi Myopathy

Miyoshi myopathy arises secondary to a mutation of the dysferlin protein gene (chromosome 2p13.3-p13.1).[37] This disorder is inherited in an autosomal recessive pattern.

Clinical description

The clinical onset is from 15 to 38 years. There is usually distal symmetric weakness of gastrocnemius and soleus, but in rare cases this can be asymmetric.[38] Upper limbs and proximal muscles are also involved. The progression

is slow, and about 30% of patients present with wheelchair confinement.

Diagnostic method

Serum CK is very high. EMG may show myopathic or neurogenic patterns. MRI shows selective involvement of the hamstring, gastrocnemius, and soleus. Muscle immunohistochemistry shows absent dysferlin.

Bethlem Myopathy

There are several loci for the collagen gene mutation—type VI, subunit α1, α2, α3 (chromosome 21q22.3, chromosome 2q37)—which result in Bethlem myopathy.[39] These occur with an autosomal dominant inheritance pattern.

Clinical description

At onset, there are contractures and congenital torticollis. Weakness is more proximal than distal. Progression is mild during childhood but may become disabling in adulthood. Other features include skin lesions similar to follicular hyperkeratosis and cardiac dysfunction with conduction abnormalities.

Diagnostic method

Serum CK could be normal or elevated. EMG shows a myopathic pattern. MRI shows selective involvement of the vastus lateralis and hamstrings. Muscle biopsy shows nonspecific myopathic changes.

INHERITED METABOLIC MYOPATHIES

Inherited metabolic myopathies are a group of relatively rare diseases and are much less common than most of the muscular dystrophies. However, improved diagnostic methods that include morphologic, biochemical, and genetic testing have resulted in an increasing number of patients being diagnosed with inherited metabolic myopathies (Table 15-7).

Mitochondrial Myopathies

Mutations in mitochondrial DNA are important causes of human disease that are transmitted by maternal inheritance. Brain, heart, and muscle tissues that show high energy expenditure and are dependent on oxidative metabolism are frequent sites of mitochondrial pathology. There are many different phenotypes, some of which predominantly affect the brain and others that often present as a neuromuscular disorder. Several mitochondrial phenotypes also show multisystem involvement. Clinical presentation of mitochondrial myopathies could be weakness, fatigue, or rhabdomyolysis. Table 15-8

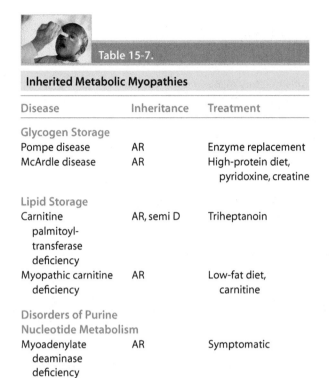

Table 15-7.

Inherited Metabolic Myopathies

Disease	Inheritance	Treatment
Glycogen Storage		
Pompe disease	AR	Enzyme replacement
McArdle disease	AR	High-protein diet, pyridoxine, creatine
Lipid Storage		
Carnitine palmitoyl-transferase deficiency	AR, semi D	Triheptanoin
Myopathic carnitine deficiency	AR	Low-fat diet, carnitine
Disorders of Purine Nucleotide Metabolism		
Myoadenylate deaminase deficiency	AR	Symptomatic

outlines the principal mitochondrial myopathies with their associated neurological features.

MELAS (Mitochondrial Encephalomyopathy, Lactic Acidosis, Stroke)

This disorder can have either a maternal inheritance or a sporadic form. The onset is in childhood. Systemic features include pigmentary retinopathy, cardiomyopathy, diabetes, pancreatitis, nephrotic syndrome, and multiple endocrine dysfunctions. The prognosis is for survival into the second to fourth decades. The most common

causes of death are cardiopulmonary failure and status epilepticus.

Diagnostic method. Serum lactic acidosis is common. The CK is usually normal. The EMG may be normal or reveal myopathic changes. MRI may show multifocal strokes. Muscle biopsy shows ragged red fibers. Genetic blood testing reveals that 80% of cases are associated with A3243G.

MERRF (Myoclonic Epilepsy; Ragged Red Fibers)

MERRF is a disorder with a myoclonic epilepsy syndrome and myopathy that has a maternal inheritance pattern. The onset is typically during late adolescence. Other features include short stature and lipomatosis. The prognosis is variable

Diagnostic method. Serum CK is normal and lactic acidosis is variable. Muscle biopsy shows ragged red fibers. Genetic blood testing reveals that 80% of cases are associated with A8344G.

Kearns-Sayre syndrome

Kearns-Sayre syndrome is a myopathic syndrome that is inherited in a sporadic fashion. The onset is during adolescence. Patients have short stature, with cardiac conduction block and thyroid dysfunction. The syndrome typically progresses to death by early adulthood.

Diagnostic method. Serum lactic acidosis is common. CSF usually has a high protein. Muscle pathology shows ragged red fibers.

Coenzyme Q10 deficiency

Coenzyme Q10 deficiency can have either a recessive or sporadic inheritance pattern. The onset is during childhood. One phenotype has an isolated myopathy weakness

Table 15-8.

Other Neurological Features in Some Mitochondrial Myopathies

	MELAS	MERRF	Kearns-Sayre	CO Q10 Deficiency	COX Deficiency Benign	COX Deficiency Fatal
Neuropathy	Yes	Yes	Yes	Yes	Yes	Yes
PEO	Yes	No	Yes	No	Yes	No
Dementia	Yes	Yes	Yes	No	No	No
Convulsion	Yes	Yes	No	No	Yes	No
Ataxia	Yes	Yes	Yes	Yes	No	No
Encephalopathy	Yes	No	No	Yes	Yes	No
Hemiparesis	Yes	No	Yes	No	No	No
Myoclonus	No	Yes	No	No	No	No
Extrapyramidal	Yes	No	No	Yes	No	No

phenotype, while another variety has recurrent myoglobinuria that is induced by mild to moderate exercise or fever. The variety with myoglobinuria also presents with seizures and cognitive impairment.

Diagnostic method. Laboratory studies reveal serum lactic acidosis and elevated serum CK. EMG may show a myopathic pattern. Muscle pathology shows fibers with mitochondrial proliferation with lipid storage and reduced coenzyme Q10 levels. The primary treatment is coenzyme Q10, 150 to 500 mg/d and riboflavin 100 mg/d.

COX deficiency (cytochrome oxidase C deficiency)

There are two infantile myopathies associated with severe COX deficiency. Both of these are inherited in an autosomal recessive pattern. The benign myopathy has an onset during infancy or childhood. The course is not progressive and there is occasional spontaneous improvement. The other form is a fatal condition that causes respiratory insufficiency and death before 1 year of age. When the kidney is affected this is referred to as Toni-Fanconi syndrome. The brain and heart are spared.

Diagnostic method

Serum lactic acidosis and elevated CK are typical. Muscle biopsy shows severe reduction in COX and ragged red fibers are usually seen.

INFLAMMATORY MYOPATHIES

Inflammatory myopathies are a heterogeneous group of muscle diseases with different pathologic mechanisms, from autoimmune conditions to specific infective forms. Table 15-9 outlines different types of myositis in children.

Juvenile Dermatomyositis

Juvenile dermatomyositis is the most common inflammatory myopathy of childhood. It is a rare systemic autoimmune myopathy that shows a high incidence of vasculopathy. Both genetic and environmental risk factors seem to have a role in the cause of juvenile dermatomyositis. The HLA B8-DRB1*0301 ancestral haplotype is a strong immunogenetic risk factor. Antecedent viral infections (coxsackie B, parvovirus, echovirus) and birth seasonality suggest that environmental stimuli are also involved. There is weakness in proximal muscles and pathognomonic skin rashes. Muscle swelling may occur. The skin shows violaceous periorbital erythema (heliotrope). This rash may also arise on the extensor surfaces of joints. The occurrence of generalized rash and ulcerations means a worse prognosis. Other skin features include ulcerations (due to complement deposition with occlusive endarteropathy of dermal vessels)

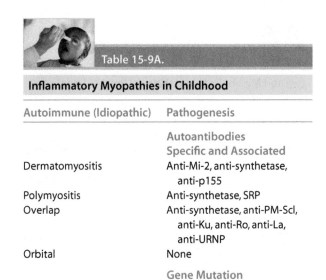

Table 15-9A.

Inflammatory Myopathies in Childhood

Autoimmune (Idiopathic)	Pathogenesis
	Autoantibodies Specific and Associated
Dermatomyositis	Anti-Mi-2, anti-synthetase, anti-p155
Polymyositis	Anti-synthetase, SRP
Overlap	Anti-synthetase, anti-PM-Scl, anti-Ku, anti-Ro, anti-La, anti-URNP
Orbital	None
	Gene Mutation
Focal	TNFRSF1A protein

and Gottron papules (intercarpal phalangeal). There are some amyopathic forms in which myositis occurs later. Even with treatment, recovery may be incomplete. Mortality is low.

Diagnostic method

Serum CK is elevated. MRI is useful to localize affected muscle prior the EMG and biopsy tests. EMG often reveals a myopathic pattern with spontaneous activity. Muscle biopsy shows mononuclear cells at perimysial, perivascular, and endomysial sites (the inflammatory infiltrate consists of B cells, CD4+ T cells, and plasmacytoid dendritic cells). Perifascicular fiber atrophy and regeneration also occur.

Treatment

Daily oral prednisone (1-2 mg/kg/d). In cases of severe vasculopathy intravenous methylprenidsolone

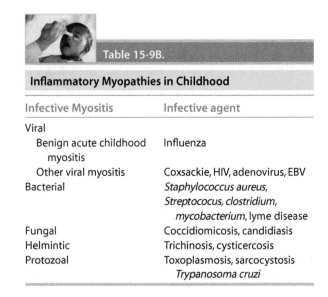

Table 15-9B.

Inflammatory Myopathies in Childhood

Infective Myositis	Infective agent
Viral	
Benign acute childhood myositis	Influenza
Other viral myositis	Coxsackie, HIV, adenovirus, EBV
Bacterial	*Staphylococcus aureus*, *Streptococus, clostridium, mycobacterium*, lyme disease
Fungal	Coccidiomicosis, candidiasis
Helmintic	Trichinosis, cysticercosis
Protozoal	Toxoplasmosis, sarcocystosis *Trypanosoma cruzi*

(30 mg/ kg/d for 3 days) may also be of benefit. Severe cases may require more aggressive immunomodulation.

Juvenile Polymyositis

Juvenile polymyositis is rare and the inflammatory infiltrate is predominantly endomysial, consisting of CD8+ and CD4+ cells as well as dendritic cells, macrophages and plasma cells.

Overlap Syndromes

Myositis associated with autoantibodies like scleroderma (PM-Scl, U1-nRNP), Sjögren syndrome (SSA/Ro), and lupus (U1-nRNP, U2- nRNP) are rare during childhood.

Focal Myositis

Focal myositis is very rare in children. Boys are more frequently affected than girls. A solitary and painful asymmetric muscle mass is found (quadriceps and gastrocnemius are the most commonly involved).

Orbital Myositis

Orbital myositis is also very rare. The course is variable, and one or more extraocular muscles is infiltrated by an idiopathic inflammatory process. Both diseases can be treated with prednisone.

INFECTIOUS MYOSITIS

Infection of muscles is uncommon in children. There are a wide range of infective agents that can produce myositis (virus, bacteria, fungi, parasites) as delineated in Table 15-9B.

Myopathic Channelopathies in Children

Myopathic channelopathies are caused by inherited mutations of ion channels and can affect different organs including muscles. Muscle diseases are outlined in Table 15-10.

Myotonia Congenital (Thomsen)

Myotonia congenita occurs secondary to a mutation of the muscle chloride channel (CLCN1). This is an autosomal dominant disorder on chromosome 7q35. There is a recessive form (Becker). Onset can be from infancy to adulthood. A parent may describe weakness instead of stiffness due to myotonia; children usually have muscle hypertrophy. There is mild weakness in the proximal muscles.

Paramyotonia Congenita

Paramyotonia congenita arises secondary to a sodium channel mutation (SCN4 A). The defect is autosomal dominant and localizes to chromosome 17q35. Onset occurs during the first decade of life. Myotonia is worse in cold temperature and with exercise. Symptoms are not progressive. Muscles of the face are more sensitive to worsening in cold temperatures.

Diagnostic method

Serum CK is usually normal. EMG shows myotonic discharges. Genetic testing may be available in specialized centers.

Treatment

For both paramyotonia congenita and myotonia congenital, treatment is symptomatic with treatment for myotonic stiffness, like phenytoin, carbamazepine, and quinine.

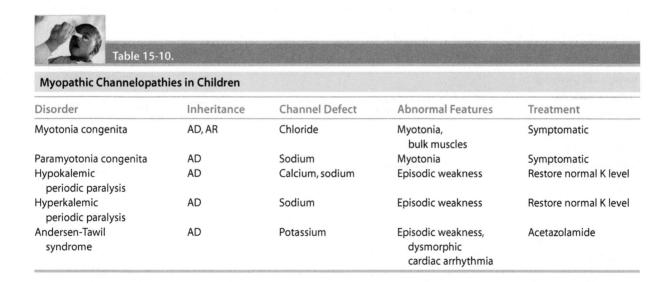

Table 15-10.

Myopathic Channelopathies in Children

Disorder	Inheritance	Channel Defect	Abnormal Features	Treatment
Myotonia congenita	AD, AR	Chloride	Myotonia, bulk muscles	Symptomatic
Paramyotonia congenita	AD	Sodium	Myotonia	Symptomatic
Hypokalemic periodic paralysis	AD	Calcium, sodium	Episodic weakness	Restore normal K level
Hyperkalemic periodic paralysis	AD	Sodium	Episodic weakness	Restore normal K level
Andersen-Tawil syndrome	AD	Potassium	Episodic weakness, dysmorphic cardiac arrhythmia	Acetazolamide

Hypokalemic Periodic Paralysis

Hypokalemic periodic paralysis is the most frequent form of periodic paralysis occurring in 1 per 100,000 children. It is usually due to a calcium channel mutation, CACNA1S, localized to chromosome 1q31. It is inherited in an autosomal dominant pattern. A sodium channel mutation, SCN4A, which is localized to chromosome 17q13 and is also autosomal dominant, also exists. Onset occurs during early childhood. The disease presents as episodic weakness of proximal muscles, which may be triggered by cold temperature, physical activity, and carbohydrate-rich meals. Attacks usually occur at night or early in the morning.

Diagnostic method

Laboratory studies may reveal a low potassium level in the serum. The EKG is often abnormal as well.

Treatment

During the attack the normal serum potassium level must be restored. As a long-term treatment, acetazolamide may be of benefit. The most important treatment is to avoid the triggering factors.

Hyperkalemic Periodic Paralysis

Hyperkalemic periodic paralysis is less common than the hypokalemic form. The hyperkalemic form is secondary to a mutation of the sodium channel (SCN4A) on chromosome 17q35. It is inherited in an autosomal dominant pattern. Onset occurs during infancy or childhood. There is episodic weakness. Attacks can occur several times during the day and are relatively brief (15-60 min). Clinical myotonia can occur between attacks. Some patient may develop a progressive myopathy as well. Attacks may be provoked by exercise, exposure to cold temperature, stress, and fasting.

Diagnostic method

A high serum potassium level should be present during an attack.

Treatment

During the attack a high sugar load may be of benefit. Thiazides, acetazolamide, and intravenous calicum gluconate may also be useful. It is important to avoid triggering factors.

ENDOCRINE MYOPATHIES IN CHILDREN

Exogenous and iatrogenic endocrinologic disorders may produce muscle dysfunction. Some of them occur in pediatric patients. Table 15-11 shows the principal endocrine disorders with muscle involvement.

Table 15-11.

Endocrine Myopathies in Children

Condition	Clinical	CK	EMG
Thyroid Dysfunction			
Hypothyroidism (Debré-Kocher-Sémélaigne)	Proximal weakness, muscle pseudo-hypertrophy	High	Myopathic
Hyperthyroidism.	Proximal weakness, bulba weakness, periodic paralysis, thyroid ophthalmopathy	Normal	Fasciculations
Parathyroid Dysfunction			
Hypoparathyroidism	Tetany, Chvostek sign	Normal or elevated	Normal
Hyperparathyroidism	Proximal weakness with brisk reflexes	Normal	Myopathic
Steroid-Induced Myopathy			
Cushing disease	Proximal weakness	Elevated	Myopathic
Exogenous steroids			
Hyperaldosteronism			
Conn syndrome	Episodic weakness, proximal weakness	Elevated	Myopathic
Growth Hormone Excess			
Acromegaly	Proximal weakness	Normal	Myopathic

Table 15-12.

Drug-Induced Myopathies

Type	Drugs	Clinical Features	CK	Biopsy
Steroid	Fluorinated prednisone	Chronic proximal weakness Acute generalized weakness	Normal	Type 2 fiber atrophy
Necrotizing	Clofibrato Gemfibrozil	Acute or chronic weakness Rhabdomyolysis	High	Necrotic fibers
Mitochondrial	Zidovudine	Acute or chronicproximal weaknes Rhabdomyolysis	Normal or elevated	Ragged red fibers
Lysosomal storage	Chloroquine	Acute or chronic weakness	High	Type 1 fiber atrophy autophagic vacuoles
Anti-microtubular	Colchicine	Acute or chronic weakness	Normal or elevated	Autophagic vacuoles
Inflammatory	Interferon-α Penicillamine Phenytoin	Acute or chronic proximal weakness	High	Inflammatory cell infiltrates

TOXIC MYOPATHIES

There are several mechanisms by which biologic toxins and drugs produce myotoxicity. Table 15-12 outlines different drug-induced myopathies according the underlying mechanism.

REFERENCES

1. Anlar B. Juvenile myasthenia: diagnosis and treatment. *Paediatr Drugs*. 2000;2:161-169.
2. Scheife RT, Hills JR, Munsat TL. Myasthenia gravis: signs, symptoms, diagnosis, immunology, and current therapy. *Pharmacotherapy*. 1981;1:39-54.
3. Evoli A, Tonali PA, Padua L, et al. Clinical correlates with anti-MuSK antibodies in generalized seronegative myasthenia gravis. *Brain*. 2003;126:2304-2311.
4. Keys PA, Blume RP. Therapeutic strategies for myasthenia gravis. *DICP*. 1991;25:1101-1108.
5. Schwendimann RN, Burton E, Minagar A. Management of myasthenia gravis. *Am J Ther*. 2005;12:262-268.
6. Mintz S, Petersen SR, MacFarland D, Petajan J, Richards RC. The current role of thymectomy for myasthenia gravis. *Am J Surg*. 1980;140:734-737.
7. Clemmens MR, Bell L. Infant botulism presenting with poor feeding and lethargy: a review of 4 cases. *Pediatr Emerg Care*. 2007;23:492-494.
8. Brook I. Infant botulism. *J Perinatol*. 2007;27:175-180.
9. Cai S, Singh BR, Sharma S. Botulism diagnostics: from clinical symptoms to in vitro assays. *Crit Rev Microbiol*. 2007;33:109-125.
10. Burke ME. Myasthenia gravis and pregnancy. *J Perinat Neonatal Nurs*. 1993;7:11-21.
11. Shillito P, Vincent A, Newsom-Davis J. Congenital myasthenic syndromes. *Neuromuscul Disord*. 1993;3:183-190.
12. D'Amico A, Bertini E. Congenital myopathies. *Curr Neurol Neurosci Rep*. 2008;8:73-79.
13. Laing NG. Congenital myopathies. *Curr Opin Neurol*. 2007;20:583-589.
14. Jungbluth H. Central core disease. *Orphanet J Rare Dis*. 2007;2:25.
15. Robinson R, Carpenter D, Shaw MA, Halsall J, Hopkins P. Mutations in RYR1 in malignant hyperthermia and central core disease. *Hum Mutat*. 2006;27:977-989.
16. Jungbluth H, Wallgren-Pettersson C, Laporte J. Centronuclear (myotubular) myopathy. *Orphanet J Rare Dis*. 2008 3:26.
17. Jackson CE. A clinical approach to muscle diseases. *Semin Neurol*. 2008;28:228-240.
18. Shibuya S, Wakayama Y, Inoue M, Kojima H, Oniki H. Merosin (laminin-2) localization in basal lamina of normal skeletal muscle fibers and changes in plasma membrane of merosin-deficient skeletal muscle fibers. *Med Electron Microsc*. 2003;36:213-220.
19. Martin PT. The dystroglycanopathies: the new disorders of O-linked glycosylation. *Semin Pediatr Neurol*. 2005;12:152-158.
20. Muntoni F, Brockington M, Blake DJ, Torelli S, Brown SC. Defective glycosylation in muscular dystrophy. *Lancet*. 2002;360:1419-1421.
21. Toda T, Chiyonobu T, Xiong H, et al. Fukutin and alpha-dystroglycanopathies. *Acta Myol*. 2005;24:60-63.
22. Hewitt JE, Grewal PK. Glycosylation defects in inherited muscle disease. *Cell Mol Life Sci*. 2003;60:251-258.
23. van Reeuwijk J, Brunner HG, van Bokhoven H. Glyc-O-genetics of Walker-Warburg syndrome. *Clin Genet*. 2005;67:281-289.
24. den Dunnen JT, Beggs AH. Multiplex PCR for identifying DMD gene deletions. *Curr Protoc Hum Genet*. 2006 May; Chapter 9:Unit 9.3.
25. Sussman M. Duchenne muscular dystrophy. *J Am Acad Orthop Surg*. 2002;10:138-151.

26. Manzur AY, Kuntzer T, Pike M, Swan A. Glucocorticoid corticosteroids for Duchenne muscular dystrophy. *Cochrane Database Syst Rev*. 2008;23:CD003725.

27. Angelini C. The role of corticosteroids in muscular dystrophy: a critical appraisal. *Muscle Nerve*. 2007;36:424-435.

28. Campbell C, Jacob P. Deflazacort for the treatment of Duchenne dystrophy: a systematic review. *BMC Neurol*. 2003;3:7.

29. Emery AE. The muscular dystrophies. *Lancet*. 2002;359: 687-695.

30. Miller TM. Differential diagnosis of myotonic disorders. *Muscle Nerve*. 2008;37:293-299.

31. Wheeler TM, Thornton CA. Myotonic dystrophy: RNA-mediated muscle disease. *Curr Opin Neurol*. 2007;20:572-576.

32. Pandya S, King WM, Tawil R. Facioscapulohumeral dystrophy. *Phys Ther*. 2008;88:105-113.

33. Wheeler MA, Ellis JA. Molecular signatures of Emery-Dreifuss muscular dystrophy. *Biochem Soc Trans*. 2008;36: 1354-1358.

34. Muchir A, Worman HJ. Emery-Dreifuss muscular dystrophy. *Curr Neurol Neurosci Rep*. 2007;7:78-83.

35. Cullington D, Pyatt JR. Emery-Dreifuss muscular dystrophy with cardiac manifestations. *Br J Hosp Med (Lond)*. 2005;66:642-643.

36. Mathews KD, Moore SA. Muscular dystrophy. *Curr Neurol Neurosci Rep*. 2003;3:78-85.

37. Bansal D, Campbell KP. Dysferlin and the plasma membrane repair in muscular dystrophy. *Trends Cell Biol*. 2004;14:206-213.

38. Udd B, Griggs R. Distal myopathies. *Curr Opin Neurol*. 2001;14:561-566.

39. Bertini E, Pepe G. Collagen type VI and related disorders: Bethlem myopathy and Ullrich scleroatonic muscular dystrophy. *Eur J Paediatr Neurol*. 2002;6:193-198.

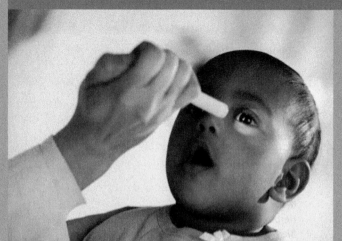

CHAPTER 16

Neuroinfectious Disease

Marvin B. Harper,
Cynthia J. Campen, Sarah M.
Kranick, Daniel J. Licht, Mark
Gorman, and Scott L. Pomeroy

MENINGITIS

Definitions and Epidemiology

Meningitis is defined as an inflammation of the lep-tomeninges by any cause. Bacteria cause meningitis by invading and replicating in the subarachnoid space and cause significant morbidity and mortality. Viral infections may also cause meningitis, mostly commonly enteroviruses, but few children with viral meningitis suffer any long-term sequelae. Therefore the focus of this chapter will be on bacterial meningitis. Figure 16-1 gives the age, organism, and specific rates of bacterial meningitis in the United States prior to the introduction of currently used conjugate vaccines (note the y-axis is a log scale). As can be seen, the greatest risk period for bacterial meningitis is in the first 6 months of life.

Overall, there has been a remarkable decline in the rate of bacterial meningitis in the developed world over the last 2 decades with the introduction of the *Haemophilus influenzae* type b conjugate vaccines, the *Streptococcus pneumoniae* conjugate vaccines, and greater use of meningococcal vaccines. *Haemophilus influenzae* type b was once the leading cause of bacterial meningitis in children but has been virtually eliminated in countries utilizing the conjugate vaccine. In the first 2 months of life, Enterobacteriaceae (eg, *E. coli*, *Klebsiella* species), group B streptococci, and occasionally *Listeria monocytogenes*, *Salmonella* species, or enterococci will cause bacterial meningitis. Infections due to *S pneumoniae* occur with increasing in frequency over the second month to become the most likely cause of bacterial meningitis, and continue to increase in frequency until 4 or 5 months of age when they begin to decline. *Neisseria meningitidis* is the most common

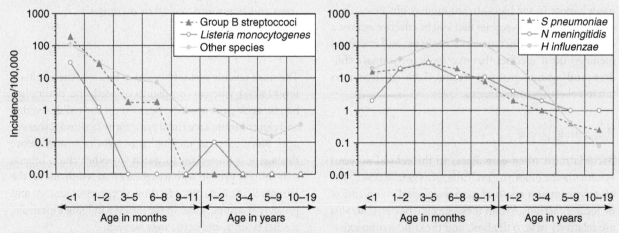

FIGURE 16-1 ■ Incidence rates of bacterial meningitis by age and pathogen prior to the introduction of the conjugate *Haemophilus influenzae* type b and heptavalent *S-pneumoniae* vaccines. (*From Wenger JD, Hightower AW, Facklam RR, Gaventa S, Broome CV, eds. Bacterial meningitis in the United States, 1986: report of a multistate surveillance study. The Bacterial Meningitis Study Group. J Infect Dis. 1990;162:1316-1323.*)

Table 16-1.

Etiology of Meningitis

Common
Enteroviruses
Neisseria meningitides
Streptococcus pneumoniae
Group B streptococci
Escherichi coli
Haemophilus influenzae
Listeria monocytogenes

Less Common
Herpes simplex
Klebsiella species (and other Enterobaceriaceae)
Lyme disease
Candida species
Salmonella species
Mycobacterium tuberculosis
Pseudomonas aeruginosa
Staphylococcus aureus
Enterococcal species

Rare
Cysticercosis
Cryptococcus
Lymphocytic choriomeningitis
Mumps
Syphilis
Amoebae

cause of bacterial meningitis by 1 year of age. *S pneumoniae* remains the second most common cause after 1 year of age, and all other pathogens trail behind considerably. These two pathogens occur more commonly in the winter months, presumably in association with common respiratory viruses that disrupt mucosal barriers, thereby allowing these colonizing pathogens to move from the nasopharynx to the bloodstream more easily. Research is ongoing to develop vaccines that will be effective against a greater number of pneumococcal serotypes and improved meningococcal vaccines that may work for younger children and against group B strains. Table 16-1 reviews microbial causes of meningitis.

Pathogenesis

Bacteria most often gain access to the central nervous system via the bloodstream. Pathogens gain access to the bloodstream as a result of nasopharyngeal colonization or local infections. When these specific bacterial strains are relatively new to the host, and the child has no existing circulating antibody against that strain, the bacteria may at least temporarily evade other host defenses and cause a transient or sustained bacteremia. Some of these bacteria may traverse the blood-brain barrier and replicate in the subarachnoid space. Once bacteria begin to replicate within the central nervous system, the human host has no adequate mechanism to recover without medical intervention.

The risk for sequelae and mortality vary significantly by age of the child, pathogen, and underlying host compromise at baseline and at presentation with meningitis. Patients may have impaired neurological function as a result of brain inflammation secondary to the bacteria and the host response to infection as well as due to cerebral hypoperfusion related to septic shock with hypotension, raised intracranial pressure, and/or disorders in local circulatory regulation including microvascular obstruction. Brain injury centers prominently on the cortex, hippocampus, and the inner ear, and the injuries are not simply the result of bacterial invasion but also occur as a result of a symphony of inflammatory mediators whose roles and control remain the focus of intense evaluation and give the promise of potential for future clinical intervention.[1]

Meningitis may also develop as the result of direct extension of pathogens from sites such as the sinuses, mastoids, dermoid sinuses, or the skull. Recurrent episodes of bacterial meningitis should prompt immunologic evaluation as well as careful anatomic evaluation of contiguous structures (eg, for congenital or traumatic bony, vascular, or dural defects).

Clinical Presentation

In practice, patients present in one of two manners. The first is easier to recognize quickly but carries a worse prognosis. Approximately 25% of patients have a short clinical course of only a few hours and present with fever and mental status changes (irritability, lethargy, confusion), and the diagnosis is not elusive. The other 75% of patients with bacterial meningitis have a more insidious clinical presentation with simple fever and nonspecific symptoms that progress over 1, 2, or more days to cause signs and symptoms typical of meningitis.

Signs and Symptoms

The most reliably present finding in bacterial meningitis is fever (98%), whereas complaints of headache, photophobia, or neck pain won't be heard until the child is verbal and can communicate these symptoms (around 2 years of age). Since bacterial meningitis is most common before this age it is important to watch for other clues. Infants may initially present with irritability that is difficult for the parents to alleviate, poor feeding, sleepiness, lethargy, and possibly vomiting. Later in the illness a bulging fontanelle, nuchal rigidity, and coma may be seen.

For an older child, where neck pain can be more easily assessed, the neck pain seen with meningitis is worsened by neck flexion. The typical child can easily touch the chin to the chest without the need to open the mouth and reluctance to do so is worrisome. Patients with meningismus will often open the mouth in an attempt to reach the chest with less neck flexion. Flexion typically causes pain at the back of the neck and moving down to the upper mid-back area. It should be noted that ibuprofen and other analgesics may temporarily resolve the neck pain despite the presence of meningitis.

Seizures occur as part of the presentation in 15% to 30% of patients, but will only rarely occur as simple (brief, nonfocal) seizures without other signs or symptoms worrisome for meningitis.[2] On the other hand, the risk of meningitis is increased significantly among febrile patients with convulsive status epilepticus (a seizure or series of seizures without recovery of consciousness between seizures lasting at least 30 minutes).[3] Therefore, if faced with a febrile patient with focal, prolonged, or recurrent seizures, or a febrile infant less than 6 months of age with any type of seizure, a lumbar puncture for CSF examination should be strongly considered.

Bacterial meningitis should be considered a medical emergency and the usual attention to airway, breathing, and circulation should be applied, as depressed mental status and associated septic shock may complicate management. The rapid institution of supportive measures and prompt administration of antimicrobials is the goal.

Differential Diagnosis

Severe pharyngitis, parapharyngeal abscess or adenitis, musculoskeletal strain, upper lobe pneumonia, cervical spine osteomyelitis, epidural abscess, and subarachnoid hemorrhage may all produce meningismus. Depressed mental status may occur as a result of encephalitis, ingestions, mass lesions of the CNS, or simple febrile seizure.

The possibility of another primary focus for infection that might also require specific therapy or follow-up should be considered. This site may be distant (eg, pyelonephritis, pleural empyema, osteomyelitis), but by causing bacteremia may have caused meningitis. In addition, a contiguous focus may also be the cause. Sinusitis, mastoiditis, osteomyelitis of the skull, or even a brain abscess may require additional intervention.

Diagnosis

While the diagnosis is simple when patients come with classic symptoms of photophobia, nuchal rigidity, severe headache, or mental status changes, this is not generally the case at the initial evaluation. There is a continuum from a complete absence of clinical signs or symptoms at the time the first bacteria cross the blood–brain barrier to severe symptoms.

The point in that continuum of symptoms when the child is seen and the rate at which the disease is progressing will determine how difficult it will be for the clinician to recognize the child as having meningitis. It is for this reason that approximately half of all patients ultimately diagnosed with bacterial meningitis will visit a clinician during the course of their illness and be sent home from the encounter without meningitis being considered.[4]

The highest risk for meningitis during childhood is in the first month or two of life and at this age the clinical signs are few. Therefore, a lumbar puncture is generally warranted in the evaluation of the febrile infant under 2 months of age. After 2 months of age the diagnosis remains a challenge, but more clinical cues are available to the clinician experienced in evaluating young children.

Children with prior antibiotic therapy during the illness can be more difficult to diagnose. Pretreated patients are less likely to have fever at examination, less likely to have altered mental status, and will have longer duration of symptoms at diagnosis.[5] Table 16-2 summarizes the pertinent history and physical exam in the evaluation of patients suspected of having meningitis. Figure 16-2 is a flow diagram for the diagnostic approach for patients being evaluated for meningitis.

Cerebrospinal fluid studies

The cerebrospinal fluid (CSF) should be sent for cell count, glucose, protein, Gram stain, and bacterial culture. A CSF fungal culture should also be performed in premature

Table 16-2.

Pertinent History and Physical Exam

Important History of Present Illness
Fever, lethargy, irritability, headache, photophobia, neck pain or stiffness, mental status changes, focal neurological deficits, seizures (especially focal, prolonged, recurrent)

Important Past Medical History
Immunocompromise, hemoglobinopathies, asplenia, chronic liver or renal disease, implanted hardware such as cochlear implants or ventriculo-peritoneal shunt, medications, allergies

Important Elements of the Physical Exam
Assessment of airway, gag reflex, vital signs, and perfusion
Head including fontanel and head circumference
Eyes (include fundoscopic exam), ears, nose, and throat
Neck
Neurological exam
Mental status: alertness, orientation
Skin examination for perfusion, petechiae, purpura

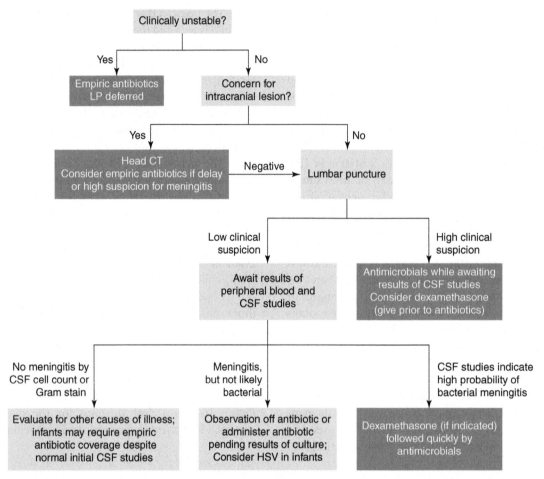

FIGURE 16-2 ■ Clinical approach to the patient with possible meningitis. The decision to administer or delay administration of dexamethasone and empiric antimicrobials until after cranial imaging, lumbar puncture, or results of blood and CSF analysis will depend on the overall clinical appearance of the child and degree of suspicion for acute bacterial meningitis. (*Reproduced with permission from Shah S.* Pediatric Practice: Infectious Disease. *New York: McGraw-Hill; 2009: Figure 16-2.*)

infants and in children with other immunocompromising conditions. Most patients with bacterial meningitis will have an elevated CSF WBC count with 80% or more polymorphonuclear cells; the CSF glucose will be low in about 50%; and the CSF protein concentration is generally elevated. The CSF culture is positive in about 80% of patients, and the culture is positive within 24 to 48 hours unless antimicrobials were given prior to lumbar puncture.

For the infant under 1 month of age with CSF pleocytosis no prediction rule can reliably exclude bacterial meningitis, and these infants should be treated as possibly having bacterial meningitis until the results of CSF culture are known. Further, not even normal CSF parameters exclude bacterial meningitis, as 10% of neonates with bacterial meningitis will not have a CSF pleocytosis,[6-8] and a majority of very low birth weight (< 1.5 kg) neonates with bacterial meningitis have no CSF pleocytosis at diagnosis (by positive CSF culture).[6]

For older infants and children with CSF pleocytosis a multicenter review of pediatric cases of bacterial

meningitis clearly demonstrated that children older than 1 month with CSF pleocytosis (and no antibiotic pretreatment) can be considered at very low risk of bacterial meningitis if the Gram stain has no organisms, the CSF absolute neutrophil count is < 1000 cells/mm^3, the CSF protein is < 80 mg/dL, the peripheral blood absolute neutrophil count is < 10,000 cells/mm^3, and there is no history of seizure before or at the time of presentation.[7] Nonetheless, even with these serially applied low-risk criteria, 2 of 121 children with bacterial meningitis had none of these risk factors for a sensitivity of 98% (95% confidence intervals: 94%-100%).

Among patients beyond the first months of life the serum procalcitonin (≥ 0.5 ng/mL), C-reactive protein (> 20 mg/L), CSF lactate, and the CSF glucose or CSF glucose to serum glucose ratio can all be helpful in distinguishing bacterial from nonbacterial causes of acute meningitis.[8-11] While not routinely available, the CSF levels of interleukin 6 (IL-6) and tumor necrosis factor (TNF) are also much higher in patients with bacterial versus aseptic meningitis.[12] Patients with bacterial meningitis have a predominance of polymorphonuclear cells before treatment. Approximately half of patients with aseptic or demonstrated enteroviral meningitis will also have a CSF polymorphonuclear cell predominance. Symptom duration does reliably result in a change in the CSF white blood profile, so serial lumbar punctures for this purpose are not recommended.[18,19]

Latex agglutination studies of the CSF for bacterial antigens do not typically provide any benefit and are not routinely recommended.[13] Polymerase chain reaction tests for bacteria are not readily available and have not shown much benefit beyond culture, but some available viral PCR tests are faster and more sensitive than viral culture and should be considered for specific etiologies. Because enteroviruses are common causes of meningitis and enterovirus polymerase chain reaction tests (EV-PCR) are now readily available, it is suggested that if the turn-around time for this test at your institution is usually < 48 hours, this test should be routinely considered. Previous studies have demonstrated a decrease in hospital length of stay when EV-PCR testing is routinely performed during enteroviral season.[14] Because it is slower than most routine bacterial culture or PCR tests, the routine use of viral culture is not recommended. Where herpes simplex meningoencephalitis is a possible concern, an HSV-PCR should be sent.

A positive Gram stain or growth of a pathogen in CSF culture definitively identifies bacterial meningitis. Unfortunately the diagnosis is more difficult to establish or exclude in the patient that has received antibiotic treatment prior to obtaining CSF for examination and culture. Pretreated patients are less likely to have a positive CSF Gram stain or culture.[5] While bacteria can be recovered in some circumstances for 1 or more days after initiation of antimicrobial therapy the CSF is sterilized in 2 hours or less with meningococcal infections, in 4 to 12 hours with pneumococcal infections, and as early as 8 hours with group B streptococcal infections.[15] Table 16-3 includes suggested studies to be ordered in the evaluation of the patient with suspected meningitis.

It should be noted that it may not be possible to safely perform a lumbar puncture, and the diagnosis will need to be a presumptive one in some patients. The lack of a definitive diagnosis should not delay treatment given the potential for significant morbidity. The lumbar puncture may need to be deferred if there are concerns of clinical instability, significantly elevated intracranial pressure (bradycardia, hypertension, irregular respirations, papilledema), or concern for intracranial lesion. The presence of thrombocytopenia (< 50,000 platelets/mm[3]) should prompt consideration for platelet transfusion prior to lumbar puncture. The presence of skin infection in the area overlying lumbar puncture should also be considered a relative contraindication

Table 16-3.

Key Considerations for Evaluation and Management of Bacterial Meningitis

Step 1. General assessment
   a. Assess vital signs and perfusion
   b. Establish vascular access
   c. Does the patient need cranial imaging?

Step 2. Laboratory studies
   a. Blood should be sent for complete cell count and culture
   b. Consider blood for electrolytes, blood urea nitrogen, creatinine, and glucose
   c. Cerebrospinal fluid should be obtained and sent for:
      ■ Gram stain
      ■ Bacterial culture
      ■ Cell count and differential
      ■ Glucose and protein
      ■ Consider sending CSF for viral studies such as enteroviral and/or herpes simplex PCR
      ■ Consider sending CSF for fungal or mycobacterial studies
   d. Consider sending lyme serology based on local epidemiology

Step 3. Treat infection
   a. Dexamethasone if appropriate
   b. Antimicrobials

Step 4. Subsequent management
   a. Follow neurological exam closely, especially cranial nerves
   b. Daily weights and strict measurement of intake and output
   c. Formal hearing evaluation
   d. Consider long-term follow-up including neuropsychiatric testing

because of the concern for inoculating bacteria from the skin site to the CSF.

Other studies

The decision to perform a lumbar puncture should not rest on the results of blood testing. Among infants, a very low or high peripheral white blood count (WBC) does increase the risk for bacterial meningitis, but 41% will have peripheral WBC values in the normal range.[16] A negative peripheral blood culture does not rule out bacterial meningitis. Among patients with confirmed bacterial meningitis, no bacterial growth is seen in blood cultures in approximately one-third of cases.[15,17-19] Despite these limitations, blood should be routinely obtained for culture from patients evaluated for suspected meningitis. A positive blood culture will influence the choice of antimicrobial therapy in cases where the CSF does not yield growth of a pathogen. Serologic tests may be helpful, and Lyme serology should be routinely ordered in the proper epidemiologic setting (eg, areas where infection is common, where there is an opportunity for exposure).

Neuroimaging does not need to be routinely ordered but should be performed during the course of therapy when patients experience unexplained changes in mental status, focal neurologic deficits, or there is other reason for concern of intracranial abscess, empyema, hemorrhage, infarct, or thrombosis.

Management

Optimize supportive care to ensure adequate oxygen delivery including consideration of adequate cerebral perfusion pressure. Patients with septic shock will require appropriate resuscitation to maintain adequate oxygen and glucose delivery to the brain. In patients without the need for additional fluids to support the circulation, intravenous fluids should provide for "maintenance" needs but should be given cautiously to avoid worsening the hyponatremia of the syndrome of inappropriate antidiuretic hormone secretion (SIADH), should it occur. Baseline and daily weight measurements and the evaluation of electrolytes may be helpful in monitoring for the development of SIADH.

When there is a high clinical suspicion for bacterial meningitis, the lumbar puncture should be done as soon as it is clinically safe and feasible, and the administration of antibiotic(s) should occur without awaiting the results of CSF studies or computed tomography (which itself is not routinely indicated unless there are focal signs or symptoms). Delays in antibiotic administration should be avoided and are associated with worsened outcome in adults.[20]

Treatment

Until an organism is isolated, patients should be treated with empiric antibiotic therapy that covers the range of potentially causative pathogens. Empiric antimicrobial coverage should rarely be narrowed based on the reading of the Gram stain alone, as errors in interpretation are common. Conversely if the Gram stain suggests an organism not well covered by empiric therapy, the coverage should be broadened awaiting the results of culture. It is important to consider *Listeria* as a potential pathogen, since optimal therapy includes the use of ampicillin, which is no longer routinely included in many empiric treatment strategies.

The initial empiric antibiotic therapy for most children is listed in Table 16-4. Dosing recommendations for these antimicrobials is listed in Table 16-5. Once the specific etiologic agent causing the meningitis is known, the treatment can be focused on that organism. Recommendations by organism (and the organism antibiotic susceptibility) are listed in Table 16-6.

Table 16-4.

Initial Empiric Therapy of Suspected Bacterial Meningitis

Age	Common Bacterial Pathogens	Initial Empiric Therapy[a]
< 2 months	Group B streptococci, *E coli* and other Enterobacteriacae, *S pneumoniae, Listeria monocytogenes*	Ampicillin plus cefotaxime[b] plus aminoglycoside
> 2 months	*N meningitides, S pneumoniae,* Haemophilus influenzae species	Dexamethasone[c] plus cefotaxime plus vancomycin

[a] *Specific doses of antimicrobials vary by age and are generally higher than for other indications. Pathogens and empiric therapy will not necessarily be the same for premature infants, immunocompromised children, and those post head trauma or surgery. Additional therapy will be guided by result of CSF Gram stain and the result of blood and CSF culture.*
[b] *Meropenem may be substituted for cefotaxime in case of allergy or the need for more broad-spectrum gram-negative coverage. If gram-positive cocci are identified, the addition of vancomycin should be considered until S. pneumoniae and S. aureus have been excluded.*
[c] *Dexamethasone should be considered if S pneumoniae or H influenzae type b are the suspected pathogens.*

Duration of antibiotic therapy varies depending on the causative organism, the time to CSF sterilization, the extent of CSF inflammation, and the patient's clinical response. In uncomplicated cases, parenteral antibiotic courses are typically of 7 days for *N meningitidis*, 7 to 10 days for *H influenzae* type b, 10 to 14 days for *S pneumoniae*, 14 to 21 days for group B streptococci, and 21 days for gram-negative organisms.

Vancomycin is a necessary component in the empiric treatment of patients with possible penicillin-resistant *Pneumococcus*. However, one retrospective study has suggested that the use of vancomycin in the first 2 hours of treatment may be associated with an increased risk for hearing loss in pneumococcal meningitis.[21] Further corroboration is needed before changes in practice can be recommended, but the priority should be to administer the dexamethasone and cefotaxime as quickly as is feasible and then administer vancomycin.

Corticosteriod therapy

Dexamethasone, when given 15 minutes prior to or simultaneously with antibiotics, appears to reduce mortality and sequelae among patients with *H influenzae* type b and *S pneumoniae* meningitis.[22] It is not known whether dexamethasone therapy has an effect on cognitive outcome. There is no demonstrated efficacy for the use of dexamethasone after antibiotics have been administered. There has been no demonstrated benefit to the use of steroids in meningococcal or neonatal meningitis.[23-25]

Table 16-5.

Drug Dosing for Bacterial Meningitis by Age for Selected Medications

Medication	0–7 Days of Age[a]	8–28 Days of Age	Infants and Children	Adult Maximum Dose
Aminoglycosides				
Gentamicin	2 mg/kg/dose q12h	2 mg/kg/dose q8h	2.5 mg/kg/dose q8h	—
Tobramicin	2 mg/kg/dose q12h	2 mg/kg/dose q8h	2.5 mg/kg/dose q8h	—
Amikacin	10 mg/kg/dose q12h	7 mg/kg/dose q8h	7 mg/kg/dose q8h	—
Ampicillin	50 mg/kg/dose q8h	50 mg/kg/dose q6h	75 mg/kg/dose q6h	12 g/d
Cefotaxime[b]	50 mg/kg/dose q8h	50 mg/kg/dose q6h	50 mg/kg/dose q6h	12 g/d
Meropenem	40 mg/kg/dose q8h	40 mg/kg/dose q8h	40 mg/kg/dose q8h	6 g/d
Vancomycin	15 mg/kg/dose q12h	15 mg/kg/dose q8h	15 mg/kg/dose q6h	—

[a] Assumes gestational age >36 weeks.
[b] Cefotaxime may be used at a dose of up to 300 mg/kg/d in pneumococcal infections.

The key steps in the evaluation and management are summarized in Table 16-3. Most authors reserve the use of dexamethasone for patients with clinical or laboratory findings highly suggestive of bacterial meningitis thought most likely to be due to *H influenzae* type b or *S pneumoniae*. Dexamethasone is not routinely recommended for the child with suspected aseptic meningitis receiving antimicrobial therapy pending the results of bacterial culture. Dexamethasone has not been adequately studied or demonstrated beneficial in the treatment of neonates with bacterial meningitis.

Additional considerations

A repeat lumbar puncture for a follow-up cerebrospinal fluid culture is not routinely recommended but should be considered when patients fail to improve within the first 24 to 48 hours or when the identified pathogen can be anticipated to be difficult to eliminate with conventional antibiotic therapy based on susceptibility testing or prior experience (eg, nosocomial gram-negative infections, resistant pneumococcus).

Consultation with an infectious diseases specialist is recommended for most cases of gram-negative meningitis, fungal meningitis, meningitis in a patient with reduced immunity or indwelling intracranial hardware, and in the treatment of organisms with reduced susceptibility to antibiotics.

Meropenem is preferred to a third-generation cephalosporin for the treatment of specific gram-negative

Table 16-6.

Treatment by Pathogen

Bacteria	Antibiotic(s) of Choice[a]
Group B streptococci	Ampicillin plus an aminoglycoside (during early therapy)
E coli	Cefotaxime plus an aminoglycoside
Listeria monocytogenes	Ampicillin plus an aminoglycoside (during early therapy)
S pneumoniae	
Cefotaxime-susceptible MIC ≤0.5 µg/mL	Cefotaxime
S pneumoniae[b]	
Penicillin nonsusceptible MIC ≥0.1 µg/mL and cefotaxime nonsusceptible MIC ≥1.0 µg/mL	Cefotaxime AND vancomycin ± rifampin
Penicillin MIC ≤0.1 µg/mL	Penicillin G or ampicillin
Penicillin MIC 0.1-1.0 µg/mL	Cefotaxime
H influenzae	Cefotaxime

[a] Specific therapy will also be guided by clinical improvement and specific susceptibility testing performed on the bacteria recovered from the patient.
[b] Consultation with an infectious disease specialist is recommended.

infections due to organisms such as *Citrobacter, Enterobacter,* or *Serratia*-related cases, which may possess the ability to express extended-spectrum beta-lactamases (ESBL) that may be induced by cephalosporin therapy.

Course and Prognosis

The mortality is associated with many factors, but overall is about 5% for *H influenzae* and meningococcal meningitis and in the vicinity of 20% for pneumococcal and *Listeria* meningitis in developed countries. The most common complications are listed in Table 16-7.

The risk for mortality and sequelae is related to the severity of disease. Not surprisingly, mortality (approximately 30%) and the rate of sequelae among survivors (approximately 70%) are very high among patients requiring mechanical ventilation during therapy of acute bacterial meningitis and are highly correlated with severity of illness at admission.[26] Mortality also increases if there is a significant neurological event during the acute phase of the illness. This may be due to general cerebral edema, hypoperfusion, loss of microcirculatory control, and vascular thromboses that cause secondary effects such as herniation and infarction.

The time course of presentation is also associated with severity of disease. Children who present and are diagnosed as having bacterial meningitis within the first 24 hours of illness are much more likely to have severe disease than those with a more insidious presentation that may develop over 2 days or more before diagnosis.[27]

Subdural effusions are commonly noted during the first week of therapy for bacterial meningitis of

Table 16-7.

Potential Complications of Meningitis

Short-Term Complications
Septic shock
SIADH
Seizures
Brain infarction
Cerebral edema
Intracranial abscess
Intracranial venous thrombosis (eg, cavernous venous
  thrombosis)
Intracranial hemorrhage
Cranial nerve palsies, most notably hearing loss

Long-Term Complications
Seizures
Cranial nerve palsies (including hearing loss)
Focal cerebral deficits (eg, hemiparesis)
Cognitive impairment

infants (approximately 30%) but do not typically require intervention.[28] Subdural empyema is a rare but important complication of meningitis, which can usually be distinguished from effusion with diagnostic imaging.[29]

Monitoring of urine output, daily weights, and serum electrolytes is prudent in the early phase in order to quickly identify hyponatremia and manage patients developing SIADH secretion. Less common complications include acute spinal cord dysfunction—myelitis.

Long-term sequelae

Hearing loss occurs in a large proportion (10%-30%, depending on pathogen) of children and is associated with severity of infection (lower CSF glucose levels, raised intracranial pressure, nuchal rigidity, *S pneumoniae* as the causative agent) with profound hearing loss in 5%.[30] Hearing loss, when it occurs, will be noted to some degree with the earliest testing.[31] While many children will experience some improvement in hearing over time, others may have further progression of hearing loss over months to years.[32] After bacterial meningitis children are more likely to have cognitive impairments such as poor linguistic and executive functions and these children are more likely to have behavioral problems than their peers.[33] As a result, even after apparent complete recovery from bacterial meningitis, children benefit from formal neuropsychiatric evaluation in addition to routine tests of hearing, as the findings may be subtle. Three percent to five percent of children will have seizures, mental retardation, and/or some degree of spasticity or paresis.[30]

Special circumstances

Patients with immunocompromise, intracranial implants including cochlear implants, ventriculoperitoneal shunts, and infants in the intensive care setting are at increased risk of meningitis including meningitis due to bacteria or fungi not typical of other children. Therefore, they should be considered separately with regard to primary prevention and optimal initial empiric therapy.

Citrobacter meningitis in the neonate, and *Citrobacter koseri* in particular, is associated with a very high rate of mortality (30%) and sequelae (75%), and is the most common cause of neonatal abscess (Figure 16-3). Infants with *Citrobacter* meningitis should have brain imaging during the course of therapy to evaluate for this complication.

Meningitis with cranial nerve palsies, appropriate local epidemiology, or protracted symptoms, should raise suspicion for Lyme disease, and depending on the cranial nerves involved, a basilar meningitis as can be seen with tuberculous or some fungal meningitis should be considered.[34] Causes of chronic meningitis are also quite varied, but pathogens such as *Brucella*, those causing Lyme disease and syphilis, cryptococci, and other

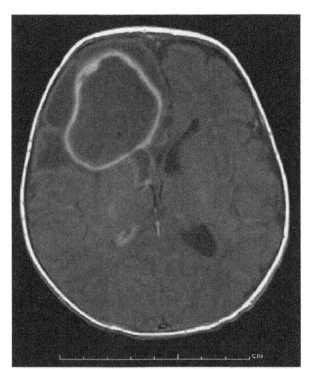

FIGURE 16-3 ■ Brain abscess complicating *Citrobacter koseri* meningitis in a 7-week-old female (T1-weighted MRI post-gadolinium image.) (*Reproduced with permission from Shah S. Pediatric Practice: Infectious Disease. New York: McGraw-Hill; 2009: Figure 16-3.*)

fungi may cause a more indolent and chronic meningitis. Noninfectious causes include malignancies, sarcoid, and autoimmune disease.

Discussion of eosinophilic meningitis (> 10 eosinophils/mm³ of CSF) is beyond the scope of this chapter, but may be seen in relation to indwelling foreign body, certain parasitic diseases, malignancies, in response to medications, and with coccidioidal meningitis.

Prevention

Chemoprophylaxis is recommended for close contacts of patients with disease due to *N meningitides* or *H influenzae* type b. Active immunization against *H influenzae* type b and *S pneumoniae* is now part of routine childhood vaccination schedules and immunization for *N meningitidis* is typically required prior to college entry in the United States.

Intrapartum ampicillin administered to women at high risk of transmitting group B streptococci to their infants is effective in reducing the risk of early-onset but not late-onset group B streptococcal disease. Women with penicillin allergy can receive clindaymycin, erythromycin, or in the absence of immediate-type hypersensitivity, a first-generation cephalosporin. Up to 20% of pregnant women require intrapartum antibiotic prophylaxis. Recurrent group B streptococcal infections occur; most of the isolates from recurrent infections are identical to the

isolates from the initial infection. Recurrent infection likely occurs as a consequence of persistent mucosal group B streptococcal colonization. Attempts to eradicate mucosal colonization with oral rifampin have met with varied success. Consultation with a pediatric infectious diseases or immunology specialist should be considered in infants with recurrent group B streptococcal infection.[35]

VIRAL ENCEPHALITIS

Encephalitis causes significant morbidity and mortality and raises difficult diagnostic and management challenges. The etiology is often elusive and, given the lack of literature on the subject, there is little information physicians can offer in the way of prognosis or etiology-specific treatment. This section defines encephalitis and describes its major causes with emphasis on the presentation, pathology, and management of viral encephalitis in pediatric populations.

Definitions and Epidemiology

Encephalitis is defined as inflammation of the brain tissue, infectious or otherwise, causing alterations in cerebral function. The patient with encephalitis often presents with fever, headache, altered mental status, behavioral changes, focal neurological signs, and seizures. Meningoencephalitis describes the clinical entity in which the inflammation extends to the subarachnoid spaces and meninges. When the spinal cord is involved in the inflammatory process, then the term "encephalomyelitis" is used. Noninfectious encephalitis is an antibody-mediated inflammation of the brain parenchyma, which may be triggered by immune response to a viral illness or tumor.

Estimating the true incidence of encephalitis is difficult, as most cases are not reported to local health departments. The most accurate estimates are those concerning the subset of arthropod-borne viral, or arboviral, encephalitides due to tracking efforts at the Centers for Disease Control (CDC), which estimates between 250 to 3000 cases occurring annually.[36] The California Encephalitis Project documented all hospitalized cases of encephalitis in California from 1991 to 1999 and found 35 to 50 cases per 100,000 people annually. Encephalitis occurred in the highest numbers in infants, followed by the elderly. A specific cause was reported in approximately 45% of the 13,939 cases; HSV accounted for 14% of all cases while arboviral disease was identified in fewer than 1% of the cases (West Nile Virus had not yet become established in California).[34]

Pathophysiology

Due to the protection of the blood–brain barrier (BBB), the lack of a lymphatic system and the absence of major histocompatibility complexes (antigen-presenting cells), the brain was historically considered an immunologically isolated organ without the same vulnerabilities to infectious agents or immune responses as other body systems. It is increasingly apparent that the BBB is a far more dynamic entity than previously thought.

The BBB is made of capillary endothelial cells, astrocytes, and pericytes with unique properties not seen in other organ systems. These anatomic differences include narrow tight junctions, lack of fenestrations, decreased transport, and a continuous basement membrane. Electrically, the surfaces of these cells are negatively charged, and therefore repel proteins and other negatively charged molecules. Specific areas within the CNS differ in their levels of BBB permeability. For example, the choroid plexus endothelium has fenestrations, allowing free entry of immune cells to the CSF. The ependymal lining of the ventricles lacks tight junctions, which permits drainage of CNS antigens into the CSF.

Diagnosis

The definitive diagnosis of encephalitis requires brain tissue, which yields a diagnosis by microscopic evaluation for inclusion bodies, isolation of the causative agent from brain tissue cultures, or detection of the infectious agent by in situ polymerase chain reaction (PCR). Detection of a serologic response or identification of the infectious agent in the CSF or other body fluids allows a presumptive diagnosis. The California Encephalitis Project reported a definitive diagnosis (brain tissue diagnosis) in 30% of cases, while a presumed diagnosis (serum, urine, or stool) was found in 12%.[38] Other sources report diagnostic rates of 50%.[39]

While isolating virus from CSF and other body fluid cultures is helpful for definitive diagnosis, this process is cumbersome and prone to contamination. PCR testing, which detects tiny portions of the DNA in the CSF, allows diagnoses to be made more quickly and reliably. Detecting antibodies for serologic testing is limited by even small doses of immunoglobulin therapy, and because it often requires both infected samples and convalescent samples, may take weeks to confirm.

Neuroimaging

All viruses affecting the central nervous system (CNS) produce similar pathologic features, including inflammation and neuronal death. Thus, most viral CNS infections appear on neuroimaging as an increase in water content of the affected tissue. On CT scan this increased water content is manifest as patchy hypodensities, and on MRI as hypointense signal on T1 and hyperintense signal on T2 and FLAIR (fluid-attenuated inversion recovery).

When imaged early in its course, viral encephalitis may first appear on MRI as restricted diffusion on diffusion-weighted imaging (Figure 16-4). Thus, acute DWI changes may be more sensitive to abnormalities than conventional T1 or T2 imaging sequences[40-42]

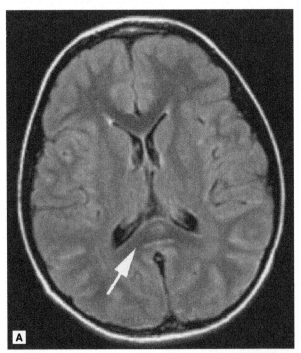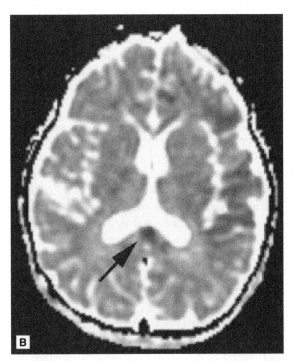

FIGURE 16-4 ■ MRI of viral encephalitis in a 7-year-old male presenting with sudden-onset status epilepticus. **(A)** Hyperintensity in the splenium of the corpus callosum (white arrow) on axial FLAIR MRI. **(B)** Restriction of water diffusion demonstrated on apparent diffusion coefficient (ADC) maps of the diffusion weight imaging (DWI) examination (black arrow). (*Reproduced with permission from Shah S. Pediatric Practice: Infectious Disease. New York: McGraw-Hill; 2009: Figure 17-1.*)

in early imaging. Later in the disease process, MRI often shows confluent areas of T2 hyperintensities involving white and gray matter, which may exert a variable amount of mass effect. When present, these hyperintensities enhance diffusely with gadolinium. While these findings fail to differentiate viral infections from one another, the asymmetry and the involvement of both white and gray matter structures help to differentiate viral encephalitis from primary metabolic/ toxic disorders or parainfectious disorders, such as acute disseminated encephalomyelitis (ADEM; Figure 16-5).

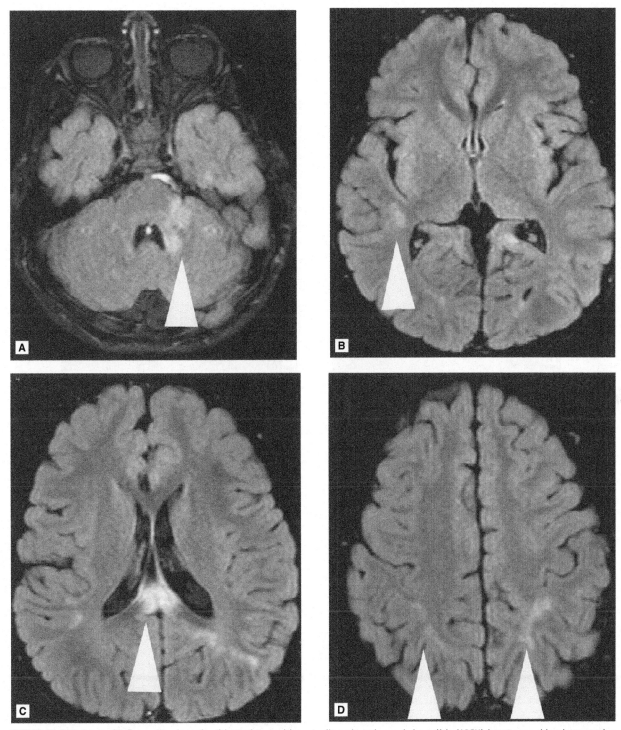

FIGURE 16-5 ■ Areas of inflammation (arrowheads) consistent with acute disseminated encephalomyelitis (ADEM) in a 9-year-old male presenting with lethargy, irritability, and left hemi-ataxia. (A) Inflammatory lesion in the left cerebellar peduncle. (B) Subcortical inflammatory white matter lesion in the right temporal lobe. (C) Prominent lesion in the splenium of the corpus callosum. (D) Multiple bilateral subcortical inflammatory white matter lesions. (*Reproduced with permission from Shah S. Pediatric Practice: Infectious Disease. New York: McGraw-Hill; 2009: Figure 17-2.*)

Though these general features apply to most viral encephalitides, certain infections show characteristic tropisms that are helpful in the differential diagnosis. Herpes simplex virus (HSV) encephalitis has been associated with hemorrhagic inflammation, frequently bilateral, of the medial temporal lobe, sylvian fissure, and orbital-frontal cortex (Figure 16-6).

In neonates, the areas of inflammation are seldom as well defined as in older children or adults, and manifest as loss of distinction of the gray–white interface on T2-weighted imaging. Echo gradient imaging reveals a hemorrhagic component corresponding to infarction on diffusion-weighted imaging in the acute phase of the disease (5 to 7 days from insult).

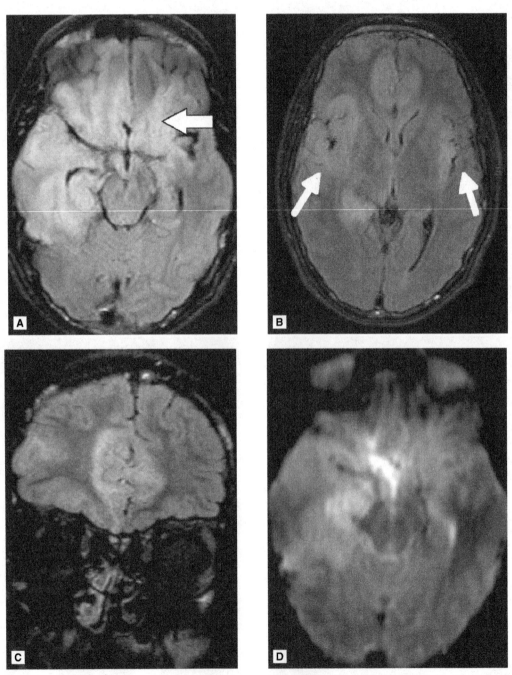

FIGURE 16-6 ■ 14-year-old male presenting with coma and status epilepticus, diagnosed with HSV encephalitis. **(A)** Axial flair demonstrating medial temporal (hippocampus) and orbitofrontal (*arrow*) involvement. **(B)** Axial flair demonstrating bilateral sylvian fissure (*arrows*) involvement. **(C)** Coronal flair demonstrating orbitofrontal and interhemispheric involvement. **(D)** Diffusion weighted imaging (*b* = 1000) demonstrating infarction (cytotoxic edema) of the right temporal lobe. (*Reproduced with permission from Shah S. Pediatric Practice: Infectious Disease. New York: McGraw-Hill; 2009: Figure 17-3.*)

Varicella-zoster virus (VZV) is an infrequent cause of encephalitis, but must be considered as a possible cause in those patients at risk either from immunocompromise or from direct inoculation via lumbar puncture. VZV is a common pathogen in other CNS infections such as transverse myelitis and cerebellitis and has been associated with transient arteriopathy of childhood and stroke.[43,44]

Other diagnostic testing

Electroencephalogram (EEG) must be considered early in the evaluation of patients with viral encephalitis, as subclinical seizures are a treatable cause of altered mental status. EEG may also disclose other nonspecific abnormalities including focal slowing or focal epileptiform discharges. Acute destructive lesions can produce periodic lateralized epileptiform discharges (PLEDS), usually in temporal leads. PLEDS are considered nonspecific but are highly suggestive of HSV encephalitis.[45]

CSF profiles in viral encephalitis typically show mildly elevated WBC counts, with a lymphocytic predominance and, later in the course, mildly elevated protein. Elevated RBC counts and xanthochromia reflect the necrotizing nature of HSV infection; however, early in the disease CSF findings can be normal. PCR is the most common method used for CSF analysis, although PCR specificity may be as low as 94%, with 98% sensitivity,[46] between 72 hours and 2 weeks of symptom onset. For this reason, patients may require repeat testing (Table 16-8).

Differential Diagnosis

The etiology of infectious viral encephalitis has changed significantly with the advent of widespread immunizations (Tables 16-9 and 16-10). The most common causes of viral encephalitis 30 years ago were measles, mumps, rubella, and varicella, which now rarely cause neurological disease. HSV is thought to be the most common diagnosable and treatable cause of viral encephalitis in both the United States and United Kingdom, with arboviruses, varicella zoster virus, Epstein-Barr virus (EBV), mumps, measles, and enteroviruses following in prevalence. A Finnish study published in 2001 found VZV to be the most common cause of diagnosed viral encephalitis, meningitis, and myelitis (29% of all confirmed agents), with HSV, enteroviruses, and influenza A making up the majority of other confirmed etiologic agents.[47] Even within this population, however, an etiologic agent was not identified in 60% of cases. In U.S. National Hospital Discharge Data, the pathogenic species was found in only 40% of cases.[48] According to the California Encephalitis Project, up to 70% of cases of encephalitis remain idiopathic.[37]

Table 16-8.

Acute Disseminated Encephalomyelitis Versus Viral Encephalitis

	ADEM	Viral Encephalitis
Age	Children >> Adults	Any
Recent vaccine	+++	–
Prodromal illness	+++	+
Fever	±	+++
Visual symptoms	±	–
Spinal cord/cerebellum involvement	±	–
CSF	Lymphocytic pleocytosis	Lymphocytic pleocytosis
	± Elevated protein	Elevated protein
	Normal glucose	± Normal glucose
	Negative cultures	± Negative cultures
	+ Elevated oligoclonal bands and myelin basic protein	– Oligoclonal bands
		– Myelin basic protein
Serum	± Leucocytosis	+++ Leucocytosis
MRI	Multiple areas of white matter hyperintensity	Focal areas (1 or 2) of white or gray matter hyperintensity
	Often bilateral	Unilateral/bilateral
	Often in deep brain structures (basal ganglia, brainstem, cerebellum, spinal cord) and optic nerves	Usually cortical

– Not present
+ Present
± Not consistently present
+++ Consistently present

Table 16-9.

Viral Encephalitides

Double-stranded DNA viruses	Adenovirus
	Cytomegalovirus
	Epstein-Barr virus
	Hepatitis B
	Herpes simplex virus 1 and 2
	Human herpesvirus 6 and 7
	Varicella zoster
Single stranded DNA virus	Parvovirus
Arboviruses (single-stranded RNA viruses)	California (La Crosse) virus
	Eastern equine virus
	St. Louis encepalitis
	West Nile virus
	Western equine virus
	Powassan
	Colorado tick fever
	Venezuelan equine
Enterovirus (single-stranded RNA viruses)	Poliovirus
	Coxsackie
	Echovirus
Other RNA viruses	Hepatitis A influenza
	Parainfluenza
	Respiratory syncytial virus
	Rotavirus
Paramyxovirus	Hendra
	Measles
	Mumps
	Nipah
Transmitted via mammals	Rabies
	Equine morbillivirus (Hendra)
	Nipah
	Lymphocytic choriomeningitis
	Encephalomyocarditis
	Vesicular stomatitis

Table 16-10.

Nonviral Causes of Encephalitis

Bacterial	*Actinomyces*
	Bartonella henselae
	Brucellosis
	Haemophilus influenzae
	Leptospirosis
	Legionella
	Mycobacterium tuberculosis
	Mycobacterium pneumoniae
	Neisseria meningitidis
	Nocardia actinomyces
	Salmonella typhi
	Streptococcus pneumoniae
	Spirochetal infections
	Treponema pallidum
	Leptospira
	Borrelia burgdorferi
	Treponema pallidum
	Tropheryma whippeli
Rickettsial	Ehrilichiosis
	Rickettsia rickettsia
	Rickettsia prowazeki
	Rickettsia typhi
	Coxiella burnetti (Q fever)
Fungal	Aspergillosis
	Candidiasis
	Coccidioides immitis
	Cryptococcus neoformans
Parasitic	*Acanthamoeba* species
	Balamuthia mandrillaris
	Cerebral malaria
	Human African trypanosomiasis
	Naegleria species
	Plasmodium species
	Schistosomiasis
	Strongyloides stercoralis
	Toxoplasma gondii
	Trypanosoma species
	Trichinella spiralis
Postimmunization encephalitis	Smallpox vaccine
	Typhoid-paratyphoid vaccine
	Influenza vaccine
	Measles vaccine
Other	*Chlamydia psittaci*
	Chlamydophila pneumoniae[a]

[a] *Formerly* Chlamydia pneumoniae.

Postinfectious encephalitis, or acute disseminated encephalomyelitis (ADEM), is the most common white matter disease in children[49] and is usually seen days to weeks after mild viral illness or immunizations. The presumed cause of ADEM is thought to be antibodies to the offending virus cross-reacting with myelin surface proteins. The inflammation results in widespread monophasic demyelination, with a full recovery expected in the majority of pediatric cases. ADEM differs from viral encephalitis in the location of lesions on imaging: ADEM has a predilection for the cerebellum and optic nerves, which is unusual for encephalitis. Spinal cord inflammation may be noted in both, but is more frequent in ADEM than in viral encephalomyelitis. Clinical progression to coma occurs more rapidly and more commonly in ADEM than in viral encephalitis.[45]

CSF profiles in ADEM and viral encephalitis are similar and typically show elevated WBC counts with a lymphocytic predominance. To distinguish the two entities a thorough history of prodromal illnesses must be combined with MRI findings as well as negative CSF, blood, nasopharyngeal swab, urine serology, and cultures (Table 16-8). ADEM is treated with immunomodulation using high-dose intravenous glucocorticoids or pooled intravenous immune globulin (IVIG). The precise mechanism of action of these latter therapies is unknown.

Paraneoplastic encephalitis typically involves the limbic area with a fulminant and progressive course. The pathophysiology is thought to involve antibodies formed against a neoplasm that cross-react to brain tissue antigens. Thus paraneoplastic disorders can be diagnosed by identifying pathologic antibodies in the CSF. Paraneoplastic disorders are rare in children, but should be considered in the differential diagnosis, as they can resemble HSV encephalitis. Ospoclonus-myoclonus, or the "syndrome of dancing eyes and dancing feet," is perhaps the most common paraneoplastic disorder and is associated with neuroblastoma, which is invariably low grade. Opsoclonus refers to unusual and exaggerated eye movements that can be elicited on visual tracking. Myoclonus is rapid, jerky, involuntary movements of the limbs or trunk.

Clinical Presentation and Management

Because the etiologic agent remains unknown in most cases of viral encephalitis, management is limited to symptomatic treatment. Tests to consider in the initial evaluation of the child with encephalitis are summarized in Table 16-11, while key clinical features of the viral encephalitides are summarized in Table 16-12. Even for diagnosable entities, very few treatment options exist. HSV and VZV should be treated with acyclovir, while cytomegalovirus (CMV) can be treated with ganciclovir (Table 16-13). In immunocompromised patients, aggressive treatment with antibiotics and antivirals is important until treatable causes of encephalitis/meningitis are ruled out.

The development of novel antiviral agents has lagged due to the research emphasis on immunization. As the majority of cases lack an isolated causative agent, the value of developing specific antiviral drugs is questionable. The use of immunomodulatory therapy, such

Table 16-11.

Laboratory Diagnosis of Viral Encephalitides

Virus	PCR CSF	PCR Serum	Serology: CSF	Serology: Serum	Culture: Pharynx	Culture: Rectum	Culture: Blood	Culture: CSF	Other
HSV 1 & 2	+++	+	±	−	−	−	−		Intranuclear inclusion bodies on pathology
VZV	+	+++	+++	+	−	−	−	+	Skin vesicle
HHV6	±	±	−	±	−	−	+	+	
EBV/CMV	+	+	+++	+++	±	−	±	±	
Adenovirus	+		±	±	+++ PCR	+		+	
Arbovirus[a]	+	+	+++	+++	−	−	+++	±	
Enterovirus	+++	+	−		+	++	±	++	
Measles virus	+	−	+ IgG	+ IgG	+	−	+	−	Urine
Rabies virus	+	−	+++	+++	−	−	−	+	Negri bodies
Mycoplasma pneumoniae				IgM	+++ PCR +++	−	−	−	
Influenza	−	−	−	±	+++ DFA +++	−	−	−	

− Not useful for diagnosis.
± Variable utility.
+ Effective.
+++ Highly reliable.
DFA, direct fluorescent antibody.
[a] Arboviruses include St. Louis encephalitis (SLE), Western Equine encephalitis (WEE), and West Nile virus (WNV).

Table 16-12.

Key Features of the Viral Encephalitides

Virus	Key Clinical or Epidemiologic Features
HSV	Common cause of encephalitis.
	Predilection for temporal lobes, sylvian fissure, orbital-frontal cortex. Associated with periodic lateralizing epileptiform discharges on EEG, vesicles on the skin, focal seizures, hemiparesis, aphasia and cranial neuropathies.
HHV-6	Rarely causes encephalitis.
	Typically occurs in infants and small children, and has a focal onset.
VZV	Uncommon cause of encephalitis.
	Typically occurs in children. Usually associated with vesicular rash, headache, vomiting, altered mental status, and seizures. Can also cause ischemic or hemorrhagic infarcts.
EBV	Rarely causes encephalitis.
	Often associated with rash or mononucleosis.
CMV	Rarely causes encephalitis.
	More common in immunocompromised patients.
EV	Common cause of CNS infection, but rarely causes encephalitis.
	Often associated with pharyngitis, gastroenteritis, and rash.
Arboviruses	Most common causes of worldwide encephalitis.
WNV	Associated with headache, vomiting, diarrhea, abdominal pain, and rash. Presents with seizures, flaccid paralysis, cranial neuropathies.
EEE	Rare cause of encephalitis, but children are most affected.
	Presents with sudden high fever, seizures, and altered mental status.
SLE	Rarely causes encephalitis.
	Presents with headache.
La Crosse	Rare cause of encephalitis, but occurs most commonly in children.
	Associated with upper respiratory illness, abdominal pain, and seizures.
Influenza	Rarely causes encephalitis in the United States.
	Presents with a prodrome of myalgias and fever, progresses to cause seizure.
Rabies	Rare in developed countries, but common throughout the world.
Encephalitic	Presents with anxiety, hydrophobia, aerophobia, hypersalivation, and seizures.
Paralytic	Presents with progressive peripheral nerve paralysis
Measles	Rarely causes encephalitis, more commonly causes SSPE.
	SSPE occurs months to years after measles infection and presents with progressive dementia, myoclonus, seizures, and ataxia.
Mumps	Rarely causes encephalitis.
	Presents with fever, headache, and a typically mild course.
	Postinfectious encephalomyelitis: occurs 7-10 days after mumps infection and is more severe. Symptoms include seizure, hemiparesis, and altered mental status.

as steroids, to treat encephalitis is compelling; however, the relative rarity of cases makes a single-center study difficult if not impossible. Acyclovir, supportive care, and rehabilitative therapies remain the only treatments at this time for viral encephalitis.

Herpes simplex virus 1 and 2

Herpes simplex virus (HSV) 1 and 2 are double-stranded DNA viruses that remain dormant in human host neurons. The clinical features distinguishing HSV 1 and 2 are few, and thus it is not clinically useful to discriminate between them.

One-third of patients with HSV encephalitis are less than 20 years of age and the majority have no prior existing conditions.[50] About half of all patients with HSV encephalitis report a viral prodrome prior to the onset of neurological symptoms, with symptoms of upper respiratory and gastrointestinal illness being the most commonly reported. Neonates who acquire HSV develop CNS infection in over 50% of cases. Infection typically occurs at the time of birth (85%), but can also occur transplacentally (5%) or in the postpartum period (10%).[45] Symptoms of HSV infection in neonates range from subtle (skin vesicles) to fulminant (fever, seizures, obtundation).

HSV infects peripheral sensory neurons and then spreads to the CNS by retrograde axonal transport. The patient invariably experiences fever, headache, and altered mental status. Focal seizures at the time of presentation

Table 16-13.

Antiviral Therapy

Antiviral Agent	Indication	Drug-Related Complications
Acyclovir	Herpes viruses	Nephrotoxic
Amantadine	Influenza A	Declining effectiveness, anticholinergic effects
Cidofovir	CMV retinitis, acyclovir-resistant herpes	Nephrotoxic
Foscarnet	Herpes viruses: CMV (including CMV retinitis), herpes simplex viruses	Hypocalcemia, renal failure
Ganciclovir	CMV	Aplastic anemia, phlebitis, nephrotoxic, teratogenesis,
Oseltamivir[a]	Influenza A and B	Stevens-Johnson syndrome, hepatitis
Ribavarin	Influenza A and B, West Nile virus Research ongoing in hepatitis B/C, polio, measles, smallpox	Nephrotoxic, teratogenesis

[a] *Currently considered first-line therapy for influenza-related complications.*

are common (75% of patients), while hemiparesis (45%), aphasia (75%), and cranial neuropathies are also seen. Infections can rapidly progress to involve greater areas of brain tissue.[45]

In the last 20 to 30 years, with the advent of acyclovir, there have been significant declines in the mortality and morbidity associated with HSV encephalitis. Prior to the use of acyclovir, approximately 70% of patients with HSV encephalitis died; this has decreased to 19% since the widespread use of acyclovir.[38] Neurological outcomes have also improved, and long-term studies demonstrate a normal outcome in 38%, moderate impairment in 9%, and severe impairment in 53%.[38,50] Outcomes were most improved in younger age-groups and in patients with shorter latency to treatment.[38] The typical dose of acyclovir is 30 mg/kg/d IV, divided every 8 hours for 14 to 21 days in children; and 60 mg/kg/d IV divided every 8 hours for 21 days in neonates.

Human herpesvirus 6 (HHV-6)

Human herpesvirus 6 (HHV-6), also known as roseola, usually infects children during infancy, with two-thirds of children seroconverting by 1 year.[51] HHV-6 encephalitis is usually focal, and thus can be confused with HSV encephalitis. Viral invasion of the CNS is a common event during primary infection, as demonstrated by the high rate of febrile seizures. It typically causes high fever, with frank encephalitis occurring only rarely.[52] The incidence of HHV-6 encephalitis is unknown.

Varicella zoster virus (VZV)

Prior to widespread vaccination campaigns, 4 million cases of primary varicella zoster virus (VZV; chickenpox) occurred annually. Rates of serious infection-related morbidity and mortality were highest in children under 10 years

of age, accounting for 60% of hospitalizations and 40% of deaths.[53] Direct infection of the CNS during a primary VZV infection is rare, but meningoencephalitis may occur by invasion of the vascular endothelium,[54] leading to primary VZV encephalitis. Occurring mostly in the pediatric population, this small-vessel vasculopathy presents with headache, fever, vomiting, altered mental status, seizure, and focal deficits. Encephalitis may also complicate reactivation of VZV (zoster or shingles), usually in elderly populations. This encephalitis, by contrast, is due to a large-vessel vasculopathy, with acute focal deficits developing weeks to months after the clinical infection. MRI findings include ischemic or hemorrhagic infarcts in the cortex and subcortical gray and white matter.

The diagnosis of VZV encephalitis is made via CSF PCR for VZV or serology for VZV specific IgM in the CSF. Treatment in children is acyclovir IV 60 mg/kg/d, divided every 8 hours for 14 days.

Epstein–Barr virus

Epstein–Barr virus (EBV) causes severe encephalitis in fewer than 1% of infected patients.[54] More often, EBV causes aseptic meningitis, cerebellitis, myelitis, or ADEM with a benign course and full recovery from the infection expected. The diagnosis of EBV is made by measuring acute and convalescent serum IgM antibodies to the EBV capsid antigen. A CSF PCR test is available, but sensitivity and specificity of this test are unknown.

Cytomegalovirus

Congenitally acquired cytomegalovirus (CMV) causes severe and permanent brain injury, but encephalitis due to CMV is relatively uncommon except in the immunocompromised child.[39] Serious CMV infections in the immunocompromised are treated with ganciclovir.

Enterovirus

The enterovirus (EV) family—including polioviruses, coxsackie viruses A and B, and echoviruses—are collectively the leading viral cause of CNS disease in children in the United States, particularly affecting neonates and immunocompromised hosts.[45] Outbreaks of EV generally occur in late summer and early fall and are often associated with pharyngitis, gastrointestinal symptoms, or rash and desquamation of the hands, feet, and mouth (herpangina). Encephalitis, meningoencephalitis, cerebellitis, and a polio-like syndrome are most often seen with EV serotypes 70 and 71, but can occur with any virus in this family.[45] The viruses can be cultured directly from the CSF, but diagnosis is usually made by CSF EV PCR, which has 96% to 100% sensitivity and >99% specificity.[51] Current treatment is symptomatic and supportive, while drug trials are ongoing.

Arbovirus

Arboviruses are the most commonly identified cause of severe encephalitis worldwide.[39] Single-stranded RNA viruses, they are usually transmitted to humans via mosquito or tick vectors, although transmission has also been reported following blood product transfusion, organ transplantation, needle sticks, transplacentally and via breast milk. Arboviruses have complex life-cycles involving birds and other mammals, with humans being dead-end hosts. After entering the bloodstream, they reach the CNS via endothelial cell infection. The infection in the brain is diffuse, and thus the sequelae are nonfocal, including altered mental status, vomiting, and fever. PCR testing has not been developed for routine use, as its sensitivity in arboviruses is poor. Evaluation of virus-specific IgM from CSF or blood is the most widely used diagnostic method.

West Nile virus

Prior to 1999 there were no reported West Nile virus (WNV) cases in the Western Hemisphere. In 2006, a total of 4256 infected individuals were reported, with 1449 cases of confirmed West Nile meningitis/encephalitis, including 165 fatalities.[55] Roughly 80% of infected individuals experience no symptoms, while 20% have mild flu-like symptoms of fever, headache, vomiting, diarrhea, abdominal pain, myalgia, and rash.[56] Neuroinvasive disease typically includes seizures, altered mental status, meningoencephalitis, acute flaccid paralysis, cranial neuropathies, movement disorders, and optic neuritis.[45,57] In patients with neuroinvasive disease, 15% progress to coma.[57] The proportion of each presenting symptom varies with location and timing within the season. WNV meningitis and encephalitis occur more commonly in adults and are uncommon in children.

Diagnosis of neuroinvasive disease is made by CSF serology. WNV IgM is detectable in more than 90% of infected individuals 1 week after symptom onset. IgM-related immunity may persist for more than 1.5 years, complicating the diagnosis of acute disease. The presence of anti-WNV IgG peaks at 4 weeks after infection and persists throughout life. Currently the treatment of WNV is supportive, though current clinical trials include passive immunization, interferon alpha, and ribavirin. Overall, mortality from WNV is roughly 2% to 14%, with encephalitis-specific mortality estimated at 12% to 24%.[45,57] In the United States, donor blood is screened for WNV.

Eastern equine encephalitis

Like WNV, eastern equine encephalitis (EEE) can cause severe disease, with 30% mortality and 30% serious neurological sequelae in survivors.[58] It is an uncommon cause of illness in North America, with only 95 cases reported between 1995 and 2005.[59] The presentation is both sudden and fulminant, with high fever, seizures, and rapid deterioration of mental status. Young children are most severely affected and have the highest rate of neurological sequelae in recovery.

St. Louis encephalitis virus

St. Louis encephalitis (SLE) virus is more common than EEE and, according to the CDC, carries a risk of serious neurological morbidity in 10% of patients and of mortality in 5%. From 1964 to 2005, there were 4478 cases in the United States, with an annual average of 128 cases.[60] While the disease is widespread throughout North America, there is a higher risk of encephalitis and serious neurological infection in low-income areas, as well as with the elderly.[61] Most individuals infected with SLE are asymptomatic, but when symptoms are present they range from simple headache to severe encephalitis.

California (La Crosse) virus

La Crosse virus is less frequent than EEE or SLE in the United States and causes a milder form of encephalitis. Between 1964 and 2005 there were 3375 cases reported to the CDC, ranging from 41 to 167 per year.[62] Most cases are asymptomatic or result in mild illness, with rare neurological sequelae and very rare mortality (<1%).[63] It is overwhelmingly a childhood disease, with over 90% of cases occurring in children under 16 years. When symptoms occur, the presentation is a sudden onset of fever, headache, upper respiratory illness, abdominal pain, and seizures.

Influenza virus

Influenza types A and B are common causes of illness, but rarely cause neurological complications in the United States. Influenza has been associated with Reye syndrome, encephalitis, transverse myelitis, acute necrotizing encephalopathy, Guillain-Barré syndrome, and seizures. The data regarding serious neurological sequelae differ by geography and strain. Japanese data shows that roughly 100 children die annually from influenza encephalitis.[64] Similarly, the mortality rates in influenza encephalopathy in Japan are as high as 25% to 37%.[65,66] A recent study suggests the prevalence of influenza encephalitis in the United States is considerably lower; this single-center, retrospective chart review found only 842 laboratory-confirmed cases of influenza A and B in children from 2000 to 2004. Of those patients, 72 children experienced influenza-related neurological complications, but the authors found no cases of influenza encephalitis or influenza-related mortality.[67] The neurological complications consisted of seizures (78%), acute encephalopathy (11%), cerebral infarction after hypotension (5%), postinfectious influenza encephalopathy (3%), and aseptic meningitis (3%).[67] From 2003 to 2004, of the 153 deaths in children from influenza reported to state health departments, 16% were associated with altered mental status and 6% were associated with encephalopathy.[68] Treatment for influenza is primarily supportive, although rimantadine and oseltamivir have been used for CNS infections.

Rabies virus

While relatively rare in the United States, rabies is an important cause of serious neurological illness and death. There were only 36 laboratory-confirmed cases in the United States from 1990 to 2001,[69] with half of those cases occurring in children and adolescents.[39] Worldwide, however, roughly 55,000 deaths occur due to rabies each year.[70] It is generally spread to humans by infected animal bites, although documented cases of rabies with no history or evidence of an animal bite exist. The virus spreads through retrograde axonal transport, causing progressive changes in mental status, seizures, cranial neuropathies, dysphagia, and paresis. Two forms of CNS rabies exist: one causes encephalitis, with seizures and fever, and eventually progresses to paralysis; the other begins with paralysis of the peripheral nerves and is associated with fever, but not seizures. The paralytic form differs from Guillan-Barré syndrome by the association with fever, and the lack of sensory deficits. Once these symptoms occur, the disease almost invariably induces cardiopulmonary failure and death, in 5 to 7 days. Diagnosis is typically made at autopsy via serologic or PCR testing of brain tissue, and histologic examination of the tissue may demonstrate Negri bodies. Viral culture may be used as a confirmatory technique. The most sensitive (100%) noninvasive antemortem diagnostic test is PCR analysis looking for rabies RNA in the saliva of the patient, with the next most sensitive (67%) test being antigen testing of hair follicles obtained by nuchal skin biopsy.[71] Additional tests include antibody testing of CSF and serum, and antigen testing of a touch impression from the cornea.

There is no treatment available for rabies after symptom onset, but presymptomatic post exposure vaccine combined with immunoglobulin administration is highly effective if given within 24 hours after exposure,[72] and may be effective for up to 72 hours after exposure, in some cases. The only case of survival documented after symptom onset occurred in a 15-year-old girl who was placed into chemical coma with ketamine, midazolam, and barbiturates. High-dose ribavirin (33 mg/kg/load plus 64 mg/kg/d) and amantidine (200 mg/kg/d) were administered for 1 week. Five months after hospitalization she had dysarthria, buccolingual choreoathetosis, intermittent dystonia, and ballismus, but was able to attend high school part-time. No formal neurocognitive testing was reported at that time.[73] As of April 2007, she planned to graduate from high school and to attend college. Her persistent neurological deficits include numbness on her thumb, in the area of the bite, abnormal tone in her left arm, and a widened running gait.[73] Further attempts to utilize this treatment strategy have failed.[74]

Measles virus

Measles is rare in the postvaccine era and progresses to encephalitis in only 0.74 per1000 cases.[39] Its more common neurological syndrome, subacute sclerosing panencephalitis (SSPE), occurs in older children and adults months to years after a primary measles infection. This clinical syndrome presents with dementia, myoclonus, ataxia, epilepsy, and motor function decline, and progresses slowly to death. The clinical features have been divided into four stages (the Jabour stages)

IA	Behavioral, cognitive, and personality changes.
IB	Myoclonic spasms.
IIA	Mental deterioration, myoclonic spasms (periodic, generalized, frequently causing drop spells).
IIB	Apraxias, agnosias, language difficulties, spasticity. Ambulation with assistance.
IIIA	Less speech, visual difficulties, myoclonic spasms frequent, ± seizures.
IIIB	No spontaneous speech, poor comprehension, blind, myoclonic spasms, bedridden, dysphagia, EEG w/ background delta, chorea, ballismus.
IV	No myoclonus, EEG low voltage with no periodic slow-wave complexes, vegetative state.[75]

SSPE findings on EEG include high-voltage (300-1500 µV) and repetitive polyphasic sharp and slow-wave complexes of 0.5- to 2-second duration recurring every 4 to 15 seconds. Rarely, the complexes can occur at intervals of 1 to 5 minutes, with the intercomplex interval shortening as the disease progresses.

Treatment for SSPE is predominantly symptomatic. Intrathecal interferon alpha initially showed promise in a case report by inducing remission for 7 to 8 years, but this initial success was followed by a severe neurocognitive decline.[76]

Mumps virus

While most cases of mumps occur in areas of the world where routine childhood vaccinations do not occur, epidemics have also been seen in vaccinated populations. In the first 10 months of 2006, there were 5783 cases of mumps reported, with a median age of 22.[77] According to the CDC, 50% to 60% of cases of mumps show a CSF pleocytosis, despite encephalitis occurring in less than 2 per 100,000 cases.[48] Mumps occurs more often in the spring and has a low mortality rate. Patients with mumps encephalitis present with mild, nonfocal symptoms of fever and headache. Diagnosis is made by CSF and serum serology with culture of the nasopharynx, CSF, urine, and saliva.

A postinfectious encephalomyelitis due to mumps may also occur, usually 7 to 10 days after infection. These patients exhibit more severe symptoms such as seizure, hemiparesis, and altered mental status. This variant carries a higher mortality rate of 10%.[45]

Emerging viruses

Nipah and Hendra viruses are both in the family Paramyxoviridae. The Nipah virus was identified in 1999 as the cause of a large outbreak of encephalitis among pig farmers in Malaysia and Singapore. The natural reservoir for Nipah virus is still under investigation, but preliminary data implicate bats of the genus *Pteropus* in Malaysia. In Malaysia and Singapore, humans were infected with Nipah virus through close contact with infected pigs. The Hendra virus, first isolated in 1994, is related but not identical to the Nipah virus. It is predominantly known to cause fatal respiratory infections in horses and humans, but a solitary case of adult encephalitis has been reported.

Prognosis

Expected outcomes vary significantly with the etiology of the viral encephalitis, but certain generalizations can be made. Young infants usually have more severe disease and therefore more significant sequelae. One study examining the prognostic indicators in 462 cases of pediatric encephalitis (including HSV, VZV, enterovirus, respiratory virus, measles, mumps, rubella, and *M. pneumoniae* etiologies) found mortality five times greater in infants compared to older children, and found that patients with significantly altered mental status had 4 times the risk of death.[79] The majority of survivors experience seizures or cognitive and focal neurological deficits, negatively affecting their quality of life. The economic

impact of encephalitis is difficult to calculate, as survivors typically require intensive supportive services and, as a group, have decreased independence as adults. Overwhelmingly, the longitudinal data on outcomes in encephalitis have focused on herpes encephalitis before the advent of acyclovir. The most recent longitudinal study examined the rehabilitation of 8 patients, including 1 child, diagnosed with encephalitis from 1990 to 1997. The study focused only on the rehabilitation scores of the patients, without mention of seizure incidence, cognitive or physical impairment, or quality of life.[80] Clearly more investigation into the outcomes of children with viral encephalitis is required before conclusions can be drawn regarding prognosis.

TRANSVERSE MYELITIS

Definitions and Epidemiology

Acute transverse myelopathy is a clinical syndrome consisting of progressive symptoms and signs reflecting sensory, motor, or autonomic dysfunction attributable to the spinal cord. This syndrome can be caused by a heterogeneous group of disorders, including acute transverse myelitis (ATM). Definitions of ATM have varied significantly in the literature.[81,82] To address this nonuniformity, the criteria proposed by the Transverse Myelitis Consortium Working Group[83] (Table 16-14) should be used to establish the diagnosis and guide the differential diagnosis and workup. The diagnosis of ATM can be further refined by determining whether there is partial or complete involvement of the spinal cord in the axial plane. Complete ATM is characterized by moderate to severe symmetric symptoms, while partial ATM is marked by milder, asymmetric symptoms.[84]

Acute transverse myelitis can be associated with more diffuse central nervous system (CNS) demyelinating disorders, systemic autoimmune disorders, or specific associated infections. Idiopathic ATM is associated with a nonspecific preceding infection or no apparent cause and constitutes the most common subgroup of pediatric ATM.

Idiopathic ATM afflicts approximately 1.34 persons per million.[85] In the pediatric age group, patients present at a mean age of 8 years with an equal gender ratio.[81,82,84,86-89] Approximately 280 cases of ATM occur in pediatric patients in the United States per year.[90,91]

Pathogenesis

Infectious agents can cause spinal cord dysfunction by directly infecting the spinal cord parenchyma (infectious myelopathy)[82] or by triggering postinfectious, immune-mediated processes. In some cases, such as human T-cell lymphotropic virus (HTLV) associated

Table 16-14.

Transverse Myelitis Consortium Working Group Diagnostic Criteria

Inclusion Criteria	Exclusion Criteria
Development of sensory, motor, or autonomic dysfunction attributable to the spinal cord.	History of previous radiation to the spine within the last 10 yr.
Bilateral signs and/or symptoms (though not necessarily symmetric).	Clear arterial distribution clinical deficit consistent with thrombosis of the anterior spinal artery.
Clearly defined sensory level	Abnormal flow voids on the surface of the spinal cord c/w AVM.
Exclusion of extra-axial compressive etiology by neuroimaging (MRI or myelography; CT of spine not adequate).	Serologic or clinical evidence of connective tissue disease (sarcoidosis, Behçet disease, Sjögren syndrome, SLE, mixed connective tissue disorder, etc.).[a]
Inflammation within the spinal cord demonstrated by CSF pleocytosis or elevated IgG index or gadolinium enhancement. If none of the inflammatory criteria is met at symptom onset, repeat MRI and lumbar puncture evaluation between 2 and 7 days following symptom onset meet criteria.	CNS manifestations of syphilis, Lyme disease, HIV, HTLV-1, *Mycoplasma*, other viral infection (eg, HSV-1, HSV-2, VZV, EBV, CMV, HHV-6, enteroviruses).[a]
	Brain MRI abnormalities suggestive of MS.[a]
Progression to nadir between 4 hr and 21 days following the onset of symptoms (if patient awakens with symptoms, symptoms must become more pronounced from point of awakening).	History of clinically apparent optic neuritis.[a]

AVM, arteriovenous malformation; SLE, systemic lupus erythematosus; HTLV-1, human T-cell lymphotropic virus-1; HSV, herpes simplex virus; VZV, varicella zoster virus; EBV, Epstein-Barr virus; CMV, cytomegalovirus; HHV, human herpes virus.
[a] Do not exclude disease-associated acute transverse myelitis.

myelitis, damage to the spinal cord may be produced by direct infection as well as the immune response to the microbe. Several agents, including cytomegalovirus (CMV) and varicella zoster virus (VZV), are associated with direct CNS infection in certain patients (many of whom are immunocompromised) and postinfectious ATM in others.

Among all cases of ATM, the preceding infection is most commonly a nonspecific upper respiratory tract infection.[81,85,89] Approximately 50% of patients report a preceding infection with an intervening symptom-free interval of 5 to 11 days.[81,85,89,90] Some cases of ATM are associated with recent vaccination, although causality is difficult to prove given the paucity of cases and the frequency with which children are vaccinated.[81,86,90,93-95]

Although the precise pathophysiology of ATM is uncertain, the frequent association with preceding infections and accumulating immunologic data support an inflammatory cause for the disorder.[81,85,96,97] Increased peripheral blood lymphocyte responses to myelin basic protein have been demonstrated in the research setting in patients with ATM.[98] None of the 6 patients who were tested in the recovery stage in this study showed significant responses to myelin basic protein, suggesting that the cellular autoimmune reaction is short-lived. In addition, the production of interleukin-6 (IL-6) by astrocytes appears to lead to nitric oxide–induced injury to

spinal cord oligodendrocytes and axons in patients with idiopathic ATM. IL-6 levels are markedly elevated in the CSF of patients with ATM and correlate with long-term disability.[96]

In a specific form of ATM that also includes optic neuritis, termed neuromyelitis optica (NMO),[99] a novel biomarker (NMO-IgG) has been detected in 73% of adult patients and several pediatric patients.[100-102] This auto-antibody targets the predominant CNS water channel protein aquaporin-4, which is concentrated in astrocytic foot processes in the blood-brain barrier. The role of NMO-IgG and aquaporin-4 in the more common, idiopathic form of ATM is uncertain.

Clinical Presentation

Seven published case series ranging in size from 9 to 50 patients disclose common symptoms in pediatric patients with ATM.[81,82,86-90] Patients universally report acute to subacute, bilateral leg weakness, which is symmetric in approximately 67% of patients.[81] Involvement of the arms occurs in about 40% of patients. Approximately 90% of patients complain of bowel and bladder dysfunction. A similar percentage of patients report sensory symptoms, including parasthesias and numbness. Back pain and fever afflict nearly 50% of patients and may prompt consideration of primary infectious etiologies, such as an epidural abscess. The symptoms of ATM develop rapidly, peaking at an average of 2 and 5 days, in 2 respective studies.[81,90]

The general examination, although usually unremarkable, may reveal signs suggestive of an underlying systemic infection or autoimmune disorder. Abdominal examination may reveal a distended bladder. On the neurological examination, the presence of any mental status changes suggests that the myelitis is a component of a more diffuse process, such as acute disseminated encephalomyelitis (ADEM). In the acute stages, muscle tone is flaccid in affected limbs. All sensory modalities should be carefully assessed. A spinal cord sensory level is usually located in the thoracic region (80%) and less commonly in the cervical (10%) or lumbar (10%) area.[85] In the acute phase, deep tendon reflexes are depressed in approximately 70% of patients and later become hyperactive. Similarly, Babinski responses may be negative early in the acute phase, but soon become positive, indicating upper motor neuron dysfunction.

Differential Diagnosis

Numerous disorders can affect the spinal cord and produce identical symptoms and signs that mimic idiopathic ATM (Table 16-15). Such conditions must be ruled out through a combination of history, physical examination, neuroimaging, and laboratory evaluation (Figure 16-7).

Isolated spinal cord dysfunction

Extra-medullary compressive lesions, including spinal epidural abscesses,[103] spinal epidural hematomas,[102] and tumors,[105] are neurosurgical emergencies that must be diagnosed rapidly for effective treatment. Intramedullary lesions that can mimic ATM include primary spinal cord tumors (most commonly astrocytomas and ependymomas),[106-108] radiation injury,[109] spinal cord infarction, and vascular malformations.[110] Direct infections of the spinal cord, typically viral in etiology, can also occur.

The initial clinical presentation of ATM can be very similar to that of Guillain-Barré syndrome. Both can present with back pain, paraparesis, and sensory abnormalities. Although typically absent in both disorders acutely, the presence of deep tendon reflexes would point strongly towards ATM. When deep tendon reflexes are absent, the presence of a spinal cord sensory level and bowel and bladder involvement is suggestive of ATM.

Spinal cord dysfunction plus additional neurological or systemic symptoms and signs

The presence of mental status changes and cerebral white matter magnetic resonance imaging (MRI) abnormalities point towards ADEM as the correct

Table 16-15.

Differential Diagnosis of Idiopathic Acute Transverse Myelitis Mimicking Conditions

Common
Traumatic spinal cord injury
Guillain-Barré syndrome

Uncommon
Extramedullary compressive lesions (epidural abscess, epidural hematoma, tumor)
Intramedullary spinal cord tumors (astrocytomas, ependymomas)
Ischemia/infarction
Direct infectious myelopathies
Vascular malformations
Radiation injury

Diffuse Central Nervous System Demyelinating Disorders

Common
Acute disseminated encephalomyelitis (ADEM)

Uncommon
Multiple sclerosis (MS)
Neuromyelitis optica (NMO)

Systemic Autoimmune Disorders

Uncommon
Systemic lupus erythematosus
Antiphospholipid antibody syndrome
Neurosarcoidosis

diagnosis. Mild, asymmetric spinal cord symptoms, previous episodes of transient neurological symptoms attributable to locations other than the spinal cord, and subclinical brain MRI lesions point towards multiple sclerosis.[111] Concurrent or preceding optic neuritis suggests NMO as a possible diagnosis.[99]

Acute transverse myelitis can also be secondary to a variety of systemic autoimmune disorders. Involvement of other organ systems, particularly the skin, lungs, kidneys, and joints, may point to a particular diagnosis, such as systemic lupus erythematosus or sarcoidosis.

Diagnosis

Neuroimaging

Every patient with suspected ATM should undergo emergent gadolinium-enhanced MRI of the entire spine in order to confirm the diagnosis and rule out alternative diagnoses, particularly compressive lesions. T1- and T2-weighted sagittal imaging of the entire spine can serve as an initial screen, followed by axial imaging in

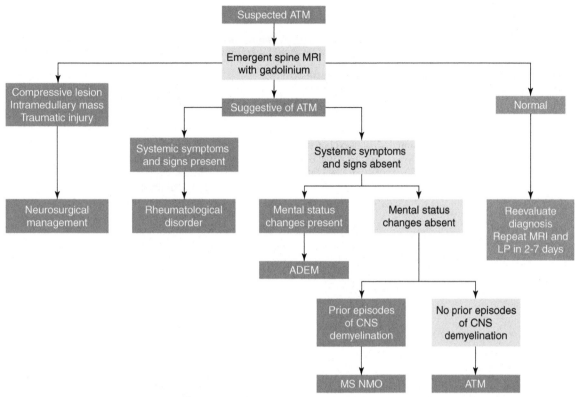

FIGURE 16-7 ■ Diagnostic algorithm for acute transverse myelitis (ATM). (Key: ADEM, acute disseminated encephalomyelitis; CNS, central nervous system; GBS, Guillain-Barré syndrome; LP, lumbar puncture; MRI, magnetic resonance imaging; MS, multiple sclerosis; NMO, neuromyelitis optica.) (*Reproduced with permission from Shah S:* Pediatric Practice: Infectious Disease. *New York: McGraw-Hill; 2009: Figure 18-1.*)

areas of suspected pathology.[112] All patients with ATM should also undergo gadolinium-enhanced MRI of the brain to assess for additional demyelinating lesions suggestive of ADEM or multiple sclerosis.

Spinal MRI in ATM typically reveals T1 isointense and T2 hyperintense signal over several contiguous spinal cord segments,[81] and may involve the entire spine.[112] Spinal cord swelling with effacement of the surrounding cerebrospinal fluid spaces may be present in severe cases. Contrast enhancement is present in as many as 74% of patients.[90] In some patients with very suggestive clinical features, the initial spine MRI may be normal and should be repeated several days later.[81,82,86] In some cases, the MRI remains normal, but does not rule out the diagnosis.[90] Higher rostral levels and number of overall spinal segments predict worse outcome.[90]

Lumbar puncture

Unless a specific contraindication exists, all patients with ATM should undergo lumbar puncture. Approximately 50% of pediatric patients with ATM have CSF pleocytosis, typically with a lymphocytic predominance.[90] Elevated CSF protein levels, either in isolation or in conjunction with pleocytosis, are also detected in about 50% of patients.[90] Glucose is typically normal.

A normal CSF profile does not rule out ATM, as this pattern is seen in approximately 25% of patients.

Additional tests

The long list of infectious, demyelinating and rheumatologic disorders potentially associated with ATM precludes diagnostic testing for every possible disorder (Table 16-16). The etiology of a direct infectious myelopathy is usually established by positive cerebrospinal fluid (CSF) culture or polymerase chain reaction (PCR) results. In postinfectious ATM, a specific etiology can be suggested by elevated acute or rising convalescent serum titers and/or isolation of the agent from systemic sources in the setting of a suggestive clinical picture. The infectious disease workup should be focused on pathogens that are common, treatable, or suggested by particular clues in the history or examination, such as environmental exposures and immune status.

Treatment

There have been no randomized, controlled treatment trials in ATM. Based on case reports and series that have suggested a beneficial effect,[97,113,114] high-dose corticosteroids have become the standard of care in ATM. In one series of 12 children with severe ATM compared to a

Table 16-16.

Diagnostic Workup for Suspected Acute Transverse Myelitis

All Patients	Suggestive of NMO	Also Consider
Neuroimaging	**Ophthalmology Consultation**	**Infectious Diseases**
Brain and spine MRI with gadolinium	Visual evoked potentials	**Blood tests**
	Formal visual field testing	Bartonella titers
Lumbar Puncture	Serum NMO-IgG	HIV antibody
Cell counts		HTLV-I antibody
Glucose, protein		Parasitic infection titers
Gram stain		RPR
Bacterial culture		
		CSF Studies
PCR testing[a]		Cryptococcal antigen
Oligoclonal bands		HTLV antibody
Ctology		Fungal culture
		VDRL
Blood Tests		
Blood cultures		**Rheumatologic Disorders**
Acute and convalescent titers[b]		Angiotensin-converting enzyme (serum, CSF)
		Anti-dsDNA
		Anti-La
		Anti-Ro
		Anti-Smith

CSF, cerebrospinal fluid; DNA, deoxyribonucleic acid; HIV, human immunodeficiency virus; HTLV, human T-cell lymphotropic virus; RPR, rapid plasma regain; VDRL, venereal disease research laboratory.
[a] *CMV, EBV, Enterovirus, HSV, Mycoplasma pneumoniae.*
[b] *Borrelia burgdorferi, CMV, EBV, Mycoplasma pneumoniae, VZV.*

historical control group of 17 patients, the use of high-dose intravenous methylprednisolone significantly increased the proportion of children walking independently at 1 month (66% compared to 18%) and with full recovery at 1 year (55% compared to 12%).[97] Although a variety of agents and courses have been used, we use intravenous methylprednisolone 30 mg/kg/dose once a day for 5 days (maximum daily dose 1 g). The need for a prednisone taper is controversial and may be based on whether full or partial recovery is achieved with the intravenous steroids. For patients who do not adequately improve with intravenous methylprednisolone, intravenous immunoglobulins[115] or plasmapheresis can be used (Figure 16-8).

As most cases are due to secondary, immune-mediated mechanisms, antimicrobial treatment is not likely to have significant benefit. However, antimicrobial therapy should be considered in cases with highly suspected or proven associated infections, such as doxycycline or levofloxacin for *Mycoplasma pneumoniae*,[116] ganciclovir for CMV,[117] and acyclovir for HSV and VZV.[118] When antimicrobials are used, agents with good CSF penetration are preferred, as direct CNS invasion may be present in some cases.

Additional treatment includes pain management, urinary bladder catheterization, bowel regimens, peptic ulcer and deep venous thrombosis prophylaxis, physical therapy, and psychosocial support. Mechanical ventilation is required in approximately 5% of patients.

Prognosis

Disability

Although the variable definitions of recovery reported in the literature preclude a definitive assessment, the prognosis for pediatric patients with ATM is generally favorable.[119] Paine and Byers' degree-of-recovery categories have been the most widely reported outcome scale but are limited by vague terminology.[89] Based on this scale, approximately 80% of pediatric patients who receive high-dose IV methylprednisolone achieve full or good recovery and 20% have a fair or poor outcome.[87,113] Among patients not treated with high-dose IV methylprednisolone, 60% have a full or good recovery, while 40% have a fair or poor outcome.[89]

One large, tertiary-referral, center-based study of 47 children with ATM, of whom 70% were treated with intravenous steroids, has cast doubt on the favorable prognosis of the disorder in childhood.[90] In this study, approximately 40% of patients were nonambulatory and 50% required bladder catheterization at a median follow up of 3.2 years. These results may have been

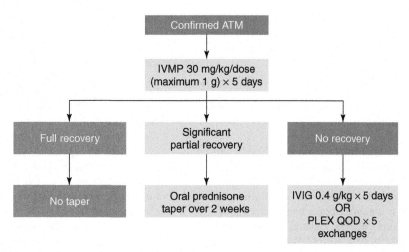

FIGURE 16-8 ■ Treatment algorithm for acute transverse myelitis (ATM). (Key: IVIG, intravenous immunoglobulin; IVMP, intravenous methylprednisolone; PLEX, plasma exchange.) (*Reproduced with permission from Shah S: Pediatric Practice: Infectious Disease. New York: McGraw-Hill; 2009: Figure 18-2.*)

influenced by a high percentage of patients less than age 3 years and patients with cervical involvement compared to other studies. Multicenter and/or population-based studies are needed to further clarify the prognosis of ATM in childhood.

During recovery, motor function returns first, with an average time to independent ambulation of 56 days in one study[81] and 25 days in a group of patients treated with high-dose IV methylprednisolone.[87] Bowel/bladder control recovers more slowly, with an average time to recovery of normal urinary function of 7 months in those patients with complete recovery.[81]

Recurrences

The overwhelming majority of pediatric patients with idiopathic ATM do not have any recurrences. In a series of 24 pediatric patients with a mean follow-up of 7 years, there were no recurrences.[81] In another study of children with a variety of initial acute demyelinating events, only 2 of 29 (7%) patients with transverse myelitis had a later demyelinating event.[120,121]

REFERENCES

1. Scheld WM, Koedel U, Nathan B, Pfister HW. Pathophysiology of bacterial meningitis: mechanism(s) of neuronal injury. *J Infect Dis.* 2002 Dec 1;186 Suppl 2:S225-33.
2. Green SM, Rothrock SG, Clem KJ, Zurcher RF, Mellick L. Can seizures be the sole manifestation of meningitis in febrile children? *Pediatrics.* 1993 Oct;92(4):527-34.
3. Chin RFM, Neville BGR, Scott RC. Meningitis is a common cause of convulsive status epilepticus with fever. *Arch Dis Child.* 2005;90:66-69.
4. Bonsu BK, Harper MB. Fever interval before diagnosis, prior antibiotic treatment, and clinical outcome for young children with bacterial meningitis. *Clin Infect Dis.* 2001;32:566-572.
5. Rothrock SG, Green SM, Wren J, Letai D, Daniel-Underwood L, Pillar E. Pediatric bacterial meningitis: is prior antibiotic therapy associated with an altered clinical presentation? *Ann Emerg Med.* 1992 Feb;21(2):146-52.
6. Doctor BA, Newman N, Minich NM, Taylor HG, Fanaroff AA, Hack M. Clinical outcomes of neonatal meningitis in very-low birth-weight infants. *Clin Pediatr (Phila).* 2001 Sep;40(9):473-80.
7. Nigrovic LE, Kuppermann N, Macias CG, et al. Pediatric Emergency Medicine Collaborative Research Committee of the American Academy of Pediatrics. Clinical prediction rule for identifying children with cerebrospinal fluid pleocytosis at very low risk of bacterial meningitis. *JAMA.* 2007 Jan 3;297(1):52-60.
8. Sormunen P, Kallio MJ, Kilpi T, Peltola H. C-reactive protein is useful in distinguishing Gram stain-negative bacterial meningitis from viral meningitis in children. *J Pediatr.* 1999 Jun;134(6):725-9.
9. Lembo RM, Marchant CD. Acute phase reactants and risk of bacterial meningitis among febrile infants and children. *Ann Emerg Med.* 1991;20:36-40.
10. Schwarz S, Bertram M, Schwab S, Andrassy K, Hacke W. Serum procalcitonin levels in bacterial and abacterial meningitis. *Crit Care Med.* 2000 Jun;28(6):1828-32.
11. Dubos F, Moulin F, Gajdos V, et al. Serum procalcitonin and other biologic markers to distinguish between bacterial and aseptic meningitis. *J Pediatr.* 2006 Jul;149(1):72-6.
12. Dulkerian SJ, Kilpatrick L, Costarino AT Jr, et al. Cytokine elevations in infants with bacterial and aseptic meningitis. *J Pediatr.* 1995 Jun;126(6):872-6.
13. Nigrovic LE, Kuppermann N, McAdam AJ, Malley R. Cerebrospinal latex agglutination fails to contribute to the microbiologic diagnosis of pretreated children with meningitis. *Pediatr Infect Dis J.* 2004 Aug;23(8):786-8.

14. Ramers C, Billman G, Hartin M, Ho S, Sawyer MH. Impact of a diagnostic cerebrospinal fluid enterovirus polymerase chain reaction test on patient management. *JAMA.* 2000 May 24-31;283(20):2680-5.

15. Kanegaye JT, Soliemanzadeh P, Bradley JS. Lumbar puncture in pediatric bacterial meningitis: defining the time interval for recovery of cerebrospinal fluid pathogens after parenteral antibiotic pretreatment. *Pediatrics.* 2001; 108:1169-1174.

16. Bonsu BK, Harper MB. Utility of the peripheral blood white blood cell count for identifying sick young infants who need lumbar puncture. *Ann Emerg Med.* 2003;41: 206-214.

17. Garges HP, Moody MA, Cotten CM, et al. Neonatal meningitis: what is the correlation among cerebrospinal fluid cultures, blood cultures, and cerebrospinal fluid parameters? *Pediatrics.* 2006 Apr;117(4):1094-100.

18. Wiswell TE, Baumgart S, Gannon CM, Spitzer AR. No lumbar puncture in the evaluation for early neonatal sepsis: will meningitis be missed? *Pediatrics.* 1995 Jun;95(6):803-6.

19. Stoll BJ, Hansen N, Fanaroff AA, et al. To tap or not to tap: high likelihood of meningitis without sepsis among very low birth weight infants. *Pediatrics.* 2004 May; 113(5):1181-6.

20. Aronin SI, Peduzzi P, Quagliarello VJ. Community-acquired bacterial meningitis: risk stratification for adverse clinical outcome and effect of antibiotic timing. *Ann Int Med.* 1998;129:862-869.

21. Buckingham SC, McCullers JA, Luján-Zilbermann J, Knapp KM, Orman KL, English BK. Early vancomycin therapy and adverse outcomes in children with pneumococcal meningitis. *Pediatrics.* 2006 May;117(5):1688-94.

22. van de Beek D, de Gans J, McIntyre P, Prasad K. Corticosteroids for acute bacterial meningitis. *Cochrane Database Syst Rev.* 2007 Jan 24;(1):CD004405.

23. Chaudhuri A. Adjunctive dexamethasone treatment in acute bacterial meningitis. *Lancet Neurol.* 2004;3: 54-62.

24. McIntyre PB, Macintyre CR, Gilmour R, Wang H. A population based study of the impact of corticosteroid therapy and delayed diagnosis on the outcome of childhood pneumococcal meningitis. *Arch Dis Child.* 2005 Apr; 90(4):391-6.

25. Grandgirard D, Leib SL. Strategies to prevent neuronal damage in paediatric bacterial meningitis. *Curr Opin Pediatr.* 2006;18:112-118.

26. Madagame ET, Havens PL, Bresnahan JM, Babel KL, Splaingard ML. Survival and functional outcome of children requiring mechanical ventilation during therapy for acute bacterial meningitis. *Crit Care Med.* 1995 Jul; 23(7):1279-83.

27. Kilpi T, Anttila M, Kallio MJ, Peltola H. Severity of childhood bacterial meningitis and duration of illness before diagnosis. *Lancet.* 1991 Aug 17;338(8764):406-9.

28. Snedeker JD, Kaplan SL, Dodge PR, Holmes SJ, Feigin RD. Subdural effusion and its relationship with neurologic sequelae of bacterial meningitis in infancy: a prospective study. *Pediatrics.* 1990 Aug;86(2):163-70.

29. Chen CY, Huang CC, Chang YC, Chow NH, Chio CC, Zimmerman RA. Subdural empyema in 10 infants: US characteristics and clinical correlates. *Radiology.* 1998 Jun;207(3):609-17.

30. Baraff LJ, Lee SI, Schriger DL. Outcomes of bacterial meningitis in children: a meta-analysis. *Pediatr Infect Dis J.* 1993; 12:389-394.

31. Richardson MP, Reid A, Tarlow MJ, Rudd PT. Hearing loss during bacterial meningitis. *Arch Dis Child.* 1997 Feb;76(2):134-8. Erratum in: *Arch Dis Child* 1997 Apr;76(4):386.

32. Woolley AL, Kirk KA, Neumann AM Jr, et al. Risk factors for hearing loss from meningitis in children: the Children's Hospital experience. *Arch Otolaryngol Head Neck Surg.* 1999 May;125(5):509-14.

33. Halket S, de Louvois J, Holt DE, Harvey D. Long term follow up after meningitis in infancy: behaviour of teenagers. *Arch Dis Child.* 2003 May;88(5):395-8.

34. Avery RA, Frank G, Glutting JJ, Eppes SC. Prediction of Lyme meningitis in children from a Lyme disease-endemic region: a logistic-regression model using history, physical, and laboratory findings. *Pediatrics.*2006 Jan;117(1):e1-7.

35. Wenger JD, Hightower AW, Facklam RR, Gaventa S, Broome CV. Bacterial meningitis in the United States, 1986: report of a multistate surveillance study. The Bacterial Meningitis Study Group. *J Infect Dis.* 1990 Dec;162(6): 1316-23.

36. Centers for Disease Control and Prevention. *Arboviral Factsheet.* 2007. Available at http://www.cdc.gov/ncidod/ dvbid/arbor/arbofact.htm.

37. Trevejo RT. Acute encephalitis hospitalizations, California, 1990-1999: unrecognized arboviral encephalitis? *Emerg Infect Dis.* 2004;10:1442-1449.

38. Lewis P, Glaser C. Encephalitis. *Pediatr Rev.* 2005;26:353-363.

39. Feigin R, Cherry J, Demmler G, SL K. Viral Encephalitis. *Textbook of Pediatric Infectious Disease.* Vol 1. 5 ed. Philadelphia: Saunders; 2004:505-517.

40. Bulakbasi N, Kocaoglu M, Tayfun C, Ucoz T. Transient Splenial Lesion of the Corpus Callosum in Clinically Mild Influenza-Associated Encephalitis/Encephalopathy. *AJNR Am J Neuroradiol.* October 1, 2006 2006;27(9):1983-1986.

41. Tsuchiya KK, Shichiro; Yoshino, Ayako; Hachiya, Junichi. MRI of influenza encephalopathy in children: value of diffusion-weighted imaging. *J Comput Assist Tomogr.* 2000;24(2):303-307.

42. Yoshikawa H, Kitamura T. Serial changes on diffusion-weighted magnetic resonance imaging in encephalitis or encephalopathy. *Pediatr Neurol.* 2006;34:308-311.

43. Gilden D. Varicella zoster virus vaculopathy and disseminated encephalomyelitis. *J Neurol Sci.* 2002;195:99-101.

44. Kleinschmidt-DeMasters B, Gilden D. Varicella-zoster virus infections of the nervous system: clinical and pathologic correlates. *Arch Pathol Lab Med.* 2001;125:770-780.

45. DeBiasi R, Tyler K. Viral meningitis and encephalitis. *Neurology Continuum.* 2006;12:58-94.

46. Lakeman F, Whitley RJ. Diagnosis of herpes simplex encephalitis: application of polymerase chain reaction to cerebrospinal fluid from brain-biopsied patients and correlation with disease. National Institute of Allergy and Infectious Diseases Collaborative Antiviral Study Group. *J Infect Dis.* 1995;171:857-863.

47. Muttilainen M, Koskiniemi M, Linnavuori K, et al. Infections of the central nervous system of suspected viral origin: A collaborative study from Finland. *Journal of Neuro Virology.* 2001;7(5):400-408.

48. Khetsuriani N, Holman R, Anderson L. Burden of encephalitis-associated hospitalizations in the United States, 1988–1997. *Clin Infect Dis.* 2002;35:175-182.

49. Silvia MT, Licht DJ. Pediatric central nervous system infections and inflammatory white matter disease. *Pediatr Clin North Am.* 2005;52:1107-1126.

50. Whitley R, Alford C, Hirsh M, et al. Vidarabine versus acyclovir therapy in herpes simplex encephalitis. *New England Journal of Medicine.* 1986;314(3):144-149.

51. DeBiasi RL, Tyler KL. Molecular methods for diagnosis of viral encephalitis. *Clin Microbiol Rev.* 2004;17:903-925.

52. Irving W, Chang J, Raymond D, Dunstan R, Grattan-Smith P, Cunningham A. Roseola infantum and other syndromes associated with acute HHV6 infection. *Arch Dis Child.* Dec 1990;65(12):1297-1300.

53. Centers for Disease Control and Prevention. *Varicella Factsheet.* 2007. Available at http://www.cdc.gov/nip/diseases/varicella/.

54. Connelly K, DeWitt L. Neurologic complications of infectious mononucleosis. *Pediatr Neurol.* 1994;10: 181-184.

55. Centers for Disease Control and Prevention. *West Nile Virus Human Case Count.* 2007. Available at http://www.cdc.gov/ncidod/dvbid/westnile/surv&controlCaseCount06_detailed.htm.

56. Mostashari F, Bunning M, Kitsutani P, et al. Epidemic West Nile encephalitis, New York, 1999: results of a household-based seroepidemiological survey. *Lancet.* Jul 28 2001;358(9278):261-264.

57. Campbell G, Marfin A, Lanciotti R, Gubler D. West Nile virus. *Lancet Infect Dis.* Sep 2002;2(9):519-529.

58. Centers for Disease Control and Prevention. *Eastern Equine Encephalitis Factsheet.* 2007. Available at www.cdc.gov.ncidod/dvbid/arbor/eeefact.htm.

59. Centers for Disease Control and Prevention. *Eastern Equine Encephalitis Human Case Count.* 2007. Available at www.cdc.gov/ncidod/dvbid/arbor/arbocase.htm.

60. Centers for Disease Control and Prevention. *St. Louis Encephalitis Case Count.* 2007. Available at www.cdc.gov/ncidod/dvbid/arbor/arbocase.htm.

61. Centers for Disease Control and Prevention. *St. Louis Encephalitis Factsheet.* 2007. Available at: www.cdc.gov/ncidod/dvbid/arbor/arbofact.htm.

62. Centers for Disease Control and Prevention. *California (La Crosse) Encephalitis Case Count.* 2007. Available at www.cdc.gov/ncidod/dvbid/arbor/arbocase.htm.

63. Centers for Disease Control and Prevention. *California (La Crosse) Encephalitis Factsheet.* 2007. Available at www.cdc.gov/ncidod/dvbid/arbor/lacfact.htm.

64. Yoshikawa H, Yamazaki S, Watanabe T, Abe T. Study of influenza-associated encephalitis/encephalopathy in children during the 1997 to 2001 influenza seasons. *J Child Neurol.* Dec 2001;16(12):885-890.

65. Morishima T, Togashi T, Yokota S, Okuno Y, Miyazaki C, Tashiro M. Encephalitis and encephalopathy associated with an influenza epidemic in Japan. *Clin Infect Dis.* 2002;35:512-517.

66. Togashi T, Matsuzono Y, Narita M, Morishima T. Influenza-associated acute encephalopathy in Japanese children in 1994-2002. *Virus Res.* 2004;103:75-78.

67. Newland JG, Laurich VM, Rosenquist AW, et al. Neurologic complications in children hospitalized with influenza: characteristics, incidence, and risk factors. *J Pediatr.* Mar 2007;150(3):306-310.

68. Bhat N, Wright J, Broder K, et al. Influenza Special Investigations Team. Influenza-associated deaths among children in the United States, 2003-2004. *New England Journal of Medicine.* 2005;15;353(24):2559-2567.

69. Centers for Disease Control and Prevention. *Rabies Case Count.* 2007. Available at http://www.cdc.gov/ ncidod/dvrd/rabies/Professional/publications/Surveillance/Surveillance01/Table2-01.htm.

70. Centers for Disease Control and Prevention. *Rabies Factsheet.* 2007. Available at www.cdc.gov/ncidod/dvrd/ rabies/.

71. Plotkin S. Rabies. *Clin Infect Dis.* 2000;30:4-12.

72. American Academy of Pediatrics. Section 3. Summaries of Infectious Diseases: Rabies. In: Pickering LK, Baker CJ, Kimberlin DW, Long SS, eds. *Red Book: 2009 Report of the Committee on Infectious Diseases.* 28th ed. Elk Grove Village, IL: American Academy of Pediatrics; 2009:552-559.

73. Willoughby R. A cure for rabies? *Sci Am.* 2007;296:88-95.

74. Centers for Disease Control and Prevention. Human rabies—Indiana and California, 2006. *MMWR Morb Mortal Wkly Rep.* 2007;56:361-365.

75. Gascon G, Yamani S, Crowell J, et al. Combined oral isoprinosine-intraventricular alpha-interferon therapy for subacute sclerosing panencephalitis. *Brain Dev.* Sep-Oct 1993;15(5):346-355.

76. Miyazaki M, Nishimura M, Toda Y, Saijo T, Mori K, Kuroda Y. Long term follow up of a patient with subacute sclerosing panencephalitis successfully treated with intrathecal interferon alpha. *Brain Dev.* 2005;27(4):301-303.

77. Centers for Disease Control and Prevention. *Mumps Factsheet.* 2007. Available at www.cdc.gov/nip/diseases/mumps/default.htm.

78. Centers for Disease Control and Prevention. *Mumps Factsheet Complications.* 2007. Available at www.cdc.gov/nip/diseases/mumps/faqs-phys-complic.htm.

79. Rautonen J, Koskiniemi M, Vaheri A. Prognostic factors in childhood acute encephalitis. *Pediatr Infect Dis J.* 1991;10:441-446.

80. Moorthi S, Schneider W, Dombovy M. Rehabilitation outcomes in encephalitis—a retrospective study 1990–1997. *Brain Inj.* 1999;13:225-229.

81. Defresne P, Hollenberg H, Husson B, et al. Acute transverse myelitis in children: clinical course and prognostic factors. *J Child Neurol.* 2003;18:401-406.

82. Knebusch M, Strassburg HM, Reiners K. Acute transverse myelitis in childhood: nine cases and review of the literature. *Dev Med Child Neurol.* 1998;40:631-639.

83. Transverse Myelitis Consortium Working Group, Proposed diagnostic criteria and nosology of acute transverse myelitis. *Neurology.* 2002;59:499-505.

84. Scott TF, Kassab SL, Singh S. Acute partial transverse myelitis with normal cerebral magnetic resonance imaging: transition rate to clinically definite multiple sclerosis. *Mult Scler.* 2005;11:373-377.

85. Berman M, Feldman S, Alter M, Zilber N, Kahana E. Acute transverse myelitis: incidence and etiologic considerations. *Neurology.* 1981;31:966-971.

86. Miyazawa R, Ikeuchi Y, Tomomasa T, Ushiku H, Ogawa T, Morikawa A. Determinants of prognosis of acute transverse myelitis in children. *Pediatr Int.* 2003;45:512-516.

87. Defresne P, Meyer L, Tardieu M, et al. Efficacy of high dose steroid therapy in children with severe acute transverse myelitis. *J Neurol Neurosurg Psychiatry.* 2001;71:272-274.

88. Dunne K, Hopkins IJ, Shield LK. Acute transverse myelopathy in childhood. *Dev Med Child Neurol.* 1986;28:198-204.

89. Paine RS, Byers RK. Transverse myelopathy in childhood. *Am J Dis Child.* 1953;85:151-163.

90. Pidcock FS, Krishnan C, Crawford TO, Salorio CF, Trovato M, Kerr DA. Acute transverse myelitis in childhood: center-based analysis of 47 cases. *Neurology.* 2007;68:1474-1480.

91. Banwell BL. The long (-itudinally extensive) and the short of it: transverse myelitis in children. *Neurology.* 2007;68:1447-1449.

92. Berger JR, Sabet A. Infectious myelopathies. *Semin Neurol.* 2002;22:133-142.

93. Kelly H. Evidence for a causal association between oral polio vaccine and transverse myelitis: a case history and review of the Literature. *J Paediatr Child Health.* 2006; 42:155-159.

94. Zanoni G, Nguyen TM, Destefani E, Masala L, Nardelli E, Tridente G. Transverse myelitis after vaccination. *Eur J Neurol.* 2002;9:696-697.

95. Fenichel GM. Neurological complications of immunization. *Ann Neurol.* 1982;12:119-128.

96. Kaplin AI, Deshpande DM, Scott E, et al. IL-6 induces regionally selective spinal cord injury in patients with the neuroinflammatory disorder transverse myelitis. *J Clin Invest.* 2005;115:2731-2741.

97. Minami K, Tsuda Y, Maeda H, Yanagawa T, Izumi G, Yoshikawa N. Acute transverse myelitis caused by Coxsackie virus B5 infection. *J Paediatr Child Health.* 2004;40:66-68.

98. Abramsky O, Teitelbaum D. The autoimmune features of acute transverse myelopathy. *Ann Neurol.* 1977; 2:36-40.

99. Wingerchuk DM, Lennon VA, Pittock SJ, Lucchinetti CF, Weinshenker BG. Revised diagnostic criteria for neuromyelitis optica. *Neurology.* 2006;66:1485-1489.

100. Lennon VA, Wingerchuk DM, Kryzer TJ, et al. A serum autoantibody marker of neuromyelitis optica: distinction from multiple sclerosis. *Lancet.* 2004;364: 2106-2112.

101. Lennon VA, Kryzer TJ, Pittock SJ, Verkman AS, Hinson SR. IgG marker of optic-spinal multiple sclerosis binds to the aquaporin-4 water channel. *J Exp Med.* 2005;202:473-477.

102. McLinskey NBA, MacAllister W, Milazzo M, Krupp L. Neuromyelitis optica in childhood. *Neuropediatrics.* 2006;26:S85.

103. Auletta JJ, John CC. Spinal epidural abscesses in children: a 15-year experience and review of the literature. *Clin Infect Dis.* 2001;32:9-16.

104. Patel H, Boaz JC, Phillips JP, Garg BP. Spontaneous spinal epidural hematoma in children. *Pediatr Neurol.* 1998; 19:302-307.

105. Pollono D, Tomarchia S, Drut R, Ibanez O, Ferreyra M, Cedola J. Spinal cord compression: a review of 70 pediatric patients. *Pediatr Hematol Oncol.* 2003;20:457-466.

106. Auguste KI, Gupta N. Pediatric intramedullary spinal cord tumors. *Neurosurg Clin North Am.* 2006;17:51-61.

107. Innocenzi G, Raco A, Cantore G, Raimondi AJ. Intramedullary astrocytomas and ependymomas in the pediatric age group: a retrospective study. *Childs Nerv Syst.* 1996;12:776-780.

108. DeSousa AL, Kalsbeck JE, Mealey J Jr., Campbell RL, Hockey A. Intraspinal tumors in children. A review of 81 cases. *J Neurosurg.* 1979;51:437-445.

109. Ullrich NJ, Marcus K, Pomeroy SL, et al. Transverse myelitis after therapy for primitive neuroectodermal tumors. *Pediatr Neurol.* 2006;35:122-125.

110. Sure U, Wakat JP, Gatscher S, Becker R, Bien S, Bertalanffy H. Spinal type IV arteriovenous malformations (perimedullary fistulas) in children. *Childs Nerv Syst.* 2000;16: 508-515.

111. Scott TF, Bhagavatula K, Snyder PJ, Chieffe C. Transverse myelitis. Comparison with spinal cord presentations of multiple sclerosis. *Neurology.* 1998;50:429-433.

112. Andronikou S, Albuquerque-Jonathan G, Wilmshurst J, Hewlett R. MRI findings in acute idiopathic transverse myelopathy in children. *Pediatr Radiol.* 2003;33: 624-629.

113. Lahat E, Pillar G, Ravid S, Barzilai A, Etzioni A, Shahar E. Rapid recovery from transverse myelopathy in children treated with methylprednisolone. *Pediatr Neurol.* 1998; 19:279-282.

114. Sebire G, Hollenberg H, Meyer L, Huault G, Landrieu P, Tardieu M. High dose methylprednisolone in severe acute transverse myelopathy. *Arch Dis Child.* 1997;76: 167-168.

115. Shahar E, Andraus J, Savitzki D, Pilar G, Zelnik N. Outcome of severe encephalomyelitis in children: effect of high-dose methylprednisolone and immunoglobulins. *J Child Neurol.* 2002;17:810-814.

116. Tsiodras S, Kelesidis T, Kelesidis I, Voumbourakis K, Giamarellou H. Mycoplasma pneumoniae-associated myelitis: a comprehensive review. *Eur J Neurol.* 2006;13:112-124.

117. Fux CA, Pfister S, Nohl F, Zimmerli S. Cytomegalovirus-associated acute transverse myelitis in immunocompetent adults. *Clin Microbiol Infect.* 2003;9:1187-1190.

118. Gilden DH, Beinlich BR, Rubinstien EM, et al. Varicella-zoster virus myelitis: an expanding spectrum. *Neurology.* 1994;44:1818-1823.

119. Pittock SJ, Lucchinetti CF. Inflammatory transverse myelitis: evolving concepts. *Curr Opin Neurol.* 2006;19:362-368.

120. Mikaeloff Y, Suissa S, Vallee L, et al. First episode of acute CNS inflammatory demyelination in childhood: prognostic factors for multiple sclerosis and disability. *J Pediatr.* 2004;144:246-252.

121. Weinshenker BG, Wingerchuk DM, Vukusic S, et al. Neuromyelitis optica IgG predicts relapse after longitudinally extensive transverse myelitis. *Ann Neurol.* 2006;59: 566-569.

CHAPTER 17

Multiple Sclerosis White Matter

Khurram Bashir

Demyelination is a process that results in either partial or complete loss of the myelin sheath following a period of normal myelin development. Demyelinating diseases may affect the central nervous system (CNS), the peripheral nervous systems (PNS), or both. CNS demyelination may occur as a result of direct damage to the myelin sheath and/or the oligodendrocytes (primary demyelination), or is secondary to axonal damage with subsequent disruption of the axon-glia interaction essential to maintain normal myelination (secondary demyelination). Acquired CNS demyelinating diseases include self-limited monophasic disorders, such as acute disseminated encephalomyelitis (ADEM), as well as chronic, recurrent conditions such as multiple sclerosis (MS) and neuromyelitis optica (NMO). On the other hand, dysmyelination is a genetic or developmental abnormality of the myelin sheath seen in various leukodystrophies such as adrenal leukodystrophy and metachromatic leukodystrophy. A discussion of dysmyelinating diseases is beyond the scope of this chapter, which focuses on childhood demyelinating diseases of the CNS. In the last few years there has been increased interest in studying childhood-onset MS, and our understanding of acquired demyelinating disorders is increasing exponentially.

MULTIPLE SCLEROSIS

Multiple sclerosis (MS) is an acquired, immune-mediated, demyelinating disease affecting the brain and the spinal cord. Despite reports of childhood-onset MS[1-3] soon after the initial descriptions of MS by Jean Marie Charcot,[4] the diagnosis of MS in childhood was disputed for a long time. In addition, early on, the misdiagnosis of a number of diseases as MS, including leukodystrophies, metabolic disorders, and tumors, and the confusion surrounding the use of various terms to describe a single disorder, cast further doubt on the existence of childhood-onset MS.[5] Although a few reports of childhood-onset MS[6,7] were still published in the literature, on the whole, childhood-onset MS was largely ignored by both the researchers and the clinicians. In fact, one of the early diagnostic criteria[8] proposed for the diagnosis of MS specifically restricted this diagnosis to patients between the ages of 10 and 50 years. The recognition of the fact that MS occurs as a distinct disease in children was brought forth by a series of articles published in the late 1950s and early 1960s.[9-11] Later publications firmly established the occurrence of MS in children under the age of 18 years, even as early as infancy.[12-15] Despite this renewed interest, the epidemiology, genetics, and natural history of pediatric-onset MS remain unclear at the present time.

Clinical Features

With an increasing number of reports being published, the clinical features of childhood-onset MS are beginning to be understood better. Despite limited natural history data, a clearer picture of this disease in children is emerging. The mean age of onset in most studies is reported to be between 8 and 14 years. Infants as young as 10 months have been reported to have findings suggestive of MS.[15] In this case, which probably represents the earliest onset of MS in published literature, a girl developed five episodes of aseptic meningitis starting at age 10 months, followed by six additional episodes to relapsing neurological deficits with variable recovery. Following her death at the age of 6 years, her brain showed multiple white matter demyelinating lesions scattered throughout the brain and brainstem, with some larger lesions demonstrating a necrotic component. Similar to MS in adults, childhood-onset MS seems to have a female preponderance, with a male-female ratio ranging from 1:1.3 to 1:3.0.[16]

The initial clinical events noted in the various case series seem to vary depending on patient population, number of patients, and the reported details of the episode. Although sensory disturbances have been suggested as the most common initial symptom in a majority of the childhood-onset MS patients,[12,17,18] other symptoms—such as motor weakness, cerebellar deficits, brainstem involvement, and optic neuritis—occur very frequently as well. In a review of the literature by Ness and associates, the reported frequency of various system involvement varied widely.[16] In childhood-onset MS patients at initial presentation, optic nerve involvement was seen in 0% to 50%, sensory involvement in 13% to 69%, motor involvement in 6% to 90%, cerebellar involvement in 4% to 80%, brainstem involvement in 6% to 60%, and spine or bladder/bowel involvement in 1% to 31%.[16] Polysymptomatic onset, which is the second most frequently encountered initial presentation in adults (after sensory complaints),[19] was seen in 10% to 67% of the patients with childhood-onset MS. Altered mental status, which is a rare initial complaint in adult-onset MS, was seen in 5% to 39% of the children with MS; this raises the possibility that some of the patients reported in these case series may have had ADEM as their initial presentation.

Optic neuritis (ON) is a frequently encountered clinically isolated syndrome (CIS) in both adults and children who go on to develop MS. Although the risk of developing clinically definite MS in adults with unilateral ON is about 38%, this risk increases to 56% in patients who have optic neuritis and demyelinating lesions on cranial MRI.[20] Long-term prospective data in children with ON is lacking. While some studies report a slightly lower risk of developing MS in children with ON,[16,21] other studies report this risk to be similar to that seen in adults.[22,23] Most studies, however, are limited because of relatively short-term follow-up while determining the subsequent risk of developing clinically definite MS. In a recent study, about one-third of the children with ON followed closely over a period of 2 years went on to develop MS.[21] In this study, bilateral ON, abnormal findings on neurological examination, and asymptomatic lesions on MRI were associated with a significantly higher risk of developing MS. Bilateral simultaneous ON is generally considered to be less likely to progress to definite MS,[24–26] but the studies by Wilejto, Lucchinetti, and their colleagues have reported a higher risk of developing MS following bilateral ON presentation.[21,27] On the other hand, bilateral sequential ON or recurrent ON are reported to increase the risk of

progressing to definite MS in children.[27] The risk of developing MS may be lower if the child has a history of an infection within 2 weeks prior to the onset of visual symptoms.[27]

Transverse myelitis in children usually presents with sensory disturbance in the extremities, which usually starts distally and then progresses, associated with weakness, gait difficulties, and bladder and bowel disturbances. A partial TM increases the risk of developing MS in adults and children alike.[28,29] Other high-risk features in children with TM that predict future development of MS include asymmetric motor and sensory findings, asymptomatic lesions on brain MRI, presence of elevated IgG index or oligoclonal bands in CSF, and abnormal visual and brainstem auditory evoked potential studies.[28]

An isolated brainstem-cerebellar syndrome (BCS) may be seen in 6% to 60% of childhood MS patients. Diplopia is probably the most frequently encountered symptom in older children presenting with BCS as their initial event,[30] while ataxia is more common in children under 10 years of age and in girls.[14] Interestingly, males are reported to present with BCS as their initial symptoms more commonly (41.4% vs. 13.2%), and also tend to demonstrate more brainstem lesions on MRI (63% vs. 40.3%) during their disease course compared to females.[31]

In a large European study of 296 patients with onset of their initial demyelinating event before age 18 years, 57% of the children developed a second clinical episode (ie, definite MS) after a mean follow-up of 2.9 years.[32] About 40% of the entire cohort presented with ADEM as their first clinical episode; and of this cohort, 29% experienced another event, thus declaring them as "definite MS." The risk of developing MS was higher in children who developed a CIS at age greater than 10 years, those who presented with ON (as opposed to TM or BCS), and those who had an initial brain MRI suggestive of demyelination. Although it is possible that some of the patients who presented with ADEM as their initial event may not meet the criteria proposed by the Internal Pediatric MS Study Group,[33] this study does support the contention that a majority of patients presenting with a CIS develop MS over a relatively short follow-up period.

The natural history of childhood-onset MS is not entirely clear. Most studies are of relatively short duration, and trying to extrapolate these short-term results to the lifetime of a patient can be problematic. The clinical classification of childhood-onset MS is based on the adult classification,[34] and at least 4 different clinical disease subtypes are identified.

■ Relapsing remitting MS (RRMS) is characterized by clearly defined disease relapses with full recovery or with sequelae and residual deficit upon recovery;

periods between disease relapses are stable, with a lack of disease progression.

■ Secondary progressive MS (SPMS) is defined as disease that has an initial relapsing-remitting disease course followed by progression with or without occasional relapses, minor remissions, and plateaus.

■ Primary progressive MS (PPMS) is defined as disease progression from the onset with occasional plateaus and temporary minor improvements.

■ Progressive relapsing MS (PRMS) is defined as progressive disease from the onset, with clear acute relapses, with or without full recovery, and periods between relapses characterized by continuing progression.

As opposed to adults, the studies of childhood-onset MS reveal a higher incidence of RRMS and a relatively low risk of PPMS.[18,35-37] More than 90% of childhood-onset MS patients present with RRMS and only 2% to 7% of young onset patients have PPMS. Generally, childhood-onset MS is believed to have a better prognosis, with relatively lower risk of progression and development of disability.[14,18,36] MS patients are also believed to have a higher risk of second relapse in the first year, higher relapse rate, shorter interval between first and second relapses, and shorter duration of relapse with more complete recovery.[16]

Patients with childhood-onset MS are also noted to have a slower disease progression compared to adults. In some natural history studies, childhood-onset MS patients took almost twice as long to reach an expanded disability status scale (EDSS)[38] of 3.0 or 4.0 as MS patients with adult onset do.[18,36] The time to reach an EDSS of 6.0 (needing assistance to ambulate) was also longer for the childhood-onset MS cases compared to adult MS patients.[36] The likelihood of changing to SPMS (14% vs. 24%), and time to conversion to SPMS (16 years vs. 7 years), also favor childhood-onset MS.[36] However, the median age of childhood-onset SPMS patients was 30 years compared to 37 years for adult-onset MS patients. This is likely a result of developing MS at an earlier age, with childhood-onset MS patients being exposed to the effects of the disease for a much longer period of time. This highlights the facts that despite a slower rate of progression, childhood-onset MS is not benign. Also, once patients switch from the RRMS to SPMS stage, the subsequent rate of progression of disease does not appear to be different between childhood-onset and adult-onset MS patients.[39] A shorter inter-relapse interval, poor recovery from the intial relapse, a greater number of relapses in the first 2 or first 5 years after disease onset, and an earlier SPMS disease course are all poor prognostic indicators.[18,32,36] Age of onset, gender, type of initial event (polysymptomatic vs. monosymptomatic), and onset of MS pre- or postpuberty do not seem to have much of an impact on the disease progression.[16]

Paraclincial Studies

All children suspected of experiencing a demyelinating event should undergo a comprehensive history and examination followed by appropriate diagnostic studies. An array of diagnostic studies is available to determine the underlying etiology, including magnetic resonance imaging (MRI), cerebrospinal fluid (CSF) analysis, evoked potential (EP) studies, and laboratory tests.

MRI is the most sensitive diagnostic study, which not only helps with the diagnosis and in determining ongoing disease activity but also as an outcome measure to assess therapeutic efficacy in clinical trials. The typical appearance of childhood-onset MS on cranial MRI is similar to that seen in adults and consists of multiple T2 hyperintense white matter lesions present in periventricular, juxta-cortical, and infra-tentorial regions (see Figure 17-1). The likelihood of finding gadolinium-enhancing lesions on a brain MRI study appears to be lower in childhood-onset cases compared to adults (13-24% vs. > 50%).[40,41] Children with MS are also more likely to demonstrate tumefactive lesions that are large in size and associated with surrounding cerebral edema without much mass effect.[42-44] Despite impressive and striking initial MRI images, these large lesions tend to resolve following treatment with glucocorticoids.[45] In very young patients, the MS lesions may appear as bilateral, diffuse, white-matter lesions with poorly defined borders.[40] Since MRI has become an important tool in establishing a diagnosis of MS and because the new adult diagnostic criteria[46] rely heavily on MRI to prove dissemination in space and time following a CIS, it is imperative to establish the utility of these adult MS MRI criteria in childhood patients. A few small studies seem to suggest that the sensitivity and specificity of the adult MS MRI criteria in childhood-onset MS are lower than seen in the adult population.[40,42] A small study has also reported increased likelihood of cerebral atrophy over a 6- to 8-year time frame.[43] Long-term studies to evaluate the predictive value of MRI in determining the disease course in childhood-onset MS are lacking.

CSF examination has been used to assist with the diagnosis of MS since the 1930s. The most specific abnormalities identified are qualitative and quantitative abnormalities of de novo immuno-globulin synthesis. An elevated IgG index and/or positive oligoclonal bands are seen in about 40% to 90% of childhood-onset MS patients.[16] A study of MS patients presenting before the age of 16 years demonstrated presence of CSF abnormalities in about 92% of patients.[42-44] The presence of IgG abnormalities alone in CSF is not sufficient to make a diagnosis of MS, as some MS patients have normal CSF; also, the CSF changes characteristic of MS are far from unique. Patients with other neurological disorders, such as

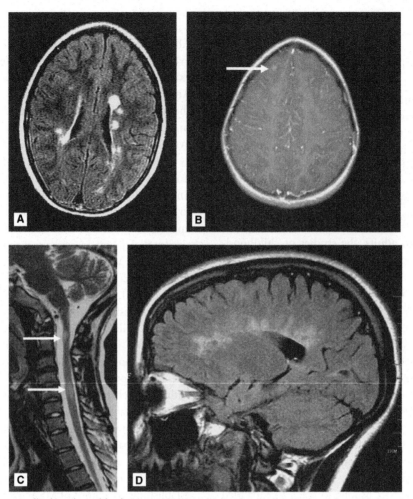

FIGURE 17-1 ■ MRI from a pediatric patient with relapsing-remitting multiple sclerosis. A: Axial FLAIR image of brain demonstrating periventricular T2 hyperintense demyelinating lesions; B: Axial T1 post-gadolinium image of brain demonstrating a left frontal lobe juxta-cortical enhancing lesion; C: Sagittal T2 images of the cervical spinal cord demonstrating two T2 hyperintense demyelinating lesions; D: Sagittal FLAIR image of the brain demonstrating periventricular T2 hyperintense demyelinating lesions. *(Images courtesy of Jayne Ness, MD, PhD.)*

ADEM, may also demonstrate oligoclonal bands and IgG synthesis abnormalities.[48,49] Other CSF abnormalities—including total protein, cell count, and myelin basic protein measurements—are nonspecific and usually normal in MS patients.

Electrophysiologic studies are useful in MS because of their objectivity, sensitivity, reproducibility, quantifiability, and standardization and comparability.[19] EP testing is used for detection of "clinically silent" lesions, thus providing objective evidence of dissemination in space. In general, EP studies of the visual system have the greatest yield and those of the brainstem auditory system the least. In one study, brainstem auditory evoked potential (BAEP) and somatosensory evoked potential (SEP) studies helped identify clinically asymptomatic lesions in only 12% of the childhood-onset MS patients.[50] Visual evoked potential (VEP) studies were reported to be abnormal in 34% of the patients with no prior history of ON. Interestingly, 84% of these patients with abnormal VEP had normal visual acuity testing on standard measures.

These MRI, CSF, and EP studies are extremely helpful in increasing the confidence in a diagnosis of MS by demonstrating characteristic abnormalities and by ruling out other potential etiologies. An important consideration when interpreting the results of these studies is to remember that there is no confirmatory diagnostic test for MS and these results should only be considered clinically significant in the appropriate clinical context.

Diagnosis

The diagnosis of childhood-onset MS has been formalized by an International Pediatric MS Study Group. The hallmark of childhood-onset MS, as in adult-onset MS, is "dissemination of neurological symptoms, of the type seen in MS, both in space and in time."[33,46] Thus, a definite diagnosis of childhood-onset MS requires one of the following[46,51]:

- Development of at least two clinical episodes of the type seen in MS separated by an arbitrarily determined interval of 30 days, if no other supportive evidence is present.
- At least 1 clinical episode (CIS) along with evidence of dissemination in space and time from MRI, CSF, and EP studies.
- As with adults, the requirement that a comprehensive evaluation of the patient has revealed "no better explanation" for the patient's symptoms.

The proposed criteria for diagnosis of dissemination in space and time established using MRI, CSF, and EP studies are outlined in Table 17-1. The major difference between the diagnosis of MS in adults and in childhood-onset MS is when the initial episode bringing the patient to medical attention is not a well-defined CIS such as optic neuritis (ON), transverse myelitis (TM), or brainstem-cerebellar syndrome (BCS) but rather ADEM. The consensus guidelines from the International

Table 17-1.

Revised MacDonald Criteria for Establishing a Diagnosis of Multiple Sclerosis

	Clinical Presentation	Additional Data Needed for MS Diagnosis
1	≥2 relapses; objective clinical evidence of ≥2 lesions	None
2	≥2 relapses; objective clinical evidence of 1 lesion	Dissemination in space, demonstrated by MRI OR ≥2 MRI lesions + positive CSF OR 2nd clinical relapse disseminated in space
3	1 relapse; objective clinical evidence of ≥2 lesions	Dissemination in time, demonstrated by MRI OR 2nd clinical relapse
4	1 relapse; objective clinical evidence of 1 lesion	Dissemination in space, demonstrated by MRI OR ≥2 MRI lesions + positive CSF AND dissemination in time, demonstrated by MRI, OR 2nd clinical relapse
5	Insidious neurological progression suggestive of MS	1 year of disease progression (retrospectively or prospectively determined) AND 2 out of 3 of the following: ■ Positive brain MRI (9 T2 lesions) OR ≥4 T2 MRI lesions and positive VEP ■ Positive spinal cord MRI (≥2 T2 lesions) ■ Positive CSF

Details of Data Requirements

Dissemination in space by MRI requires at least 3 of the following:
- At least 1 gadolinium-enhancing lesion or 9 T2 hyperintense lesions (if there is no gadolinium-enhancing lesion)
- At least 1 infratentorial lesion
- At least 1 juxtacortical lesion
- At least 3 periventricular lesions

Dissemination in time by MRI requires 1 of the following:
- Presence of a new gadolinium-enhancing lesion on an MRI scan made more than 3 months after the initial event, provided it is not a site consistent with the initial clinical event
- Presence of a new T2 hyperintense lesion developing at any time after the reference scan made at least 30 days following the initial clinical event

Positive CSF requires 1 of the following:
- Positive oligoclonal bands (preferably using isoelectric focusing technique)
- Elevated IgG index

Positive VEP requires
- Prolongation of P100 latencies consistent with MS

Pediatric MS Study Group[33] state that "in the special circumstance of a child whose initial clinical demyelinating event was diagnosed as ADEM, a second non-ADEM demyelinating event alone is not sufficient for a diagnosis of MS." In this instance, it is incumbent upon the neurologist to establish dissemination in space and in time by demonstrating either of the following:

■ Two clinical events separated from the initial ADEM event by at least 3 months.
■ At least one clinical event and development of new T2 lesions on MRI at least 3 months after the second non-ADEM event.

The rational for this is that the first demyelinating event following the initial ADEM may still be a continuation of the sentinel episode and may represent a monophasic illness rather than a chronic recurrent disease process. The Study Group did acknowledge that in rare cases ADEM may be recurrent (recurrent ADEM with similar clinical presentation) or multiphasic (recurrent ADEM with new clinical features), in which case a diagnosis of MS cannot be made with confidence (Figure 17-2).

Differential Diagnosis

One of the major caveats noted in establishing a diagnosis of MS since the initial Schumacher criteria and subsequently reaffirmed in all the proposed diagnostic criteria is the absence of any other potential neurological or systemic disease process that may potentially explain the patient's neurological symptoms.[8,33,46,52] This, then, requires a low threshold for suspecting other causes, and a comprehensive clinical evaluation by the neurologist. This is especially important in the case of a young child, especially those 10 years of age or younger, because of the immense physical, psychological, and financial cost that a diagnosis of an incurable, chronic, and disabling disease like MS carries. The differential diagnosis of MS in children is more varied and involves conditions that are not of clinical significance in adults, raising special challenges. Also, the differential diagnosis varies depending on the age of the child. The broad categories of diseases that need consideration when evaluating a child with MS include ADEM, leukodystrophies, and metabolic, nutritional, endocrine, vascular, neoplastic, inflammatory, infectious, and genetic disorders. Therefore, any atypical clinical, MRI, or CSF features should lead to a detailed examination and diagnostic evaluation to confidently rule out other potential etiologies. Some of the differential diagnoses that need consideration at different ages during MS evaluation are listed in Table 17-2. Since the differential diagnosis is extensive and the potential for misdiagnosis significant, the specific evaluation required for an individual patient needs to be tailored based on clinical history and examination while maintaining a low threshold for more detailed testing in atypical cases.

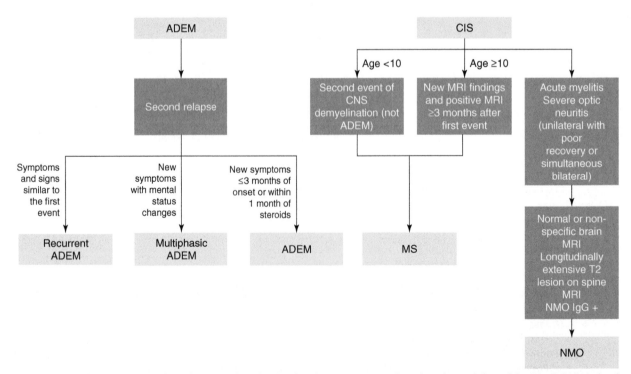

FIGURE 17-2 ■ Diagnostic scheme for pediatric CNS demyelinating disorders. (ADEM, acute disseminated encephalomyelitis; CIS, clinically isolated syndrome; MRI, magnetic resonance imaging; MS, multiple sclerosis; NMO, neuromyelitis optica.) *(Reproduced with permission from Krupp LB, Banwell B, Tenembaum S. Consensus definitions proposed for pediatric multiple sclerosis and related disorders. Neurology. 2007;68(suppl 2):S7-S12.[33])*

Table 17-2.

Differential Diagnoses to be Considered in Patients with Suspected Pediatric-Onset MS

Differential Diagnosis of Childhood-Onset MS		
≤1 Year	**≤10 Years**	**≤18 Years**
Genetic disorders	Genetic disorders	Other demyelinating disorders
▪ Aminoacidopathies	▪ Aminoacidopathies	▪ ADEM
▪ Organic acidopathies	▪ Organic acidopathies	▪ NMO
Infections	Other demyelinating disorders	Infections
▪ Meningitis	▪ ADEM	▪ Meningitis
▪ Encephalitis	▪ NMO	▪ Encephalitis
▪ Brain abscess	Infections	▪ Brain abscess
▪ HIV	▪ Meningitis	▪ Neuroborreliosis/Lyme disease
Dysmyelinating disorders	▪ Encephalitis	▪ HIV
▪ Pelizaeus-Merzbacher disease	▪ Brain abscess	▪ HTLV
Metabolic leukoencephalopathies	▪ Neuroborreliosis/Lyme disease	▪ Neurosyphilis
▪ ALD	▪ HIV	▪ PML
▪ MLD	▪ Neurosyphilis	▪ Parasitic infection[a]
▪ Krabbe disease	▪ SSPE	Neoplasms
Mitochondrial disorders	▪ Parasitic infection[a]	▪ CNS lymphoma
▪ Kearn-Sayre syndrome	Neoplasms	▪ Glial tumors (astrocytoma)
▪ Leigh disease	▪ CNS lymphoma	▪ Medulloblastoma
Miscellaneous	▪ Glial tumors (astrocytoma)	Systemic inflammatory disorders
▪ Langerhans cell histiocytosis (Letterer-Siwe disease)	▪ Medulloblastoma	▪ SLE
▪ Hemophagocytic lymphohistiocytosis (familial type)	Dysmyelinating disorders	▪ Sarcoidosis
	▪ ALD	▪ Sjögren syndrome
	▪ MLD	▪ Behçet disease
	▪ Krabbe disease	▪ Primary CNS angiitis
	▪ Pelizaeus-Merzbacher disease	Dysmyelinating disorders
	Metabolic leukoencephalopathies	▪ ALD
	▪ Refsum disease	▪ MLD
	▪ Alexander disease	▪ Krabbe disease
	▪ Fabry disease	Metabolic leukoencephalopathies
	▪ Myelinopathia centralis diffusa	▪ Wilson disease
	▪ Leukoencephalopathy with brainstem and spinal cord involvement and elevated white matter lactate	▪ Leukoencephalopathy with brainstem and spinal cord involvement and elevated white matter lactate
	Mitochondrial disorders	Mitochondrial disorders
	▪ Kearns-Sayre syndrome	▪ LHON
	▪ Leigh disease	▪ MELAS
	Gastrointestinal disorders	▪ MERRF
	▪ Celiac disease	▪ Kearns-Sayre syndrome
	Vascular disorders	Nutritional deficiencies
	▪ Moyamoya disease	▪ Vitamin B_{12} deficiency
	Miscellaneous	▪ Vitamin E deficiency
	▪ Migraine headache	▪ Folate deficiency
	▪ Radiation leukoencephalopathy	Gastrointestinal disorders
	▪ Chemotherapy-induced changes[b]	▪ Celiac disease
	▪ Langerhans cell histiocytosis (Hand-Schüller-Christian syndrome)	Vascular disorders
	▪ Hemophagocytic lymphohistiocytosis (sporadic type)	▪ Moyamoya disease
		▪ CADASIL
		▪ Anti-phospholipid antibody syndrome

(Continued)

Table 17-2. (*Continued*)

Differential Diagnoses to be Considered in Patients with Suspected Pediatric-Onset MS

	Differential Diagnosis of Childhood-Onset MS	
≤1 Year	≤10 Years	≤18 Years
		Miscellaneous
		■ Migraine headache
		■ Radiation leukoencephalopathy
		■ Chemotherapy-induced changes[b]
		■ Langerhans cell histiocytosis (localized eosinophilic granuloma)

ADEM, acute disseminated encephalomyelitis; ALD, adrenal leukodystrophy; CADASIL, cerebral autosomal dominant arteriopathy with subcortical infarcts and leukoencephalopathy; HIV, human immunodeficiency virus; HTLV, human T-cell lymphotropic virus; LHON, Leber hereditary optic neuropathy; MELAS, mitochondrial encephalopathy with lactic acidosis and stroke-like episodes; MERRF, myoclonic epilepsy with ragged red fibers; MLD, metachromatic leukodystrophy; NMO, neuromyelitis optica; PML, progressive multifocal leukoencephalopathy; SLE, systemic lupus erythematosis; SSPE, subacute sclerosing panencephalitis.
[a]Parasitic infections to be considered in a case of childhood-onset MS include cysticercosis, echinococcosis, amoebiosis, sparganosis, and myiasis; these need to be considered in children from endemic areas or those who have traveled to endemic regions.
[b]Chemotherapy agents known to cause acute or subacute CNS involvement are methotrexate, cyclosporine, and cytosine-arabinoside.

Treatment

The organization of the delivery of care to adult MS patients can be categorized as

- Pharmacologic management
  - Treatment of acute demyelinating relapses
  - Treatment of the underlying disease
  - Treatment of symptoms
- Nonpharmacologic management
- Psychosocial management
- Patient and family education

The treatment of relapses with glucocorticoid therapy, ACTH, or oral prednisone was initially employed in the 1950s and formally tested in the late 1960s. In the first randomized trial of a treatment for an unpredictable disease it was shown that recovery from a relapse was accelerated, but the natural history of the disease was unaltered.[53] The ability to alter the natural history of MS began in 1993, when interferon beta-1b (IFNβ-1b; Betaseron) was proven to reduce the relapse rate and accumulation of MRI lesions in RRMS. Since then other agents, intramuscular IFNβ-1a (Avonex), subcutaneous IFNβ-1a (Rebif), glatiramer acetate (GA; Copaxone), mitoxantrone (Novantrone), and natalizumab (Tysabri) have become available for use in MS patients. Symptom management was attempted by Charcot and others in the mid-19th century and continues to expand with the mostly unapproved new, or off-label use of medications. A number of clinical trials strongly suggest that early treatment for MS is extremely important in reducing further clinical and MRI disease activity and preventing neurological disability.[54]

Glucocorticoids have been the mainstay of therapy for an MS relapse since the late 1960s. Adrenocorticotropic hormone (ACTH) was the first agent to offer rapid recovery from relapses.[53] Intravenous methylprednisolone (IVMP) has been shown to be effective in the treatment of MS relapses, with recovery being more rapid and consistent than that seen with ACTH.[55-57] Oral prednisone is probably also effective and is substituted for IVMP by some clinicians primarily because of its easier route of administration. In general, glucocorticoid therapy is reserved for relapses that are severe enough to result in significant neurological impairment; while milder relapses can be managed expectantly. The most frequently used protocols consist of an initial steroid pulse with 3 to 5 days of IVMP with or without an oral prednisone taper. Despite a European study demonstrating efficacy over a 5-year period,[58] most studies do not demonstrate effectiveness of chronic glucocorticoid therapy in preventing disease activity or accumulation of disability.[59] The most common side effects of glucocorticoids are a metallic taste in mouth, insomnia, mood changes, increased appetite, weight gain, hypertension, and hyperglycemia. In pediatric populations, prolonged glucocorticoid use may also cause growth retardation and possibly osteopenia. Therapeutic plasma exchange (TPE) or plasmapharesis is a treatment modality that nonselectively removes plasma components that are potentially pathogenic in immune-mediated diseases. Several initial, small, uncontrolled clinical trials demonstrated results that were mixed and difficult to interpret. However, a double-blind, crossover study by Weinshenker and colleagues showed that TPE resulted in clinically significant improvement in about 40% of patients with severe acute steroid unresponsive inflammatory demyelinating episodes.[60] In managing severe demyelinating relapses, TPE should be considered as a therapeutic option for patients who do not respond to high-dose glucocorticoids. Both these treatments are generally well tolerated in children, with the adverse effect profile similar to that seen in adults. The complications of TPE include those associated with insertion of a central venous catheter and those associated with the procedure itself. The most common complications of TPE include bleeding, infections, coagulopathy, hypotension, paresthesias, urticaria, and in rare instances, anaphylactic reactions. The vast majority of these complications are mild and easily tolerated by patients. Intravenous immunoglobulins (IVIg) is sometimes used as a treatment for glucocorticoid unresponsive relapses; however, its long-term use as a maintenance therapy has not been established.[61]

Disease-modifying agents (DMA) that are currently available for use in adults with MS include IFNβ (subcutaneous IFNβ-1b, subcutaneous IFNβ-1a, and intra-muscular IFNβ-1a), a synthetic polypeptide (glatiramer acetate), a humanized monoclonal antibody (natalizumab), and an anthracenedione derivative (mitoxantrone). Interferon beta was the first agent to be evaluated for and proven to be effective in altering the natural history of MS. Although the exact mechanism underlying its therapeutic effectiveness in MS is not clear, it appears to work through matrix metalloproteinases (MMP), especially MMP-9, found in the endothelial lining of the blood–brain barrier. Subcutaneous IFNβ-1b (Betaseron) was the first drug to receive regulatory approval for use in the United States based on phase III study results that demonstrated reduction in clinical relapses and MRI disease activity.[62,63] Subsequently, IFNβ-1b has been shown to be effective in CIS and in SPMS patients with ongoing relapses.[64-67] Intramuscular IFNβ-1a

(Avonex) has been shown to delay disability progression, relapse rate, MRI disease activity, cerebral atrophy, and conversion to definite MS from CIS.[68-71] Subcutaneous IFNβ-1a (Rebif) reduces relapse rate, development of new and active MRI lesions, and disability progression in MS patients.[72,73] Glatiramer acetate, a random polymer of four amino acids (L-glutamic acid, L-alanine, L-lysine, and L-tyrosine in fixed proportions of 1.9:6.0:4.7:1.0, respectively) has been proven to decrease annualized relapse rate and MRI disease activity in RRMS patients.[74,75] Natalizumab, a humanized monoclonal antibody, decreases the frequency of relapses, progression of disability, and MRI activity both as monotherapy and in combination with intramuscular IFNβ-1a.[76,77] Natalizumab is generally considered a second-line agent after patients have failed IFNβ or GA treatment because of the development of potentially serious adverse effects including progressive multifocal encephalopathy (PML) and melanoma.[78,79] Mitoxantrone is a chemotherapeutic agent approved for patients with worsening RRMS, SPMS, and PRMS. It has been shown to reduce relapses, accumulation of disability, and MRI disease activity with a reasonable side effect profile. The side effect profile of mitoxantrone—including cardiotoxicity, acute myelocytic leukemia, and restrictive lifetime use (maximum lifetime dose is 140 mg/m^2)— limits the use of this agent to a selected group of patients. Other agents used as treatments to favorably alter the course of MS include azathioprine, methotrexate, cyclophosphamide, rituximab, and alemtuzumab. The common indications, dosage, dosing regimen, adverse effects, and monitoring of these agents are outlined in Table 17-3.

Table 17-3.

Currently Available Immunomodulatory and Immunosuppressive Disease-Modifying Therapies for MS

	IFN β-1b	IFN β-1a SC	IFN β-1b IM	GA	Natalizumab	Mitoxantrone
Trade Name	Betaseron	Rebif	Avonex	Copaxone	Tysabri	Novantrone
Source	E-coli	CHO cells	Mammalian cells	Synthetic	Monoclonal Ab	Anthracene-dione derivative
Dose	250 μg	22 μg/44 μg	30 μg	20 mg	300 mg	12 mg/m²
Route	SC	SC	IM	SC	IV	IV
Regimen	Every other day	3 times a week	Weekly	Every day	Every 4 weeks	Every 3 months
Indication(s)	CIS, Relapsing MS	CIS, Relapsing MS	Relapsing MS	RRMS	Relapsing MS	Worsening RRMS, SPMS, PRMS
Common side effects	FLS, ISR	FLS	FLS, ISR	ISR, systemic reaction	PML, HSR, infections	Infections, CHF, AML
Laboratory monitoring	CBC, LFT, TFT	CBC, LFT, TFT	CBC, LFT, TFT	None	CBC	CBC, LFT, RFT, LVEF

AML, acute myelocytic leukemia; CBC, complete blood count; CHF, congestive heart failure; CHO, Chinese hamster ovary; CIS, clinically isolated syndrome; FLS, flu-like symptoms; IFN β-1a SC, interferon beta-1a subcutaneous; IFN β-1a IM, interferon beta-1a intramuscular; IFN β-1b, interferon beta-1b; ISR, injection site reaction; PML, progressive multifocal leukoencephalopathy; HSR, hypersensitivity reaction; LFT, liver function test; LVEF, left ventricular ejection fraction; PML, progressive multifocal leukoencephalopathy; PRMS, progressive relapsing multiple sclerosis; RFT, renal function test; TFT, thyroid function test; RRMS, relapsing-remitting multiple sclerosis; SPMS, secondary progressive multiple sclerosis.

The experience with these agents in childhood MS is very limited. There are no randomized controlled trials in childhood MS with any of the DMA approved for adults with MS. Single case reports and retrospective reviews of the safety and tolerability of IFNβ-1b in small numbers of children with MS have been reported. In summary, these reports demonstrate that these agents are safe, tolerated well, and cause relatively mild adverse effects.[61] Small case series and a web-based survey of MS children suggest that GA is well tolerated and the side effects are relatively minor and similar to those seen in adults. Mitoxantrone has anecdotally been used in adolescents with worsening MS with acceptable safety and stabilization of disease.[80] There are no data available regarding the use of natalizumab or other chemotherapeutic agents for the treatment of MS in children. Although most children treated with immunomodulatory agents seem to have the same adverse effects as adults, the long-term benefit of these drugs in childhood MS is not clear. The issues of appropriate dosage and dosing regimen; efficacy; effect(s) on growth and development, both physical and emotional; effect(s) on the immature central nervous system and immune system; and long-term safety; remain unresolved and need to be addressed.

MS causes a wide variety of symptoms in both adult and pediatric MS patients. These symptoms that either occur in the setting of an acute relapse or as chronic ongoing problems have a devastating effect on the quality of life of MS patients. Identifying and treating these symptoms constitutes a major part of the management of MS. The use of pharmacologic agents even in adult MS care is largely based on anecdotal reports or small case series. There are few, if any, controlled clinical trials of agents used in symptomatic management of MS. Thus, most agents prescribed for the management of MS-associated symptoms have not been approved by the FDA for this particular indication and thereby constitute "off-label use." Nonpharmacologic management strategies, including alternative and complimentary therapies, constitute a major component of symptomatic treatment of MS symptoms. Table 17-4 outlines some of the common MS symptoms and frequently used treatments for these symptoms.

ACUTE DISSEMINATED ENCEPHALOMYELITIS

Acute disseminated encephalomyelitis (ADEM) is an acute immune-mediated inflammatory episode involving the central nervous system. ADEM usually occurs following an infection or vaccination. Although at times the terms "postinfectious encephalomyelitis" or "postvaccinal encephalomyelitis" are used to describe these clinical entities, these encephalomyelites and idiopathic ADEM have the same expected course and neuropathologic changes. Acute hemorrhagic leukoencephalitis and acute necrotizing hemorrhagic leukoencephalitis probably represent the most severe forms of ADEM.

Acute disseminated encephalomyelitis is a rare disorder that usually has a monophasic presentation and clinical course. ADEM has been reported to occur at all ages, but appears to be more common in the pediatric age group, with 5- to 8-year-old children developing it most frequently.[81] It has been described in all racial and ethnic groups and in both genders.[81] Some case series suggest a higher male-to-female ratio among pediatric patients.[82,83] Its frequency following certain infections and immunizations has been reported as 1 case in several hundreds to thousands of exposures. Some studies suggest a seasonal increase in the incidence of ADEM in spring and winter months. ADEM is very frequently (50-100% of the time) preceded by symptoms and signs of infection, usually a nonspecific upper respiratory tract infections.[81] Other infections linked to subsequent development of ADEM include varicella, mumps, rubella, enterovirus, Epstein-Barr virus, human herpes virus-6, human lymphotrophic virus type-I, adenovirus, influenza A and B, herpes simplex, *Listeria, Mycoplasma pneumoniae,* leptospirosis, and Rocky Mountain spotted fever.[19]

An increased risk of ADEM has also been reported to occur within 4 weeks of a vaccination[84] with immunization for rabies, measles, pertussis, rubella, Japanese B encephalitis, influenza, typhoid, and hepatitis B, and with tetanus antitoxin, among others.[19] The etiology of ADEM is not known, but it probably is due to the activation of immune cells directed against myelin antigen(s), due to direct damage to oligodendrocytes, or as a result of a nonspecific immune system activation. The target of this immune attack is most likely a myelin protein such as myelin basic protein (MBP), proteolipid protein (PLP), or myelin oligodendrocyte glycoprotein (MOG). ADEM is pathologically very similar to experimental allergic encephalomyelitis (EAE). Neuropathologic examination shows a severely edematous brain with prominent vasculature in the white matter and perivenular region. Acute lesions appear to be of similar age, predominantly involve the white matter, are well-demarcated, surround small- and medium-size veins, and microscopically contain perivascular mononuclear cells, reactive microglia, lipid-laden macrophages, variable myelin damage, and relatively preserved axons. Older lesions have a more marked astrocytic gliosis and myelin loss. In more severe cases, acute lesions contain a significant hemorrhagic component, warranting the terms "acute hemorrhagic leukoencephalitis" or "necrotizing leukoencephalitis"; this is associated with fibrinoid vascular necrosis, exudation of blood components including fibrin into perivascular regions, tissue necrosis, a polymorphonuclear lymphocytic infiltration, and myelin loss with some axonal loss.

Table 17-4.

Symptomatic Treatment of Select MS Symptoms

1. **Fatigue**
   - Positive attitude, active life-style, exercise, scheduled rest, regular sleep, energy conservation, cool environment
   - Amantadine, Modafinil, Pemoline, Sertraline, Fluoxetine, Methylphenidate, Dextroamphetamine, Selegiline
2. **Depression**
   - Patient and family education, fostering a good doctor-patient rapport, MS support group, psychotherapy, suicide preventive measures
   - SSRI (Citalopram, Fluoxetine, Sertraline, Escitalopram), SNRI (Venlafaxine, Duloxetine), Tri-cyclic antidepressants (Amitriptyline, Nortriptyline, Desipramine), Others (Bupropion)
3. **Pain/Dysesthesia/Allodynia**
   - Biofeedback, physical therapy, TENS Unit, local nerve blocks, acupuncture
   - Tri-cyclic antidepressants (Amitriptyline, Nortriptyline), Anti-convulsants (Carbamazepine, Gabapentin, Pregabalin, Levetiracetam), SNRI agents (Duloxetin), Others (Capsaicin, Mexiletine, NSAIDs, Tizanidine, Tramadol)
4. **Paroxysmal Symptoms**
   - Maintaining cool environment, biofeedback, TENS unit, acupuncture
   - Anti-convulsants (Carbamazepine, Gabapentin, Pregabalin, Levetiracetam), Others (Baclofen, Diazepam, Misoprostol)
5. **Spasticity/Muscle Spasms**
   - Identify and treat precipitating factors (UTI), physical therapy, regular stretching exercises, assistive devices for prevention of contractures, hydrotherapy, local nerve or motor point blocks, posterior rhizotomy, tenotomy/myotomy
   - Baclofen, Tizanidine, Dantrolene, Botulinum-A toxin, Intrathecal Baclofen, Clonazepam, Clonidine, Diazepam, Gabapentin
6. **Ataxia/Tremor/Vertigo**
   - Weighted bracelets, braces, head-rest for wheelchair, physical therapy (Frenkel's exercises), assistive devices, neurostimulatory devices (DBS), stereotactic thalamotomy, vestibular exercises
   - Propranolol, Primidone, Clonazepam, Buspirone, Isoniazid plus Pyridoxine, Diazepam, Ondansetrone, Pramipexole, Meclizine, Scopolamine transdermal patch, Chlorpromazine, Dimenhydrinate
7. **Detruser Muscle Hyperreflexia**
   - Rule out UTI and BPH, scheduled voiding, fluid restriction, biofeedback, condom catheters, adult diapers, indwelling catheter, supra-pubic cystostomy, urology referral for refractory problems
   - Hyoscyamine, Imipramine, Oxybutynin, Tolterodine, Solifenacin, Trospium, Darifenacin, Oxybutynin patch, Baclofen, Desmopressin, Dicyclomine, Flavoxate, Propantheline
8. **Urinary Hesitency and Retention**
   - Rule out UTI, scheduled voiding, intermittent self catheterization, external stimuli (rectal stimulation, rubbing thighs together, pulling on pubic hair), Credé maneuver, acidification of urine, suprapubic cystostomy
   - Bethanecol, Tamsulosin, Terazosin, Doxazosin, Methenamine Mandelate, Phenoxybenzamine
9. **Constipation**
   - High fiber diet, adequate fluid intake, regular exercise, bowel training (scheduled evacuation), digital stimulation, digital disimpaction
   - Bisacodyl, Docusate, Glycerin suppositories, Lactulose, Mini-enema, Polyethylene glycol, Casanthranol and Docusate, Magnesium hydroxide, Senna, Sodium phosphate enema, Sorbitol
10. **Erectile Dysfunction**
    - Tactile or oral stimulation, vacuum erectile devices, prosthetic penile implants, sex therapy, psychotherapy, behavioral therapy
    - Sildenafil, Vardenafil, Tadalafil, Prostaglandin E1, Phentolamine, Yohimbine, Trazodone, Fluoxetine, Bupropion

Clinically, ADEM presents with acute onset of fever, malaise, headache, nausea and/or vomiting, neck stiffness, seizures, somnolence, and behavioral changes frequently leading to encephalopathy, stupor, and coma. These symptoms are commonly associated with focal neurological deficits that include visual loss, weakness, ataxia, sensory disturbances, cranial nerve palsies, dysarthria, aphasia, extrapyramidal movement disorders, and bowel/bladder dysfunction. The typical clinical course is one of acute presentation and rapid progression with development of maximum deficits in less than a week.[83] Although these clinical features may be seen in both pediatric-onset and adult-onset cases, prolonged fever, headaches, seizures, and even status epilepticus occur more frequently in the children.[81] Paresthesias and acute polyradiculoneuropathy tend to be rare in children and common in adult-onset ADEM. ADEM is typically a monophasic illness that gradually improves over days to weeks to sometimes months, but may leave permanent, mild to moderate, residual neurological deficits. Occasionally ADEM symptoms may recur within 3 months following glucocorticoid treatment and recovery; this is usually termed "recurrent ADEM." In 5% to 20% of cases, the patients develop "multiphasic ADEM," where clinical symptoms and MRI abnormalities reoccur following an initial episode that had resolved completely on follow-up clinical and MRI examinations. Some of these patients with multiphasic ADEM may progress to RRMS while others do not.[81] In the more aggressive cases, increased intracranial pressure with resultant herniation, and/or respiratory failure from brainstem involvement, may result in death.

Imaging studies using MRI usually demonstrate multiple lesions of T2-weighted hyperintensity in the white matter of the cerebrum, cerebellum, brainstem, and spinal cord. As opposed to MS, ADEM lesions are large, patchy, poorly circumscribed areas, with gadolinium-enhancement noted in 30% to 100% of the patients (Figure 17-3).[81] These lesions tend to occur in the periventrcular and subcortical white matter, brainstem, cortical and subcortical gray matter, and extensive regions of the spinal cord. Some large lesions may show evidence of hemorrhage, which usually denotes a more aggressive course and is sometimes termed acute hemorrhagic encephalomyelitis. Various patterns of T2-weighted and gadolinium-enhancing lesions have been reported but none seem to correlate with the clinical prognosis.[81] Spinal cord MRI abnormalities are seen in 11% to 28% of the pediatric ADEM patients; these generally occur in

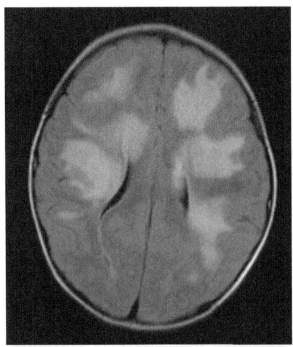

FIGURE 17-3 ■ MRI from a pediatric patient with acute disseminated encephalomyelitis: A: Axial proton density image of brain demonstrating bilateral white matter T2 hyperintense large demyelinating lesions. (*Images courtesy: Jayne Ness, MD, PhD.*)

the thoracic region, and as opposed to MS, demonstrate longitudinally extensive, gadolinium-enhancing lesions associated with cord edema.[81] Cranial MRI abnormalities tend to completely resolve on follow-up imaging studies in 50% to 75% of the affected individuals within 6 months.[85] In addition to conventional MRI studies, newer MRI techniques such as MR spectroscopy (reduced N-acetyl aspartate and elevated lactate levels), perfusion-weighted MRI (reduced or normal perfusion pattern), PET scanning (diffusely decreased cerebral metabolism), and SPECT scanning using 99m Tc-HMPAO or acetazolamide (focal areas of hypoperfusion) may be helpful in differentiating ADEM lesions from infectious, neoplastic, or vascular processes.[81] CSF may be normal but usually shows an elevated opening pressure, lymphocytic pleocytosis, normal glucose, and an increased protein and MBP. IgG index is rarely abnormal, and OCB, if present, is usually transient. CSF cultures and serologic testing are typically negative but PCR technology may assist in identifying the inciting agent. EP studies have a limited role in the evaluation of ADEM. An electroencephalogram (EEG) usually reveals nonspecific diffuse slowing. Additional laboratory investigations should include CSF cultures and acute and convalescent titers for infectious agents, serology for connective tissue diseases, and other appropriate studies to identify the inciting etiology.

ADEM shares clinical and MRI features with a number of infectious, inflammatory, demyelinating, and other disorders; the following diseases should be considered in the differential diagnosis of ADEM:

- Infectious disorders such as acute viral encephalitis; bacterial, Lyme, syphilitic, tuberculous, or cryptococcal meningitis; cysticercosis; coccidiomycosis; toxoplasmosis; intracranial parenchymal or epidural abscesses; and multiple septic emboli from subacute bacterial endocarditis.
- Demyelinating disorders such as leukodystrophies, MS, Marburg variant of MS, Balo concentric sclerosis, Schilder disseminated sclerosis, and Devic neuromyelitis optica.
- Inflammatory disorders such as vasculitis, polyarteritis nodosa, Churg-Strauss disease, Wegener granulomatousis, neuro-Beçhet syndrome, Sjögren syndrome, and systemic lupus erythematosis.
- Neoplastic disorders such as primary CNS neoplasms including gliomas, and brain metastases.
- Other disorders such as cerebral venous thrombosis, acute necrotizing encephalopathy, extra-pontine myelinolysis, and metabolic disorders.

These disorders need to be considered and ruled out when evaluating a patient for ADEM.

There is no standard or widely accepted, proven treatment for ADEM. The management consists of supportive care, reduction of increased intracranial pressure if present, treatment of infection if clinically suspected at presentation, and, once infection is excluded, high-dose glucocorticoid therapy. For patients who do not respond to glucocorticoid agents, courses of therapeutic plasma exchange (TPE) or intravenous immunoglobulin (IVIg) may be tried. Immunization against a triggering virus, when available, should be done as the risk of ADEM following immunization is usually markedly lower compared to that after primary infection with the same virus. With or without treatment, between half and three-quarters of pediatric ADEM patients recover completely or almost completely.[81] The most common long-term residual complications of ADEM include focal weakness, ataxia, visual loss, behavioral and cognitive problems, and seizures.

NEUROMYELITIS OPTICA

Neuromyelitis optica (NMO), or Devic disease, is an idiopathic, inflammatory, necrotizing demyelination of the CNS, clinically characterized by simultaneous or successive involvement of optic nerves and spinal cord. Eugène Devic, in 1884, presented a case of "myélite subaiguë compliquée de névrite optique" that summarized the cardinal neurpathologic features and coined the term "neuropticomyélite."[86,87] Other terms used to describe this condition in the literature include neuro-myélite, neuromyélite optic aiguë, acute optic neuromyelitis, neuromyelitis optica of Devic-Gault, Devic disease, ophthalmo-neuromyelitis, optic encephalomyelitis, ophthalmoencephalomyelopathy, and disseminated myelitis with optic neuritis. The debate over NMO as a variant of MS versus a separate disease entity started soon after the original descriptions and continues to date; however, most experts now believe it to be a distinct clinicopathologic entity.

NMO is a relatively rare disease, with its incidence and prevalence currently not known. It is probably under-diagnosed because of the confusion regarding its association with MS. The geographic and socioeconomic distribution of NMO is quite different from that of MS, with NMO being more prevalent in the tropics, among those in the lower socioeconomic strata, and in the Asian and African populations. The gender ratio among the reported cases seems to suggest a slightly higher incidence among females (female-male ratio = >1.4:1). Most cases are sporadic and may present at any age including the pediatric age group. An underlying hereditary component in the pathogenesis of NMO is also suggested by cases of the disease in siblings and monozygote twins. The etiology and pathogenesis of NMO is poorly understood. The temporal association with preceding viral infections in some cases and the isolation of human herpesvirus species from the neural

tissue of NMO patients suggests either an infectious or infection-induced immune-mediated etiology for NMO. Frequent association with a variety of immune-mediated connective tissue disorders and frequent presence of autoantibodies (anti-cardiolipin, anti-thyroglobulin, anti-microsomal, anti-parietal cell, antinuclear, and anti-smooth muscle antibodies) in NMO patients imply an underlying immunopathogenic mechanism. Antibodies to astrocytic glial fibrillary acidic protein (GFAP), and T-cell lines sensitive to glial S100 beta protein, have also been isolated from patients with NMO. Based on these observations, NMO is possibly the phenotypic clinical expression of a systemic immune-mediated process involving the CNS. The optic nerve and spinal cord presumably contain antigens that are targets for this neuroimmunologic process.

NMO patients may present with unilateral (40-45%) or simultaneous bilateral (25-30%) optic neuritis (ON), transverse myelitis (TM) (10-15%), or simultaneous ON and TM (10-15%). The interval between relapses is generally less than 3 months. The deficits noted in ON and TM associated with NMO tend to be severe and recovery is usually incomplete with permanent neurological deficits persisting in most patients. Death usually results from respiratory paralysis or the complications of severe neurological disability and bedbound status. According to one retrospective study, NMO may present as a rapidly progressive disease invariably resulting in severe disability and death, as a relapsing disease with attacks of ON and TM occurring at unpredictable intervals with varying degrees of recovery, or as a monophasic illness followed by variable, usually poor, recovery.[88] In this series, patients with relapsing disease were generally females, were older at the time of first symptoms, had a longer inter-attack interval (>3 months), had an associated systemic immune-mediated disorder, and generally had a better prognosis. A more benign form of NMO with near complete or total recovery and no relapses or long-term sequelae has been reported in the pediatric population.[89] In a recent series of 58 patients with NMO spectrum disorders, median age was reported to be 12 years.[90] There were more African-American patients than Caucasians, Hispanics, or Native Americans, and 88% were females. About 16% of the patients demonstrated brain abnormalities at the time of their initial presentation. The clinical course was relapsing in 93% and monophasic in the rest over a fairly short, 1-year follow-up period. About 40% of the patients had associated antoantibodies to other systemic autoimmune disorders. After a median follow-up of 12 months, only 6% had normal neurological examination and about half of the patients had significant neurological disability.

NMO is a clinical diagnosis supported by imaging and paraclinical studies. A number of diagnostic criteria based on characteristic clinical, laboratory, imaging, and

Table 17-5.

Proposed Diagnostic Criteria for Neuromyelitis Optica

Definite NMO	Requires Both Absolute and at Least Two Supportive Criteria
Absolute criteria	1. Optic neuritis 2. Acute myelitis
Supportive criteria	1. Normal or nonspecific white matter changes on cranial MRI at disease onset (not meeting radiologic diagnostic criteria for dissemination in space for MS) 2. Longitudinally extensive (≥ 3 vertebral segments in length) T2 signal abnormality 3. Presence of NMO IgG antibody
NMO Spectrum Disorder	**Includes the Following**
	1. Definite NMO 2. Single or recurrent episodes of longitudinally extensive acute myelitis 3. Single bilateral simultaneous or recurrent episodes of optic neuritis 4. Optic-spinal MS ("Asian MS") 5. Optic neuritis or longitudinally extensive myelitis associated with systemic autoimmune disease 6. Optic neuritis or longitudinally extensive myelitis associated with "specific" NMO brain lesions (hypothalamic, thalamic, brainstem)

pathologic features have been suggested to distinguish "pure" NMO from MS.[91-94] A more recent set of criteria have been proposed not only to assist with the diagnosis of NMO but also to identify clinical presentations at high risk of developing into NMO.[88] These criteria are detailed in Table 17-5.[95] It is, however, important to realize the limitations of these criteria, as they are derived from a retrospective data set from a tertiary referral clinic. Spinal cord MRI in NMO patients typically demonstrates hyperintense signal on T2-weighted images and swelling and cavitation on T1-weighted images extending 3 or more spinal segments in length (Figure 17-4B). Cranial MRI is usually normal or may demonstrate nonspecific white matter abnormalities; thalamic and brainstem lesions have been reported in some patients (Figure 17-4A).[88] MRI of the orbits may reveal optic

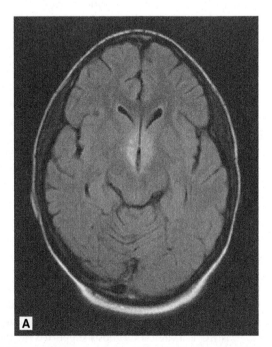
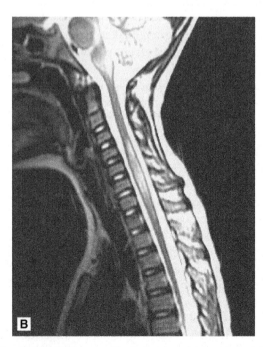

FIGURE 17-4 ■ MRI from a pediatric patient with Devic's neuromyelitis optica: A: Axial FLAIR image of brain demonstrating hypothalamic T2 hyperintense lesions; B: Sagittal T2 images of the cervical spinal cord demonstrating a longitudinally extensive T2 hyperintense demyelinating lesion.

nerves with abnormal T2W signal and gadolinium enhancement. CSF studies may be normal or may show mildly elevated protein and pleocytosis (cell count >50 WBC/mm^3 or >5 neutrophils/ mm^3), with a predominance of lymphocytes in the acute phase; IgG synthesis is normal and oligoclonal bands are absent in most cases. Visual and somatosensory EPs are expected to be abnormal, reflecting lesions of the optic nerves and spinal cord, respectively. Pathologic studies demonstrate demyelination, perivascular and parenchymal infiltration of inflammatory cells, edema, tissue necrosis and cavitation, arterial hyalinization, and astrogliosis limited to the optic nerves and the spinal cord. Recently a serologic marker, the so-called "NMO IgG antibody," has been described in more than half of patients with clinical diagnosis of NMO.[96] This autoantibody binds to an astrocytic water channel aquaporin-4 in the CNS. This antibody has also been shown to predict relapses in patients who present with initial episodes of severe optic neuritis or longitudinally extensive myelitis.[97,98] The frequency of NMO IgG in pediatric CNS inflammatory demyelinating disorders appears to be about 78% for definite NMO and 20% for recurrent optic neuritis or myelitis.[99]

The prognosis for neurological recovery and long-term survival in NMO is poor but has improved some in the recent years because of the recent advancements in technology and supportive care. The acute episodes are usually treated with high-dose glucocorticoid therapy with variable benefit and with some patients exhibiting glucocorticoid dependency. Other therapeutic approaches, such as immunosuppressants, IVIg, TPE, and lymphocytopharesis, have been used over the years with little success. Combined therapy with oral prednisone and azathioprine may be of some benefit in preventing long-term disability and recurrences. Recently, an anti-CD20 monoclonal antibody, rituximab, has been reported in small series of NMO patients to be an effective therapy in preventing more exacerbations and increasing disability.[100,101]

REFERENCES

1. Müller E. "Die multiple Sklerose des Gehirns und Rückenmarks." *In: Ihre Pathologie und Behandlung, klinisch bearbeitet.* Jena: Gustav Fischer; 1904.
2. Marie P. De la sclerose en plaques. *Rev Med.* 1883;536.
3. Schupfer F. Uber die inflantile Herdsklerose mit Betrachtungen uber sekundare Degenerationen bei disseminier Sklerose. *Monatsschr Psychiatr Neurol.* 1902;12:60-122.
4. Charcot J. Histologie de la sclerose en plaques. *Gaz Hop.* 1968;41:554-566.
5. Hanefeld F. Pediatric multiple sclerosis: a short history of a long story. *Neurology.* 2007;68(suppl 2):S3-S6.
6. Rimbaud L RH, Geraud G. De la sclerose en plaques chez l'enfant. *Rev Neurol.* 1938;69:477-482.
7. Carter H. Multiple sclerosis in childhood. *Am J Dis Child.* 1946;71:138-149.
8. Schumacher GA, Beebe G, Kibler RF, et al. Problems of experimental trials of therapy in multiple sclerosis: report by the panel on the evaluation of experimental trials of therapy in multiple sclerosis. *Ann NY Acad Sci.* 1965;122:552-568.
9. Gall JC Jr., Hayles AB, Siekert RG, Keith HM. Multiple sclerosis in children; a clinical study of 40 cases with onset in childhood. *Pediatrics.*1958;21:703-709.
10. Low NL, Carter S. Multiple sclerosis in children. *Pediatrics.* 1956;18:24-30.
11. Isler W. Multiple Sklerose im Kindesalter. *Helv Pediatr Acta.* 1961;16:412-431.
12. Duquette P, Murray TJ, Pleines J, et al. Multiple sclerosis in childhood: clinical profile in 125 patients. *J Pediatr.* 1987;111:359-363.
13. Ruggieri M, Polizzi A, Pavone L, Grimaldi LM. Multiple sclerosis in children under 6 years of age. *Neurology.* 1999;53:478-484.
14. Ruggieri M, Iannetti P, Polizzi A, Pavone L, Grimaldi LM. Multiple sclerosis in children under 10 years of age. *Neurol Sci.* 2004;25(suppl 4):S326-S335.
15. Shaw CM, Alvord EC Jr. Multiple sclerosis beginning in infancy. *J Child Neurol.* 1987;2:252-256.
16. Ness JM, Chabas D, Sadovnick AD, Pohl D, Banwell B, Weinstock-Guttman B. Clinical features of children and adolescents with multiple sclerosis. *Neurology.* 2007;68 (suppl 2):S37-S45.
17. Cole GF, Stuart CA. A long perspective on childhood multiple sclerosis. *Dev Med Child Neurol.* 1995;37:661-666.
18. Boiko A, Vorobeychik G, Paty D, Devonshire V, Sadovnick D. Early onset multiple sclerosis: a longitudinal study. *Neurology.* 2002;59:1006-1010.
19. Bashir KWJ. *Handbook of Multiple Sclerosis.* Philadelphia: Lippincott Williams & Wilkins; 2001.
20. Beck RW, Trobe JD, Moke PS, et al. High- and low-risk profiles for the development of multiple sclerosis within 10 years after optic neuritis: experience of the optic neuritis treatment trial. *Arch Ophthalmol.* 2003; 121:944-949.
21. Wilejto M, Shroff M, Buncic JR, Kennedy J, Goia C, Banwell B. The clinical features, MRI findings, and outcome of optic neuritis in children. *Neurology.* 2006;67:258-262.
22. Riikonen R, Donner M, Erkkila H. Optic neuritis in children and its relationship to multiple sclerosis: a clinical study of 21 children. *Dev Med Child Neurol.* 1988;30:349-359.
23. Mizota A, Niimura M, Adachi-Usami E. Clinical characteristics of Japanese children with optic neuritis. *Pediatr Neurol.* 2004;31:42-45.
24. Morales DS, Siatkowski RM, Howard CW, Warman R. Optic neuritis in children. *J Pediatr Ophthalmol Strabismus.* 2000;37:254-259.
25. Parkin PJ, Hierons R, McDonald WI. Bilateral optic neuritis. A long-term follow-up. *Brain.* 1984;107:951-964.
26. Hwang JM, Lee YJ, Kim MK. Optic neuritis in Asian children. *J Pediatr Ophthalmol Strabismus.* 2002;39:26-32.
27. Lucchinetti CF, Kiers L, O'Duffy A, et al. Risk factors for developing multiple sclerosis after childhood optic neuritis. *Neurology.* 1997;49:1413-1418.
28. Adams C, Armstrong D. Acute transverse myelopathy in children. *Can J Neurol Sci.* 1990;17:40-45.

29. Scott T, Weikers N, Hospodar M, Wapenski J. Acute transverse myelitis: a retrospective study using magnetic resonance imaging. *Can J Neurol Sci.* 1994;21:133-136.

30. Ghezzi A, Deplano V, Faroni J, et al. Multiple sclerosis in childhood: clinical features of 149 cases. *Mult Scler.* 1997;3:43-36.

31. Gusev E, Boiko A, Bikova O, et al. The natural history of early onset multiple sclerosis: comparison of data from Moscow and Vancouver. *Clin Neurol Neurosurg.* 2002;104:20-207.

32. Mikaeloff Y, Suissa S, Vallee L, et al. First episode of acute CNS inflammatory demyelination in childhood: prognostic factors for multiple sclerosis and disability. *J Pediatr.* 2004;144:246-252.

33. Krupp LB, Banwell B, Tenembaum S. Consensus definitions proposed for pediatric multiple sclerosis and related disorders. *Neurology.* 2007;68(suppl 2):S7-S12.

34. Lublin FD, Reingold SC. Defining the clinical course of multiple sclerosis: results of an international survey. *Neurology.* 1996;46:907-911.

35. Ghezzi A, Pozzilli C, Liguori M, et al. Prospective study of multiple sclerosis with early onset. *Mult Scler.* 2002;8:115-118.

36. Simone IL, Carrara D, Tortorella C, et al. Course and prognosis in early-onset MS: comparison with adult-onset forms. *Neurology.* 2002;59:1922-1928.

37. Pinhas-Hamiel O, Sarova-Pinhas I, Achiron A. Multiple sclerosis in childhood and adolescence: clinical features and management. *Paediatr Drugs.* 2001;3:329-336.

38. Kurtzke JF. Rating neurologic impairment in multiple sclerosis: an expanded disability status scale (EDSS). *Neurology.* 1983;33:1444-1452.

39. Confavreux C, Vukusic S, Adeleine P. Early clinical predictors and progression of irreversible disability in multiple sclerosis: an amnesic process. *Brain.* 2003;126:770-782.

40. Mikaeloff Y, Adamsbaum C, Husson B, et al. MRI prognostic factors for relapse after acute CNS inflammatory demyelination in childhood. *Brain.* 2004;127:1942-1947.

41. Korteweg T, Tintore M, Uitdehaag B, et al. MRI criteria for dissemination in space in patients with clinically isolated syndromes: a multicentre follow-up study. *Lancet Neurol.* 2006;5:221-227.

42. Hahn CD, Shroff MM, Blaser SI, Banwell BL. MRI criteria for multiple sclerosis: Evaluation in a pediatric cohort. *Neurology.* 2004;62:806-808.

43. Balassy C, Bernert G, Wober-Bingol C, et al. Long-term MRI observations of childhood-onset relapsing-remitting multiple sclerosis. *Neuropediatrics.* 2001;32:28-37.

44. McAdam LC, Blaser SI, Banwell BL. Pediatric tumefactive demyelination: case series and review of the literature. *Pediatr Neurol.* 2002;26:18-25.

45. Banwell B, Shroff M, Ness JM, Jeffery D, Schwid S, Weinstock-Guttman B. MRI features of pediatric multiple sclerosis. *Neurology.* 2007;68(suppl 2):S46-S53.

46. Polman CH, Reingold SC, Edan G, et al. Diagnostic criteria for multiple sclerosis: 2005 revisions to the "McDonald criteria." *Ann Neurol.* 2005;58:840-846.

47. Pohl D, Rostasy K, Reiber H, Hanefeld F. CSF characteristics in early-onset multiple sclerosis. *Neurology.* 2004;63:1966-1967.

48. Dale RC, de Sousa C, Chong WK, Cox TC, Harding B, Neville BG. Acute disseminated encephalomyelitis, multiphasic disseminated encephalomyelitis and multiple sclerosis in children. *Brain.* 2000;123:2407-2422.

49. Hynson JL, Kornberg AJ, Coleman LT, Shield L, Harvey AS, Kean MJ. Clinical and neuroradiologic features of acute disseminated encephalomyelitis in children. *Neurology.* 2001;56:1308-1312.

50. Pohl D, Rostasy K, Treiber-Held S, Brockmann K, Gartner J, Hanefeld F. Pediatric multiple sclerosis: detection of clinically silent lesions by multimodal evoked potentials. *J Pediatr.* 2006;149:125-127.

51. Poser CM, Paty DW, Scheinberg L, et al. New diagnostic criteria for multiple sclerosis: guidelines for research protocols. *Ann Neurol.* 1983;13:227-231.

52. McDonald WI, Compston A, Edan G, et al. Recommended diagnostic criteria for multiple sclerosis: guidelines from the International Panel on the Diagnosis of Multiple Sclerosis. *Ann Neurol.* 2001;50:121-127.

53. Rose AS, Kuzma JW, Kurtzke JF. Cooperative study in the evaluation of therapy in multiple sclerosis: ACTH vs. placebo—final report. *Neurology.* 1970;20:1-59.

54. DeAngelis T, Lublin F. Multiple sclerosis: new treatment trials and emerging therapeutic targets. *Curr Opin Neurol.* 2008;21:261-271.

55. Beck RW. Corticosteroid treatment of optic neuritis—a need to change treatment practices. *Neurology.* 1992;42:1133-1135.

56. Barnes D, Hughes RAC. Oral versus intravenous corticosteroids in acute relapses of multiple sclerosis—reply. *Lancet.* 1997;349:1697.

57. Barnes D, Hughes RAC, Morris RW, et al. Randomised trial of oral and intravenous methylprednisolone in acute relapses of multiple sclerosis. *Lancet.* 1997;349:902-906.

58. Zivadinov R, Rudick RA, De Masi R, et al. Effects of IV methylprednisolone on brain atrophy in relapsing-remitting MS. *Neurology.* 2001;57:1239-1247.

59. Frohman EM, Shah A, Eggenberger E, Metz L, Zivadinov R, Stuve O. Corticosteroids for multiple sclerosis: I. Application for treating exacerbations. *Neurotherapeutics.* 2007;4:618-626.

60. Weinshenker BG, O'Brien PC, Petterson TM, et al. A randomized trial of plasma exchange in acute central nervous system inflammatory demyelinating disease. *Ann Neurol.* 1999;46:878-886.

61. Pohl D, Waubant E, Banwell B, et al. Treatment of pediatric multiple sclerosis and variants. *Neurology.* 2007;68 (suppl 2):S54-S65.

62. Group TIMSS. Interferon beta-1b is effective in relapsing-remitting multiple sclerosis. I. Clinical results of a multicenter, randomized, double-blind, placebo-controlled trial. *Neurology.* 1993;43:655-661.

63. Paty DW, Li DKB, Group UMMS, Group IMSS. Interferon beta-1b is effective in relapsing-remitting multiple sclerosis. II. MRI analysis results of a multicenter, randomized, double-blind, placebo-controlled trial. *Neurology.* 1993;43:662-667.

64. Kappos L, Weinshenker B, Pozzilli C, et al. Interferon beta-1b in secondary progressive MS: a combined analysis of the two trials. *Neurology.* 2004;63:1779-1787.

65. Panitch H, Miller A, Paty D, Weinshenker B. Interferon beta-1b in secondary progressive MS: results from a 3-year controlled study. *Neurology.* 2004;63:1788-1795.

66. Placebo-controlled multicentre randomised trial of interferon beta-1b in treatment of secondary progressive multiple sclerosis. European Study Group on interferon beta-1b in secondary progressive MS. *Lancet.* 1998;352: 1491-1497.

67. Comi G, Filippi M, Barkhof F, et al. Effect of early interferon treatment on conversion to definite multiple sclerosis: a randomised study. *Lancet*. 2001;357:1576-1582.

68. Jacobs LD, Cookfair DL, Rudick RA, et al. Intramuscular interferon beta-1a for disease progression in relapsing multiple sclerosis. *Ann Neurol*. 1996;39:285-294.

69. Cohen JA, Cutter GR, Fischer JS, et al. Benefit of interferon beta-1a on MSFC progression in secondary progressive MS. *Neurology*. 2002;59:679-687.

70. Rudick RA, Fisher E, Lee JC, Simon J, Jacobs L. Use of the brain parenchymal fraction to measure whole brain atrophy in relapsing-remitting MS. Multiple Sclerosis Collaborative Research Group. *Neurology*. 1999;53:1698-1704.

71. Jacobs LD, Beck RW, Simon JH, et al. Intramuscular interferon beta-1a therapy initiated during a first demyelinating event in multiple sclerosis. CHAMPS Study Group. *N Engl J Med*. 2000;343:898-904.

72. Group PPoRaDbIb-aSiMSS. Randomised double-blind placebo-controlled study of interferon β-1a in relapsing/remitting multiple sclerosis. *Lancet*. 1998;352:1498-1504.

73. Li DK, Zhao GJ, Paty DW. Randomized controlled trial of interferon-beta-1a in secondary progressive MS: MRI results. *Neurology*. 2001;56:1505-1513.

74. Johnson KP, Brooks BR, Cohen JA, et al. Copolymer 1 reduces relapse rate and improves disability in relapsing-remitting multiple sclerosis: results of a phase III multicenter, double-blind, placebo-controlled trial. *Neurology*. 1995;45:1268-1276.

75. Comi G, Filippi M, Wolinsky JS. European/Canadian multicenter, double-blind, randomized, placebo-controlled study of the effects of glatiramer acetate on magnetic resonance imaging—measured disease activity and burden in patients with relapsing multiple sclerosis. European/Canadian Glatiramer Acetate Study Group. *Ann Neurol*. 2001;49:290-297.

76. Rudick RA, Stuart WH, Calabresi PA, et al. Natalizumab plus interferon beta-1a for relapsing multiple sclerosis. *N Engl J Med*. 2006;354:911-923.

77. Polman CH, O'Connor PW, Havrdova E, et al. A randomized, placebo-controlled trial of natalizumab for relapsing multiple sclerosis. *N Engl J Med*. 2006;354:899-910.

78. Kappos L, Bates D, Hartung HP, et al. Natalizumab treatment for multiple sclerosis: recommendations for patient selection and monitoring. *Lancet Neurol*. 2007;6:431-441.

79. Mullen JT, Vartanian TK, Atkins MB. Melanoma complicating treatment with natalizumab for multiple sclerosis. *N Engl J Med*. 2008;358:647-648.

80. Krupp LB, Macallister WS. Treatment of pediatric multiple sclerosis. *Curr Treat Options Neurol*. 2005;7:191-199.

81. Tenembaum S, Chitnis T, Ness J, Hahn JS. Acute disseminated encephalomyelitis. *Neurology*. 2007;68(suppl 2):S23-S36.

82. Murthy SN, Faden HS, Cohen ME, Bakshi R. Acute disseminated encephalomyelitis in children. *Pediatrics*. 2002;110:e21.

83. Tenembaum S, Chamoles N, Fejerman N. Acute disseminated encephalomyelitis: a long-term follow-up study of 84 pediatric patients. *Neurology*. 2002;59:1224-1231.

84. Leake JA, Albani S, Kao AS, et al. Acute disseminated encephalomyelitis in childhood: epidemiologic, clinical and laboratory features. *Pediatr Infect Dis J*. 2004;23:756-764.

85. Richer LP, Sinclair DB, Bhargava R. Neuroimaging features of acute disseminated encephalomyelitis in childhood. *Pediatr Neurol*. 2005;32:30-36.

86. Devic M. Myelite aigue dorso-lumbaire avec nevrite optique: autopsie. *Congres francais du Medicine*. 1894;1: 434-490.

87. Devic M. Myelite subaigue compliquee de nevrite optique. *Bull Med (Paris)*.1895;8:1033-1034.

88. Wingerchuk DM, Hogancamp WF, O'Brien PC, Weinshenker BG. The clinical course of neuromyelitis optica (Devic's syndrome). *Neurology*. 1999;53:1107-1114.

89. Jeffery AR, Buncic JR. Pediatric Devic's neuromyelitis optica. *J Pediatr Ophthalmol Strabismus*. 1996;33:223-229.

90. McKeon A, Lennon VA, Lotze T, et al. CNS aquaporin-4 autoimmunity in children. *Neurology*. 2008;71:93-100.

91. Mandler RN, Davis LE, Jeffery DR, Kornfeld M. Devic's neuromyelitis optica: a clinicopathological study of 8 patients. *Ann Neurol*. 1993;34:162-168.

92. O'Riordan JI, Gallagher HL, Thompson AJ, et al. Clinical, CSF, and MRI findings in Devic's neuromyelitis optica. *J Neurol Neurosurg Psychiatry*. 1996;60:382-387.

93. Fazekas F, Offenbacher H, Schmidt R, Strasser-Fuchs S. MRI of neuromyelitis optica: evidence for a distinct entity. *J Neurol Neurosurg Psychiatry*. 1994;57:1140-1142.

94. Filippi M, Rocca MA, Moiola L, et al. MRI and magnetization transfer imaging changes in the brain and cervical cord of patients with Devic's neuromyelitis optica. *Neurology*. 1999;53:1705-1710.

95. Wingerchuk DM, Lennon VA, Pittock SJ, Lucchinetti CF, Weinshenker BG. Revised diagnostic criteria for neuromyelitis optica. *Neurology*. 2006;66:1485-1489.

96. Lennon VA, Wingerchuk DM, Kryzer TJ, et al. A serum autoantibody marker of neuromyelitis optica: distinction from multiple sclerosis. *Lancet*. 2004;364: 2106-2112.

97. Weinshenker BG, Wingerchuk DM, Vukusic S, et al. Neuromyelitis optica IgG predicts relapse after longitudinally extensive transverse myelitis. *Ann Neurol*. 2006; 59:566–569.

98. Matiello M, Lennon VA, Jacob A, et al. NMO-IgG predicts the outcome of recurrent optic neuritis. *Neurology*. 2008;70:2197-2200.

99. Banwell B, Tenembaum S, Lennon VA, et al. Neuromyelitis optica-IgG in childhood inflammatory demyelinating CNS disorders. *Neurology*. 2008;70:344-352.

100. Cree BA, Lamb S, Morgan K, Chen A, Waubant E, Genain C. An open label study of the effects of rituximab in neuromyelitis optica. *Neurology*. 2005;64:1270-1272.

101. Jacob A, Weinshenker BG, Violich I, et al. Treatment of neuromyelitis optica with rituximab: retrospective analysis of 25 patients. *Arch Neurol*. 2008;65(11):1443-8.

CHAPTER 18

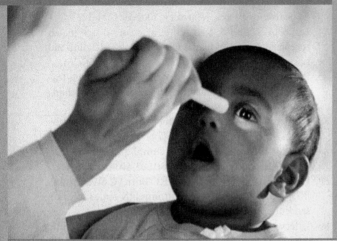

Stroke

Paul R. Carney, James D. Geyer, Matthew A. Saxonhouse, and Camilo R. Gomez

DEFINITIONS AND EPIDEMIOLOGY

Stroke in the pediatric population is being identified more frequently, and its effects, once thought to be limited, are now being recognized as more serious. Estimates of incidence range between 2 and 8 per 100,000, with neonates being disproportionately affected. A recent population-based study found that perinatal arterial ischemic stroke (PAS) was recognized in 1 in 2300 term infants.[1] The rise in diagnosis of stroke is in part attributable to improved diagnostic techniques and to greater survival of susceptible children.[2,3] Definitions and epidemiology of specific types of stroke in children are detailed below in the discussion of differential diagnosis.

In the past, it was felt that children generally recover from stroke with minimal long-term deficit (due to plasticity of the young brain). Recent studies reveal, however, that only 31% of children with ischemic stroke recovered to a normal neurological examination. Approximately 17% had persistent cognitive deficits. Disability can include physical, cognitive, behavioral, and psychiatric sequelae. Despite significant advances in management, stroke continues to be one of the leading causes of death among children.

The relative lack of controlled clinical trials significantly limits the current treatment guidelines, and the evidence-based interventions established for adults cannot be directly extrapolated to pediatric patients. Differences in the hemodynamic and coagulation pathways as well as in the significant risk factors that contribute to cerebrovascular events distinguish the two. For instance, atherosclerosis is one of the most common sources of adult stroke but rarely contributes to stroke risk in the pediatric population.[3]

PATHOGENESIS

Ischemic strokes occur secondary to insufficient cerebral oxygen delivery. This may occur because of occlusion of a vessel secondary to plaque formation (more common in adults), fibromyscular dysplasia, or vascular dissection. Cardioembolic sources of stroke are more common in children. Hematologic sources of stroke include hyperviscosity syndromes, sickle cell disease, and leukemia. Each of these disorders is discussed in much greater detail in the following sections.

Intracranial hemorrhage also occurs in several distinct subtypes. Subarachnoid hemorrhage may arise secondary to aneurysm rupture or trauma. Subdural and epidural hematomas often occur secondary to traumatic injury. Parenchymal hemorrhages may be related to a number of etiologies including trauma, abuse, collagen vascular diseases, and ischemic stroke.

CLINICAL PRESENTATION

In order to know appropriately manage stroke patients (see "Management" later in the chapter), the acutely presenting pediatric stroke patient must be recognized in a timely fashion. Unfortunately, the average delay between symptom onset and first diagnostic study is 28.5 hours, largely prohibiting the institution of hyperacute interventions.[4] This delay stems from the often nonspecific symptoms with which pediatric stroke patients present. Neonates with underlying stroke frequently present with seizures as well as lethargy and apnea, whereas older children may present with more focal neurological deficits such as speech abnormalities, visual or sensory changes, or hemiparesis.[5]

DIFFERENTIAL DIAGNOSIS

The differential diagnosis can be vast, including infections and metabolic imbalances. A few key stroke masqueraders should also be considered. Familial hemiplegic migraine is characterized by family history and EEG pattern of unilateral slow background rhythm.[5] Postictal or "Todd" paralysis is a consideration when focal weakness occurs after a seizure, and can closely mimic stroke. Patients should be treated with the urgency of an acute cerebral infarction until proven otherwise.

Physicians must be aware of predisposing conditions and risk factors to have the index of suspicion required to diagnose stroke. This involves awareness of three main categories of cerebrovascular events: arterial ischemic, hemorrhagic, and sinovenous thrombosis. Risk factors overlap for stroke subtypes, but treatment may differ.

Perinatal Stroke

Definitions and epidemiology

A number of ischemic and hemorrhagic insults may affect the developing fetal or neonatal brain. It is therefore important for the clinician to be aware of the different types of events that can cause perinatal stroke, as the evaluation, management, and expected outcome may be related to the type of lesion. Perinatal arterial ischemic stroke refers to a cerebrovascular event occurring during fetal or neonatal life, before 28 days after birth, with pathologic or radiologic evidence of focal arterial infarction of brain.[6] Sinovenous thrombosis describes thrombosis in one or more of the cerebral venous sinuses and may be associated with secondary hemorrhage.[7] Primary hemorrhagic stroke and other types of intracranial hemorrhages that tend to affect near-term and term infants tend to be associated with specific risk factors responsible for the hemorrhage. Periventricular hermorrhagic infarction, a lesion that mainly affects preterm infants, is a serious complication of germinal matrix-intraventricular hemorrhage.

Clinical presentation

Although these lesions tend to have significant overlap in terms of being hemorrhagic or ischemic, the effects of these types of events on the neonate may result in immediate or eventual death, with other long-term complications including cerebral palsy, epilepsy, blindness, behavioral disburbances, and congnitive dysfunction. Despite the type of lesion, symptoms may be subtle and are often nonspecific. The acute and chronic manifestations of perinatal stroke are reviewed in Table 18-1.

Table 18-1.

Acute and Chronic Manifestations of Perinatal Stroke

Signs of Acute Stroke

Anemia

Apnea

Encephalopathy

Focal neurological symptoms are typically difficult to identify

Murmurs, bruits, tachypnea, and absent distal pulses may suggest cardiac anomalies

Placental thrombosis may suggest infectious or embolic disease

Poor feeding

Seizures

Skin lesions may suggest infections or embolic disease

Thrombocytopenia

Signs of Chronic Infarction

Behavioral problems

Cerebral palsy

Cognitive dysfunction

Cognitive impairments

Delayed milestones

Early hand preference may be indicative of hemiparesis

Epilepsy

Head circumference

Hemiparesis

Language dysfunction

Perinatal Arterial Ischemic Stroke

Definitions and epidemiology

Perinatal arterial ischemic stroke, occurring more frequently in the near-term and term infant, has a prevalence ranging from 17 to 93 per 100,000 live births.[7-10] Most lesions occur in the left hemisphere within the distribution of the middle cerebral artery. Rarely, multifocal lesions occur but tend to be embolic in origin.[7]

Pathogenesis

A wide range of risk factors have been implicated in the etiology of perinatal arterial ischemic stroke, and these are listed in Table 18-2.[7,9,11-13] However, some studies report no finding of an obvious precipitating event in as many as 25% to 77% of cases.[14-16] The difficulty with identifying a specific risk factor for the development of the lesion is that neonates often have multiple risk factors present, making it likely that a combination of environmental risk factors interacting with genetic vulnerabilities is often responsible for the ischemic event.[6] The exact role of genetic thrombophilias in the pathogenesis of perinatal arterial ischemic stroke is yet to be defined,[17] but disorders such as factor V

Table 18-2.

Risk Factors Associated with Perinatal Arterial Ischemic Stroke

African American race
Anemia
Bacterial meningitis
Birth asphyxia
Birth trauma
Cesarean delivery
Chorioamnionitis
Congenital heart disease
Hereditary endotheliopathy with retinopathy nephropathy and stroke (HERNS)
History of infertility
Inherited or acquired prothrombotic disorders
  Factor V Leiden mutation, prothrombin 20210 promoter mutation, hyperhomocystinemia, elevated lipoprotein a, antiphospholipid antibody syndrome, protein C deficiency, protein S deficiency, antithrombin III deficiency, methylene-tetrahydrofolate reductase deficiency
Male sex
Maternal diabetes
Oligohydramnios
Polycythemia (hyperviscosity)
Preeclampsia
Primiparity
Prolonged rupture of membranes

Table 18-3.

Causes of Perinatal Intracranial Hemorrhage

Alloimmune thrombocytopenia
Arteriovenous malformation
Birth asphyxia
Cerebral tumor
Coagulation factor deficiencies
  Factor V deficiency
  Factor X deficiency
  Congential fibrinogen deficiency
  Hemophilia (factors VIII and IX)
Coarctation of the aorta
Congenital arterial aneurysm
Extracorporeal membrane oxygenation
Hyperhomocystinemia
Hypoprothrombinemia
Maternal factors
  Idiopathic thrombocytopenic purpura
  Warfarin use
  Substance abuse
  Von Willibrand disease
Vitamin K deficiency

stroke are reviewed in Table 18-1. Figure 18-1 reveals a multifocal infarction on diffusion-weighted MRI involving the pons and temporal lobe.

Leiden mutation, the prothrombin 20210 promoter mutation, hyperhomocystinemia, elevated lipoprotein (a) levels, antiphospholipid antibodies, and relative protein C deficiency have been described with increased frequency in infants who have perinatal arterial ischemic stroke when compared with healthy control subjects.[18-24] Other genetic thrombophilias have also been implicated and are provided in Table 18-3. Further studies are required to better define the potential role of infantile thrombophilia in the pathogenesis and outcome of perinatal arterial ischemic stroke, but experts in the field do recommend a comprehensive thrombophilia assessment for all infants presenting with perinatal arterial ischemic stroke, regardless of other risk factors present.[17,25]

Clinical presentation

The difficulty with identifying perinatal arterial ischemic stroke in the neonate is that symptoms tend to be nonspecific and often are difficult to identify. In many cases, the symptoms may not become evident until quite some time after the stroke. The acute and chronic manifestations of perinatal arterial ischemic

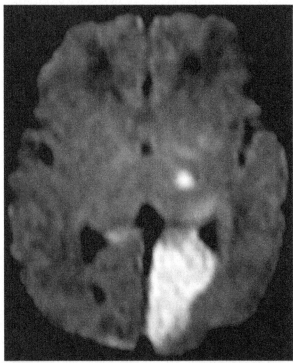

FIGURE 18-1 ■ Axial diffusion-weighted images (b = 1000) demonstrate multiple areas of high signal in the left occipital lobe and left thalamus.

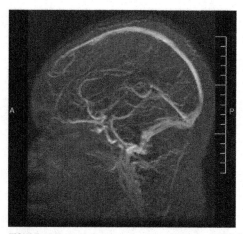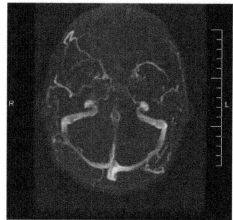

FIGURE 18-2 ■ Magnetic resonance venogram (MRV) in a normal individual.

Sinovenous Thrombosis

Clinical presentation

Most cases of sinovenous thrombosis occur in term infants and present with nonspecific clinical features as listed in Table 18-1. The superficial and lateral sinuses are most frequently involved, and venous infarction has been reported in up to 30% of cases.[26] An example of magnetic resonance venography (MRV) in a normal patient is shown in Figure 18-2.

Pathogenesis

Risk factors for the development of sinovenous thrombosis are similar to those for perinatal arterial ischemic stroke and are listed in Table 18-3, although a significant number of cases are reported as idiopathic.[16]

Hemorrhage

Definitions and epidemiology

Primary hemorrhagic stroke and other types of intracranial hemorrhage include subdural, primary subarachnoid, intracerebellar, intraventricular hemorrhage, and other miscellaneous types such as focal hemorrhages into the thalamus, basal ganglia, brainstem, or spinal cord.[4]

Periventricular hemorrhage (PVHI) is a venous hemorrhagic infarct in the drainage area of the periventricular terminal vein.[27,28] A complication mainly associated with prematurity, a recent study found that 1% of infants less than 2500 g met the diagnostic criteria for PVHI, with the highest percentage (9.9%) being those less than 750 g.[28]

Pathogenesis

The majority of these types of hemorrhages tend to be antepartum or during the stresses of delivery and associated with specific risk factors as outlined in Table 18-3. Intrapartum risk factors associated with the development of PVHI include emergent cesarean section, low Apgar scores, and need for respiratory resuscitation;

while postnatal factors include pneumothorax, pulmonary hemorrhage, patent ductus arteriosus, acidosis, hypotension requiring pressure support, and significant hypercarbia.[28] Although an exact cause/effect relationship of these risk factors and correct knowledge of when these events occur has been difficult to prove, it is felt that disturbances in systemic and cerebral hemodynamics occurring around the intrapartum and early neonatal period are important in the development of PVHI.[28]

Clinical presentation

Figure 18-3 shows a hemorrhage in the thalamic region on CT. In general, primary subarachnoid hemorrhages are more frequently seen in the premature infant but tend to be clinically benign; in contrast to intracerebellar

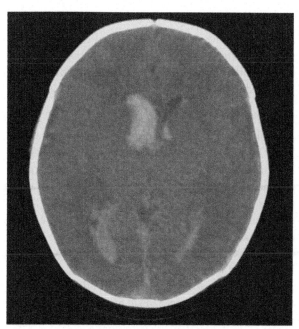

FIGURE 18-3 ■ CT head with a right thalamic hemorrhage. There is also some apparent hypodensity in the right hemisphere.

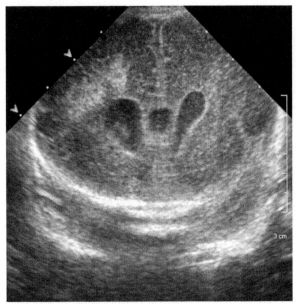

FIGURE 18-4 ■ Ultrasonography with PVHI.

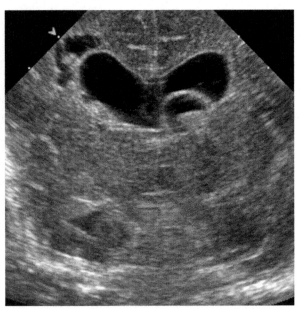

FIGURE 18-5 ■ Ultrasonography with PVHI.

hemorrhages which, although also more frequently observed in premature infants, tend to be serious.[27] Subdural and other miscellaneous types of hemorrhages tend to affect full-term infants, and their outcome is variable. Although intraventricular hemorrhages tend to predominately occur in premature infants (discussed later), they have been reported to occur in term infants as well.

PVHI usually accompanies a large germinal matrix-intraventricular hemorrhage.[28] See Figures 18-4 and 18-5 for examples of PVHI.

Arterial Ischemic Stroke

Definitions and epidemiology

Arterial ischemic stroke can be related to a number of vascular, hematologic, cardiac, and metabolic risk factors. Potential causes of ischemic stroke in children are presented in Table 18-4.

Pathogenesis

Arterial dissection most commonly occurs after trauma. These injuries occur more frequently in boys than girls. Traumatic dissection can result from head or cervical trauma, including whiplash, shaken baby, or intraoral trauma such as falling with a pencil in the mouth.[2] Rarely, dissection occurs atraumatically due to a connective tissue disease such as fibromuscular dysplasia. See Table 18-5.

The C1-2 vertebral level is the most common location for a vertebral artery dissection. Artery to artery embolism from the site of endothelial injury is the usual pathogenic mechanism for infarction.[29] In one meta-analysis, 15% of posterior circulation and 5% of anterior circulation dissections were followed by recurrent ischemic events.[30]

Diagnosis

Diagnosis is made via characteristic findings on MRI and MRA of the head and neck, extracranial vascular ultrasound, or cerebral angiography. Because C1-2 is the most common location for a vertebral artery dissection, findings of a double lumen, intimal flap, or bright crescent on T1 fat suppression images confirm the diagnosis. Also, the finding of occlusion or segmental narrowing of an artery within 6 weeks of a known trauma, or of vertebral artery occlusion at the C2 vertebral level even without trauma, should raise the possibility of dissection.[31]

Cardiac Causes of Stroke

Definitions and epidemiology

Cardiac risk factors rise in importance in pediatric stroke relative to the adult population. Congenital heart disease is one of the major risk factors for stroke in pediatric patients. The Canadian Pediatric Ischemic Stroke Registry reported that 19% of children with arterial ischemic stroke had heart disease.[2] The risk is particularly high during surgical procedures.[32] Right-to-left shunting can lead to hypoxia and polycythemia, creating a hyperviscous state. Infective endocarditis additionally poses risk for embolic stroke, and patent foramen ovale is a risk for thromboembolic strokes due to venous-arterial communication. PFO (patent foramen ovale) is three times more prevalent in pediatric stroke patients than in the general population.[2]

Vasculitis

Definitions and epidemiology

Vasculitis is another source of stroke risk in the pediatric population. Primary vasculitides include those affecting

Table 18-4.

Causes of Ischemic Stroke in Children and Young Adults

Cardiac embolism, patent foramen ovale
Connective tissue disease (Ehlers-Danlos syndrome, Menkes
   syndrome, homocystinuria)
Fabry disease (alpha-galactosidase A deficiency)
Fibromuscular dysplasia
Hypercoaguable state (primary)
   ATIII deficiency
   Protein C deficiency
   Protein S deficiency
   Dysfibrinogenemia
   Factor XII deficiency
   Antiphospholipid antibodies
   Fibrinolytic abnormalities
   Activated protein C resistance, factor V Leiden mutation
    (gene on 1q23)
   Hyperhomocysteinemia (gene on 1q36)
   CADASIL (gene on 19p13)
   Recurrent subcortical infarcts with spared U fibers
   MTHFR polymorphism
Hypercoaguable state (secondary)
   Malignancy
   Pregnancy
   Oral contraceptives
   Disseminated intravascular coagulation
   Nephrotic syndrome
   Dehydration
Hyperlipidemia
Migraine (diagnosis of exclusion)
Mitochondrial myopathy (MELAS)
Moyamoya disease (large-vessel occlusions)
Organic acidemia
Platelet abnormalities
   Myeloproliferative disease
   Diabetes mellitus
   Heparin-induced thrombocytopenia
Rheology
   Homocystinuria (cystathione synthase deficiency)
   Polycythemia vera
   Sickle cell disease
   Thrombotic thrombocytopenia purpura
Vascular dissection (trauma, strangulation, arthritis)
Vasculitis
   Infectious
   Necrotizing
    PAN, Wegener syndrome, Churg-Strauss syndrome,
     lymphomatosis
   Collagen vascular disease
    SLE, RA, Sjögren disease, scleroderma
   Systemic disease
    Behçet disease, sarcoid, ulcerative colitis
   Giant-cell arteritis
    Takayasu syndrome, temporal
   Hypersensitivity (drug, chemical)
   Neoplastic
   Primary CNS vasculitis
Vasospasm (cocaine)

Table 18-5.

Causes of Arterial Dissection

Traumatic
Cervical trauma, including whiplash, shaken baby
Head trauma
Intraoral trauma such as falling with a pencil (or popsicle) in
   the mouth
Trauma related to tonsillectomy

Nontraumatic
Ehlers-Danlos syndrome
Fibromuscular dysplasia
Klippel-Feil syndrome
Marfan disease

large and medium vessel such as Takayasu arteritis, and those affecting small vessels such as primary CNS angiitis and Wegener. Unique to children is the importance of secondary, postinfectious vasculitis. Varicella zoster infection was detected in the preceding 12 months in 31% of children in one study of acute ischemic stroke as opposed to 9% of healthy controls.[33]

Clinical presentation

Strokes caused by postinfectious vasculitis typically involved the basal ganglia with typical vascular abnormalities of focal stenosis of the distal internal carotid and proximal segments of anterior cerebral (A1), middle cerebral (M1), and posterior cerebral artery (P1).[31,33] Other pathogens including HIV and CMV may produce similar vasculitis and stroke risk. Radiation to the brain can also be a risk factor for secondary vasculitis.[2]

Moyamoya

Moyamoya is a vascular condition with risk of recurrent stroke. Primary moyamoya disease is an autosomal dominant disease most common in Japanese patients, hence the Japanese name meaning "puff of smoke." This describes the angiographic blush that occurs due to extensive collateralization in response to occlusion of large intracranial arteries, often with bilateral carotid artery occlusion. Moyamoya syndrome can also occur secondary to sickle cell disease, Down syndrome, cranial radiation, or neurofibromatosis.[2,5,31]

Sickle Cell Disease

Definitions and epidemiology

Sickle cell disease (SCD) is one of the most prevalent hematologic risk factors for pediatric stroke. An astounding (9%) of patients with SCD will have an acute ischemic stroke by the age of 14, and approximately 20% will have

MRI evidence of silent ischemic insults.[31] Risk is greatest in the younger years (ages 2-8), and two-thirds will have a recurrent event if untreated.[34,35]

Pathogenesis

The sickled erythrocytes can cause thrombosis in large blood vessels or occlusion of small blood vessels leading to hypoperfusion in watershed areas.[2]

Other Hematologic Conditions

Further hematologic variables relevant to ischemic stroke include high concentrations of lipoprotein (a), protein C deficiency, and factor V Leiden mutation.[36] These hypercoaguable states are most highly associated with risk of recurrent stroke.[35,36] Other prothrombotic states include positivity for antiphospholipid antibodies including anticardiolipin antibodies and lupus anticoagulant, protein S deficiency, factor V Leiden mutation, prothrombin gene mutation (G20210A), and antithrombin III deficiency.[2] Extensive discussion of each of these is beyond the scope of this chapter. Hyperviscosity or "sludging effect" can also be caused by dehydration, thrombocytosis, and polycythemia. Malignancies including leukemia and lymphoma can also create hypercoaguable states with increased risk of stroke. Several chemotherapeutic agents have also been implicated in cerebral infarction, including adriamycin, asparaginase, and methotrexate. Severe anemia, often seen in developing countries, can result in cerebral infarction secondary to the poor oxygen-carrying capacity.

Other etiologies to consider are toxic or iatrogenic sources such as cocaine or oral contraceptive pills. Metabolic sources of stroke risk include homocysteinuria, ornithine transcarbamylase deficiency, and MELAS (mitochondrial encephalopathy with lactic acidosis and stroke-like episodes). CADASIL and hyperhomocyteinemia can lead to endothelial damage and platelet aggregation and are treated with folate and vitamin B.[2] MELAS is a heritable mitochondrial disease that presents in childhood with proximal muscle weakness, episodic vomiting and lactic acidosis, migraine headaches, and stroke-like episodes. The areas of infarction can be inconsistent with any single vascular distribution. Diagnosis is made by muscle biopsy finding ragged red fibers, and the disease is usually progressive. Hearing and visual loss may occur as well.[2] Neurocutaneous diseases of childhood such as (Sturge-Weber and NF1) can be associated with increased risk of stroke.

Hemorrhagic Stroke

Hemorrhagic stroke in children, in contrast to adults, occurs with equal frequency to ischemic stroke.[2] Trauma and bleeding diathesis are important risk factors for hemorrhagic stroke. Risk factors for hemorrhagic stroke are outlined in Table 18-6. Vascular malformations such

Table 18-6.
Risk Factors for Hemorrhagic Stroke
Alagille syndrome
Aneurysm
Antiplatelet agents
Aphetamines
Autoimmune disorders
Cocaine
Ephedra
Hypertension
Infection
Leukemia
Sickle cell disease
Surgery
Telangiectasias
Thrombocytopenia
Trauma
Vascular malformations (see Figure 18-6)
Vasculitis
Warfarin

as aneurysm or AVM may result in an intracerebral hemorrhage (see Figure 18.6).

Aneurysm in Subarachnoid Hemorrhage

Definitions and epidemiology

Intracranial aneurysms are common in the general population. The prevalence of unruptured intracranial

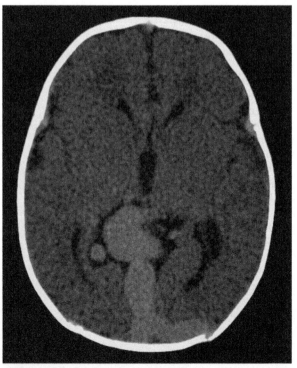

FIGURE 18-6 ■ Axial MRI with a large AVM.

aneurysms has been largely determined through autopsy studies and through angiographic series. In adults, the prevalence ranges from 0.2% to 9%, with a mean of approximately 2%. The prevalence is thought to be lower in children.

The incidence of aneurysm rupture or subarachnoid hemorrhage (number of aneurysm ruptures/ 100,000 population/year) varies depending upon factors such as the population being studied (Finnish and Japanese persons have a greater disposition) or the age distribution of the population (a younger population will have a lower incidence). The incidence of aneurysmal subarachnoid hemorrhage ranges from approximately 7 to 21 per 100,000 persons per year, with an average of 10 per 100,000 persons per year. In the United States alone, there are approximately 28,000 new patients with subarachnoid hemorrhage each year. The incidence of subarachnoid hemorrhage has remained stable over the last three decades.

Aneurysms are relatively uncommon in children and become more common with increasing age, with a peak incidence occurring between the ages of 50 and 60. There is a clear female gender predilection (approximately 1.6 times higher incidence in females). Smoking and hypertension may predispose to aneurysm formation and/or rupture.

Although most cases of subarachnoid hemorrhage are sporadic, in those families with a history of subarachnoid hemorrhage in more than one family member, the prevalence of unruptured aneurysms in other family members is markedly increased (a fourfold to tenfold increased prevalence). Autosomal polycystic kidney disease is unequivocally associated with a higher prevalence of intracranial aneurysms. Other conditions that may predispose to intracranial aneurysm formation include connective tissue disorders such as Ehlers-Danlos syndrome type IV, $\tilde{\alpha}_1$-antitrypsin deficiency, Marfan syndrome, neurofibromatosis I, and pseudoxanthoma elasticum, although the association is less well determined in some of these conditions.

Clinical presentation

ICH is suggested by the rapid onset of neurological dysfunction and signs of increased intracranial pressure (ICP), such as headache, vomiting, and decreased level of consciousness.

The symptoms of ICH are related primarily to the anatomic location and pressure resulting from the expanding hematoma. Findings such as hypertension, tachycardia, or bradycardia (Cushing response), and abnormal respiratory patterns, are common effects of elevated ICP and brainstem compression.

Diagnosis

Confirmation of ICH cannot rely solely on the clinical exam and requires the use of emergent CT scan or MRI.

Widespread use of non-enhancing CT scan of the brain has dramatically changed the diagnostic approach of this disease, becoming the method of choice to evaluate the presence of ICH. CT scan evaluates the size and location of the hematoma, extension into the ventricular system, degree of surrounding edema, and anatomic disruption. Contrast-enhanced CT scan is not done routinely in most centers, but may prove helpful in predicting hematoma expansion and outcome. MRI techniques such as gradient-echo (GRE, T2*) are highly sensitive for the diagnosis of ICH but may be more difficult to obtain in the pediatric patient (often requiring sedation). Sensitivity of MRI for ICH is 100%. MRI and CT are equivalent for the detection of acute ICH, but MRI is significantly more accurate than CT for the detection of chronic ICH.

Further discussion of unruptured aneurysms and subarachnoid hemorrhage is undertaken in the chapters on these disorders.

DIAGNOSIS

The child presenting with acute stroke will require careful history and physical examination including perinatal history and developmental milestones. As mentioned above, diagnosis of acute stroke in childhood can be challenging. The physician must have a high index of suspicion. Stroke should not be considered an "adult disease" but a neurological disorder with different manifestations in different age groups. Table 18-7 highlights many of the physical findings associated with stroke in the pediatric age group.

Table 18-7.

Signs of Acute Stroke

Common Signs and Symptoms[a]
Aphasia
Dysarthria
Gait disturbance/ataxia
Hemianopsia/vision loss
Hemiparesis
Unilateral numbness

Rare Signs and Symptoms[a]
Aprosodia (emotional loss)
Cognitive dysfunction
Seizure

Other Notes
Focal neurological symptoms are typically difficult to identify
Murmurs may suggest cardiac anomalies
Respiratory failure
Seizures
Skin lesions may suggest infections or embolic disease

[a] The gradation of symptoms, from benign to life-threatening, is not as important in this context, since relatively mild or seemingly benign symptoms may be related to potentially life-threatening stroke.

MANAGEMENT

Two sets of guidelines have recently been proposed that may help guide neurologists and generalists treating pediatric stroke. In the United States, the ACCP guidelines (American College of Clinical Pharmacy) published in *Chest* addressed both neonatal and childhood arterial ischemic stroke and cerebral sinus venous thrombosis.[37] The Scottish Intercollegiate Guidelines from the UK (UK Royal College of Physicians pediatric working group) addressed pediatric patients 1 month to 18 years of age.[38] Both sets of guidelines contain review of the literature and input from pediatric hematologists. The UK guidelines add the involvement of pediatric neurologists. The two sets of guidelines have several areas of agreement, and also variation on several points.

Initial Stabilization

Clearly the most crucial initial interventions are those of stabilizing airway, breathing, and circulation. Adequate oxygenation and ventilation are crucial to reducing the metabolic demand of the ischemic brain. Oxygen should be applied via 100% mask and intubation performed for hypoxia, failure to protect airway, decompensated shock, status epilepticus, or GCS less than 8.[39] Core temperature should be kept between approximately 36°C and 37°C.[39] Normoglycemia should be maintained, and seizures should be treated aggressively. Cardiac monitoring with telemetry or Holter monitor should be applied, and initial laboratories sent to evaluate glucose, electrolytes, liver function tests, complete blood count (WBC, Hct, platelets), coagulation profile (PT/PTT/INR), erythrocyte sedimentation rate, ANA, and toxicology screen. This can help identify a metabolic acidosis, which can be seen in MELAS; a concurrent infection; or gross hematologic abnormalities. Generally, a chest radiograph and electrocardiogram are obtained due to the significance of cardiac disease to risk of pediatric stroke.

Because a key initial branch point in the approach to stroke is the distinction between a hemorrhagic and an ischemic event, CT of the head should be performed immediately. Although MRI with diffusion-weighted imaging is better equipped to detect the acute ischemic event, the study takes longer and often requires sedation of the child. CT, although insensitive to infarction in the first 2 days and inferior for evaluating the posterior fossa, is more readily available and quickly obtained. A negative CT scan acutely does not rule out ischemia, however, and requires follow-up imaging in 24 to 48 hours.

Imaging

When MRI is performed after the CT, diffusion imaging helps age the stroke. Perfusion and proton magnetic

Table 18-8.

Signs of Chronic Infarction

Behavioral problems
Cerebral palsy
Cognitive dysfunction
Cognitive impairments
Delayed milestones
Early hand preference may be indicative of hemiparesis
Epilepsy
Head circumference
Hemiparesis
Language dysfunction

resonance spectroscopy images are variations that can help determine the territory of ischemia in addition to infarction (Table 18-8). MR angiography is a noninvasive way to detect vascular occlusions or abnormalities, but may overestimate the degree of stenosis (Table 18-9). MRI and MRA should be obtained in arterial ischemic or hemorrhagic strokes. In the latter, arterial venous malformations or aneurysms may be detected and possibly amenable to treatment. When dissection is suspected, fat suppression MRI of the neck or MRA of the cervical arteries can make

Table 18-9.

Diagnostic Testing

MRI
MRA
MRV (if suspected venous infarction)
Cardiac ECHO
EKG
Laboratory testing
   Sickle cell prep
   CBC
   Comprehensive metabolic profile
Laboratory testing (hypercoagulopathy studies)
   ATIII
   Protein C
   Protein S
   Fibrinogen
   Factor XII
   Antiphospholipid antibodies
   Activated protein C resistance
   Factor V Leiden mutation
   Homocysteine level
   CADASIL
   MTHFR polymorphism
Follow-up head CT if sudden neurological change (risk of
   secondary hemorrhage)

the diagnosis. Carotid Doppler ultrasonography can quickly evaluate for dissection in suspected cases. Conventional angiography is the "gold standard," as therapeutic interventions may be possible with the procedure, but due to it being more time-consuming and invasive, it is usually reserved for those cases in which MRA is nondiagnostic. MR venography is useful for detecting cerebral sinus thromboses, especially in patients with unexplained lethargy, seizures, or infarction with headache.

Cardiac evaluation

An echocardiogram should be obtained to evaluate for congenital heart disease or for an embolic source arising from valvular abnormalities, dilated cardiomyopathy, or abnormalities involving the proximal great vessels. A bubble contrast study with agitated saline should be part of the evaluation to detect intracardiac shunting due to a PFO. A transthoracic echocardiogram is less invasive, but a transesophageal echocardiogram allows visualization of the aortic arch and ascending aorta.[2]

Laboratory Evaluation

If the initial tier of investigations fails to identify a cause for stroke, further evaluation is indicated for known hypercoagulable states (Table 18-4). These investigations should be made 3 to 6 months after the acute stroke.[5] Hemoglobin electrophoresis is used to detect sickle cell disease; and arterial pyruvate, CSF, and arterial lactate are used to evaluate for mitochondrial disease. Lipid profile and serum and urine homocysteine can help detect a predisposition to thrombosis. HIV testing should also be considered.[2]

Sickle Cell Disease Management

Sickle cell disease (SCD) is the only area of pediatric stroke for which clear evidence-based guidelines exist. In patients with sickle cell disease, both guidelines suggest exchange transfusion to HbS less than 30%, and intravenous hydration is indicated. Transcranial Doppler ultrasound is used to screen periodically for increased cerebral flow suggesting need for exchange. The STOP trial in 1998 was aborted early due to a clear demonstration of 92% relative risk reduction in stroke with exchange transfusion for cerebral blood flow velocities greater than 200 mL/sec on transcranial Doppler.[34,40] This has led to clear recommendations by the American Academy of Neurology for screening SCD patients with transcranial Doppler ultrasound.[41] The frequency of screening has not been established. Sicklers with frequent transfusions are at risk for iron overload, and alternative therapies including hydroxyurea can also be considered in the chronic maintenance of patients with sickle cell disease.

Anticoagulants

In general, the treatment guidelines suggested in *Chest* recommend unfractionated or low molecular weight heparin for 5 to 7 days regardless of etiology, and the UK guidelines suggest aspirin 5 mg/kg acutely. Neither guideline recommends the use of alteplase. Specific situations merit further interventions as follows:[33]

Perinatal arterial ischemic stroke

Management of perinatal arterial ischemic stroke is mainly supportive. Current guidelines from the American College of Chest Physicians suggest that neonates with proven cardioembolic stroke should receive treatment with unfractionated heparin or LMWH.[37] The guidelines do not recommend anticoagulant therapy for neonates with non-cardioembolic stroke. However, the guidelines do not mention if the number of blood vessels affected should be taken into consideration or if noncardiac-related embolism warrants anticoagulation. In addition, there is a lack of information on how to properly anticoagulate neonates who are found to have a genetic thrombophilia.

Sinovenous thrombosis

Management of neonates with sinovenous thrombosis is controversial and limited by the fact that there are no current clinical trials evaluating the use of anticoagulation. Current guidelines from the American College of Chest Physicians recommend the use of either low-molecular weight heparin or unfractionated heparin only for neonates with sinovenous thrombosis but without large ischemic infarctions or evidence of intracerebral hemorrhage due to the theoretical risk of bleeding. Radiologic monitoring and initiation of anticoagulation only if extension occurs is recommended for the remainder of cases.[38] Longer-term anticoagulation with warfarin for at least 3 to 6 months may be necessary for older patients with venous thrombosis. Follow-up imaging of the venous thrombosis is necessary prior to discontinuation of treatment.

Arterial dissection

Both guidelines recommend anticoagulation for 3 to 6 months after dissection. The *Chest* guidelines specify 5 to 7 days of unfractionated (UFH) or low molecular weight heparin (LMWH) followed by LMWH or warfarin for 3 to 6 months, while the UK guidelines generally suggest anticoagulation for up to 6 months or until vessel healing.

Vasculitis

Vasculitis is usually acutely treated with steroids, with consideration for long-term immunosuppression. The *Chest* guidelines suggest aspirin 2 to 5 mg/kg/day after initial UFH or LMWH for 5 to 7 days in patients with other vasculopathies. The UK guidelines recommend continued aspirin 1 to 3 mg/kg/day after 5 mg/kg on the first day.

Cardiogenic embolism

The guidelines both support anticoagulation for cardiogenic embolism, and the *Chest* guidelines recommend UFH or LMWH for 5 to 7 days followed by LMWH or warfarin for 3 to 6 months. The doses of UFH and LMWH for the treatment of stroke are not fully developed for adults, much less for children. In general, the usual weight-based nomograms are used in adults, and this would seem reasonable in the treatment of children as well. The most important consideration is to avoid bolus therapy. Bolusing these agents results in a transient but severely elevated PTT, which could in turn increase the risk of intracranial hemorrhage.

Hemorrhagic Stroke

Hemorrhagic stroke or intracerebral hemorrhage requires close observation, likely in the intensive care unit. Tight control of blood pressure is vital. The target blood pressure should be identified after consultation between the neurologist and the neurosurgeon. If significant mass effect is present, surgical evacuation or craniotomy for decompression may be indicated. Children should be emergently transported to a tertiary care center if necessary.

EEG monitoring

Continuous electroencephalographic (cEEG) monitoring has been shown to detect nonconvulsive seizures or status epilepticus in 28% of stuporous or comatose ICH patients, a finding consistent with studies of patients with other types of severe acute brain injury. Moreover, ictal activity detected by cEEG after ICH is associated with neurological deterioration and increased midline shift. It is our practice to perform surveillance cEEG monitoring for at least 48 hours in all comatose ICH patients.

Anticonvulsant therapy

The 30-day risk of clinically evident seizures after ICH is approximately 8%. Convulsive status epilepticus may be seen in 1% to 2% of patients, and the risk of long-term epilepsy ranges from 5% to 20%. Lobar location is an independent predictor of early seizures. Acute seizures should be treated with intravenous lorazepam (0.05-0.1 mg/kg) followed by an intravenous loading dose of fosphenytoin (20 mg/kg). Critically ill patients with ICH may benefit from prophylactic antiepileptic therapy, but no randomized trial has addressed the efficacy of this approach. Some centers prophylactically treat ICH patients with large supratentorial hemorrhages and depressed level of consciousness during the first week, based on evidence that

this practice reduces the frequency of seizures from 14% to 4% during the first 7 days after severe traumatic brain injury. The AHA guidelines recommend antiepileptic medication for up to 1 month, after which therapy should be discontinued in the absence of seizures. This recommendation is supported by the results of a recent study that showed that the risk of early seizures was reduced by prophylactic AED therapy. Further detail regarding the selection of appropriate antiepileptic medications is reviewed in Chapter 3.

Temperature management

Fever after ICH is common, particularly after IVH, and should be treated aggressively. Sustained fever after ICH has been shown to be independently associated with poor outcome, and even small temperature elevations have been shown to exacerbate neuronal injury and death in experimental models of ischemia. As a general standard, acetaminophen and cooling blankets should be given to all patients with sustained fever in excess of 38.3°C (101.0°F), but evidence for the efficacy of these interventions in neurological patients is meager. Newer adhesive surface cooling systems (Arctic Sun, Medivance, Inc.) and endovascular heat exchange catheters (Cool Line System, Alsius, Inc.) have been shown to be much more effective for maintaining normothermia. However, clinical trials are needed to determine if these measures improve clinical outcome.

Nutritional support

As is the case with all critically ill neurological patients, enteral feeding should be started within 48 hours to avoid protein catabolism and malnutrition. A small-bore nasoduodenal feeding tube may reduce the risk of aspiration events.

REFERENCES

1. Schulzke S, Weber P, Luetschg J, Fahnenstich H. Incidence and diagnosis of unilateral arterial cerebral infarction in newborn infants. *J Perinat Med.* 2005;33:170-175.
2. Carlin TM, Chanmugam A. Stroke in children. *Emerg Med Clin North Am.* 2002;20:671-685.
3. DeVeber G, Adams C, Andrew M, et al. Canadian Pediatric Ischemic Stroke Registry. *Can J Neurol Sci.* 1995;22(suppl 1): S24.
4. Gabis LV, Yangala R, Lenn NJ. Time lag to diagnosis of stroke syndromes. *Pediatr Infect Dis J.* 2000;19:624-628.
5. Kirkham FJ. Stroke in childhood. *Arch Dis Child.* 1999; 81:85-89.
6. Nelson KB. Perinatal ischemic stroke. *Stroke.* 2007; 38(2 suppl):742-745.
7. Chalmers EA. Perinatal stroke—risk factors and management. *Br J Haematol.* 2005;130:333-343.
8. de Veber G. Canadian Pediatric Ischaemic Stroke Registry. *Pediatr Child Health.* A17. 2000.

9. Lee J, Croen LA, Backstrand KH, et al. Maternal and infant characteristics associated with perinatal arterial stroke in the infant. *JAMA.* 2005;293:723-729.

10. Lynch JK, Hirtz DG, DeVeber G, Nelson KB. Report of the National Institute of Neurological Disorders and Stroke workshop on perinatal and childhood stroke. *Pediatrics.* 2002;109:116-123.

11. Hunt RW, Inder TE. Perinatal and neonatal ischaemic stroke: a review. *Thromb Res.* 2006;118:39-48.

12. Miller V. Neonatal cerebral infarction. *Semin Pediatr Neurol.* 2000;7:278-288.

13. Wu YW, Lynch JK, Nelson KB. Perinatal arterial stroke: understanding mechanisms and outcomes. *Semin Neurol.* 2005;25:424-434.

14. Fullerton HJ, Wu YW, Sidney S, Johnston SC. Risk of recurrent childhood arterial ischemic stroke in a population-based cohort: the importance of cerebrovascular imaging. *Pediatrics.* 2007;119:495-501.

15. Govaert P ME, Zecic A, Roelens F, Oostra A, Vanzieleghem B. Perinatal cortical infarction within middle cerebral artery trunks. *Arch Dis Child Fetal Neonatal Ed.* 2000;82: F59-F63.

16. de Veber GA AM, Andrew M. Cerebral thromboembolism in neonates: clinical and radiographic features. *Blood.* 1998;92:2959.

17. Kenet G, Nowak-Gottl U. Fetal and neonatal thrombophilia. *Obstet Gynecol Clin North Am.* 2006;33:457-466.

18. Harum KH, Hoon AH Jr., Kato GJ, Casella JF, Breiter SN, Johnston MV. Homozygous factor-V mutation as a genetic cause of perinatal thrombosis and cerebral palsy. *Dev Med Child Neurol.* 1999;41:777-780.

19. Varelas PN, Sleight BJ, Rinder HM, Sze G, Ment LR. Stroke in a neonate heterozygous for factor V Leiden. *Pediatr Neurol.* 1998;18:262-264.

20. Thorarensen O, Ryan S, Hunter J, Younkin DP. Factor V Leiden mutation: an unrecognized cause of hemiplegic cerebral palsy, neonatal stroke, and placental thrombosis. *Ann Neurol.* 1997;42:372-375.

21. Hagstrom JN, Walter J, Bluebond-Langner R, Amatniek JC, Manno CS, High KA. Prevalence of the factor V leiden mutation in children and neonates with thromboembolic disease. *J Pediatr.* 1998;133:777-781.

22. Gunther G, Junker R, Strater R, et al. Symptomatic ischemic stroke in full-term neonates : role of acquired and genetic prothrombotic risk factors. *Stroke.* 2000;31:2437-2441.

23. Hogeveen M, Blom HJ, Van Amerongen M, Boogmans B, Van Beynum IM, Van De Bor M. Hyperhomocysteinemia as risk factor for ischemic and hemorrhagic stroke in newborn infants. *J Pediatr.* 2002;141:429-431.

24. Golomb MR, MacGregor DL, Domi T, et al. Presumed pre- or perinatal arterial ischemic stroke: risk factors and outcomes. *Ann Neurol.* 2001;50:163-168.

25. Nowak-Gottl U, Duering C, Kempf-Bielack B, Strater R. Thromboembolic diseases in neonates and children. *Pathophysiol Haemost Thromb.* 2003;33:269-274.

26. Wu YW, Hamrick SE, Miller SP, et al. Intraventricular hemorrhage in term neonates caused by sinovenous thrombosis. *Ann Neurol.* 2003;54:123-126.

27. JJ V. *Neurology of the Newborn.* 4th ed. Philadelphia: Saunders; 2001.

28. Bassan H, Feldman HA, Limperopoulos C, et al. Periventricular hemorrhagic infarction: risk factors and neonatal outcome. *Pediatr Neurol.* 2006;35:85-92.

29. Fullerton HJ, Claiborne Johnston S, Smith WS. Arterial dissection and stroke in children. *Neurology.* 2001; 57:1155-1160.

30. Kirkham F, Sebire G, Steinlin M, Strater R. Arterial ishaemic stroke in children. *Thromb Haemost.* 2004; 92:697-706.

31. Sebire G, Fullerton H, Riou E, deVeber G. Toward the definition of cerebral arteriopathies of childhood. *Curr Opin Pediatr.* 2004;16:617-622.

32. DeVeber G. Arterial ischemic strokes in infants and children: an overview of current approaches. *Semin Thromb Hemost.* 2003;29:567-573.

33. Askalan R, Laughlin S, Mayank S, et al. Chickenpox and stroke in childhood: a study of frequency and causation. *Stroke.* 2001;32:1257-1262.

34. Adams FJ, McKie VC, Hsu L, et al. Prevention of first stroke by transfusion in children with sickle cell anemia and abnormal results on transcranial Doppler ultrasonography. *N Engl J Med.* 1998;339:5-11.

35. Jordan LC. Stroke in childhood. *Neurologist.* 2006;12:94-102.

36. Lynch JK. Cerebrovascular disorders in children. *Curr Neurol Neurosci Rep.* 2004;4:129-138.

37. Monagle P CA, Massicotte P, Chalmers E, Michelson AD. Antithrombotic therapy in children: the seventh ACCP conference on antithrombotic and thrombolytic therapy. *Chest.* 2004;126:645-687.

38. DeVeber G. In pursuit of evidence-based treatments for paediatric stroke: the UK and *Chest* guidelines. *Lancet Neurol.* 2005;4:432-436.

39. Hutchison JS, Ichord R, Guerguerian A, deVeber G. Cerebrovascular disorders. *Semin Pediatr Neurol.* 2004;11:139-146.

40. Adams RJ, McKie VC, Brambilla DJ, et al. Stroke prevention trial in sickle cell anemia. *Control Clin Trials.* 1998;19:110-129.

41. Sloan MA, Alexandrov AV, Tegeler CH, et al. Assessment: transcranial Doppler ultrasonography: report of the Therapeutics and Technology Assessment Subcommittee of the American Academy of Neurology. *Neurology.* 2004;62: 1468.

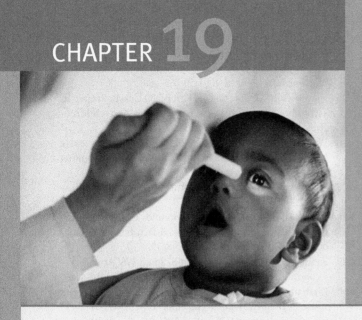

CHAPTER 19

Traumatic Brain Injury

Jose A. Pineda and Jeffrey R. Leonard

DEFINITIONS AND EPIDEMIOLOGY

Traumatic brain injury (TBI) is a leading cause of death and disability among children and young adults.[1,2] Unintentional injuries (ie, car accidents and falls) are the leading cause of death for children 1 to 14 years of age.[3] Among such injuries, TBI is a leading cause of injury-related morbidity and mortality.[4] Furthermore, despite modern automobile design and injury prevention campaigns, important causes of TBI have increased in recent years.[5] In addition to unintentional injuries, child abuse remains a significant problem and constitutes the leading cause of serious head injury in infants.[6] With nearly half a million children affected each year, TBI is a serious public health problem.[7]

Traditionally, TBI severity has been defined using the Glasgow Coma Scale (GCS). The GCS, shown in Table 19-1, was developed in order to standardize the neurological assessment of adult patients with traumatic brain injury.[8] It was specifically designed to be easily performed based upon clinical data and to have a low rate of inter-observer variability. Despite its limitations when applied to children,[9,10] the GCS is widely used for the initial assessment and for monitoring progress of pediatric TBI. A pediatric version of the GCS also seems to be a reliable tool for predicting the need for acute intervention in preverbal children with TBI.[11]

The GCS score is determined by adding the values for eye opening, verbal response, and motor response. Possible values range from 3 to 15. Note that this scale rates the best response only. In patients who are intubated, in whom assessment of best verbal response cannot be performed, notation of this is made in the GCS score by adding a "T" to the end of the score. In patients who are intubated, the best possible score would therefore be 11T. For patients 4 years old or younger, the Pediatric Glasgow Coma Scale is recommended (Table 19-2).

Table 19-1.

Glasgow Coma Scale (GCS)

Eye opening	Verbalization	Motor response
4: Spontaneous	5: Oriented	6: Obeys
3: To speech	4: Confused	5: Localizes pain
2: To pain	3: Inappropriate	4: Withdraws to pain
1: No response	2: Incomprehensible	3: Decorticate posturing (flexor)
	1: No response	2: Decerebrate posturing (extensor)
		1: No response

Table 19-2.

Pediatric Glasgow Coma Scale

Eye opening	Verbalization	Motor response
4: Spontaneous	5: Coos, babbles	6: Normal spontaneous movement
3: To voice	4: Irritable	5: Withdraws to touch
2: To pain	3: Cries to pain	4: Withdraws to pain
1: No response	2: Moans to pain	3: Decorticate posturing
	1: No response	2: Decerebrate posturing
		1: No response

Certain numerical values of the Glasgow Coma Scale have been used to define the severity of TBI:

Mild traumatic brain injury	GCS 14-15
Moderate traumatic brain injury	GCS 9-13
Severe traumatic brain injury	GCS 3-8

Both severe and mild to moderate TBI represent significant neurological diseases for children. Although mild to moderate traumatic brain injury very infrequently will result in severe disability or death, outcomes are variable and long-term sequelae have been reported.

PATHOGENESIS

Although our understanding of the mechanisms of damage to the immature brain after TBI remains quite limited, it is becoming clear that mechanisms of cellular injury and death in the immature brain are different from those described to date in the mature brain. Just as comprehensive evaluations of outcome describe functional differences, modern biomechanical and biochemical techniques have demonstrated that cellular and molecular responses to injury differ in the immature brain. That such differences exist seems intuitive given critical periods of vulnerability for the developing nervous system. As an example, better characterization of cerebral blood flow before and after injury is needed to enable appropriate strategies that will optimize oxygen delivery to the brain in children.

Pathologic changes that occur following trauma may be considered to occur in two stages. Damage that occurs at the time of the injury is referred to as the primary injury. This includes damage to axons, neurons, and cerebral blood vessels that occurs as a result of the force of the injury—that is, shear and strain forces that result in tearing of delicate cerebral structures. This injury may result in diffuse axonal injury, intracerebral/subdural/epidural hematomas (from disruption of cerebral or dural blood vessels), or cortical contusions. Injury to the brain that occurs at any time after the initial impact of the traumatic event is termed the secondary injury. Events that may result in secondary injury to the brain and that have been shown to adversely affect outcome include hypoxia, hypotension, and hyperthermia. These types of injuries are preventable by caregivers, and their prevention may result in significant improvements in outcome. Figure 19-1 illustrates the concept of primary and secondary injury. Secondary injury may irreversibly damage brain tissue that was weakened by, but survived, the primary injury.

CLINICAL PRESENTATION

Mild and Moderate Traumatic Brain Injury

Mild head injury is a term first described by Rimel and associates and was taken to mean GCS 13 to 15 in a 1981 article.[12] Although minor, head injuries not associated with a loss of consciousness constitute one of the most common public health problems. A certain number of children with minor head injuries (GCS 14-15) who have also lost consciousness are found to have significant intracranial pathology requiring neurosurgical procedures. With that in mind, a number of authors have attempted to redefine mild TBI since that original article. Because of the immense magnitude of the

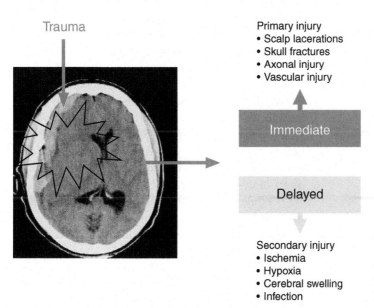

Trauma

Primary injury
• Scalp lacerations
• Skull fractures
• Axonal injury
• Vascular injury

Immediate

Delayed

Secondary injury
• Ischemia
• Hypoxia
• Cerebral swelling
• Infection

FIGURE 19-1 ■ Current classification of primary and secondary insults to the brain after trauma. Primary injury can only be avoided by effective prevention. Delayed injury can go on for days and constitutes a therapeutic target for current and future surgical and intensive care strategies.

problem, numerous organizations, including the American Academy of Pediatrics, the American Academy of Family Physicians, and the American Academy of Neurology, have come up with practice parameters that address different aspects of mild pediatric head injury.[13,14]

Concussion is an entity that is commonly seen in pediatric patients with mild to moderate head injury. It is defined as a trauma-induced alteration in mental status that may or may not involve loss of consciousness.[14] Patients with a concussion experience an immediate loss of consciousness, suppression of reflexes, transient cessation of breathing, and amnesia. The reflexes return and the patient begins to reconnect with the surrounding environment. The time to recovery is variable and may take several hours to days. The duration of the amnestic period, particularly anterograde amnesia, is probably the most reliable indicator of the presence of pathologic lesions. Postconcussive emesis in children is another worrisome problem in the acute setting. It can affect nearly one-half of patients and usually resolves within a few hours. Postconcussive emesis has not been associated with an increasing frequency of intracranial lesions.[15] Concussions also occur without a defined loss of consciousness. Sports-related concussions are another common entity that primary care physicians, pediatric neurologists, and pediatric neurosurgeons have to deal with every day. Most children will recover from a sports-related concussion though recovery may take time, up to several months after the injury. The symptoms following a concussion are divided into three categories. Somatic complaints include headaches, fatigue, sleep disturbance, balance problems, and sensitivity to light and noise. Emotional and behavioral problems can manifest as irritability, lowered frustration tolerance, increased emotionality, depression, anxiety, and other personality changes. The last, and some feel the most important, category, especially in the school-age child is cognitive problems. Children may have slowed thinking, poor concentration, distractibility, trouble with learning and memory, and other problem-solving difficulties.

Severe Traumatic Brain Injury

Severe TBI in children carries a mortality of 8% to 22%.[16,17] Approximately seven children between the ages of 0 to 14 years die every day, and many more suffer permanent disabilities as a result of TBI.[4]

Severe TBI is defined as a GCS score of 8 or less. By definition, children with severe TBI present with significant abnormalities in their neurological exam including coma, abnormal breathing (including at times apnea), focal neurological deficits, seizures, and even signs of herniation. Evolving brain edema or intracranial bleeding can result in acute deterioration of the child's neurological exam. Consideration should always be given to extracranial injuries, since such injuries can result in secondary injury to the brain.

DIAGNOSIS

Mild and Moderate Traumatic Brain Injury

In the pediatric head injury population, the most common clinical situation will be the child who rapidly regains consciousness after an injury. By the time the child is examined, the child will commonly have a GCS score of 13 to 15 or a mild head injury. The child also has a defined risk for having an intracranial injury. The Glasgow Coma Scale has long been considered a reliable indicator of severity of injury.

A number of tools have been developed to aid in the assessment of concussion. One of the most commonly used tools is the Standard Assessment of Concussion. It has been extensively validated and has significant normative data. The concussion symptom index has also been used, especially in athletes with normative data in high school as well as college athletes.[18] Additionally, neuropsychological testing is one of the most important tools for detecting deficits in pediatric TBI, especially in patients with mild TBI. In sports-related concussion, the baseline use of neuropsychological testing has been used to determine return-to-play parameters in the absence of postconcussive symptoms.

Skull radiographs have a limited role in the diagnosis of intracranial injury following either mild or moderate pediatric head injury. Given the low predictive value of skull radiographs, the American Academy of Pediatrics recommends that cranial computed tomography (CT) scanning is the desirable imaging modality.[13] Over 5 million children present to emergency rooms across the country with this diagnosis, and CT scanning of each of these patients, while considered the gold standard, would overwhelm the facilities and expose countless children to pointless radiation. Because of the higher degree of intracranial injury associated with a GCS score of less than 15, the authors recommend that any patient with a GCS less than 15 undergo a head CT. Another potential high-risk category is the patient who presents with a focal neurological deficit. The frequency of an intracranial injury in this population has been reported to be 11%.[19]

While the utility of computed tomography after minor head injury has been extensively studied, and different clinical criteria for predicting intracranial injury have been identified (Table 19-3), CT scanning can be associated with increased risk for long-term cancer, the need for sedation to accomplish the scan, and a prolonged ED evaluation, and this in turn has lead to

Table 19-3.

Different Clinical Criteria for Predicting Intracranial Injury

Author	No of Patients	Imaging Modality	No of Patients with Intracranial Injury	Associated Factors
Quayle et al.[20]	322	CT	27	Skull fracture, signs of basilar skull fracture, loss of consciousness for more than 5 min, altered mental status, focal neurological abnormality
Hennes et al.[21]	55	CT	37	Altered mental status, evidence of elevated intracranial pressure, seizures, and focal deficits
Rivara et al.[22]	98	CT	49	Abnormal GCS, altered consciousness, focal neurological deficit
Dietrich et al.[23]	322	CT	39	Loss of consciousness, amnesia, GCS less than 15, and focal neurological deficit
Rammundo et al.[24]	300	CT	53	Suspicion for child abuse, focal motor deficit, papillary asymmetry

multiple studies attempting to identify clinical predictors of intracranial injury. Boran and associates studied 421 patients with a GCS of 15 and were able to determine injuries found by either CT or plain radiographs. Intracranial lesions were found in 8.8% of the patients. They were able to determine that the only clinical parameters associated with an increase in intracranial lesion were posttraumatic seizures and loss of consciousness.[15] In NEXUS (National Emergency X-Radiography Utilization Study), a large study looking at 1666 pediatric blunt trauma patients, CT was found to detect significant intracranial injury in 138, or 8.3%, of the patients. These authors also attempted to utilize a modification of the University of California-Davis Pediatric Head Injury Rule to identify patients with an intracranial injury. The sensitivity of their tool was found to be only 90.4%, with 13 children being misclassified as low risk.

Posttraumatic sequelae, especially in those patients with mild head injury, are significant, with upward of 15% of patients experiencing disabling symptoms up to 1 year after injury. Many of these patients do not have abnormalities on CT imaging. Limitations of CT scanning in detecting injury has lead to the use of magnetic resonance imaging (MRI) to detect diffuse axonal injury (DAI) and deliver prognostic information in cases of mild to moderate TBI. DAI is a type of injury characterized by significant axonal damage or shearing in brain regions such as the corpus collosum, parasagittal white matter, and gray-white matter junctions. Diffusion tensor imaging measures the microscopic random translational motion of water molecules within tissue. Wilde and others studied children with DTI and uninjured controls, and their data suggested that DTI may serve

as an indicator for predicting outcome in pediatric patients with TBI.[25] Magnetic resonance spectroscopy (MRS) is another imaging modality that is currently being used at some centers in the evaluation of patients with TBI. MRS has been shown to detect biochemical alterations, yet its value in providing truly valuable prognostic information in patients with mild to moderate TBI remains to be determined.

Severe Traumatic Brain Injury

Motor vehicle accidents and falls constitute the most common causes of severe TBI. In infants, the most common cause of severe TBI is child abuse, and a higher index of suspicion for intracranial injury may be required owing to an inconsistent clinical history.

The diagnosis of severe TBI is usually made based on the history and initial clinical findings. Once the diagnosis is made, children with severe TBI require close and continuous neurological monitoring, as their condition may rapidly deteriorate. In addition to abnormal neurological findings, including a GCS score of 8 or less, children with severe TBI can have signs of skull fractures, such as raccoon eyes, retro-orbital hematomas, and palpable abnormalities of the skull. The initial clinical diagnosis is usually confirmed by a CT scan in the acute phase, although children with severe brain injury can present with an initially normal brain CT. The initial scan is important because it may identify injuries that are amenable to surgical treatment, such as intracranial hematomas. Patients with a history of severe TBI and an abnormal CT scan are at increased risk of developing increased intracranial pressure.

While CT continues to be the primary diagnostic imaging modality in severe TBI, advanced MRI techniques, including diffusion tensor imaging and MR spectroscopy, are promising techniques with increased sensitivity, better prognostic capabilities, and also insights into the pathophysiology of brain injury after trauma.

Shaken Baby Syndrome

Shaken baby syndrome (SBS) is an important category of TBI in children, and children victims of SBS can present with signs and symptoms of severe TBI. In fact, SBS is the most common cause of traumatic brain injury in infants. As an entity, SBS provokes significant medical legal issues and requires careful attention to the etiology of the injury. Patients with SBS are difficult to evaluate because they often present with symptoms only, and if trauma is reported, it is usually minor. A patient's clinical presentation can vary significantly depending on the severity of the injury. Symptoms can range from mild lethargy and seizures to coma and even death.

Computed tomography is usually the initial diagnostic study. CT findings include subdural as well as subarachnoid hemorrhage. These are often thin, exerting no mass effect, but cover the entire hemisphere. In cases where the injury is severe, patients can present with diffuse loss of gray-white differentiation on CT scan, reflecting widespread cortical loss.[26] Once the child has been stabilized and is not felt to be in a life-threatening situation, most major children's hospitals have a child protection service responsible for the complete medical workup of this patient. Workup includes a skeletal survey to assess for the presence of new or old fractures. Ophthalmology also must assess the child for the presence of retinal hemorrhages. Disorders such as coagulopathies and metabolic disorders need to be ruled out.

TREATMENT

Mild to Moderate Traumatic Brain Injury

Initial evaluation of head-injured patients should always be performed according to the trauma protocols, with assessment of the ABCs and a focused history and physical exam. Life-threatening injuries should be assessed and supersede all other concerns. Once the child is deemed stable, then especially in patients with mild head injuries, a detailed physical exam is important. Concussion is probably one of the most important entities in pediatric TBI. Clinicians generally accept that no two concussions are exactly alike, making it necessary to individualize care within the parameters of their situation

and rational clinical practice. Although no specific therapies for concussion-related symptoms currently exist, a number of experts have provided guidelines on the management of concussions as related to timing for return to play (Table 19-4).[27]

The overall incidence of posttraumatic seizure ranges between 5.5% and 21%. Seizures are usually classified based on the time to occurrence. The incidence of posttraumatic seizure also varies with decreasing GCS, as one might expect. Children with mild TBI have a seizure risk of approximately 2% to 6%. This increases to 12% to 27% in patients with moderate TBI, and the incidence of posttraumatic seizures also increases with younger age. The interval between the head injury and the first seizure can vary. Immediate seizures have a better prognosis in determining whether or not someone will be at risk for developing posttraumatic epilepsy. In contrast, the occurrence of a single late posttraumatic seizure has been used to define posttraumatic epilepsy. Inflicted (SBS) versus noninflicted TBI patients also differ in the rates of posttraumatic epilepsy. Victims of SBS have a rate of 48% to 65%, much higher than the 15% to 17% seen in patients after noninflicted trauma. This is most likely owing to the higher incidence of subdural hematomas in patients with SBS.[28]

Severe Traumatic Brain Injury

Treatment of patients with severe traumatic brain injury (GCS score of 8 or less) remains controversial. Much remains to be learned about the pathophysiology of brain injury and strategies for brain resuscitation in children. Although implementation of trauma programs and access to pediatric intensive care have improved outcome, there is only limited evidence behind treatment guidelines for children suffering severe TBI and there are no specific pharmacologic therapies available. Current treatment strategies are largely supportive.

Nevertheless, significant progress has been made over the past two decades. Despite the lack of class I evidence that demonstrates long-term, significant efficacy for any given treatment modality or intervention, mortality and morbidity from TBI have improved for both children and adults. Guidelines for in-hospital treatment of severe head injury in adults were published in 1997, and a revision of such document became recently available. Guidelines for prehospital management of traumatic brain injury in adults and children were also published in 2000 by the Brain Trauma Foundation (www.braintrauma.org). Finally, in July 2003 the *Guidelines for the Acute Medical Management of Severe Traumatic Brain Injury in Infants, Children and Adolescents* were published.[29] The purpose of these documents was to upgrade practice parameters from opinion to guidelines that are supported by the best evidence available. It is important to note that most recommendations in this

Table 19-4.

Different Clinical Criteria for Predicting Intracranial Injury

Guidelines for Return to Play following Concussion	Guidelines		Concussion Severity		
			1	2	3
Concussion Symptoms <15 min, no PTA	Cantu	1	Return to play when asymtomatic	Return to play in 2 wk when asymtomatic for 1 wk	Terminate season; may resume next year
	Colorado	1	Return to play when asymtomatic for 20 min	Return to play when asymtomatic for 1 wk	Stop participation; may return in 3 mo
	AAN	1	Return to play when asymtomatic for 15 min	Return to play when asymtomatic for 1 wk, 2nd concussion– terminate activity	
PTA <30 min and no LOC	Cantu	1	Return to play when asymtomatic for 1 wk	Return to play in 2 wk when asymtomatic for 1 wk; consider termination of season	Terminate season; may return next season
	Colorado	2	Return to play when asymtomatic for 1 wk	Return to play when asymtomatic for 1 mo	Terminate season; may return next season
Concussion Symptoms >15 min	AAN	2	Return to play when asymtomatic for 1 wk	Return to play in 2 wk if asymtomatic	
PTA >30 min <24 h and LOC <5 min	Cantu	2	Return to play when asymtomatic for 1 wk	Return to play in 1 mo when asymtomatic for 1 wk; consider termination of season	Terminate season; may return next season
	Colorado	2	Transport to hospital, return to play 1 mo after injury when asymtomatic for 2 wk	Terminate season; discourage return	
PTA >30 min <24 h and LOC for seconds	AAN	3	Transport to hospital, return to play when asymtomatic for 1 wk	Return to play after 1 mo	
PTA >24 h and LOC >5 min	Cantu	3	Return to play 1 mo after injury when asymtomatic for 1 wk	Terminate season	
	Colorado	3	Transport to hospital, return to play 1 mo after injury when asymtomatic for 2 wk	Terminate season; discourage return	
	AAN	3	Return to play when asymtomatic for 2 wk	Return to play when asymtomatic for 1 mo	

document are at the "option" level, given the lack of clinical evidence to support guideline and standard-of-care level recommendations. Upgrading practice parameters to standards of care—the strongest recommendation a guideline can make—will require new knowledge acquired through carefully planned clinical research.

Over the past years a significant amount of laboratory and human evidence has accumulated that demonstrates the impact of physiologic variables such as temperature, glucose level, and blood pressure on outcome. Protocols or guidelines focused in controlling such variables from the scene to the intensive care unit are likely to impact outcome. Also, standardized management of patients may improve the quality of clinical trials testing new therapies in pediatric head injury.

The main goal of current management protocols is to focus on normalizing physiologic variables that impact outcome after brain injury, both in children and adults. Therapeutic interventions known to decrease intracranial pressure (ICP) with a safe therapeutic profile are included. Second-tier therapies shown to be beneficial but also associated with significant side effects (ie, pentobarbital coma) are offered as treatment options for cases of persistent intracranial hypertension.

Management Protocol

Clinical judgment should be used to individualize patient management. As previously discussed, many aspects of care can only be considered treatment options. Treatment pathways apply to all patients admitted with severe TBI caused by

- Accidental trauma (blunt or penetrating trauma to the head)
- Gunshot wounds to the head
- Nonaccidental head trauma

Secondary insult prevention

The objective of intensive care management of severe traumatic brain injury is to prevent secondary insults to the traumatized brain. This may be achieved by direct and focused attention to those insults known to be associated with poor neurological outcome. This includes (1) prevention of cerebral ischemia and hypoxia and (2) prevention of cerebral hyperthermia.

Cerebral ischemia

Cerebral ischemia may occur as a direct result of inadequate cerebral perfusion, decreased oxygen or glucose supply, increased metabolic demand of the brain, or from increased cerebral vascular resistance.

Cerebral perfusion

Inadequate perfusion may have a direct and deleterious effect on the pathophysiology of brain injury. Cerebral perfusion is described in terms of cerebral perfusion pressure (CPP). CPP is calculated as the difference between mean arterial pressure (MAP) and mean intracranial pressure (ICP). That is, CPP = MAP – ICP. Current recommended guidelines suggest that CPP should be maintained around 60 mm Hg in adult patients. CPP values should be interpreted in the context of other perfusion indexes if those are available.

- Lower threshold levels of 50 mm Hg (2-6 years), 55 mm Hg (7-10 years), and 60 mm Hg (11-16 years) have been recommended for children. For adolescents, a minimum CPP of 60 mm Hg is recommended. Patients with CPP below these thresholds can experience a worse outcome.
- Optimal CPP levels for children lesser than 2 years of age have not been established, but several studies demonstrate that a CPP of 40 mm Hg or less is associated with higher mortality and worse outcome in children of any age.[30] We therefore consider 45 mm Hg a critical threshold for CPP in children less than 2 years of age.

Mean arterial pressure

Mean arterial pressure (MAP) is an important determining factor in the CPP equation. One of the difficulties we face in caring for the patient with a severe head

Table 19-5.

Age-Appropriate Mean Arterial Pressure (MAP)

Age (yr)	Normal MAP (mm Hg)
1-2	53-59
3-4	61-65
5-6	67-69
7-8	70-72
9-10	73-75
11-12	75-77
13-14	77-79
15-17	80-84

injury is determining an appropriate MAP. Factors to consider include patient age[31] and preexisting hypertension. Age-appropriate MAP (Table 19-5) should be maintained and adjustments of MAP to maintain CPP above critical thresholds may be necessary.

It is also important to note that early systolic hypotension has also been associated with poor outcome after TBI in multiple pediatric clinical studies. Different definitions of hypotension have been used. A recent study described an association between early hypotension and outcome using the 75th percentile for age-appropriate systolic blood pressure (AASBP) as the threshold for hypotension. Maintaining AASBP from the initial stabilization phase is important and may influence outcome in children with traumatic brain injury.[32] Hypotension is harmful after pediatric neurotrauma and should be avoided with appropriate volume resuscitation and vasopressor support.

Intracranial pressure

The skull is a rigid structure containing cerebrospinal fluid (CSF), blood, and brain tissue. After TBI the normal balance between these intracranial contents may be disturbed, resulting in increasing pressure within the skull. Importantly, even infants and neonates with open fontanels can develop increased ICP once the intracranial volume expansion overwhelms the compliance of the immature skull and meninges. Elevated ICP has been shown to have definite prognostic implications in children with severe brain injury. In addition, it is generally held that treatment of elevated ICP may improve outcome in the patient with severe TBI. Measurement of ICP enables (1) calculation of CPP; (2) monitoring progress; and (3) assessment of treatment effectiveness. Indications for ICP monitoring in children with severe TBI include

- Patients with a GCS of 3 to 8 after initial resuscitation, who have an abnormal CT scan on admission (ie, hematoma, contusion, compressed basal cisterns, or edema).

- The treating physician may choose to monitor ICP in certain patients for whom serial neurological examination is precluded by sedation/analgesia or anesthesia. ICP monitoring is appropriate in children with severe TBI and a normal CT scan if motor posturing is noted on admission. ICP monitoring should be considered in children with severe TBI and a normal CT scan for those who are noted to have hypotension on admission and in children whose neurological exam does not improve or deteriorates. The presence of open fontanels and/or sutures in an infant with severe TBI does not preclude the development of intracranial hypertension or negate the utility of ICP monitoring.

The following methods are commonly used to monitor ICP in children with severe traumatic brain injury:

- *Ventriculostomy.* Placement of a ventriculostomy catheter and transduction of the fluid column is the mainstay of ICP monitoring. Placement of a catheter within the ventricle also offers a treatment option for raised ICP by allowing CSF drainage. When measuring the pressure, it is necessary to always close off the drainage system prior to recording the pressure readings. Problems with monitoring ICP by ventriculostomy and a transduced fluid column include difficulty with insertion, particularly if the ventricles are small; variable accuracy, because fluid-filled columns are subject to poor waveform, especially if the ventricles are small or collapsed; mechanical problems such as air bubbles, blood clots, or debris in tubing; and infection.
- *Ventriculostomy with built-in microsensor.* New-generation ventriculostomy catheters do not require transduction of a fluid column. They have a built-in miniaturized strain gauge transducer in the tip of the catheter, which gives continuous accurate ICP readings even while simultaneously/continuosly draining CSF.
- *Intraparenchymal bolt.* This may be the ideal method of monitoring ICP if the ventricular system is not accessible. A pressure sensor is introduced into the brain parenchyma and held in place by a bolt secured into the skull.

ICP management

Normal adult ICP values range from 5 to 15 mm Hg. Normal ICP values tend to be lower in infants and younger children (Table 19-4). Increased ICP in children with severe TBI correlates with worse outcome and also decreased cerebral blood flow.[33] Careful management of the patient with ICP monitoring is important, as good ICP control may improve outcome. Basic measures aimed at maintaining adequate venous drainage from the head are safe and simple, and promote normal ICP. Overly tight cervical collars as well as circumferential taping of the endotracheal tube can restrict venous drainage from the head, which may increase ICP. Cervical flexion or extension and lateral head rotation can alter cerebral venous outflow. Maintaining neutral head alignment promotes venous drainage. As demonstrated in Figure 19-2, the effect of cerebral venous outflow on ICP can be significant. Elevating the head of the bed (HOB) 30 degrees by flexing the patient at the hips—not at the abdomen—will also promote venous drainage. However, there may be instances when raising the HOB is contraindicated. If CPP is low, it will be preferable to position the patient in a supine position to increase CPP. To avoid orthostatic hypotension, HOB elevation should be considered with euvolemic patients only. Additionally, in patients with a spine not cleared, the reverse Trendelenburg position can be used to elevate the head without disrupting the spinal alignment.

The currently recommended threshold for treatment of elevated intracranial pressure is 20 mm Hg. In small children, 15 mm Hg might be more appropriate, but data supporting this lower threshold are lacking. Interpretation and treatment of intracranial pressure based on this threshold value should be made in conjunction with careful attention to maintaining CPP above critical values.

There are many causes of raised ICP that are not directly related to intracranial pathology. These factors should be excluded and/or treated prior to initiating other treatments. These factors include

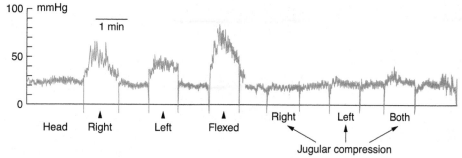

FIGURE 19-2 ■ Effect of head position and jugular compression on ICP. (*Reproduced with permission from Hulme A, Cooper R. The effects of head position and jugular vein compression (JVC) on intracranial pressure (ICP): a clinical study. In: Beks JWF, Bosch DA, Brock M, eds. Intracranial Pressure III. Berlin: Springer-Verlag; 1976:259-263.*)

1. Hyperthermia
2. Hypoxemia
3. Agitation and pain
4. Shivering
5. Resistance to mechanical ventilation
6. Seizures

For children with persistent intracranial hypertension, the methods described in the following sections may result in substantial reductions in ICP, improved cerebral perfusion, and may improve clinical outcome.

Sedation and analgesia.

If patients are inadequately sedated the sympathetic nervous system is overactive. This may result in significant increases in intracranial blood volume. After TBI, the brain's ability to compensate for this increase in blood volume is impaired and the intracranial pressure will rise. It is important to ensure that adequate sedation and analgesia are given to avoid this situation. We recommend midazolam and fentanyl as first-line therapy. If the level of sedation and analgesia is not optimal, morphine may be substituted for fentanyl, but should be used carefully in patients with abnormal renal function. Sedatives and analgesics should be carefully titrated to avoid hemodynamic instability. In compliance with current published recommendations from the FDA, continuous infusions of propofol should not be used for continuous sedation in the pediatric intensive care unit. Exceptions for short periods of sedation (ie, less than 6 hours) can be made at the discretion of the neurocritical care team and require appropriate hemodynamic and biochemical monitoring for indicators of propofol side effects (ie, hypotension, bradycardia, lactic acidosis, lipemia, evidence of rhabdomyolysis).

Neuromuscular blockade.

Neuromuscular blockade (NMB) can potentially reduce mean airway pressure, which can facilitate cerebral venous outflow, prevent shivering or posturing, and reduce metabolic demands. In contrast, NMB carries the risk of masking seizures, cardiovascular side effects, and immobilization stress (if inadequate sedation and analgesia); increases the risk of pneumonia in adult patients with TBI; and increases length of stay in the ICU.[34] After careful consideration of the potential benefit and risk, NMB can be considered as second-tier therapy for persistent intracranial hypertension (ICP > 20 mm Hg) and/or perfusion deficits (low CPP or brain tissue oxygen tension). Since there are no validated tools to monitor NMB in comatose patients with acute brain injury, we recommend that NMB agents be discontinued periodically, for example, every 24 hours. If no benefit is noted, NMB can be discontinued. If the patient becomes difficult to ventilate or ICP increases, NMB can be reinstituted and evaluated again (Figure 19-3). Considering the potential risk associated with the use of NMB, we recommend avoiding this strategy if no benefit on ICP or the ability to mechanically ventilate can be demonstrated.

Cerebrospinal fluid (CSF) drainage.

If a ventriculostomy is present, CSF may be drained intermittently or continuously. The reservoir is placed above the external auditory canal at a predetermined height. Overdrainage of CSF should be avoided as it could collapse the ventricles. Lumbar puncture should not be done in acute TBI owing to risk of herniation. The addition of lumbar drainage can be considered as an option only in the case of refractory intracranial hypertension with a functioning ventriculostomy, open basal cisterns, and no evidence of a major mass lesion or shift on

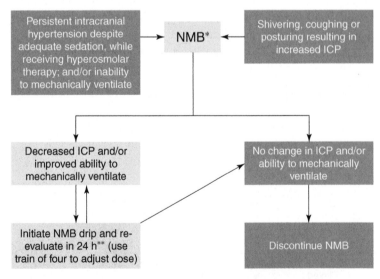

*NMB, neuromuscular blockade. Use vecuronium unless the patient has abnormal renal or hepatic function (cisatricurium for patients with abnormal renal/hepatic function).
**To evaluate effect of NBM, discontinue infusion and evaluate for increases in ICP and/or difficulty to mechanically ventilate It may be neccesary to discontinue NMB earlier than 24 hours after initiation if a neurological exam is needed.

FIGURE 19-3 ■ Algorithm describing an organized approach to the use of neuromuscular blockade in children with severe TBI. Clinical judgment should be used to individualize patient management. Aspects of care included in this algorithm constitute treatment options.

imaging studies. In pediatric patients with refractory intracranial hypertension, controlled lumbar drainage has been successful in lowering ICP.[35]

Hyperosmolar therapy. Mannitol is an osmotic diuretic and an effective treatment for patients with increased ICP caused by cerebral edema. Mannitol decreases ICP by several proposed mechanisms, including shifting fluid from the brain to the intravascular space and decreasing CSF production. Mannitol may also improve cerebral blood flow by reducing blood viscosity. When treating patients with mannitol, hypotension caused by dehydration and hypovolemia should be avoided. Osmolar gap measurements correlate with mannitol levels better than serum osmolarity and should be maintained below 20.[36,37] Using osmolar gap calculations also avoids confusion when using mannitol and hypertonic saline concurrently. Hypertonic saline is effective to control increased ICP after severe head injury. A continuous infusion administered on a sliding scale (the minimum dose required to control ICP should be used) is recommended (Figure 19-4). Serum sodium of 150 to 160 mEq/L, and a serum osmolality level of 360 mOsm/L, appear to be tolerated with hypertonic saline, although cases of renal failure have been reported.[38] Until more safety and efficacy information becomes available, serum sodium levels greater than 165 mEq/L should be avoided. Rapid changes in serum sodium in children with hypernatremia can result in worsening intracranial hypertension.

The long-standing acceptance, safety, and limited evidentiary support of the efficacy of mannitol therapy should be weighted against the limited clinical experience but reasonably good performance of hypertonic saline.

Hyperventilation. In the past, hyperventilation was often employed as a means to reduce high ICP. Current practice now supports avoiding hyperventilation unless signs of herniation are exhibited. Hyperventilation lowers ICP by causing vasoconstriction and decreasing cerebral blood flow (CBF). For every 1 mm decrease in PCO_2 there is a 3% decrease in CBF. Accordingly, PCO_2 should be kept at 35 to 40 mm Hg. The caregiver should anticipate the need for $ETCO_2$ monitoring. In the setting of hyperventilation as a second-tier therapy to treat refractory intracranial hypertension, perfusion indexes such as brain tissue PO_2, jugular bulb hemoglobin oxygen saturation, and/or cerebral blood flow (CBF) should be monitored. Although hyperventilation-induced cerebral ischemia remains a controversial topic, the use of prophylactic aggressive hyperventilation has been associated with worse outcome in adult patients with TBI.[39]

Cerebral Oxygenation

Cerebral hypoxia can exacerbate the deleterious effects of acute traumatic brain injury. Despite aggressive treatment for ICP and CPP, cerebral hypoxia can be persistent.

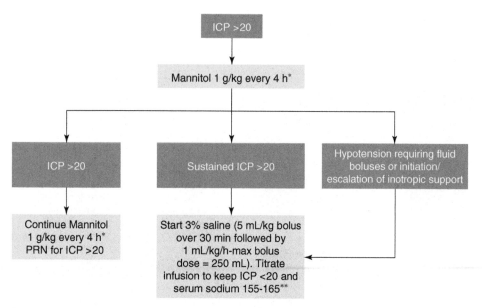

*Keep osmolar gap <20; **Osmolar gap = (measured osmolality) − (calculated osmolality); Calculated osmolality = 1.86 (Na + K) + (BUN/2.8) + (glucose/18) + 10**

**Keep serum osmolarity less than 360 mOsm/L. If sodium >165, titrate infusion down by 0.25 mL/kg/h every 12 h. Avoid changes in serum sodium of >10 meq/24 h. Note that increases in ICP can occur with decreasing serum Na$^+$ even during hypernatremic states. Wean 3% saline solution by 0.25 mL/kg/h every 12 h to avoid sudden changes in serum sodium and potential rebound intracranial hypertension.

FIGURE 19-4 ■ Use of hyperosmolar therapy for the treatment of intracranial hypertension. Clinical judgment should be used to individualize patient management. Aspects of care included in this algorithm constitute treatment options.

Depth and duration of brain tissue hypoxia has been associated with increased mortality in severe TBI patients.[40]

We now have the ability to measure brain tissue oxygen pressure ($PbtO_2$) continuously by a small probe placed into brain tissue and secured to the skull by a bolt. The $PbtO_2$ monitor measures intraparenchimal oxygen and temperature and is intended to be used in conjunction with other monitors to help indicate the perfusion status of cerebral tissue. It is intended to provide data additional to that obtained by current clinical practice in cases where ischemia or hypoxia is a concern. Indications for $PbtO_2$ monitoring are the same as for ICP monitoring and include any patient with a GCS of 3 to 8, an abnormal CT scan of the brain, and/or abnormal clinical exam. The use of both ICP and $PbtO_2$ monitors and therapy directed at $PbtO_2$ is associated with reduced patient death following severe TBI.[41] These associations are also supported by neuropathology and physiology preclinical data on the consequences of low $PbtO_2$ values.

Normal human brain has a critical $PbtO_2$ between 15 and 20 mm Hg, below which infarction of tissue may occur. In clinical practice, a target $PbtO_2$ of 25 to 35 mm Hg has been adopted. Table 19-6 outlines some of the underlying factors that may be responsible for abnormal values.

Table 19-6.

Factors that may be Responsible for Abnormal $PbtO_2$ Values

$PbtO_2 < 25$ mm Hg

Decreased oxygen delivery:	Increased oxygen demand:
Hypotension/hypovolemia	Inadequate sedation—pain, agitation
Hypoxia	Shivering
Increased ICP	Fever
Anemia	Seizures
Vasospasm	

$PbtO_2 < 35$ mm Hg
Hyperdynamic circulation
Excessive oxygen administration

$PbtO_2$ values must be interpreted in conjunction with other monitoring parameters and the clinical situation.

The most common clinical scenario will be a low $PbtO_2$ (<25 mm Hg). It is important to ensure that the monitor is functioning normally and that the probe is correctly connected and calibrated (Figure 19-5). Consideration can be given to placing patient on 100%

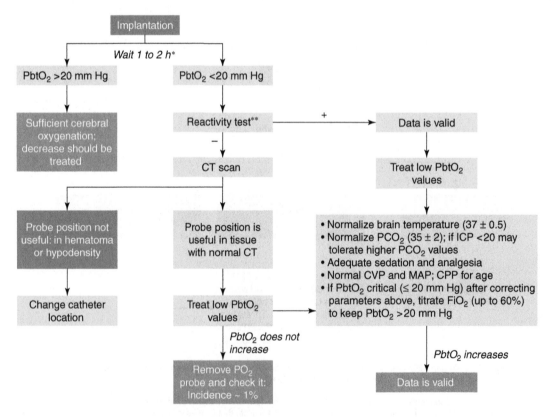

* Probe stabilization period
** Increase 100% FiO_2 for 15 min and observe for increase in $PbtO_2$ (+ test)

FIGURE 19-5 ■ Brain tissue oxygen tension ($PbtO_2$) management algorithm. Suggestions for exclusion of micro-hemorrhage/abnormal tissue artifact and management of critical $PbtO_2$ values are included. Clinical judgment should be used to individualize patient management. Aspects of care included in this algorithm constitute treatment options.

FiO$_2$ for 15 minutes as a temporary intervention while underlying causes are investigated. The main priority is to optimize other parameters in order to decrease FiO$_2$ and increase PbtO$_2$: Is the patient adequately sedated? Is the patient hydrated and hemodinamically stable? Does the patient have significant anemia? Is the patient hyperthermic?

Is the patient being hyperventilated? There may be other parameters that are outside the goal of management range, such as high ICP. Additional management suggestions are shown in the severe TBI management flow sheet (Figure 19-6). After considering and attempting to correct all relevant parameters, attempts can be made to

Pediatric severe TBI management flow sheet

CHECK
- Patient position (head neutral, elevated HOB 30°)
- Equipment functioning properly (good waveform)
- No recent interventions (respiratory, nursing)
- Exclude seizure activity

FLUID THERAPY, VASOPRESSORS
- Maintain CVP 5 to 10 mm Hg (NS for fluid resuscitation)
- Use D5W/NSaline for maint. Adjust dextrose concentration to maintain serum glucose 80-150 mg/dL
- Maintain Hb >10, HCT >33 (Use packed RBC's)
- Once volume loaded use inotropic/vasopressor support

SEDATION AND ANALGESIA
- Sedate to sedation score of 4
- Midazolam
- Fentanyl or
- Morphine
- Avoid hypotension secondary to sedative/analgesic agents

CSF DRAINAGE OPTIONS
- Initial settings and changes to draining level per pediatric neurosurgery service
- Drain CSF for 15 min, then re-evaluate ICP. If persistent CPP deficit or ICP >20, consider continuous CSF drainage with intermittent reading of ICP (close drain for 5 min to obtain reading)

HYPEROSMOLAR THERAPIES
- Use mannitol if normotensive (see osmolar therapy algorithm for dose, scheduling and labs)
- Hypertonic saline (3%): Use before mannitol if patient hemoynamically unstable (see osmolar therapy algorithm for dose, scheduling and labs).

CONSIDER 2nd tier therapy
- Check perfusion indices—is there evidence of hyperemia? (PbtO$_2$ >35 mm Hg)
  -If hyperemic, consider transient controlled hyperventilation (PCO$_2$ 25-35 mm Hg) to normalize perfusion indices (keep PbtO$_2$ >20 mm Hg)
  - Consider low dose barbiturates.
- Not hyperemic
  - Is the patient salvageable?
    (a) Assess: Mechanism of injury, best GCS, age, pupil reactivity, CT scan
    (b) Frontal focal contusions with initial good GCS consider decompressive craniectomy
    (c) Barbiturate therapy: Pentobarbital infusion to burst suppression

Flow chart:

GCS ≤8 → Surgery as indicated

Art line, ETCO$_2$, CVP, ICP monitor, and Licox (PbtO$_2$, Tbt) as indicated

Goals of management:
1. Maintain adequate MAP (age specific)
2. Fluids to maintain CVP 5 to 10 mm Hg
3. Na+ >140
4. Hb >10 g/dL, HCT>33
5. Adequate sedation and analgesia
6. Brain/core temperature 37 ± 0.5°C
7. O$_2$ sat >96%, PaCO$_2$ 37 ± 2 mm Hg (tolerate higher if normal ICP)
8. 25 mm Hg <brain PO$_2$ (PbtO$_2$) <35 mm Hg

CPP deficit (see text for CPP values for age) → CHECK

Low MAP / ICP >20 mm Hg for 5 min

Fluid therapy, vasopressors / Sedation and analgesia

Consider repeating CT scan ← ICP >20 mm Hg for 5 min

Check perfusion indices

PbtO$_2$ <20 / PbtO$_2$ >20

- Confirm data is valid and correct abnormal/critical values (see PbtO$_2$ algorithm)
- Check CVP/PCWP and CPP
- Is CPP appropriate:
- Ensure adequate sedation
- Titrate PCO$_2$ to 35 ± 2 mm Hg

Persisting CPP deficit ICP >20 mm Hg

Drain CSF if ventriculostomy present

Persisting CPP deficit ICP >20 mm Hg

Hyperosmolar therapies

Persisting CPP deficit ICP >20 mm Hg

Consider 2nd tier therapy

FIGURE 19-6 ■ This management algorithm focuses on a set of goals and relies on the coordinated input of a number of monitored variables to provide a method for identifying underlying pathophysiology and assisting in directing management.

correct critical PbtO$_2$ values by titrating the FiO$_2$ to keep the patient's PbtO$_2$ lesser than 20 mm Hg. When titrating FiO$_2$ for prolonged periods of therapy, it is suggested that the FiO$_2$ be kept greater than or equal to 60%. In the context of low brain oxygenation, glucose control (serum glucose 80-180) is important after TBI because of the deleterious effects of hyperglycemia or hypoglycemia in the setting of brain ischemia.

Cerebral Hyperthermia

Elevated temperature can contribute to worsening brain injury after severe TBI. A number of trials are looking at hypothermia as a management technique to improve outcome after traumatic brain injury. It has been reported to be effective in some centers, but at present this treatment has not been proven to be effective in a multicenter trial. While the efficacy of hypothermia after severe TBI in children remains to be determined, our management approach does include temperature control aimed at maintaining normothermia. Brain temperature can now be measured continuously. The brain temperature probe comes as part of the PbtO$_2$ setup and does not require any additional equipment. Our current management strategy is to maintain a brain temperature of 37 ± 0.5°C. This we achieve by active cooling as required. If brain temperature monitoring is not available, continuous temperature monitoring using either an esophageal, rectal, or Foley catheter temperature probe is recommended. Oral and axillary temperature measurements are discouraged, especially when using external cooling. Fever is combated aggressively because of the impact that high temperature can have in outcome after several types of brain injury, including trauma. While attempting to normalize brain/core temperature, shivering remains an issue. Shivering is considered a problem not only because it is uncomfortable to patients but also because it can increase ICP. Pharmacologic and nonpharmacologic interventions to avoid shivering should be attempted in order to assure effective temperature regulation and prevent raises in ICP. Such interventions may include transient use of neuromuscular blockade.

A Coordinated Target-Specific Management Approach

The primary concern when taking care of children with severe TBI is maintaining adequate cerebral perfusion— "perfuse it or lose it"—while optimizing relevant physiologic and clinical variables such as temperature and level of sedation. The initial monitoring setup may include an arterial line and central venous line if hemodynamically indicated; ICP monitor—ventriculostomy or intraparenchymal microsensor; pulse oximetry;

end- tidal CO$_2$, and the PbtO$_2$ and temperature probes. The risk/benefit ratio of all monitoring devices and therapeutic interventions should be carefully analyzed by the multidisciplinary team usually involved in the complex care of this fragile patient population.

REFERENCES

1. MacKenzie, EJ: Epidemiology of injuries: current trends and future challenges. *Epidemiol Rev.* 2000;22:112.
2. Prins, ML and Hovda, DA: Developing experimental models to address traumatic brain injury in children. *J Neurotrauma.* 2003;20:123.
3. Centers for Disease Control and Prevention: America's Children in Brief: Key National Indicators of Well-Being, 2006. *Centers for Disease Control and Prevention, National Center for Health Statistics, National Vital Statistics System.* 2006;
4. Keenan, HT and Bratton, SL: Epidemiology and outcomes of pediatric traumatic brain injury. *Dev Neurosci.* 2006; 28:256.
5. Scheidler, MG, et al: Risk factors and predictors of mortality in children after ejection from motor vehicle crashes. *J Trauma.* 2000;49:864.
6. Zenel, J and Goldstein, B: Child abuse in the pediatric intensive care unit. *Crit Care Med.* 2002;30:S515.
7. Langlois, JA, et al: The incidence of traumatic brain injury among children in the United States: differences by race. *J Head Trauma Rehabil.* 2005;20:229.
8. Jennett, B and Bond, M: Assessment of outcome after severe brain damage. *Lancet.* 1975;1:480.
9. Jankowitz, BT and Adelson, PD: Pediatric traumatic brain injury: past, present and future. *Dev Neurosci.* 2006;28:264.
10. Reilly, PL, et al: Assessing the conscious level in infants and young children: a paediatric version of the Glasgow Coma Scale. *Childs Nerv Syst.* 1988;4:30.
11. Holmes, JF, et al: Performance of the pediatric glasgow coma scale in children with blunt head trauma. *Acad Emerg Med.* 2005;12:814.
12. Rimel, RW, et al: Disability caused by minor head injury. *Neurosurgery.* 1981;9:221.
13. The management of minor closed head injury in children. Committee on Quality Improvement, American Academy of Pediatrics. Commission on Clinical Policies and Research, American Academy of Family Physicians. *Pediatrics.* 1999;104:1407.
14. Kelly, JP and Rosenberg, JH: The development of guidelines for the management of concussion in sports. *J Head Trauma Rehabil.* 1998;13:53.
15. Boran, BO, et al: Evaluation of mild head injury in a pediatric population. *Pediatr Neurosurg.* 2006;42:203.
16. Mendelson, KG and Fallat, ME: Pediatric injuries: prevention to resolution. *Surg Clin North Am.* 2007;87:207.
17. Ducrocq, SC, et al: Epidemiology and early predictive factors of mortality and outcome in children with traumatic severe brain injury: experience of a French pediatric trauma center. *Pediatr Crit Care Med.* 2006;7:461.
18. Kirkwood, MW, et al: Pediatric sport-related concussion: a review of the clinical management of an oft-neglected population. *Pediatrics.* 2006;117:1359.

19. Duus, BR, et al: Prognostic signs in the evaluation of patients with minor head injury. *Br J Surg.* 1993;80:988.

20. Wilde, EA, et al: Diffusion tensor imaging in the corpus callosum in children after moderate to severe traumatic brain injury. *J Neurotrauma.* 2006;23:1412.

21. Duhaime, AC and Partington, MD: Overview and clinical presentation of inflicted head injury in infants. *Neurosurg Clin N Am.* 2002;13:149.

22. Statler, KD: Pediatric posttraumatic seizures: epidemiology, putative mechanisms of epileptogenesis and promising investigational progress. *Dev Neurosci.* 2006; 28:354.

23. Harmon, KG: Assessment and management of concussion in sports. *Am Fam Physician.* 1999;60: 887.

24. Adelson, PD, et al: Guidelines for the acute medical management of severe traumatic brain injury in infants, children, and adolescents. Chapter 1: Introduction. *Pediatr Crit Care Med.* 2003;4:S2.

25. Adelson, PD, et al: Guidelines for the acute medical management of severe traumatic brain injury in infants, children, and adolescents. Chapter 8. Cerebral perfusion pressure. *Pediatr Crit Care Med.* 2003;4:S31.

26. Haque, IU and Zaritsky, AL: Analysis of the evidence for the lower limit of systolic and mean arterial pressure in children. *Pediatr Crit Care Med.* 2007;8:138.

27. Vavilala, MS, et al: Blood pressure and outcome after severe pediatric traumatic brain injury. *J Trauma.* 2003;55: 1039.

28. Adelson, PD, et al: Guidelines for the acute medical management of severe traumatic brain injury in infants, children, and adolescents. Chapter 6. Threshold for treatment of intracranial hypertension. *Pediatr Crit Care Med.* 2003;4:S25.

29. Hsiang, JK, et al: Early, routine paralysis for intracranial pressure control in severe head injury: is it necessary? *Crit Care Med.* 1994;22:1471.

30. Levy, DI, et al: Controlled lumbar drainage in pediatric head injury. *J Neurosurg.* 1995;83:453.

31. Garcia-Morales, EJ, et al: Osmole gap in neurologic-neurosurgical intensive care unit: Its normal value, calculation, and relationship with mannitol serum concentrations. *Crit Care Med.* 2004;32:986.

32. Gondim Fde, A, et al: Osmolality not predictive of mannitol-induced acute renal insufficiency. *J Neurosurg.* 2005;103:444.

33. Dominguez, TE, et al: Caution should be exercised when maintaining a serum sodium level >160 meq/L. *Crit Care Med.* 2004;32:1438.

34. Muizelaar, JP, et al: Adverse effects of prolonged hyperventilation in patients with severe head injury: a randomized clinical trial. *J Neurosurg.* 1991;75:731.

35. Figaji, AA, et al: Brain tissue oxygen tension monitoring in pediatric severe traumatic brain injury : Part 1: Relationship with outcome. *Childs Nerv Syst.* 2009;

36. Stiefel, MF, et al: Reduced mortality rate in patients with severe traumatic brain injury treated with brain tissue oxygen monitoring. *J Neurosurg.* 2005;103:805.

37. Quayle, KS, et al: Diagnostic testing for acute head injury in children: when are head computed tomography and skull radiographs indicated? *Pediatrics.* 1997;99:E11.

38. Hennes, H, et al: Clinical predictors of severe head trauma in children. *Am J Dis Child.* 1988;142:1045.

39. Rivara, F, et al: Poor prediction of positive computed tomographic scans by clinical criteria in symptomatic pediatric head trauma. *Pediatrics.* 1987;80:579.

40. Dietrich, AM, et al: Pediatric head injuries: can clinical factors reliably predict an abnormality on computed tomography? *Ann Emerg Med.* 1993;22:1535.

41. Ramundo, ML, et al: Clinical predictors of computed tomographic abnormalities following pediatric traumatic brain injury. *Pediatr Emerg Care.* 1995;11:1.

CHAPTER 20

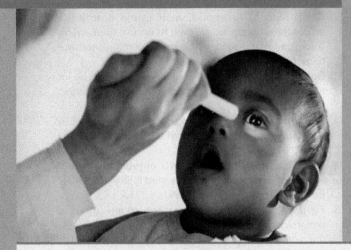

Toxic and Metabolic Encephalopathies

Edgard Andrade and Ronald Sanders

Metabolic disorders and disorders caused by exposure to a toxic agent portend a good prognosis, leading most of the time to a full recovery when recognized and treated promptly. Despite significant advances in critical care in the last 30 years, leading to improved survival of affected patients, little advance has been made in the treatment of acute neurological problems in the pediatric population. Metabolic disorders represent an exception to this statement, due to the development of new diagnostic techniques combined with a better understanding of the pathophysiology of such disorders, which have lead to the application of life-saving therapeutic tools and reducing the severity of brain injury. Examples include hemodialysis for the treatment of urea cycle disorders[1] (eg, citrulinemia). In addition, significant advances in communication have made more readily available consultative expertise through academic centers worldwide. Access to the Internet has allowed most practitioners managing patients with a toxic or metabolic encephalopathy to maintain the highest standards of treatment, reduce injury, improve survival, and reverse changes in the penumbra zone of the affected areas of the brain.

This chapter is an approach to the different etiologies causing a metabolic derangement leading to a toxic or metabolic encephalopathy, and classified according to the age of the patient. Also, this chapter provides a wide overview of the pathogenesis, clinical approach, and treatment of patients affected with such disorders.

DEFINITIONS

Toxic and metabolic encephalopathies refers to a group of disorders characterized by changes in the level of consciousness due to an exogenous or endogenous substance causing a metabolic derangement in the normal neuronal activity and leading to a transient or permanent damage of neuronal pathways (see Figure 20-1). The source of the injurious substrate can be from (1) a malfunctioning organ such as the liver or kidney, (2) an outside source such as a poisoning, or (3) deregulation of internal homeostasis as seen in primary or secondary electrolyte disturbances. Either pathway leads to compromise of autoregulation of the blood-brain barrier or internal brain homeostasis. Several etiologies are included in this syndrome and classified in two groups: congenital and acquired disorders.[2] Causes of acquired disorders are listed in Table 20-1 and include exogenous poisoning (eg, methanol, ethanol, and ethylene glycol), diabetes mellitus, uremia, and late-onset congenital enzymatic deficiencies. Causes of congenital disorders leading to a toxic metabolic encephalopathy can be divided into early and late onset, based on the clinical presentation, and include organic acidurias, congenital glycosylation disorders, and neurotransmitter deficiencies[3] (Table 20-2). For better understanding, definitions of several terms used when describing patients with altered mental status have been summarized in Table 20-3.

In the newborn, differential diagnosis considerations include two categories: disorders of glucose/ion metabolism and genetically programmed congenital errors of the metabolism. Disorders of glucose/ion metabolism are generally correctable if suspected and diagnosed promptly. Three important disorders in this category are (1) salt-wasting syndromes, (2) congenital hypothyroidism, and (3) vitamin D-dependent rickets. There are two different groups of genetically programmed congenital errors of metabolism that we classify based on clinical presentation: (1) acute-onset neurological derangement and (2) static encephalopathies of prenatal onset such as peroxysomal disorders. Several classifications

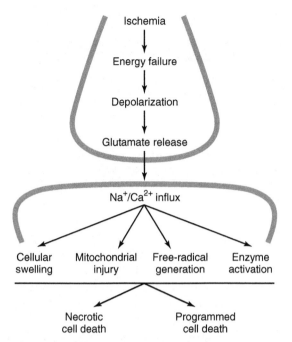

Ischemia

↓

Energy failure

↓

Depolarization

↓

Glutamate release

↓

Na⁺/Ca²⁺ influx

Cellular swelling | Mitochondrial injury | Free-radical generation | Enzyme activation

Necrotic cell death | Programmed cell death

FIGURE 20-1 ■ Pathogenesis of ischemic neuronal death. Ischemia deprives the brain of metabolic substrates, especially glucose, making it impossible for cells to carry out energy-dependent functions such as the maintenance of trans-membrane ion gradients. Loss of these gradients depolarizes cell membranes, leading to the influx of calcium through voltage-gated calcium channels and triggering the release of neurotransmitters such as glutamate from presynaptic nerve terminals. Glutamate binds to receptors on the postsynaptic neuronal membrane to activate the influx of sodium and calcium. This sets in motion a cascade of biochemical events that causes cellular swelling, injures mitochondria, generates toxic free radicals, and activates proteases, nucleases, and other enzymes. Depending on the severity and duration of ischemia, neurons may die rapidly, from necrosis, or more gradually, from programmed cell death or apoptosis. Necrotic cell death is characterized by shrinkage of the nucleus (pyknosis), early loss of membrane integrity, structural changes in mitochondria, and eventually cellular lysis. Programmed cell death (PCD) depends on the synthesis of new proteins. Apoptosis, one form of PCD, is associated with margination of nuclear chromatin, relative preservation of cell membrane and mitochondrial integrity, and the formation of membrane-bound extracellular blebs (apoptotic bodies). Necrosis and PCD can coexist in different regions of an ischemic lesion. (*Reproduced with permission from Aminoff MJ, Greenberg, DA, Simon RP: Clinical Neurology, 6ed. McGraw-Hill, Inc. New York, 2005. Figure 9-3.*)

have been attempted to better grade the severity of the symptoms. We have developed our own classification based on clinical findings and degree of impairment (Table 20-4).

Table 20-1.[4]

Acquired Causes of Metabolic Encephalopathy

Diabetes mellitus
Uremia
Liver failure[5]
Sepsis
Infectious etiologies such as HIV and hepatitis A, B, C, and D

Table 20-2.

Congenital Causes of Metabolic Encephalopathy

Urea cycle disorders
Disorders of congenital glycosylation
Congenital neurotransmitter deficiency

PATHOGENESIS

Disorders of Glucose and Ion Metabolism

Disorders of glucose and ion metabolism should be considered in the differential diagnosis of patients with altered level of consciousness. Under normal circumstances, glucose is the main source of energy for the brain. The brain is extremely susceptible to hypoglycemia. This is due to the fact that brain glucose is only 25% of the total blood glucose. Besides, there are no significant sources of stored glucose in the form of glycogen, as happens in cardiac or skeletal muscle. The central nervous system better tolerates hyperglycemia than hypoglycemia. However, hyperglycemia can cause significant neurological symptoms.

After having a load of glucose, the pancreas releases large amounts of insulin that regulate the glucose metabolism. Several other mechanisms are triggered after food ingestion, including storage of glucose in the liver as glycogen (glycogenosis). The human body has enough glycogen to maintain the blood glucose concentration between 80 and 100 mg/dL for 24 to 36 hours after having a last meal. Then, generation of glycogen (gluconeogenesis) takes over as the main mechanism for glucose control. Alanine and glutamate as well as lactic and pyruvic acid are well-known substrates for energy formation in this setting. The liver is the main organ involved in the process of maintaining glucose during starvation. After the hepatic sources for glucose have been depleted, the kidneys and other organs could contribute up to 50% of basal glucose. This explains why several organs are clinically involved during the severe hypoglycemic stage.

Table 20-3.

Altered Level of Consciousness: Definitions

Lethargy: Inability to maintain the arousal state.
Obtundation: Responsive to verbal or tactile stimuli
Stupor: Responsive to pain
Coma: Unresponsive to any stimuli, including pain

Table 20-4.

Clinical Staging of Metabolic Encephalopathy

System	Mild	Moderate	Severe
Upper cortical function	Lethargy/obtundation	Stupor	Coma
Brainstem	Hypertension/tachycardia	Hypotension	Absent protective reflexes
White matter symptoms	Hyper/hyporeflexia	Hyper/hypotonia	Spasticity, contractures
Gray matter symptoms	—	Clinical seizures	Subclinical seizures

The mean cerebral blood flow is 50 mL/100 g of brain tissue. This flow provides large amounts of glucose to the brain if the peripheral glycemia is between 5 and 6 mmol/L. A cerebrospinal glucose transporter protein maintains appropriate CSF glucose level. Once in the brain, the glucose is metabolized into ATP by two main pathways: glycolisis and the Krebs cycle. Detailed review of both processes is beyond the scope of this chapter. However, faulty glycolitic mechanisms are responsible for significant systemic and neurological symptoms. A congenital disorder characterized by seizures and developmental delay has been identified—glucose transporter deficiency. In this disorder, cerebrospinal fluid (CSF) glucose is low due to a faulty glucose transporter protein. A ketogenic diet appears to be one of the main therapeutic tools available for better seizure control in this population. However, a ketogenic diet does not appear to modify other aspects of the disorder, such as developmental delay. Genetic testing is available for patients suspected to have glucose transporter deficiency.

Hypoglycemia

The most common causes of hypoglycemia are (1) overuse of glucose, as seen in carnitine deficiency, sepsis, prediabetic state, and oral hypoglycemic abuse; (2) underproduction of glucose, as seen in enzymatic disorders[6] (glucose-6-phosphatase deficiency, glycogen phosphorylase deficiency, glycogen synthetase deficiency, pyruvate carboxylase deficiency, and phosphoenolpyruvate carboxykinase deficiency); and (3) hormonal imbalances (eg, growth hormone). Maternal use of hypoglycemic medications or neonatal sepsis are the most common causes in the newborn period. Salycilate overdose and alcohol intoxication should be ruled out in the teenage population. There are three hypoglycemic syndromes: acute, subacute, and chronic.

1. Patients presenting in the acute state are usually restless and complain of dizziness or nervousness. Most of the time, patients presenting with an acute hypoglycemic state have a past history of diabetes mellitus. The most common cause of hypoglycemia in this group of patients is due to overdose of insulin or oral hypoglycemic medications. Symptoms usually resolve with a loading dose of IV glucose.

2. The subacute syndrome is characterized by obtundation, slowness of thought process, and amnesia. It is not uncommon to find hypothermia. The diagnosis is confirmed by checking the blood glucose during one of the episodes.

3. Chronic hypoglycemia is an uncommon situation, and when suspected, an insulinoma or excessive use of antihyperglycemic medications should be considered. Unlike the two prior groups, patients with chronic hypoglycemia usually do not respond to boluses of intravenous glucose.

Hyperglycemia

The most common cause of hyperglycemia in the pediatric population is diabetic ketoacidosis (DKA). This condition is usually triggered by an infection in an otherwise well-controlled diabetic type I patient, or can present as new-onset hyperglycemia in an otherwise previously healthy patient, prompting a visit to the emergency room due to obtundation or other changes in the level of consciousness. In addition to polyurea and polydipsia, symptoms include anorexia, nausea, vomit, dehydration, and coma. This is a disorder of severe deficit of insulin. In the absence of insulin, the body's peripheral glucose uptake and glycogen formation are inhibited, leading to excessive lypolisis, glycogenolysis, and hyperglycemia. Treatment with insulin enhances entry of glucose in to the cell, glycogen formation, and reduction of the rate of ketone body formation. Supportive treatment is based on the judicious correction of hypernatremia and dehydration. An excessively rapid correction of hypernatremia and hyperosmolarity may lead to cerebral edema. It is believed that a clinically silent form of cerebral edema may be present in most cases of DKA. When clinically indicated, further evaluation, including placement of an intracranial pressure monitor, should be considered to better guide therapy. The treatment of cerebral edema in this particular setting is based in decreasing the elevated intracranial pressure, including intubation, mechanical ventilation, elevation of the head, hyperoxygenation, and measures aiming to avoid Valsalva maneuvers such as treating constipation and avoiding excessive gag or suction stimuli to the throat or the trachea. The use of manitol to facilitate osmogenic diuresis is one of the pharmacologic tools available when treating patients with cerebral edema.

Disorders of Sodium Metabolism

When hyponatremia is confirmed, serum osmolarity must also be checked, since hyponatremia and hypoosmolarity are both frequently associated. Causes include renal loss (renal disease, adrenal insufficiency), gastrointestinal losses (diarrhea, vomit), sequestration (peritonitis), hemodilution, sickle cell disease, hyperosmosis, hyperglycemia, and inappropriate secretion of antidiuretic hormone (SIADH). In addition to hyponatremia, the diagnosis of SIADH should be suspected in the normovolemic or hypervolemic patient with documented normal renal function.

Water restriction is usually the treatment for mild cases. More severe cases require hypertonic solutions and diuretic treatment. Excessive overcorrection may lead to hypernatremia and central pontine myelonolisis (CPM). This last disorder is characterized by acute demyelination of the pontine structures due to fast correction of hyponatremia. Patients with CPM develop a myriad of symptoms including changes in sensorium, lower cranial nerve palsies, and diffuse weakness. Serial and frequent serum electrolytes monitoring and avoidance of excessive administration of hypertonic, hypernatremic solutions are needed to prevent this irreversible and permanent complication. Brain MRI typically show areas of demyelination in the mamillary bodies and around the fourth ventricle (see Figure 20-2).

Hyperosmolarity

Hyperosmolarity should be suspected in diabetic patients or in an otherwise healthy person presenting with severe dehydration and acute intracranial bleeding. Bleeding occurs due to tearing of the bridging vessels at the level of the dural sinuses. The deficit of water should be estimated carefully and replacement therapy should be started promptly, bearing in mind that a fast correction

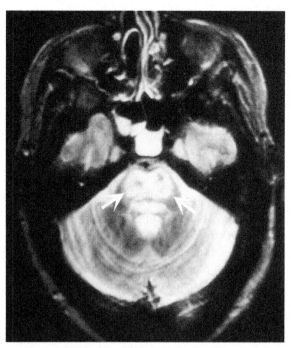

FIGURE 20-2 ■ Central pontine myelinolysis. Axial T2-weighted MR scan through the pons reveals a symmetric area of abnormal high signal intensity within the basis pontis (arrows).(*Reproduced with permission from Fauci AS, Kasper DL, Braunwald E, Hauser SL, Longo DL, Jameson JL, Loscalzo J: Harrison's Principles of Internal Medicine, 17th ed. McGraw-Hill, Inc. New York, 2008. Figure 269-6.*)

may lead to brain swelling. In general, it is recommended to attempt correction by the oral route, aiming to replace the deficits slowly.

Disorders of Calcium Metabolism

This group of disorders is usually associated with a deficient parathyroid gland function. In normal circumstances, about 50% of the serum calcium is bound to protein and therefore considered metabolically in quiescent form. The other 50% is ionized and therefore metabolically active. Hyperthyroidism may be associated with hypercalcemia and should be part of the differential diagnosis when evaluating patients with idiopathic hypercalcemia. Symptoms of hypercalcemia range from altered consciousness, weakness, and nausea and vomitting to coma. The most common causes of hypercalcemia are sarcoidosis, thiazide diuretics, vitamin D intoxication, and excessive calcium intake. Treatment includes hydration, diuresis, and supportive treatment.

Hypothyroidism is usually associated with hypocalcemia. Clinically, patients complain of paresthesias around the mouth and fingers, cramps, headaches, and seizures. The presence of positive Chvostek and Trousseau signs documented in the physical examination should raise the index of suspicion. Chovstek sign consists of tapping the thenar region and looking for a spasmodic contracture of the hand. Trousseau sign is usually elicited in the hypocalcemic patient when the cuff of a blood pressure monitoring device is applied to the arm and inflated above the diastolic pressure until a tonic contracture of the arm is present. Both findings are indicative of hypocalcemia. Treatment is based in administration of calcium to correct the deficit.

Hypothyroidism can also present clinically as idiopathic intracranial hypertension, formerly known as pseudotumor cerebri. Postural headaches, sixth cranial nerve palsy, and blunted optic disk borders are typical findings. Optic disk edema is a common finding. Figure 20-3 shows blunting of the optic disc borders and elevation of retinal blood vessels. Patients may complain of having blurry or double vision and early morning headaches. The pathophysiology of benign increased intracranial pressure syndrome is not well understood, but a mismatch between excessive CSF production by the choroid plexus and deficient CSF reabsorption mechanisms has been postulated. The diagnosis is suspected when the patient has a focal neurological exam such as optic disk edema or sixth cranial nerve palsy and has a normal brain MRI. The spinal tap is both diagnostic and therapeutic. An opening spinal pressure above 25 ml H20, within the right clinical setting, is confirmatory. Then, drainage of cerebro-spinal fluid is the treatment of choice. The aim is to drain enough CSF to bring the

Table 20-5.

Causes of Increased Intracranial Pressure Syndrome

Infectious	Systemic Disorders
Lyme disease	Iron deficiency anemia
Rocky Mountain spotted fever	Systemic lupus erythematosus
Cat scratch disease	Leukemia
	Malnutrition
Metabolic	Guillain-Barré syndrome
Hyperthyroidism	
Hypoparathyroidism	**Drugs**
Pregnancy	Vitamin A deficiency/excess
Adrenal insufficiency	Oral contraceptive pills
Diabetic ketoacidosis	INH
	Vitamin D deficiency
	Thyroid replacement hormones
	Corticosteroids

closing pressure to half the opening pressure. A comprehensive list of etiologies causing idiopathic increased intracranial pressure is given in Table 20-5. In nearly 60% of the cases, the cause is not established (idiopathic). When established, the treatment should be aimed to treat the cause. Early diagnosis and treatment should be established promptly to prevent further injury to the optic nerve and subsequent permanent blindness. Carbonic anhydrase inhibitors such as acetazolamide are usually the first line of therapy by decreasing the production of CSF. Other potential options are loop diuretics such as furosemide or corticosteroids such as prednisone. Patients with idiopathic intracranial pressure that fail medical treatment should be referred to the neurosurgeon for a decompressive procedure of the optic nerves such as optic nerve fenestration. Consultative expertise obtained from a neuro-opthalmologist should also be sought to better guide the therapy.

CLINICAL PRESENTATION

Toxic and metabolic encephalopathy should be considered in the differential diagnosis of patients with altered mental status. Patients may present with a myriad of symptoms including lethargy, obtundation, stupor, or coma. Lethargy is defined as an inability to maintain arousal. Obtundation is characterized by significant altered level of consciousness that is responsive at least to verbal stimuli. Stupor is a more significant abnormal level of consciousness in which patients are only responsive to pain. Coma implies full unresponsiveness to any type of stimuli (Table 20-6). Patients with toxic encephalopathy present with the acute onset of symptoms. Changes in sensorium, cognitive decline, jaundice, headaches, anemia,

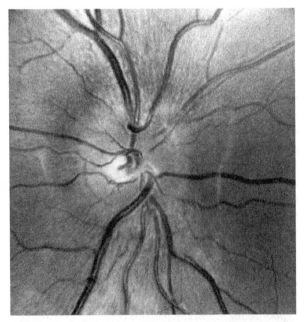

FIGURE 20-3 ■ Mild papilledema. The disk margins are blurred superiorly and inferiorly by the thickened layer of nerve fibers entering the disk. (*Reproduced, with permission, from Vaughan DG, Asbury T, Riordan-Eva P [editors]: General Ophthalmology, 15th ed. Originally published by Appleton & Lange. Copyright © 1999 by The McGraw-Hill Companies, Inc.*)

Table 20-6.

Glasgow Coma Scale

Eye Opening

Spontaneously	4
To verbal commands	3
To nociceptive stimuli	2
No response	1

Best Motor Response

Follows commands	6
Localizes painful stimuli	5
Withdraws to painful stimuli	4
Abnormal flexion	3
Abnormal extension	2
No response	1

Verbal Response

Oriented	5
Confused	4
Makes inappropriate words	3
Makes incomprehensive sounds	2
No response	1

Table 20-7.[7]

Etiology of Toxic and Metabolic Encephalopathies

Ion Metabolism
Hyponatremia
Hypernatremia
Hyperkalemia
Hypocalcemia
Hypomagnesemia

Glucose Homeostasis
Hypoglycemia
Diabetic ketoacidosis

Metabolic Disorders Due to Inborn Errors of Metabolism
Nonketotic hyperglycinemia
Glycogen storage disease
Mitochondrial disorders: acyl carnitine deficiency
Pyruvic dehydrogenase deficiency
Urea cycle disorders (citrullinemia)

Renal Disorders
Uremia (chronic, acute)
Dialysis
Hypertension

Endocrine Disorders
Hypothryroidism
Thyroid storm (hyperthyroidism)
Adrenal insufficiency
Hyperparathyroidism

Epilepsy
Subclinical seizures
Postictal state

Migraine
Occipital migraines

Toxic
Substance abuse
Prescription drugs
Over-the-counter drug abuse
Ciguatera toxin

Infectious Disorders
Bacterial infections: meningitis, toxic shock syndrome, and cat scratch disease
Viral infections: enterovirus, measles, and West Nile virus encephalitis
Others: Lyme disease, Rocky Mountain spotted fever

and seizures are usual common clinical scenarios. More focal neurological findings are seen in selected cases. For example, patients with homocystinuria are at increased risk of stroke and therefore may present with acute, new onset hemiparesis or visual complaints. The differential diagnosis is listed in Table 20-7.

Drug Overdose

Toxic exposure to a drug, whether accidental or intentional, should always be suspected in the patient presenting with altered mental status or in coma. Accidental poisoning is commonly seen in the toddler who finds readily available bottles of medications in the surroundings. Intentional poisoning due to a suicidal plan is most often seen in the teenage patient. The most common toxic substances abused are alcohol, salycilates, acetaminophen, benzodiazepines, barbiturates, and antidepressants. Serum screening tests are the best way to confirm an overdose. Patients with suspected ethylene glycol toxicity would have the history of antifreeze exposure. The blood level predicts the toxicity. Similar situations occurs with acetaminophen, digoxin, lithium, salicylates, and theophylline. Methanol poisoning is a special consideration. Patients have the history of consumption of alcohol that has been fraudulently altered. Symptoms include blindness and coma. Methanol is

metabolized by the enzyme alcohol dehydrogenase into formaldehyde, a more deleterious byproduct, causing a wide range of demyelinating effects in the nervous system. The optic nerve is particularly sensitive to the effects of formaldehyde and therefore blindness is a common complication. Treatment is aimed to block the alcohol dehydrogenase. IV alcohol is available as a first-line therapy in such patients.

Congenital Inborn Errors of Metabolism

Maple syrup urine disease

Maple syrup urine disease is an autosomal recessive disorder of the metabolism of amino acids due to absence or faulty functioning of the branching-chain alpha ketoacid dehydrogenase enzyme and leading to toxic accumulation of alpha-amino acids valine, leucin, and isoleucin. There are five different forms, but the neonatal presentation has the worst prognosis. Patients present with changes in level of consciousness after the first week of life.[8] Then, seizures, hypotonia, and poor oral intake are present. Brain imaging will demonstrate edema of the white matter. Ketoacidosis, hypoglycemia, and ketonuria are typical laboratory findings. Histopathology evaluation shows spongiform degeneration of white matter. The diagnosis is suspected when high levels of valine, leucin, and isoleucin are found during an acute exacerbation. Measurement of enzyme activity in fibroblasts is diagnostic. During acute crisis, treatment is supported by removal of the excessive concentration of amino acids using hemodialysis or peritoneal dialysis. Long-term treatment includes a valine-restriction diet, avoidance of catabolic stress, and good nutritional support.

Organic acidopathies

Branched-chain amino-acidopathies are autosomal recessive disorders of the metabolism of propionate and methyl malonate and their cofactors biotin and cobalamin. Onset of clinical symptoms ranges from the neonatal period to early infancy, and includes various forms of hypoglycemia, metabolic acidosis, hyperamonemia, seizures, and coma.[9] Other features include growth failure, abnormal liver function test, neutropenia, thrombocytopenia, and cardiovascular collapse. The pathogenesis of this disease is due to accumulation of a substrate in the toxic ranges. Lack of energy production is the result of a deficient supply of highly efficient energetic compounds for gluconeogenesis and limited availability of free CoA for mitochondrial fatty acid oxidation. The diagnosis is suspected when a neonate or a young child presents with metabolic acidosis, hypoglycemia, hyperamonemia, and ketosis. Further enzymatic testing using skin fibroblast cultures can confirm the diagnosis. The treatment consists of glucose administration, protein restriction, and cardiovascular and respiratory support in the critical care settings. Cofactor supplementation is useful to reverse the pathogenic process. Carnitine and glycine supplementation will improve clearance of the toxic metabolites.

DIAGNOSIS

The presentation of a delirious child to the emergency room should prompt expeditious and organized evaluation due to the potential for deterioration if not diagnosed and treated promptly. The diagnosis should be based on a carefully obtained history and detailed physical and neurological examinations as well. A systematic approach is a must in order to avoid missing an important part of the differential diagnosis. The following questions should be entertained:

1. Timing of the onset of symptoms
2. Provoking or precipitating factors
3. History of toxic ingestions or availability of medications or other substances potentially injurious (eg, prescription medications for other adults living in the same household where the child has been lately seen)
4. Significant past medical history (migraines, epilepsy)
5. Travel history
6. Infectious contacts with a history of encephalopathy
7. Any genetic or metabolic disorders in the family.

The physical exam should be complete, including the vital signs and general appearance of the patient. Findings that should be sought during the physical and neurological exam include the following:

1. Glasgow coma scale score (Table 20-6)
2. Presence of raccoon eyes (suggests injury to the anterior fossa)
3. Presence of retro-auricular bleeding or oozing bloody material per auditory canal (suggests injury to the middle fossa)
4. Nose bleeding or drainage of spinal fluid by nose (injury to the anterior fossa)
5. Scalp tenderness

Clinical History

Children with altered mental status required prompt assessment and treatment because of the risk of rapid deterioration if intervention is not well organized, adequate, and fast. The clinical history is the cornerstone for the correct diagnosis of a delirious child. A diagnostic algorithm has been provided in Figure 20-4 as an attempt to better guide the diagnostic approach when assessing a patient with suspected toxic or metabolic encephalopathy. The following pertinent questions should be considered when assessing a patient with altered mental status:

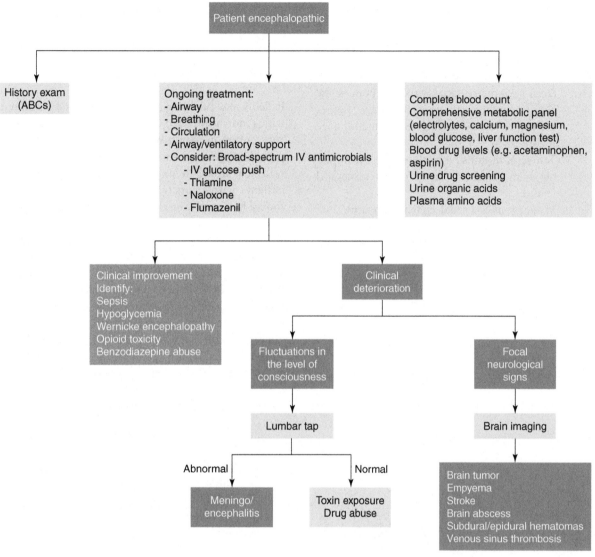

FIGURE 20-4 ■ Diagnostic algorithm for the encephalopathic patient.

1. Prior events leading to the current presentation
2. History of accidental drug exposure, including prescribed or over-the-counter medications available in the home's cabinets
3. Travel history to rural areas
4. Symptoms of systemic illness such as rash, jaundice, malaise, bony tenderness, joint pain, diffuse pain, or fever
5. Prior intercurrent illness (vomiting, diarrhea, cough, runny nose, congestion)
6. History of seizures, migraines
7. Other family members with similar symptoms
8. History of trauma
9. Symptoms suggestive of increased intracranial pressure such as headaches, blurry vision, vomiting, changes in personality, or changes in the level of consciousness

Physical Exam

The physical exam should be tailored according to the patient's age, and should look for the following signs:

1. Complete vital signs, including oxygen saturation
2. Testing of mental status (orientation in time, place, and person; short- and long-term memory; affect, counting, paraphrasing errors; fund of knowledge)
3. Signs of child abuse or neglect (poor hygiene, old fractures, retinal hemorrhages, hematomas, or other skin manifestations of physical abuse)
4. Signs of meningitis such as neck rigidity, Kernig sign (pain and resistance to extending the knees with the leg flexed), or Brudzinski sign (spontaneous flexion at the hips when passively flexing the neck)

5. Careful eye exam looking for papilledema
6. Judicious cranial nerve examination looking for nystagmus, size and reactivity of the pupils to direct and consensual light stimuli, internuclear opthalmoplegias, cranial nerve paresis, facial asymmetry, facial weakness, poor palate elevation, poor gag, poor sucking response, corneal reflex, swallowing, and coughing (see Figure 20-5)
7. Testing of motor strength looking for hemiplegia, hemiparesis, or other focal neurological features
8. Plantar response and deep tendon reflexes
9. Frontal release signs such as palmo-mental reflex (look for oral movements, upon hand stroking), sucking response

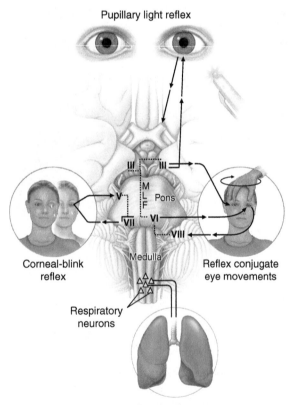

FIGURE 20-5 ■ Examination of brainstem reflexes in coma. Midbrain and third nerve function are tested by pupillary reaction to light, pontine function by spontaneous and reflex eye movements and corneal responses, and medullary function by respiratory and pharyngeal responses. Reflex conjugate, horizontal eye movements are dependent on the medial longitudinal fasciculus (MLF) interconnecting the sixth and contralateral third nerve nuclei. Head rotation (oculocephalic reflex) or caloric stimulation of the labyrinths (oculovestibular reflex) elicits contraversive eye movements. (*Reproduced with permission from Fauci AS, Kasper DL, Braunwald E, Hauser SL, Longo DL, Jameson JL, Loscalzo J: Harrison's Principles of Internal Medicine, 17th ed. McGraw-Hill, Inc. New York, 2008. Figure 268-3.*)

DIFFERENTIAL DIAGNOSIS AND TREATMENT

Inborn Errors of Metabolism

Patients may present with an acute decompensation or with a more protracted clinical syndrome. Seizures are a very common symptom, especially in the neonatal period.[10] Sepsis is the most important differential diagnosis that always should be considered and ruled out in patients with neonatal seizures. Bacterial etiologies should be always considered when assessing an unconscious or poorly responsive baby. Group B streptococcal sepsis is one of the most feared infections in the neonatal period. There are two syndromes: early (less than 2 weeks of age) and late (older than 2 weeks of age). Presenting symptoms and signs are fever or hypothermia, lethargy, seizures, bulging fontanel, and tachypnnea. The patient rapidly deteriorates into septic shock. However, features that help distinguish sepsis from a congenital metabolic disorder are the presence of hyperamonemia, hypoglycemia, and acidosis.

Inherited metabolic disorders characterized by encephalopathy are the following:

1. Pyruvic dehydrogenase deficiency
2. Pyruvate carboxylase deficiency
3. Disorders of hepatic glycogenolisis or gluconeogenesis
4. Respiratory chain disorders
5. Ornithine carbamoylase deficiency
6. Glycogen storage disease
7. Carnitine deficiency

Patients with **glycogen storage diseases** present clinically with hypoglycemic encephalopathy and lactic acidosis. Glucose 6-phosphatase deficiency (type I glycogenosis) is an autosomal recessive disorder. Glucose 6-phosphatase catalyzes the final steps of gluconeogenesis and glycogenosis to produce glucose. Its role is of the utmost importance to maintain glucose homeostasis. Accumulation of its precursor, glucose 6-phosphate, leads into lactic acidemia. Diagnosis is based on determination of enzymatic levels in hepatic tissue, since enzyme is not present in skin fibroblasts. Acute decompensation requires judicious glucose maintenance through intravenous fluids. Long-term treatment requires nocturnal infusions of enteral glucose and frequent, daytime, highly enriched carbohydrate meals.

Fructose 1–6 biphosphatase deficiency is another autosomal recessive disorder presenting clinically as metabolic encephalopathy, lactic academia, and hypoglycemia. This disorder is due to defective gluconeogenesis. In addition to the brain, the liver is also involved. Therefore diagnosis is similar to that for type I glycogenosis. Treatment includes glucose supplementation, sucrose supplementation, and fructose restriction.

Pyruvate dehydrogenase complex deficiency is a disorder of congenital lactic acidemia.[11] Several enzymes could be affected in this disorder. E1 component defect is the most common enzymatic disorder in this group and is inherited as an X-linked dominant trait. Clinically, there is evidence of intrauterine growth retardation, brain dysgenesis (partial and complete agenesis of the corpus callosum), and facial dysmorphology. Fulminant lactic acidosis is a presenting form in the neonatal period. Survivors may develop necrotic changes, and cavitations in the cerebral cortex, basal ganglia, and brainstem.[12] Palliative treatment is based on the use of a ketogenic diet, carnitine supplementation, and thiamine.[13]

Pyruvic carboxylase is a critical pathway in the generation of citric acid during gluconeogenesis. A faulty pyruvic carboxylase enzyme produces marked substrate deficiency for the neurotransmitter pool needed for the synthesis of glutamate and GABA. Severe lactic acidosis, citrullinemia, and hyperamonemia are common findings during acute exacerbations. Diffuse atrophy, both cortical and subcortical, or cystic encephalomalacia, are common radiographic and hystopathologic findings due to neuronal death and arrested myelination.[14,15]

Respiratory chain disorders have in common a defective oxidative phosphorylation pathway. External opthalmoplegia, cardiomyopathy, lactic acidosis, and encephalopathy are common features. Treatment is symptomatic.[16,17]

Medium-chain acyl-CoA dehydrogenase deficiency is an autosomal recessive disorder of the beta-oxidation of fatty acids. Carnitine has two functions: carrying long-chain fatty acids into the mitochondria and modulation of acyl-CoA and esterification of toxic acyl-CoA byproducts. The process of transferring fatty acids inside the inner mitochondrial layer requires the conversion of acyl-CoA and the presence of carnitine palmytoil transferase. If the carnitine concentration is low, toxic levels of acyl-CoA accumulate, leading to mitochondrial dysfunction and poor energy generation. Clinical symptoms include poor exercise tolerance or recurrent episodes of hypoglycemia during acute stress (eg, infection). Poor tolerance to brief periods of hypoglycemia is also a common feature. Proximal weakness is another presenting feature. Although it is less frequent, cardiomyopathy could be a first presenting symptom. Cardiovascular collapse and sudden infant death syndrome (SIDS) have also been reported. However, medium-chain acyl-CoA dehydrogenase deficiency is not an important cause of SIDS. The diagnosis is suspected when low levels of ketone bodies are found in urine during an acute exacerbation along with an elevated concentration of aspartate aminotransferase,

aspartate amino transferase, and lactate dehydrogenase levels. Enzyme deficiency analysis is available. Genetic testing and mutation analysis confirm the diagnosis.

Disorders of Sodium Metabolism and Osmolality

Hypernatremia may be secondary to excessive overhydration with hypertonic solutions or due to excessive water loss during dehydration. It could be seen during periods of acute gastroenteritis, vomiting, and diarrhea. Excessive use of hypertonic solutions could cause iatrogenic hypernatremia.

Nonketotic hyperglycemic coma and diabetic ketoacidosis (DKA) are two complications seen in patients with diabetes mellitus. Nonketotic hyperglycemic coma is an unusual disorder in children and therefore will not be discussed in this chapter. **Diabetic ketoacidosis** is the most common complication of poorly controlled diabetes mellitus. It could also be seen in children with undiagnosed symptomatic hyperglycemia. An intercurrent infectious illness or poor compliance with insulin therapy are the most common triggering factors. Symptoms include polydypsia, lethargy, polyurea, polyphagia, and dehydration. A progressive change in the level of consciousness rapidly ensues, leading to coma if no intervention is provided promptly. Several degrees of cerebral edema are almost universally seen in patients presenting emergently with diabetic ketoacidosis. The mortality rate is 10%, and judicious correction of hyperglycemia, acidosis, and hyponatremia are indicated to improve survival. The diagnosis is established by the presence of hyperglycemia (blood glucose level above 400), acidosis (pH below 7.25 and serum bicarbonate less than 15 mmol/L), and the presence of serum and urine ketones. The treatment is targeted to correct hyperglycemia and fluid deficit during 48 hours. The sodium deficit should be calculated and corrected by half during the first 12 hours of treatment. The other half of the sodium deficit is corrected in the remaining 36 hours. The other issue is to avoid excessive administration of hypotonic fluids because of the risk of worsening the subsequent and ongoing cerebral edema, leading eventually to a brain herniation syndrome if not recognized and treated aggressively. Venous sinus thrombosis and intracranial hemorrhage are also potential complications seen in patients with DKA, and brain imaging should be considered in patients with focal neurological signs. Computed brain tomography taken at 24 hours and at 72 hours after the onset of the symptoms demonstrate an area of infarct in the territory of the left Middle Cerebral Artery (see Figure 20-6).

Hypoglycemia is usually due to insulin overdose. In the neonate, hypoglycemia is due to poor glucose

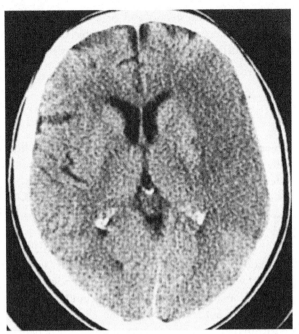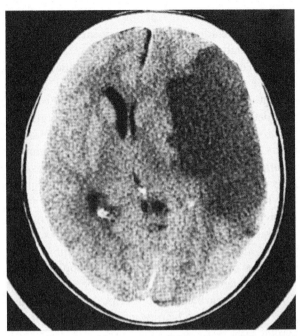

FIGURE 20-6 ■ Massive ischemic infarct of left cerebral hemisphere mainly in the distribution of the superior division of the middle cerebral artery. CT scans taken 24 h (left) and 72 h (right) following the onset of neurologic symptoms. The second scan demonstrates marked swelling of the infarcted tissue and displacement of central structures. (*Reproduced with permission from Ropper AH, Samuels MA: Adams & Victor's Principles of Neurology, 9th ed. McGraw-Hill, Inc. New York, 2009. Figure 34-18.*)

regulation. Sepsis should be suspected in the neonate with symptomatic hypoglycemia. Certain inborn error of the metabolism could initially present with hypoglycemia. However, it is not clinically symptomatic until serum glucose levels drop below 50 mg/dL. Dizziness and tremors progressing to delirium, syncope, and loss of consciousness are the usual presenting symptoms. The diagnosis should be suspected in the jittery or obtunded neonate. Also the diagnosis should be considered in the older patient with a history of diabetes mellitus and presenting with significant altered mental status. Bedside glucometers are readily available for easy and fast diagnosis. Final confirmation is achieved by immediately testing peripheral blood glucose in a recently drawn serum sample. If the patient is symptomatic, IV fluid replacement with a dextrose solution should be administered promptly.

Hyponatremia can be due to two different causes: (1) sodium loss or (2) water retention due to syndrome of inappropriate antidiuretic hormone secretion (SIADH). This complication can be seen in head trauma, meningitis, or intracranial hemorrhage. Clinically, the patient is obtunded or lethargic. Hyponatremia is the hallmark of SIADH. In this disorder, there is an excessive secretion of antidiuretic hormone (ADH), leading to water retention and causing secondary hyponatremia and hypoosmolarity. As a consequence, there is less fluid

filtered into the glomeruli. Urine osmolality is high but not higher than plasma osmolality, and this is an important diagnostic key. Therefore, urine and serum osmolality and serial urine sodium levels should be routinely checked in patients with hyponatremia to confirm the diagnosis. Treatment involves fluid restriction by as much as 50% of the daily recommended allowance.

Sodium loss due to vomiting, diarrhea and dehydration may cause significant disturbances in the level of consciousness leading to hyponatremia and encephalopathy. The patients are usually lethargic. Symptoms may rapidly progress to seizures and coma. The diagnosis is confirmed by measuring serum and urine sodium concentrations. The treatment is targeted to slow correction of hyponatremia up to 130 mEq/L but no more than 0.5 mEq/L per hour for the first 48 hours, using a sodium chloride solution. Fast correction could lead to central pontine myelinolisis, a permanent injury due to coagulation necrosis of the pontine structures.

Hypernatremia can be iatrogenic or due to dehydration. Excessive administration of hypertonic and hypernatremic solutions may lead to iatrogenic hypernatremia, and if this is not recognized, could lead to significant brain injury or death. In addition, patients with vomiting and diarrhea can develop hypernatremic dehydration, especially if there is a restriction of fluid intake. Symptoms are irritability, lethargy, seizures, and coma. Treatment is aimed to correct the hypernatremia slowly. The patient is usually symptomatic when the serum sodium level is above 160 mmol/L. Rapid hypernatremia correction could lead to excessive water retention and cerebral edema with all the potential complications including transtentorial or uncal herniation and death. Therefore, it is recommended to correct the intravascular volume deficit slowly with the use of hyponatremic or normo-natremic solutions. Patients with hypernatremic dehydration are at higher risk for other complications such as venous sinus thrombosis. This complication should be ruled out in the patient with focal neurological signs. Magnetic resonance venography is a useful brain imaging procedure available to exclude this condition.

Renal Disorders

Acute uremic encephalopathy is a complication seen in patients with renal disease. The patient develops symptoms during several days in the setting of abnormal kidney function and elevated creatinine levels. Usually the patient has the history of hemolytic uremic syndrome, or acute renal insufficiency. Lethargy, irritability, and lack of coherence are common symptoms. The physical exam is significant for asterixis, fasciculations, and cramps. Without intervention, patients may develop seizures and become comatose. The diagnosis is suspected when the patient present with acute renal failure and significant acute mental status changes. The severity of the abnormal kidney function does not correlate with the abnormalities of the central nervous system. Elevated ammonia levels, hyperkalemia, and hypercalcemia may contribute to the symptoms. Electroencephalography (EEG) shows diffuse slowing and disorganization of the background and periodic triphasic waves. Measures aimed to correct the electrolyte abnormalities, such as hemodialysis, are the cornerstone of treatment of this population. Prognosis is usually good once the kidney function has normalized

Chronic uremic encephalopathy is a common complication in patients with end-stage renal disease. Patients develop symptoms during weeks or months, and typically have other complications such as hyperthyroidism, hypercalcemia, hyperostosis, and growth failure. Common neurological symptoms are progressive developmental delay in all four domains (fine motor, gross motor, speech, and social). Other common early findings are fine tremors, hyperreflexia, and hypotonia. The symptoms may progress to diffuse myoclonus and fasciculation. Nerve conduction velocities are prolonged. The EMG shows slow amplitude potentials. The EEG shows diffuse slowing of the background activity and multifocal epileptiform discharges. Symptoms may progress to a vegetative state through the years and eventually death. Treatment is aimed to correct the electrolyte abnormalities. Long-term hemodialysis is the most important intervention available to treat the patients.

Hypertensive encephalopathy is a neurological emergency characterized by sudden and uncontrolled high blood pressure above the limits of cerebral blood flow autoregulation. Headaches, nausea, vomiting, and dizziness are common symptoms. Then, visual complaints and progressive changes in the level of consciousness ensue. However, due to the lack of specificity of such complaints, other differential diagnosis should be considered including uremic encephalopathy, meningitis, and sepsis. The patient's blood pressure will be high, and the treatment should be aimed to control the hypertensive crisis with antihypertensive medications. If not controlled, the patient may develop focal neurological signs and seizures. Other findings in the neurological exam are optic disk edema and retinal hemorrhages. Emergent brain imaging is indicated to rule out intracranial hemorrhage in the presence of a new onset focal neurological sign. Brain MRI will show areas of increased signal intensity in the occipital regions, which is indicative of cerebral edema. The patient should be admitted to the critical care unit, where appropriate therapy is started with intravenous antiepileptic medications for seizure control and antihypertensive medications for aggressive blood pressure control. In addition, measures to diminish cerebral edema and to treat elevated intracranial pressure should be considered, if clinically indicated.

Endocrine Disorders

Hashimoto encephalopathy is a disorder characterized by recurrent encephalopathy. Patients will present with headaches, obtundation, stupor, and intractable seizures. The neurological examination may show focal signs early in the disease that can be easily confused with transient ischemic attacks. The child is euthyroid, but further serologic testing will show elevated titers of antithyroid antibodies such as anti-thyroglobulin and anti-microsomal antibodies. Spinal fluid analysis will reveal elevated protein with a normal cell count and opening pressure. Treatment with corticosteroids is helpful in controlling the acute exacerbation and for the long term as well. It is important to look for a secondary autoimmune disorder, since frequently patients will have evidence of other organ involvement.

Adrenal insufficiency can be a lethal cause of encephalopathy in children. The patient may have the history of sepsis, adrenal gland bleeding, or abrupt corticosteroid withdrawal such as seen in patients receiving prednisone for myasthenia gravis or Duchenne muscular dystrophy. Vomiting, malaise, and lethargy, progressing to unresponsiveness and coma, are common findings. Treatment involves aggressive fluid replacement therapy, close monitoring of electrolyte imbalances, and corticosteroid replacement.

Hypocalcemic seizures are one of the manifestations of hypoparathyroidism. The symptoms may be present as early as in the neonatal period or during early infancy. It is important to check total and free calcium, magnesium, and vitamin D levels in an otherwise healthy baby presenting with new-onset seizures. The patient may present with focal seizures, and hypocalcemia is usually recognized during serologic screening. Antiepileptic medications do not have a role in the treatment of hypocalcemic seizures. Treatment is heavily supported in correcting hypocalcemia with calcium supplementation.

Hypercalcemia can cause agitation, mania, or psychosis but will not cause obtundation or coma. Patients will complain of weakness and the physical exam will reveal findings indicative of myopathy. Changes in mental status will be noticed with serum calcium levels above 11 mg/dL. Seizures are not presenting symptoms in patients with hypercalcemia.

Undiagnosed hyperthyroidism can present clinically as a thyroid storm. The patients will have significant changes in the personality such as mania, agitation, delirium, and paranoia. Other symptoms include diarrhea, vomiting, weight loss, and cardiac arrhythmias. Thyroid storm is a life-threatening disorder that requires fast intervention. The patients may quickly become obtunded and comatose.

Hypothyroidism may present with constipation, cold skin, and menstrual irregularities. The patient's physical exam is significant for psychomotor slowing and cognitive deficits. Focal neurological findings are lower cranial nerve neuropathies and ataxia. Other manifestations of central nervous system disease are seizure and coma. The peripheral nervous system is also affected, and peripheral neuropathy or myopathy are common findings. Thyroid replacement therapy is the cornerstone in the treatment of this population.

Patients with severe liver dysfunction, as a rule, will have a varying form of hepatic encephalopathy.[18] The most common causes are viral hepatitis with marked liver involvement, Reye disease due to ingestion of aspirin, or accidental poisoning (eg, acetaminophen).[19] The pathophysiology of encephalopathy is due to the severe liver dysfunction with subsequent release of several toxins from the portal circulation to the systemic circulation and causing end-organ symptoms. High excretion of branched-chain amino acids that work as false neurotransmitters and elevated serum ammonia concentrations are particularly important in the pathogenesis of the encephalopathy.[20] A second syndrome affecting the posterior columns of the spinal cord due to deficient vitamin E can also be seen in patients with liver

dysfunction. Ataxia, areflexia, and gaze paresis are the most common symptoms. Patients with liver failure will present with abdominal pain, jaundice, acholia, and dark urine. Early symptoms of hepatic encephalopathy are changes in the affect and obtundation. Asterixis, a tremor of the hands that is elicited by stroking the fingers with the hand extended and the wrist flexed, is seen at this stage. The symptoms may worsen if the patient developed other complications such as gastrointestinal bleeding, bacterial infection, sepsis, excessive protein ingestion, or using hepatotoxic medications. Then, symptoms may progress to seizures, coma, and decerebrate posturing.[21] Serologic test results typical of liver failure are hyperbilirubinemia, elevated transaminases, prolonged prothrombin time, hyperammonemia, and hypoalbuminemia. The EEG will show lack of a dominant posterior rhythm, diffuse slowing and attenuation of the background, and triphasic waves. In mild cases, treatment is supportive until regeneration and normalization of liver function are achieved. More severe cases require supportive treatment until a liver transplant is available.[22] Measurements aiming to minimize liver injury and removal of excessive ammonia levels are also recommended, and include dietary modifications, bowel enemas, and avoidance of hepatotoxic drugs.[23]

REFERENCES

1. Enns GM, Berry SA, Berry GT, Rhead WJ, Brusilow SW, Hamosh A. Survival after treatment with phenylacetate and benzoate for urea-cycle disorders. *N Engl J Med.* 2007; 356:2282-2292.

2. Smith W, Kishnani P S, Lee B, et al. Urea cycle disorders: clinical presentation outside the newborn period. *Crit Care Clin.* 2005;21 (suppl):S9-S17.

3. Filiano JJ. Neurometabolic diseases in the newborn. *Clin Perinatol.* 2006;33:411-479.

4. Lockwood AH. Toxic and metabolic encephalopathies. In: Bradley WG, Fenichel GM, Marsden CD., eds. *Neurology in Clinical Practice: Principles of Diagnosis and Management.* Vol. 2. Woburn, MA: Butterworth-Heinemann; 2000:1475-1493.

5. Cochran JB, Losek JD. Acute liver failure in children. *Pediatr Emerg Care.* 2007; 23:129-135.

6. Koeberl DD, Kishnani PS, Chen YT. Glycogen storage disease types I and II: treatment updates. *J Inherit Metab Dis.* 2007;30:159-164.

7. Fenichel GM. Altered states of consciousness. In: *Clinical Pediatric Neurology: A Sign and Symptom Approach.* 5th ed. Vol. 1. Philadelphia: Elsevier; 2005:47-75.

8. Kerruish NJ, Robertson SP. Newborn screening: new developments, new dilemmas. *J Med Ethics.* 2005;31: 393-398.

9. Sethi R, Barshop B, Stucky ER. Vomiting-again? *J Hosp Med.* 2007;2:189-193.

10. Riviello JJ Jr, Ashwal S, Hirtz D, et al. Practice parameter: diagnostic assessment of the child with status epilepticus

(an evidence-based review): report of the Quality Standards Subcommittee of the American Academy of Neurology and the Practice Committee of the Child Neurology Society. *Neurology*. 2006;67:1542-1550.

11. Carrozzo R, Piemonte F, Tessa A, et al. Infantile mitochondrial disorders. *Biosci Rep*. 2007;27: 105-112.

12. Barkovich AJ. An approach to MRI of metabolic disorders in children. *J Neuroradiol*. 2007;34:75-88.

13. Mori M, Yamagata T, Goto T, Saito, S, Momoi M Dichloroacetate treatment for mitochondrial cytopathy: long-term effects in MELAS. *Brain Dev*. 2004;26:453-458.

14. Barkovich AJ. MR imaging of the neonatal brain. *Neuroimaging Clin N Am*. 2006;16:117-135, viii-ix.

15. Cecil KM. MR spectroscopy of metabolic disorders. *Neuroimaging Clin N Am*. 2006;16:87-116, viii.

16. Wong LJ. Diagnostic challenges of mitochondrial DNA disorders. *Mitochondrion*. 2007;7:45-52.

17. Stacpoole PW, Kerr DS, Bunch ST, et al. Controlled clinical trial of dichloroacetate for treatment of congenital lactic acidosis in children. *Pediatrics*. 2006;117:1519-1531.

18. Cochran JB, Losek LD. Acute liver failure in children. *Pediatr Emerg Care*. 2007;23:129-135.

19. Bucuvalas J, Yazigi N, Squires RH Jr. Acute liver failure in children. *Clin Liver Dis*. 2006;10:149-168, vii.

20. Gheorghe L, Iacob R, Vadan R, Iacob S, Gheorghe C. Improvement of hepatic encephalopathy using a modified high-calorie high-protein diet. *Rom J Gastroenterol*. 2005;14:231-238.

21. Borg M. Symptomatic myoclonus. *Neurophysiol Clin*. 2006;36:309-318.

22. Morioka D, Kasahara M, Takada Y, et al. Current role of liver transplantation for the treatment of urea cycle disorders: a review of the worldwide English literature and 13 cases at Kyoto University. *Liver Transpl*. 2005;11:1332-1342.

23. Singh, RH, Rhead WJ, Smith W, Lee B, King LS, Summar, M. Nutritional management of urea cycle disorders. *Crit Care Clin*. 2005;21(suppl):S27-S35.

CHAPTER 21

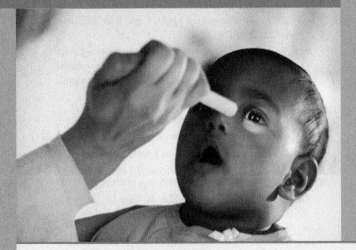

Genetic Testing For Neurological Disorders

Aditi I. Dagli and
Charles A. Williams

Many of the neurological disorders discussed in this book have a genetic etiology that can be diagnosed and/or confirmed by chromosomal or molecular testing. Due to advances in genetic technology, the range of testing options has increased dramatically in the last few years. Deciding which test to perform and how to interpret the results can be daunting. Accordingly, in this chapter we review the different types of clinically available genetic tests. These can be employed for general screening or for confirmation of a clinically diagnosed condition. The general portfolio of such testing is illustrated in Table 21-1, and this chapter will review these types of tests.

ROUTINE CHROMOSOME STUDY

A routine chromosome study (karyotype) involves evaluating the chromosomes during the metaphase period of cell mitosis, and the test is usually performed on blood cells. Lymphocytes are grown in culture and stained with a dye such as Giemsa to obtain a distinct pattern of light and dark bands. This banding pattern is unique to each of the 46 chromosomes, and helps to identify them on microscopic examination (Figure 21-1). A routine chromosome study can identify extra or missing chromosomes (eg, Down [47, XY+21] and Klinefelter [47, XXY] syndromes) as well as detect large inversions, translocations, deletions, duplications, and extra fragments (eg, marker chromosomes). The visual resolution of this study, however, is only at the 10 to 20 million base pair level (Table 21-2). Higher-resolution tests are available (as discussed below in Array-Based Comparative Genomic Hybridization) that detect much smaller changes in the chromosome.

Individuals who present with developmental delay and/or mental retardation should prompt the clinician to consider ordering at least a routine chromosome study.

Table 21-1.

Common Types of Genetic and/or Metabolic Tests That May Be Obtained During a Neurological Evaluation

Chromosome-Based Tests
Routine G-banded analysis
Single FISH probe study (eg, for Angelman syndrome)
Multiple probe FISH study (eg, subtelomeres)
Array-based comparative genomic hybridization (CGH)

Molecular Mutation-Based Tests
Single mutation study
Multiple mutation screens (eg, Charot-Marie-Tooth multigene panel)
Complete gene sequencing and/or gene deletion study (eg, Neurofibromatosis, type)
Trinucleotide repeat analysis (eg, for Fragile X)
DNA methylation study (eg, to rule out Prader-Willi syndrome)
Single nucleotide polymorphism (SNP) analysis (eg, to rule out uniparental disomy)

Mitochondrial-Based Tests
Mitochondrial DNA (mtDNA) sequence analysis
Southern blot study for mtDNA deletions and duplications
Electron transport function (ETF) assays

Metabolic Testing
Urine organic acids
Plasma amino acids
Plasma acylcarnitine profile

Other Tests
Enzyme Assay (eg, Lysosomal Enzymes)

A chromosome study is especially indicated when a developmentally delayed child has any of these associated conditions:

Chromosome 6

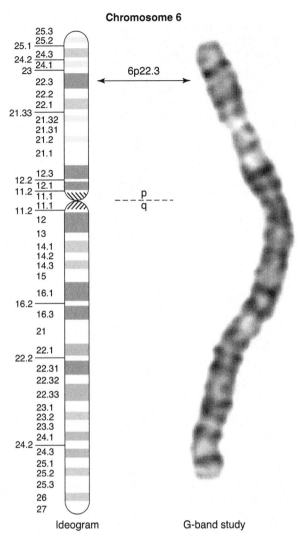

6p22.3

FIGURE 21-1 ◼ Illustration of how chromosome 6 appears on a routine G-banded chromosome study. This is compared to a high-resolution diagram of chromosome 6 that shows the numeral position of each band. The horizontal *arrows* indicate a common band on each chromosome.

Ideogram   G-band study

◾ Single or multiple malformations
◾ Seizures
◾ Dysmorphic facial features
◾ Short stature
◾ Autism
◾ Family history of mental retardation

FLUORESCENCE IN-SITU HYBRIDIZATION (FISH)

Fluorescence in-situ hybridization (FISH) detects the presence or absence of a large DNA sequence involving a particular gene or chromosome region. In this technique, test DNA is first separated into single strands and then hybridized with a fluorescent-labeled DNA probe

Table 21-2.

Sensitivity of Different Genetic Tests to Detect DNA Changes.

Type of test	Detection size*
Routine chromosome study	10-20 million
Individual FISH	3-5 million
Subtelomere FISH panel	3-5 million per probe
Array-based CGH:	
Low resolution (~1200 probes)	400,000-1.5 million
High resolution (~10-90,000 probes)	(30,000-300,0000)
Gene analysis:	
Gene deletion, gene duplication testing	30,000-800,0000 depending on gene
Point mutation analysis	1
Panel of common mutations	1 (for each mutated region)
Complete gene sequencing	1 (over length of the gene)

*= level of sensitivity, in base pairs of DNA
Resolution power is indicated at the DNA base pair level

(usually 0.3-1.0 Mb in size) that is complementary to the region of interest. If the area under study is present, the labeled DNA will bind to it. This can be visualized as a fluorescent spot under the microscope, as illustrated in Figure 21-2 for the 1p36.3 microdeletion condition. This deletion is usually not detected on a routine chromosome study.[1] During the last decade, the development of FISH led to the identification of various "microdeletion syndromes" (Table 21-3).[2–4] However, to be able to judiciously order the appropriate FISH study, one must be aware of the clinical phenotypes of the specific microdeletion syndromes. To overcome this limitation, FISH screening panels have been developed to test simultaneously for multiple microdeletion syndromes.[5] An example of this is the subtelomere FISH panel that can detect minute rearrangements in the subtelomeric regions of all the chromosomes. Subtelomeric deletions or duplications are responsible for some cases of unexplained developmental delay that were otherwise not diagnosed by a routine karyotype.[6]

ARRAY-BASED COMPARATIVE GENOMIC HYBRIDIZATION

Array-based comparative genomic hybridization (array-CGH) can detect alterations in copy number of DNA sequences for specific chromosome regions.[7] In this technique, the DNA of the patient and a normal control are labeled with fluorescent dyes (green and red, respectively) and both DNAs are hybridized to normal cloned

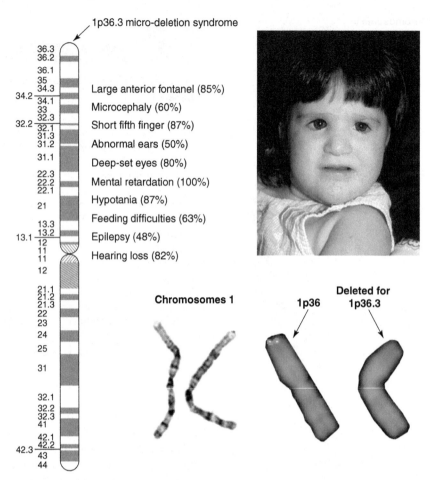

1p36.3 micro-deletion syndrome

Large anterior fontanel (85%)
Microcephaly (60%)
Short fifth finger (87%)
Abnormal ears (50%)
Deep-set eyes (80%)
Mental retardation (100%)
Hypotania (87%)
Feeding difficulties (63%)
Epilepsy (48%)
Hearing loss (82%)

Chromosomes 1

1p36   Deleted for 1p36.3

FIGURE 21-2 ■ Illustration of how a subtelomere FISH study of region 1p36.3 (lower right panel) can detect a small microdeletion at the terminal portion of the p arm. A normal G-banded chromosome pair is also illustrated. Typical clinical features of the 1p36.3 microdeletion syndrome are listed, accompanied by a photograph of an affected child.

Table 21-3.

Classical and Newly Identified Microdeletion Syndromes and Where They Map on the Chromosomes

Syndromes	Deletion Region	Duplication phenotype?
Classical:		
Angelman	15q11.2-q13 (maternal)	Yes
DiGeorge/Velocardio-Facial	22q11.2	Yes
Smith-Magenis	17p11.2	Yes
Williams	7q11.2	Yes
Prader-Willi	15q11.2-q13 (paternal)	No
More Recently Identified:		
McDermid-Phelan	22q13.3	No
1p36.3 syndrome	1p36.3	No
17q23.3 syndrome	17q23.3	No

Some of these regions can also be associated with abnormal clinical phenotypes due to duplications

DNA fragments embedded in a silicon target chip. The exact locations of these DNA fragments on the chromosomes are known. The DNA sequences from both sources compete for their targets on the chip, and images of both fluorescent signals are then captured. Regions equally represented in both samples appear yellow (because both the red and green fluorochromes are detected), deleted regions appear red, and amplified regions are green (Figure 21-3). In this way, a global overview of gains and losses throughout the entire test genome is obtained.[8] Microarray analysis can identify deletions and duplications of the loci represented on the microarray chip, with the resolution being a function of the number and size of target fragments used and the genomic distance between each of the fragments.[9] Using array-CGH, detection rates for chromosome abnormalities range from 5% to 17% in individuals with developmental delay who have had prior routine cytogenetic testing.[9–11] Figure 21-4 illustrates the utility of this test in a case of identical twins that otherwise had normal chromosome study and extensive FISH testing. Because

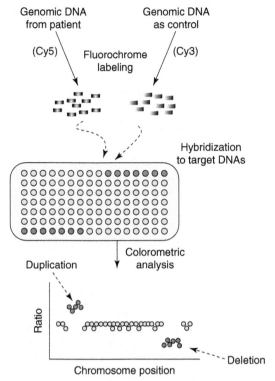

of the high sensitivity of array-CGH, false positives can occur due to the presence of genomic regions of duplications and deletions that are evolutionarily derived and are of no clinical consequence (often termed copy number variants). In such cases, the parents must be tested to see if they too carry the copy number variation. Array-CGH will not be able to detect balanced translocations because in these situations there is no loss or gain of chromosome material.

MUTATION TESTING/SEQUENCE ANALYSIS

Molecular genetic testing reviewed herein includes tests to detect mutations, gene deletions, abnormal number of nucleotide repeats, abnormal DNA methylation, and uniparental disomy. A mutation in a gene can have different effects, and some of the common changes are illustrated in Figure 21-5. A pathogenic mutation either eliminates the protein that the gene codes for, or affects the structure and ultimately the function of the translated protein. Gene mutations can be identified either by targeted mutation analysis (searching for common known mutations) or by sequence analysis of the entire coding region of the gene. These can be achieved by using techniques

FIGURE 21-3 ■ Basic steps of an array-based CGH analysis. See text for detail. Colored circles indicate duplication, normal amount, or deletion of targeted regions. (Cy5 and Cy3 are cyanine dyes used for labeling.)

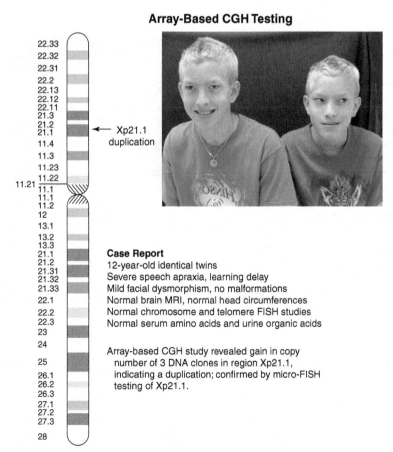

Array-Based CGH Testing

Case Report
12-year-old identical twins
Severe speech apraxia, learning delay
Mild facial dysmorphism, no malformations
Normal brain MRI, normal head circumferences
Normal chromosome and telomere FISH studies
Normal serum amino acids and urine organic acids

Array-based CGH study revealed gain in copy
  number of 3 DNA clones in region Xp21.1,
  indicating a duplication; confirmed by micro-FISH
  testing of Xp21.1.

FIGURE 21-4 ■ Illustration of how CGH testing is able to detect a small region of duplicated DNA on the X chromosome, identified by the study of one of the twins, both with learning delay and mild craniofacial abnormalities.

Nucleotide mutations and their effects

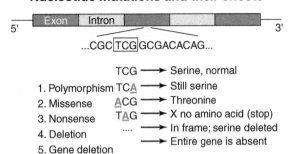

1. Polymorphism TC<u>A</u> → Still serine
2. Missense <u>A</u>CG → Threonine
3. Nonsense T<u>A</u>G → X no amino acid (stop)
4. Deletion .... → In frame; serine deleted
5. Gene deletion → Entire gene is absent

TCG → Serine, normal

FIGURE 21-5 ■ Illustration of the prototypical structure of a gene indicating the 5′ starting position and the 3′ terminal portion. A DNA sequence comprising part of an active coding region (exon) is illustrated and a codon is boxed to indicate that 3 nucleotides code for the amino acid, serine. Numbers 1 through 5 illustrate the types of mutations and normal variants caused by different nucleotide substitutions.

such as Southern blot analysis or polymerase chain reaction (PCR). In Southern blot analysis, restriction fragment enzymes are used to break the DNA into fragments of different size. The DNA fragments are loaded onto an agarose gel and separated by applying an electric current. If the test DNA has mutations, bands with abnormal lengths are formed. PCR is a method that allows the DNA region of interest to be amplified in an exponential manner using a DNA polymerase enzyme and an amplification reaction that is repeated over and over again, producing multiple copies of the DNA region of interest (eg, 20 cycles will produce over 100,000 copies). The PCR product can be analyzed by several methods. For sequence analysis of the gene, nucleotides tagged to fluorescent dyes are added to the PCR reaction, and a laser within an automated DNA sequencing machine is used to analyze the DNA for sequence changes.

DNA sequencing can provide unequivocal diagnosis when a known pathogenic mutation is identified, as illustrated in the case of Sotos syndrome (Figure 21-6), in which the child is found to have a missense mutation. The mutation is determined to be pathogenic because this sequence variant has also been identified in other cases of Sotos syndrome. However, some missense mutations can be normal variants, so extra care is needed in interpreting this type of mutation change. This caveat becomes especially important when multiple genes are sequenced as part of a test panel. For example, the Charcot-Marie-Tooth group of disorders (ie, the hereditary sensory neuropathies) is caused by mutations in many different genes.[12] Genetic screening for these genes can detect several missense mutations of unknown significance, and unless the missense mutation has previously been shown to be pathogenic, the

Sotos Syndrome (Cerebral gigantism)

Clinical features

Increased birth weight and length
Somatic overgrowth in childhood
Macrocephaly, dilation of ventricles
Prominent forehead and chin
Down-slanting palpebral fissures
Poor coordination
Large hands and feet
Mild developmental delay
Advanced bone age

Mutation test result in patient

2003: RI9884Q (5951G→A), a missense mutation in a functionally important domain of the NSD1 gene

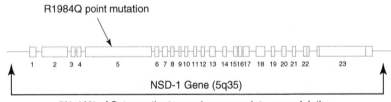

R1984Q point mutation

NSD-1 Gene (5q35)

5%-10% of Sotos patients may have complete gene deletion.

FIGURE 21-6 ■ Mutation analysis detected a missense mutation in this girl. The Sotos gene (NSD-1) is indicated in the lower part of the illustration. The lower line with bracketed arrows illustrates that a significant portion of individuals with Sotos syndrome can have complete deletion of the gene. Unless special methods are employed, DNA sequence analysis of the Sotos gene would not detect a complete gene deletion, as it would sequence only the normal gene allele.

Table 21-4.

Differential Diagnosis of Genetic Conditions

Condition	Location	Gene	% Deleted
Neurofibromatosis, Type 1	17q11.2	NF1	10
Sotos syndrome	5q35.3	NSD1	5-10
Rubinstein-Taybi	16p13.3	CREBE	5
Tuberous sclerosis 2	16p13.3	TSC2	2-5
PTEN macrocephaly syndromes	10q23.3	PTEN	10

These genetic conditions may be encountered during a neurological evaluation of a child with learning disability, seizures, and/or clinical dysmorphism. The percentage of individuals with complete gene deletions is listed at right.

significance of these mutations may be difficult to determine. Furthermore, it should be stressed that gene sequencing may not be able to detect a complete gene deletion, as only the normal allele present would be amplified and sequenced. Accordingly, in certain disorders, studies to detect gene deletions should also be pursued when the sequence testing does not identify a mutation (Table 21-4). For example, in the Sotos syndrome, 10% of individuals can have a complete gene deletion but this can be diagnosed using a FISH probe for the NSD1 gene region.[13,14]

UNSTABLE REPEAT EXPANSIONS

Normally, some genes have stable repeating sequences within their nucleotide structure. Up to a certain number of repeats is considered normal; beyond this, the individual is at risk of either developing disease or passing an expansion on to his or her offspring that will cause disease in them. There are over 40 neurological disorders that have been linked to what are called "unstable" repeat expansions.[15] Fragile X syndrome, which causes mild to severe mental retardation (MR), is caused by an unstable trinucleotide expansion in the FMR1 gene (Figure 21-7). The diagnosis of fragile X syndrome should be considered in boys with MR or autism who have nonspecific physical examination findings. In premutation carrier females, the number of triplet repeats can expand during gametogenesis and can cause transmission of a full mutation to an offspring. Full mutation causes moderate MR in males and can cause mild MR in females. Premutation carrier females can develop premature ovarian failure, and carrier males, in late adulthood, can develop fragile X-associated tremor/ataxia characterized by late-onset, progressive cerebellar ataxia and intention tremor.[16] Fragile X syndrome and other repeat expansion disorders can be diagnosed using PCR or Southern blotting. See Table 21-5 for a list of common pediatric repeat expansion disorders.

The Fragile X Syndrome

Affects 1/2000 males

Physical features
Relatively large cranium
Elongated face with prominent jaw
Large, flexible ears
Large testes (post-pubertal)
IQ variable: LD to severe MR

Behaviors
Eye avoidance behavior
Autistic-like features, shyness
Cluttered, perseverative speech

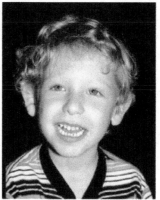

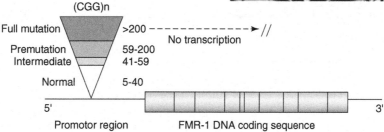

Large CGG repeats cut off DNA transcription of the FMR-1 gene.

FIGURE 21-7 ■ Illustration of a boy with the fragile X syndrome who has more than 200 CGG repeats. Clinical features are indicated. The diagram illustrates the general structure of the fragile X gene and the *triangle* illustrates various classes of expansions.

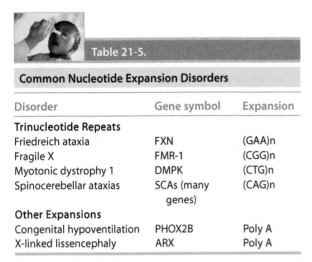

Table 21-5.

Common Nucleotide Expansion Disorders

Disorder	Gene symbol	Expansion
Trinucleotide Repeats		
Friedreich ataxia	FXN	(GAA)n
Fragile X	FMR-1	(CGG)n
Myotonic dystrophy 1	DMPK	(CTG)n
Spinocerebellar ataxias	SCAs (many genes)	(CAG)n
Other Expansions		
Congenital hypoventilation	PHOX2B	Poly A
X-linked lissencephaly	ARX	Poly A

These disorders may be encountered in neurological practice. Gene symbols are listed as is the type of expansion, indicating what nucleotides are repeated.

DNA METHYLATION STUDIES

Genomic imprinting is a phenomenon in which expression of a gene on a particular chromosome depends on the parent of origin of the chromosome. This effect is achieved by silencing the gene derived from one parent. This silencing is associated with changes in DNA methylation of the imprinted gene/gene region during gametogenesis. A clinical disorder can occur if the child does not inherit the active copy of the gene. In such cases, the active gene is typically disrupted by a microdeletion. This disruption can be caused by other mechanisms such as uniparental disomy. Such absence is detected by an abnormal DNA methylation pattern for the gene of interest (Fig. 21-8).

DNA methylation testing identifies most cases of Angelman and Prader-Willi syndrome

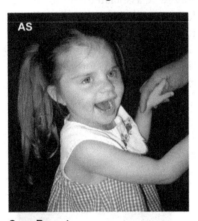

Case Report

The girl with Angelman syndrome had developmental delay, ataxia, happy disposition, and a seizure disorder.

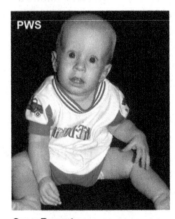

Case Report

The boy with Prader-Willi syndrome had severe neonatal muscular hypotonia, hypoplastic scrotal sac, small penis, and a narrow bitemporal region of the face.

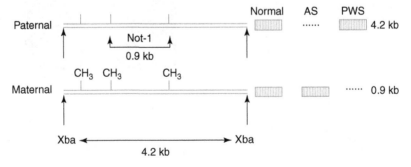

DNA methylation testing of 5'SNRPN gene (15q11–q13)

FIGURE 21-8 ■ Illustration of two individuals, one affected with Angelman and the other with Prader–Willi syndrome. The maternal and paternal regions of 15q11.2-13 illustrate how restriction enzymes can generate different size fragments that can be used to distinguish microdeletions or other abnormalities in the paternal or the maternal chromosome. For Angelman syndrome, absence of the maternal 15q11.2-13 region (or imprinting problems that interfere with appropriate methylation of this region) will result in smaller fragment sizes due to the action of the Not-1 enzyme on the paternal region. The reverse is the case with Prader–Willi syndrome. This and related methodologies are important initial screening tests for these conditions.

UNIPARENTAL DISOMY STUDIES

Uniparental disomy (UPD) means that both chromosomes of a pair are derived from the same parent.[17] For example, in Prader-Willi syndrome, about 30% of cases are caused by maternal UPD for chromosome 15. UPD can be detected by PCR using parent-specific short tandem repeat markers and more recently single nucleotide polymorphism (SNP) microarrays.[18] Parental blood samples must be tested along with the child's sample, and the UPD is thus confirmed when a child fails to inherit alleles from one parent for one specific chromosome.[19]

DISORDERS OF MITOCHONDRIAL FUNCTION

In oxidative phosphorylation, ATP is produced by the enzymes of the mitochondrial respiratory chain. The respiratory chain is arranged in five complexes that are embedded in the inner mitochondrial membrane (Figure 21-9). The genes that code for the various components of the mitochondrial respiratory chain are present on the nuclear as well as the mitochondrial genome. Of the 87 protein components of the respiratory chain, 13 are encoded by genes in the mitochondrial genome. Respiratory chain dysfunction often leads to symptoms in multiple organs or systems, and this reflects the ubiquitous importance of ATP.[20]

In a neonate or young infant, the neurological presentation of a disorder of mitochondrial function can be one of poor feeding, muscle hypotonia, decreased arousal, abnormal movements, and seizures. Laboratory testing often shows impressive lactic acidosis. Presentations in later childhood include gaze paralysis, external ophthalmoplegia (from brainstem involvement), weakness, ataxia, seizures, myoclonus, and stroke-like episodes. Other types of multiorgan involvement can occur. Many individuals display a cluster of symptoms described as clinical syndromes, such as MELAS (mitochondrial encephalopathy with lactic acidosis), MERRF (myoclonic epilepsy with ragged red ribers), and NARP (neurogenic weakness with ataxia and retinitis pigmentosa).[20]

Homoplasmy is a state in which thousands of copies of mitochondrial DNA (mtDNA) in each of our cells are identical, as would be expected for someone having a normal mitochondrial genome. However, most individuals with mitochondrial disorders due to mutations in the mtDNA have a mixture of normal and abnormal mtDNA in their cells; this is termed heteroplasmy. This may be an explanation for the varied clinical phenotypes seen in individuals with the same mtDNA abnormality.[21]

Genetic testing for mitochondrial disorders includes molecular testing to look for mutations in genes present on the mitochondrial or nuclear genome. For molecular testing for mtDNA, Southern blot analysis will detect deletions or duplications, while targeted mutation analysis looks for known common mutations. Sequencing of the entire mtDNA (18,000 bps) can also be performed. If an abnormality is found, it will confirm the diagnosis, but if no abnormality is found the diagnosis cannot be excluded.

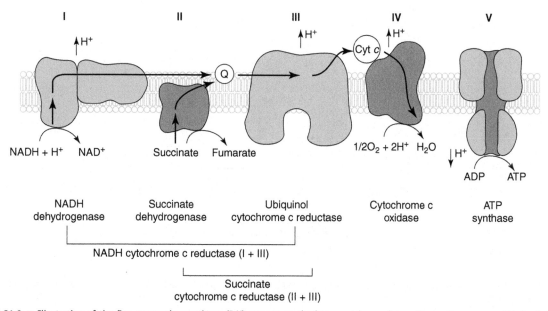

FIGURE 21-9 ■ Illustration of the five enzymatic complexes (I-V) present on the inner matrix membrane. Enzymatic assay can involve individual enzyme analysis or a combination of enzyme analyses (eg, I + III assay) as illustrated. The *arrows* indicate the flow of electrons. (Q, conenzyme Q.)

The child in the Figure 21-10 was found to have a point mutation in the gene coding for one of the subunits of complex V (ATP synthase) in 65% of his mtDNA in blood, which indicates that he is heteroplasmic in blood for this mutation. He has mental retardation, ataxia, and muscle weakness, and had been diagnosed with cerebral palsy before the mtDNA mutation was discovered. Mutation analysis in his case tested only for a panel of common mtDNA mutations (eg, mutations associated with NARP, MELAS, and MERRF), and a point mutation was indeed identified. Currently, the entire mtDNA can be sequenced, although in clinical practice this is rarely done. There is also limited testing for nuclear gene mutations.

Electron transport function (ETF) studies are usually performed on fresh or flash-frozen muscle or liver tissue. ETF studies measure the consumption of oxygen by mitochondria in the presence of various substrates.

Mitochondrial Mutation in ATP Synthase Gene

Case report

Normal birth, no problems
Negative family history
Walked at 2.5 y, clumsy walking thereafter
4 y: IQ ~50-60,
Diagnosis: "cerebral palsy"
Examination at 8.5 y: positive Gower sign
Normal retina and hearing examinations
Normal MRI, EEG, chromosomes, and
Fragile X

MtDNA testing

T8993G mutation in complex V
(ATP synthase) in 65% of mtDNA in blood

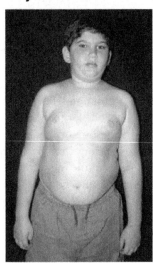

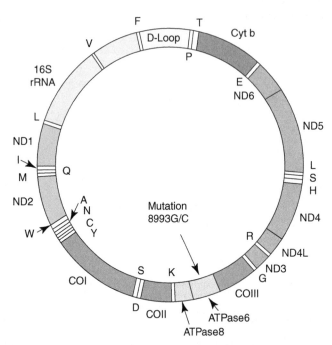

FIGURE 21-10 ■ Presentation of a case involving a child with learning delay, clumsy gait, and mild muscle weakness. DNA mutation analysis in peripheral blood identified a common mutation in one of the subunits (6) of the ATP synthase gene. The circular genome of mitochondrial DNA is illustrated. Single letters (eg, A, N, W, Y) represent transfer RNA genes. Other components of various mitochondrial ETF enzymes, or other mitochondrial structural proteins, are labeled.

- Complex I: Impaired respiration with NADH-producing substrates
- Complex II: Impaired respiration with FADH$_2$-producing substrates
- Complex III and IV: Impaired respiration with NADH and FADH$_2$ substrates
- Complex V: Impaired respiration with various substrates and correction with addition of an uncoupling agent, suggesting abnormality in phosphorylation[20]

ETF studies provide evidence for either focal or general impairment of the respiratory chain. However, the ETF enzymatic phenotype (eg, a 50% reduction in complex I and III activities) is usually not sufficient to confirm the clinical suspicion of a mitochondrial disorder. In such cases, additional mitochondrial or nuclear DNA testing is needed and careful clinical correlation is required.

BIOCHEMICAL TESTING

Biochemical testing often includes serum amino acids, lactate, pyruvate, and acylcarnitine profile determinations. Urine screening can include testing for organic acids, mucopolysaccharides, and oligosaccharrides. Selected neurotransmitters can be measured on CSF, but these tests are not generally included under the rubric of metabolic testing. Serum amino acid, acylcarnitine profile, and urine organic acid screening tests provide a reasonable first approach for evaluation of a child presenting with episodic illness or failure to thrive. These will detect most biochemical disorders associated with defects in amino acid, organic acid, and fatty acid metabolism.

When a particular disorder is suspected based on an abnormal metabolic profile, enzyme assays can be performed to confirm the diagnosis. However, in some cases the clinician may decide to proceed to confirmatory DNA testing or may elect to first perform DNA testing prior to enzyme confirmation. Identification of the mutation(s) in the affected individual then allows other family members to be tested for affected or carrier status. Enzyme analysis is not usually the best method to detect carrier status, as the carrier can produce enough enzyme activity so as to overlap the range of activity for normal controls.

Lysosomal storage diseases are usually neurodegenerative diseases and include Niemann–Pick disease, mucopolysaccharidoses, Krabbe disease, Gaucher disease, and metachromatic leukodystrophy. When a lysosomal enzyme is significantly reduced, its substrate accumulates in the cell, leading to the disorder. Enzyme panels are available to screen for various lysosomal disorders, and based on clinical features and other supporting tests, individual patients are screened for selected ones. The panel usually includes a list of enzymes and many of them can be ruled out clinically.

INHERITANCE PATTERNS AND NEUROGENETIC TESTING

The clinical evaluation involves obtaining a detailed family history to identify familial inheritance patterns. Recognizing a specific inheritance pattern can help focus the clinical differential diagnosis and guide clinical testing. For example, the hereditary spastic parapareses (SPG disorders) can be inherited in an autosomal dominant, autosomal recessive, or X-linked recessive manner, and each has a different set of associated genes.[22] Identifying the inheritance pattern can thus help focus the diagnosis and limit the extent of genetic testing.

The most important inheritance patterns are illustrated in Figure 21-11 and summarized below.

- *Autosomal dominant:* Only one abnormal allele is required to cause disease. With every pregnancy, the affected parent has a 50% chance of transmitting the abnormal allele to the offspring.
- *Autosomal recessive:* Two abnormal alleles are required to cause disease. Parents of the affected child are usually unaffected and are carriers. With each pregnancy, the parents have a 25% chance of having an affected child and a 50% chance that the child will be a carrier.
- *X-linked recessive:* Caused by a mutation in a gene on the X chromosome. All males who carry the mutation express the phenotype. Carrier females do not generally express the phenotype. Due to the process of X chromosome inactivation, carrier females could

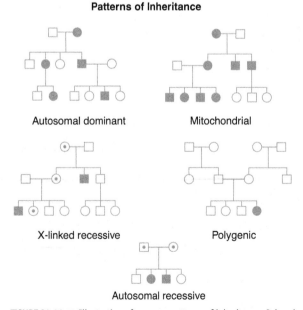

Patterns of Inheritance

Autosomal dominant

Mitochondrial

X-linked recessive

Polygenic

Autosomal recessive

FIGURE 21-11 ▪ Illustration of common patterns of inheritance. Colored *boxes* or *circles* represent affected status and centered *dots* represent carrier status.

have varying degrees of clinical expression. The probability that a carrier female can transmit the mutated gene to her children is 50% at each pregnancy. The females who inherit the mutation will be carriers and males who inherit it will be affected.

■ *Mitochondrial inheritance:* The mitochondrial genome is different from the nuclear genome because it is only transmitted by the mother to her offspring. A mother carrying the mutation will transmit it to 100% of her offspring, but they may or may not be symptomatic depending usually on the percentage of mutant mtDNA and the age of the individual.

■ *Polygenic inheritance:* Also known as multifactorial inheritance, and probably caused by the influence of multiple genes that act in confluence with environmental factors. Examples of such inheritance include cleft lip with or without cleft palate and spina bifida. Although polygenic traits disorders can occur in multiple family members, no recognizable pattern of inheritance is typically observed. A risk of 3% to 10% can usually be assessed for first-degree relatives (eg, siblings, children) of an affected individual.

ONLINE RESOURCES

There are excellent online resources that provide current information about genetic disorders. Two important ones are listed here:

■ OMIM (Online Mendelian Inheritance in Man): www.ncbi.nlm.nih.gov/omim/
This is a database of genetic disorders and their genes that show a Mendelian inheritance pattern.
■ Genetests:
www.ncbi.nlm.nih.gov/sites/GeneTests/?db=Gene Tests
This site contains disease reviews and a directory of genetic testing laboratories.

REFERENCES

1. Battaglia A. Del 1p36 syndrome: a newly emerging clinical entity. *Brain Dev.* 2005;27:358.
2. Devriendt K, Vermeesch JR. Chromosomal phenotypes and submicroscopic abnormalities. *Hum Genomics.* 2004; 1:126.
3. Shaw CJ, Lupski JR. Implications of human genome architecture for rearrangement-based disorders: the genomic basis of disease: *Hum Mol Genet.* 2004;13:1, R57-64.
4. Schwartz S, Graf MD. Microdeletion syndromes. Characteristics and diagnosis: *Methods Mol Biol.* 2002;204:275-290.
5. Ligon AH, Beaudet AL, Shaffer LG. Simultaneous, multilocus FISH analysis for detection of microdeletions in the diagnostic evaluation of developmental delay and mental retardation: *Am J Hum Genet.* 1997;61:51.
6. Ravnan JB, Tepperberg JH, Papenhausen P, et al. Subtelomere FISH analysis of 11 688 cases: an evaluation of the frequency and pattern of subtelomere rearrangements in individuals with developmental disabilities: *J Med Genet.* 2006;43:478.
7. Weiss MM, Hermsen MA, Meijer GA, et al. Comparative genomic hybridisation: *Mol Pathol.* 1999;52:243.
8. Oostlander AE, Meijer GA, Ylstra B. Microarray-based comparative genomic hybridization and its applications in human genetics: *Clin Genet.* 2004;66:488.
9. Shaffer LG, Bejjani BA. Medical applications of array CGH and the transformation of clinical cytogenetics: *Cytogenet Genome Res.* 2006;115:303.
10. Engels H, Brockschmidt A, Hoischen A, et al. DNA microarray analysis identifies candidate regions and genes in unexplained mental retardation: *Neurology.* 2007; 68:743.
11. Veltman JA. Genomic microarrays in clinical diagnosis: *Curr Opin Pediatr.* 2006;18:598.
12. Zuchner S, Vance JM. Mechanisms of disease: a molecular genetic update on hereditary axonal neuropathies: *Nat Clin Pract Neurol.* 2006;2:45.
13. Faravelli F. NSD1 mutations in Sotos syndrome: *Am J Med Genet C Semin Med Genet.* 2005;137:24.
14. Niikawa N. Molecular basis of Sotos syndrome: *Horm Res.* 2004;62(suppl):360.
15. Pearson CE, Nichol Edamura K, Cleary JD. Repeat instability: mechanisms of dynamic mutations: *Nat Rev Genet.* 2005;6:729.
16. Saul RA and Tarleton JC. FMR1-related disorders. GeneReviews at GeneTests: Medical Genetics Information Resource. http://www.genetests.org. University of Washington, Seattle; 1997–2007.
17. Engel E. A new genetic concept: uniparental disomy and its potential effect, isodisomy: *Am J Med Genet.* 1980; 6:137.
18. Bruce S, Leinonen R, Lindgren CM, et al. Global analysis of uniparental disomy using high density genotyping arrays: *J Med Genet.* 2005;42:847.
19. Shaffer LG, Agan N, Goldberg JD, et al. American College of Medical Genetics statement of diagnostic testing for uniparental disomy: *Genet Med.* 2001;3:206.
20. Munnich A, Cormier-Daire RA V, Rustin R. Clinical presentation of respiratory chain deficiency. In: Scriver CR, Sly WS, Valle D, Vogelstein B, eds. *The Online Molecular and Metabolic Bases of Inherited Disease.* New York: McGraw-Hill; 2001:2261.
21. Chinnery P. Mitochondrial disorders overview. GeneReviews at GeneTests: Medical Genetics Information Resource. http://www.genetests.org. University of Washington, Seattle, 2006.
22. Fortini D, Cricchi F, Di Fabio R, et al. Current insights into familial spastic paraparesis: new advances in an old disease: *Funct Neurol.* 2003;18(1):43.

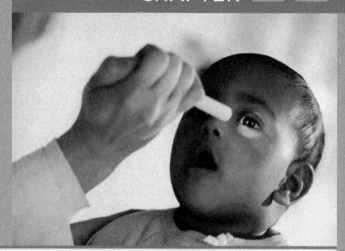

CHAPTER 22

Neurocutaneous Syndromes

Paul R. Carney and James D. Geyer

TUBEROUS SCLEROSIS

Definitions and Epidemiology

Tuberous sclerosis is a genetic disease occurring in approximately 1 in 10,000 people. It is inherited in an autosomal dominant pattern isolated to chromosome 9, and in rare instances chromosome 16.[1,2] Though autosomal dominant, there is variable penetrance.[3]

Pathogenesis

Tuberous sclerosis is associated with a variety of central nervous system findings. Cortical tubers are the hallmark finding on imaging and pathologic specimens. These consist of giant cells, gliosis, disorganized myelin, and hamartomas. Heterotopic islands of gray matter in the deep white matter are commonly seen.[4] Subependymal giant-cell astrocytomas can occur and may result in clinical findings secondary to the associated mass effect.[5]

Clinical Presentation/Diagnosis

Tuberous sclerosis was initially defined by Voigt's classical triad of epilepsy, adenoma sebaceum, and mental deficiency. Unfortunately, this classic triad is present in only one-third of patients.[4]

The primary diagnostic criteria for tuberous sclerosis includes adenoma sebaceum, which occur in 90% of patients above 4 years of age. Ungual fibromas typically appear at puberty. Cerebral cortical tubers are an integral component of tuberous sclerosis. Subependymal nodules, also called "candle gutterings," may be seen on imaging studies but may be absent in the very young patient. Fibrous forehead plaques also increase in frequency with increasing age.

There are also a number of secondary criteria for the diagnosis of tuberous sclerosis. Infantile spasms occur in three-quarters of patients and usually start at 4 to 7 months of age. In these patients, the EEG may show hypsarrhythmia.[6]

Ash leaf spots occur in 90% of patients. They are hypomelanotic lesions and may be the earliest skin manifestation of tuberous sclerosis. These lesions require a Wood lamp for diagnosis (Figure 22-1).

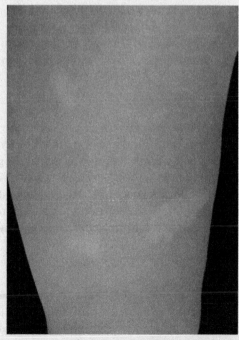

FIGURE 22-1 ■ Hypomelanotic ash leaf macules on the lower leg of a child with tuberous sclerosis complex. (*Reproduced with permission from Wolff K, Goldsmith LA, Katz SI, Gilchrest BA, Paller AS, Lefferell DJ. Fitzpatrick's Dermatology in General Medicine. 7th ed. New York: McGraw-Hill; 2008: Figure 141-2.*)

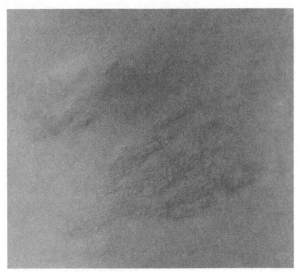

FIGURE 22-2 ■ The Shagreen patch in tuberous sclerosis complex is a firm, bumpy plaque that is usually located on the lower back. (*Reproduced with permission from Wolff K, Goldsmith LA, Katz SI, Gilchrest BA, Paller AS, Lefferell DJ. Fitzpatrick's Dermatology in General Medicine. 7th ed. New York: McGraw-Hill; 2008: Figure 141-7.*)

Shagreen patches are another dermatologic manifestation of tuberous sclerosis. These lesions are subepidermal fibrous patches that have the appearance of orange peel. While they may occur in various locations, they are most common in the lumbosacral region (Figure 22-2).

A number of other physical findings may occur including retinal hamartomas, retinal phakomas, bilateral renal cysts, angiolipomas of the kidney, cardiac rhabdomyosarcomas, and renal failure. Renal failure is the most common cause of death in tuberous sclerosis.[7]

Diagnostic Tests

Neuroimaging is the primary diagnostic study for tuberous sclerosis. Cortical tubers are typically hypodense on CT and measure 5 mm to 3 cm. Candle gutterings appear on the walls of the lateral ventricles and are fequently calcified. Subependymal giant-cell astrocytomas occur most frequently at the foramen of Monro and can cause hydrocephalus secondary to obstruction.

Treatment

The treatment of tuberous sclerosis remains symptomatic. The patients who develop obstructive hydrocephalus from a subependymal giant cell astrocytoma near the foramen of Monroe may require lesion resection or shunt placement. The treatment of infantile spasms is reviewed in detail in Chapter 3.

Adrenocorticotropic hormone and additional antiepileptic drugs are the mainstays of therapy.

NEUROFIBROMATOSIS TYPE I (PERIPHERAL)

Definitions and Epidemiology

Neurofibromatosis type I is a relatively common genetic disease. It is inherited in an autosomal dominant pattern isolated to chromosome 17.

Pathogenesis

Neurofibromatosis (NF) type I is the "peripheral type" of neurofibromatosis, meaning that there are peripheral and external manifestations of the disease. Neurofibromas are the hallmark feature of NF type I. These are typically benign but can undergo malignant degeneration in 2% to 5% of patients.[8] Cutaneous tumors are common and consist of loosely arranged elongated connective tissue cells. Café-au-lait spots are hyperpigmented lesions that arise because of an increased number of melanosomes in a normal number of melanocytes.

Clinical Presentation/Diagnosis

Neurofibromatosis type I has numerous peripheral or external manifestations. Café-au-lait spots may occur in an isolated fashion in normal individuals but suggest NF-I when there are 6 or more. Axillary freckles are another common dermatologic manifestation. These findings are more pronounced as the child ages. Lisch nodules are white hamartomas in the iris.

Multiple cutaneous tumors known as molluscum fibrosum are frequently seen (Figure 22-3). Multiple subcutaneous tumors also develop, including firm nodules and plexiform neuromas. The plexiform neuromas have the feel of a "bag of worms" (Figure 22-4).

Central nervous system lesions are also common.[9] Neuromas, including acoustic neuromas and trigeminal neuromas, arise frequently. Spinal root tumors may result in radicular findings. Optic gliomas occur frequently but usually have a slowly progressive course. In rare cases, the optic glioma may have a more malignant course. In some cases, obstructive hydrocephalus can develop from glial overgrowth.

Intellectual impairment occurs in approximately 40% of patients. Hyperactivity is also a commonly reported problem. Seizures are much more common in NF-I patients than in the general population, with a 20-fold increased rate.

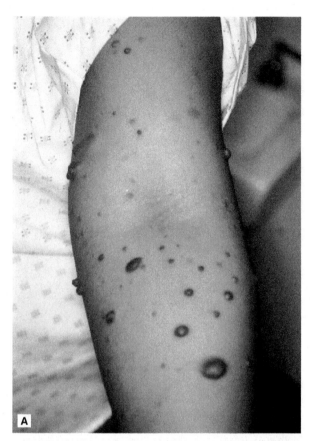

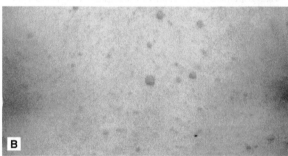

FIGURE 22-3 ■ **(A)** Cutaneous neurofibromas with overlying hyperpigmentation. **(B)** Multiple cutaneous neurofibromas. (*Reproduced with permission from Wolff K, Goldsmith LA, Katz SI, Gilchrest BA, Paller AS, Lefferell DJ. Fitzpatrick's Dermatology in General Medicine. 7th ed. New York: McGraw-Hill; 2008: Figures 142-3 and 142-4.*)

A number of other disorders are associated with NF-I including bone cysts, pathologic bone fractures (pseudoarthrosis), pheochromocytoma, scoliosis, precocious puberty, and syringomyelia. Cardiac manifestations have also been reported.[10]

Treatment

There is no primary treatment for NF-I. Management is supportive and directed at the comorbid conditions and complications such as seizures, intracranial tumors, and hydrocephalus.

NEUROFIBROMATOSIS TYPE II (CENTRAL)

Definitions and Epidemiology

Neurofibromatosis type II (NF-II) is genetic disease that is less common than NF-I. It is inherited in an autosomal dominant pattern isolated to chromosome 22.[11]

Pathogenesis

Neurofibromatosis type II is the "central type" of neurofibromatosis, meaning that there is a lack of peripheral and external manifestations of the disease.[11,12]

Clinical Presentation/Diagnosis

Neurofibromatosis type II does not have peripheral or external manifestations. Café-au-lait spots and neurofibromas are absent.[11] Bilateral acoustic neuromas are commonly seen in NF-II. The neuromas usually grow on the vestibular portion of CN VIII. The first symptom is hearing loss secondary to compression on the cochlear component of CN VIII. Meningiomas also frequently occur.

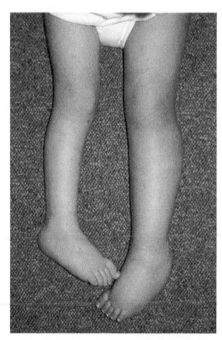

FIGURE 22-4 ■ Plexiform neurofibroma of left lower extremity leading to leg length discrepancy. (*Reproduced with permission from Wolff K, Goldsmith LA, Katz SI, Gilchrest BA, Paller AS, Lefferell DJ. Fitzpatrick's Dermatology in General Medicine. 7th ed. New York: McGraw-Hill; 2008: Figure 142-5.3.*)

Treatment

There is no primary treatment for NF-II. Management is supportive and directed at the comorbid conditions and complications such as seizures and intracranial tumors.

STURGE-WEBER SYNDROME (ENCEPHALOTRIGEMINAL ANGIOMATOSIS)

Definitions and Epidemiology

Sturge-Weber syndrome is a relatively rare disorder that occurs in a sporadic fashion.[13,14]

Pathogenesis

Sturge-Weber syndrome develops secondary to leptomeningeal angiomas.[13] Calcifications of the blood vessel walls and calcification of the underlying cortex create the classic imaging findings associated with the disorder. The occipital lobe is most frequently affected.

Clinical Presentation/Diagnosis

The classic dermatologic finding associated with Sturge-Weber syndrome is the port wine nevus of the face. This is usually unilateral but in rare cases may be bilateral.[15] The extent of the nevus usually mirrors the extent of the intracranial involvement. Nearly all nevi that involve the upper eyelid have associated cerebral lesions (Figure 22-5).

There is usually a contralateral hemiparesis associated with contralateral hemiatrophy. Mental retardation is commonly present. Seizures are a frequent complication and are often intractable.

Glaucoma is also a common comorbid condition.

Diagnostic Tests

Routine x-rays may reveal "tram-line calcifications" by age 2 years. These occur secondary to calcification of the cortex. Neuroimaging with CT scan of the head also reveals the calcifications. Cerebral atrophy in the affected region is common. The calvarial diploe is often thickened. MRI also reveals the atrophy and may also display gyriform enhancement.

Seizures are a common complication of Sturge-Weber syndrome. The interictal EEG reveals decreased potentials over affected area. Interictal epileptiform discharges may also occur.

Treatment

There is no primary treatment for Sturge–Weber syndrome. Management is supportive and directed at the

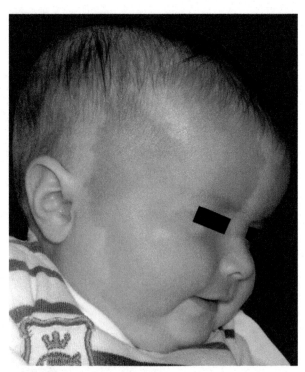

FIGURE 22-5 ■ Extensive right facial capillary malformation involving the ophthalmic and maxillary branches of the trigeminal nerve in a 6-month-old girl affected with Sturge-Weber syndrome. *(Reproduced with permission from Wolff K, Goldsmith LA, Katz SI, Gilchrest BA, Paller AS, Lefferell DJ. Fitzpatrick's Dermatology in General Medicine. 7th ed. New York: McGraw-Hill; 2008: Figure 173-4A.)*

comorbid conditions and complications such as seizures and glaucoma.

FAMILIAL TELANGIECTASIA (RENDU-OSLER-WEBER SYNDROME)

Definitions and Epidemiology

Familial telangiectasia is genetic disease inherited in an autosomal dominant pattern. A defect in blood vessel walls results in mechanical fragility of the vessels. The primary clinical features are angiomas in the skin, CNS, GI tract, GU tract, and mucous membranes (Figure 22-6). These angiomas can result in bleeding, including intracranial hemorrhage.

INCONTINENTIA PIGMENTI

Definitions and Epidemiology

Incontinentia pigmenti is genetic disease. It is inherited in an X-linked dominant pattern.

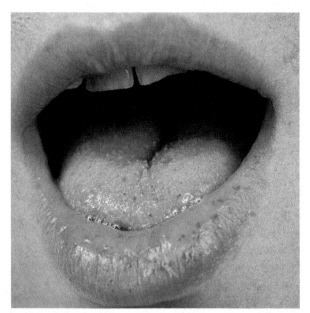

FIGURE 22-6 ■ Rendu-Osler-Weber syndrome. Note the punctuate and splinter-like telangiectasia on the lips and tongue. (*Reproduced with permission from Wolff K, Goldsmith LA, Katz SI, Gilchrest BA, Paller AS, Lefferell DJ. Fitzpatrick's Dermatology in General Medicine. 7th ed. New York: McGraw-Hill; 2008: Figure 151-12.*)

Pathogenesis

The cerebral pathology includes atrophy and microgyria. Focal necrosis in white matter also develops over time.

Clinical Presentation/Diagnosis

Dermatologic lesions begin as linear vesiculobullous lesions and progress to hyperkeratosis and hyperpigmentation with linear streaks and whorls (Figure 22-7).

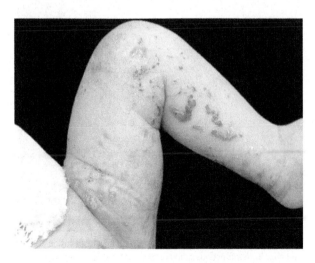

FIGURE 22-7 ■ Incontinentia pigmenti in a 2-week-old baby. Note the verrucous lesions. (*Reproduced with permission from Wolff K, Goldsmith LA, Katz SI, Gilchrest BA, Paller AS, Lefferell DJ. Fitzpatrick's Dermatology in General Medicine. 7th ed. New York: McGraw-Hill; 2008: Figure 73-14A.*)

There is often a slate-gray pigmentation.[4] Alopecia is also a common finding.

Neurological manifestations include delayed motor development and mental retardation. Spastic hemiparesis or paraparesis is a common complication, further adding to the difficulty in caring for the patient. The microgyria and the areas of necrosis raise the risk of seizures. Episodes of recurrent encephalomyelitis have also been associated with incontinentia pigmenti.[16]

Diagnostic Tests

Laboratory studies are nonspecific, but eosinophilia is a common finding, occurring in approximately 65% of patients.[16]

Treatment

There is no primary treatment for incontinentia pigmenti. Management is supportive and directed at the comorbid conditions and complications such as seizures.

VON HIPPEL-LINDAU DISEASE (HEMANGIOBLASTOMA OF THE CEREBELLUM)

Definitions and Epidemiology

Von Hippel-Lindau disease is a relatively rare disorder that occurs in a familial fashion. The inheritance pattern is autosomal dominant.

Pathogenesis

The primary pathologic feature of von Hippel-Lindau disease is the presence of cerebellar hemangioblastomas. These are multicystic tumors. Retinal hemangioblastomas are also a common finding. Hepatic cysts, pancreatic cysts, renal tumors, and pheochromocytomas frequently develop and complicate the clinical course.[17]

Clinical Presentation/Diagnosis

Most patients present with ataxia. The cerebellar hemangiomas can impair cerebellar function by mass effect and altered perfusion. Furthermore, the hemangioma can cause obstructive hydrocephalus with the typical associated features.

Diagnostic Tests

From a laboratory perspective, polycythemia occurs because of increased erythropoietin production.

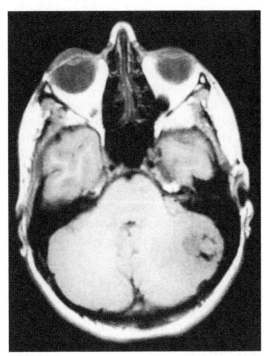

FIGURE 22-8 ■ Hemangioblastoma. MRI in the axial plane shows the vascular tumor in the left cerebellar hemisphere. (*Reproduced with permission from Ropper AH, Brown RH, eds. Adams and Victor's Principles of Neurology. 8th ed. New York: McGraw-Hill; 2005: Figure. 31-13.*)

Neuroimaging with contrast-enhanced brain MRI is the primary modality for the diagnosis of von Hippel-Lindau disease (Figure 22-8).

Treatment

There is no primary treatment for von Hippel-Lindau disease. Management is supportive and directed at the comorbid conditions and complications such as hydrocephalus.

ATAXIA-TELANGIECTASIA (LOUIS-BAR SYNDROME)

Definitions and Epidemiology

Ataxia-telangiectasia is an autosomal recessive disease with a mutation in the ATM gene (leads to defect in DNA repair) on chromosome 11. Symptoms of ataxia-telangiectasia typically begin during infancy.

Pathogenesis

Cerebellar degeneration is the hallmark pathologic feature. There is loss of myelinated fibers in the posterior columns, spinocerebellar tracts, and in the peripheral nerves. Degeneration occurs in the dorsal roots, sympathetic ganglia, and the anterior horn cells. Loss of pigmented cells occurs in the substantia nigra and in the locus ceruleus. Lewy bodies can be seen in the pigmented cells.

Clinical Presentation/Diagnosis

Development is typically normal for the first few years. Then there is progressive truncal ataxia, usually resulting in the patient being wheelchair-bound by age 12 years. The hallmark oculocutaneous telangiectasias usually appear between age 3 and 5 years, well after the onset of ataxia. Ocular symptoms include nystagmus, oculomotor dyspraxia, and absent optokinetic nystagmus. Other symptoms include dysarthria, dystonia, athetosis, myoclonic jerks, polyneuropathy, and cognitive dysfunction (Figure 22-9).[4]

Ataxia-telangiectasia is also associated with cancer, typically leukemias and lymphomas. The average age of death is 20 years and is usually from infection or neoplasm.

Diagnostic Tests

Diagnostic studies reveal elevated AFP and CEA levels (alpha-fetoprotein and carcinoembryonic antigen), and

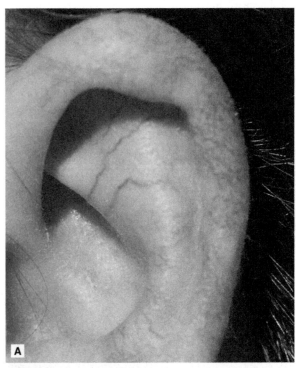

A

FIGURE 22-9 ■ **A.** Ataxia-telangiectasia. Telangiectases inside and on the helix. **B.** Noninfectious granulomatous dermatitis of a patient with ataxia-telangiectasia. These persistent lesions tend to ulcerate. (*Reproduced with permission from Wolff K, Goldsmith LA, Katz SI, Gilchrest BA, Paller AS, Lefferell DJ. Fitzpatrick's Dermatology in General Medicine. 7th ed. New York: McGraw-Hill; 2008: Figures 144-10 and 144-11.*)

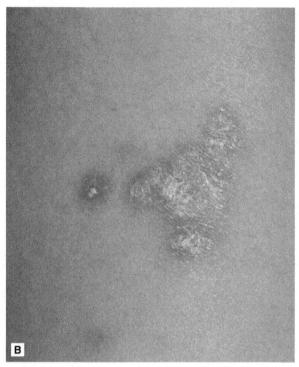

FIGURE 22-9 ■ *(Continued)*

decreased or absent IgA levels. Fibroblasts can be screened for increased x-ray sensitivity and radioresistant DNA synthesis. The associated immunodeficiency leads to recurrent respiratory infections.

Treatment

There is no primary treatment for ataxia-telangiectasia. Management is supportive and directed at the comorbid conditions and complications.

REFERENCES

1. Curatolo P, ed. *Tuberous Sclerosis Complex: From Basic Science to Clinical Phenotypes.* International Child Neurology Association. London: Mac Keith Press; 2003.

2. Hennel SJ, Ekert PG, Volpe JJ, et al. Loss of heterozygosity on chromosome 16p13.3 in hamartomas from tuberous sclerosis patients. *Nat Genet.* 1994;6:193.

3. Berberich MS, Hall BD. Penetrance and variability in tuberous sclerosis. *Birth Defects.* 1979;15:297.

4. Geyer J, Keating J, Potts D, Carney P, eds. *Neurology for the Boards.* 3rd ed. Philadelphia, PA: Lippincott Williams & Wilkins; 2006:277-281.

5. Goh S, Butler WE, Thiele EA. Subependymal giant cell tumors in tuberous sclerosis complex: diagnosis and management. *Neurology.* 2004;63:1457.

6. Curatolo P, Seri S, Verdecchia M, et al. Infantile spasms in tuberous sclerosis complex. *Brain Dev.* 2001;23:502.

7. Franz DN. Non-neurologic manifestations of tuberous slerosis complex. *J Child Neurol.* 2004;19:690.

8. Evans DG, Baser ME, McGaughran J, et al. Malignant peripheral nerve sheath tumours in neurofibromatosis 1. *J Med Genet.* 2002;39:311.

9. DiPaolo DP, Zimmerman RA, Rorke LB, et al. Neurofibromatosis type 1: pathologic substrate of high signal intensity foci in the brain. *Radiology.* 1995;195:721.

10. Friedman JM, Arbiser J, Epstein JA, et al. Cardiovascular disease in neurofibromatosis1: report of the NF1 Cardiovascular Task Force. *Genet Med.* 2002;4:105.

11. Evans DG. Neurofibromatosis type 2: genetic and clinical features. *Ear Nose Throat J.* 1999;78:97.

12. Baser ME, Wallace AJ, Strachan T, et al. Clinical and molecular correlates of somatic mosaicism in neurofibromatosis 2. *J Med Genet.* 2000;37:542.

13. Alexander GL. Sturge–Weber syndrome. In: Vinken PJ, Bruyn GW, eds. *Handbook of Clinical Neurology.* New York: American Elsevier; 1972.

14. Chao DHC. Congenital neurocutaneous syndromes in childhoold. III. Sturge-Weber disease. *J Pediatr.* 1959; 55:635.

15. Bebin EM, Gomez MR. Prognosis of Sturge-Weber syndrome: comparison of unihemispheric and and bihemispheric involvement. *J Child Neurol.* 1988;3:181.

16. Brunquell P. Recurrent encephalomyelitis associated with incontinentia pigmenti. *Pediatr Neurol.* 1987;3:174.

17. Atuk NO, McDonald T, Wood T, et al. Familial pheochromocytoma hypercalcemia and von Hippel-Lindau disease. *Medicine.* 1979;58:209.

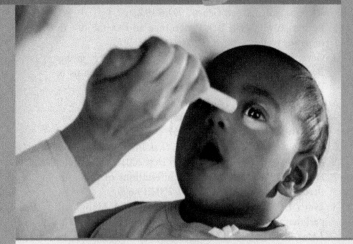

CHAPTER 23

Metabolic Disorders

James D. Geyer, Paul R. Carney, and Stephenie C. Dillard

Metabolic disorders include a wide array of diseases affecting a number of important pathways that frequently result in neurological consequences. The advances in biochemistry and molecular genetics have revealed much about these disorders. As with most technological advances, as the disorders are better defined, more closely related variants emerge. This further complicates the clinical and diagnostic picture for the pediatrician and subspecialist alike. The introductory section of Chapter 24 discusses these issues in greater detail. The same factors apply to the metabolic disorders, and there is considerable overlap between these two categories of disease.

An often overlooked component of the management of these disorders is a coordinated genetic counseling program. This is more than simply advising a family that a disease is hereditary. There should be coordinated genetic, reproductive, and medical counseling and management.[1]

GLYCOGEN STORAGE DISEASES

Table 23-1 gives an overview of the glycogen storage diseases (GSDs).

Acid Maltase Deficiency—Pompe Disease

Biochemistry and clinical characteristics

Acid maltase deficiency (AMD), or Pompe disease (Box 23-1), is an autosomal recessive (AR) glycogen storage disease with several different manifestations.[2] Infantile AMD manifests itself within weeks of birth. The clinical manifestations include floppy baby syndrome, generalized and bulbar weakness, macroglossia, cardiomegaly, and hepatomegaly. The symptoms progress to death by age 2 years.

Table 23-1.

Glycogen Storage Disease Quick Reference Table

Type	Eponym	Defect	Involved Tissue	Special Features
I	Von Gierke	Glucose-6-phosphatase	Liver, kidney	Hypoglycemic seizures
II	Pompe	Acid maltase	Generalized	Floppy baby
III	Forbe	Debranching enzyme	Generalized	
IV	—	Transglucosidase	Generalized	
V	McArdle	Muscle phosphorylase	Muscle	Cramps, weakness
VI	—	Liver phosphorylase	Liver, WBC	Hypoglycemia
VII	Tarui	Phosphofructokinase	Muscle, RBC	Cramps, weakness
VIII	—	Phosphorylase kinase	Liver	

Adapted with permission from Geyer J, Keating J, Potts D, Carney P, eds. Neurology for the Boards. 3rd ed. Philadelphia, PA: Lippincott Williams & Wilkins; 2006.

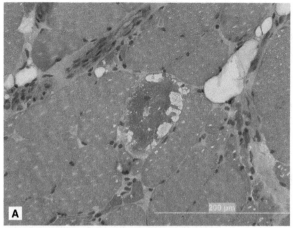

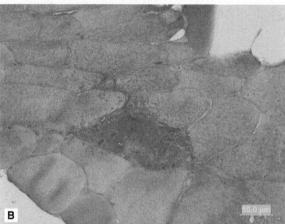

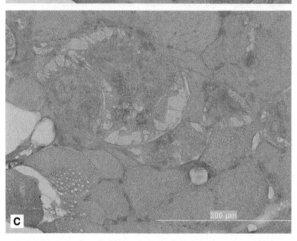

FIGURE 23-1 ■ Muscle biopsy in Pompe disease reveals one or more vacuoles within many muscle fibers **(A)** that stain intensely red **(B)** on periodic acid-Schiff (PAS) stain, showing that they are filled with glycogen **(C)**. (*Reproduced with permission from Amato A, Russell J, eds.* Neuromuscular Disorders. *New York: McGraw-Hill; 2008:601, Figure 26-2.*)

Box 23-1. Pompe Disease

Common Name: Pompe disease
Inheritance: Autosomal recessive
Metabolic Defect: Acid maltase deficiency
Clinical Pattern: Infantile AMD: floppy baby syndrome, generalized and bulbar weakness, macroglossia, cardiomegaly, and hepatomegaly, progressing to death by age 2 years.

Adult AMD, on the other hand, usually starts in the twenties or thirties. The clinical presentation is different in this population, with the primary findings being respiratory weakness more prominent than limb-girdle weakness and intracranial aneurysms secondary to glycogen accumulation in vessels.

Evaluation and pathology

The evaluation of AMD reveals increased creatine kinase (CK) with a normal ischemic exercise test. The needle EMG reveals evidence of myopathy and electrical myotonia without clinical myotonia. There is a vacuolar myopathy with accumulation of PAS-positive material in lysosomes on microscopic evaluation (Figure 23-1).

Management

Enzyme replacement may offer an effective treatment for infantile-onset Pompe disease.[3,4]

Muscle Phosphorylase Deficiency— McArdle Disease

Biochemistry and clinical characteristics

Muscle phosphorylase deficiency, or McArdle disease (Box 23-2), is an autosomal recessive glycogen storage disease.[5,6] In childhood, it manifests itself with exercise intolerance. In adulthood, cramps and myalgias are more common complaints. Symptoms typically resolve with rest, but permanent weakness occurs in approximately one-third of patients. Acute muscle necrosis can occur but is rare.[7]

Evaluation and pathology

The evaluation of muscle phosphorylase deficiency reveals increased creatine kinase (CK) in 90% of patients. The ischemic exercise test is positive with no rise in serum lactate after ischemic exercise. Myoglobinuria with exercise occurs in half the patients. The needle EMG is usually normal. Subsarcolemmal glycogen deposits (blebs) that are PAS positive, intermyofibrillar vacuoles, and immunohistochemical stains showing absent staining for phosphorylase, are evident on microscopic evaluation (Figure 23-2).

Box 23-2. McArdle Disease

Common Name: McArdle disease
Inheritance: Autosomal recessive
Metabolic Defect: Muscle phosphorylase deficiency
Clinical Pattern: Exercise intolerance. In adulthood, cramps and myalgias are more common. Symptoms typically resolve with rest.

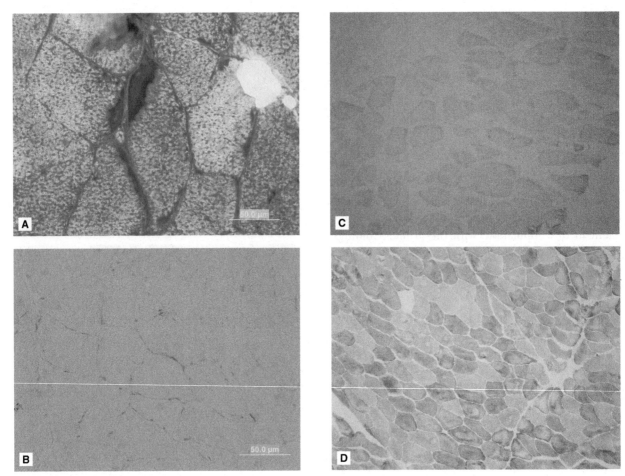

FIGURE 23-2 ■ Scattered muscle fibers have small foci of increased glycogen deposition in subsarcolemmal regions in McArdle disease **(A)**, periodic acid-Schiff (PAS) stain. When diastase is added to the PAS stain, the abnormal accumulations are no longer evident, suggesting that the deposits were glycogen **(B)**. Myophosphorylase stain demonstrates absent myophosphorylase activity **(C)** compared to a healthy control biopsy **(D)**. (*Reproduced with permission from Amato A, Russell J, eds.* Neuromuscular Disorders. *New York: McGraw-Hill; 2008:76, Figure 3-6.*)

Management

Creatine supplementation may offer some treatment benefit for skeletal muscle function in McArdle disease.[8]

Muscle Phosphofructokinase Deficiency—Tarui Disease

Biochemistry and clinical characteristics

Muscle phosphofructokinase deficiency, or Tarui disease (Box 23-3), is an autosomal recessive glycogen storage disease. Tarui disease begins in childhood with premature fatigue, weakness, and stiffness induced by exercise.

Box 23-3. Tarui Disease

Common Name: Tarui disease
Inheritance: Autosomal recessive
Metabolic Defect: Muscle phosphofructokinase deficiency
Clinical Pattern: Premature fatigue, weakness, stiffness induced by exercise, myalgias, and cramps. Symptoms typically resolve with rest.

Myalgias and cramps are common. Symptoms typically resolve with rest.[9,10]

Evaluation and pathology

The evaluation of muscle phosphofructokinase deficiency reveals increased creatine kinase (CK) levels.[11] The ischemic exercise test is positive, with no rise in serum lactate after ischemic exercise. A mild hemolysis can also occur. The needle EMG is usually normal but some patients have myopathic changes. Subsarcolemmal glycogen deposits (blebs) that are PAS positive, intermyofibrillar vacuoles, and immunohistochemical stains showing absent staining for phosphofructokinase, are the most common findings on microscopic evaluation.

AMINO ACID METABOLISM

Organic Amino Acidurias

A number of disorders involving amino acid metabolism result in similar symptoms and can be identified via urinary organic acid analysis. A number of different disorders exist and are similar though not directly related. The most important consideration is to recognize the general classification of the disorder by its symptom complex. The urinary organic acid panel can be obtained to identify the exact metabolic defect.[12]

All the organic acidurias are inherited in an autosomal recessive fashion and begin during infancy. A number of characteristics are common to the organic acidurias including vomiting, anorexia, lethargy, ketoacidosis, dehydration, hyperammonemia, neutropenia, and failure to thrive.[13,14] Several neurological manifestations also arise, including seizures, hypomyelination, mental retardation, and coma. Without treatment, these are potentially life-threatening disorders.

Hyperammonemia and hyperglycinemia are common amongst the amino acudurias. Urine and serum organic acid panels can be used to identify the specific disorder.[15]

Specific organic acidurias

Proprionic acidemia is associated with hypotonia, infantile spasms, hypsarrhythmia, and myoclonus in addition to the signs and symptoms common to all the organic acidurias. Treatment includes a diet low in valine, isoleucine, methionine, and threonine. Carnitine supplementation is also necessary.[16,17]

Methylmalonic aciduria typically becomes symptomatic in the first week of life with vomiting, hypotonia, and metabolic acidosis. This may be followed by spascticity, dystonia, strokes, chorea, and developmental delay. The principle treatment is supplemental vitamin B_{12}. If the patient does not respond to Vitamin B_{12}, then a low-protein diet with supplemental L-carnitine may be required.[16,17]

Patients with isovaleric aciduria typically have a strong odor of urine and stale perspiration. Pancytopenia may also complicate the clinical course. Oral glycine supplements are the primary treatment.

Glutaric Acidurias

Just as in the organic aminoacidurias, the family of glutaric acidurias is composed of several unrelated diseases.

Glutaric aciduria type I

Biochemistry and clinical characteristics. Glutaric aciduria type I (Box 23-4) is an autosomal recessive disorder that begins in infancy. The condition presents with a variety of manifestations. Some patients present with an early neurodegenerative disorder with hypotonia, chorea, and seizures. Others have relatively normal early development until the deterioration is suddenly triggered. Macrocephaly is present in 70% and developmental delay is common.[16,17]

Box 23-4. Glutaric Aciduria Type I

Common Name: Glutaric aciduria type I
Incidence: 1:100,000
Inheritance: Autosomal recessive
Metabolic Defect: Glutaryl-CoA dehydrogenase deficiency
Clinical Pattern: Variable. Hypotonia, chorea, seizures, macrocephaly, and developmental delay are common.

Evaluation and pathology. The evaluation of glutaric aciduria type I reveals abnormal urine and serum organic acids. Enzyme assays are also helpful in the diagnosis. Neuroimaging reveals cortical atrophy, gliosis in the caudate and putamen, and atrophy of the caudate.

Management. Treatment consists of a low-protein diet, carnitine supplements, and riboflavin supplements. The diet should, however, be high in calories and low in lysine and tryptophan.

Glutaric aciduria type II

Biochemistry and clinical characteristics. Glutaric aciduria type II (Box 23-5) is also an autosomal recessive (AR) disorder that has several different courses depending on the subtype. There are three subtypes: neonatal with congenital abnormalities, neonatal without congenital abnormalities, and late-onset form. Neonatal glutaric aciduria type II presents with severe metabolic acidosis, cardiomyopathy, and hypoglycemia. The physical features associated with glutaric aciduria type II include macrocephaly, high forehead, flat nasal bridge, and malformed ears.

Evaluation and pathology. The evaluation of glutaric aciduria type II reveals abnormal urine and serum organic acids. Enzyme assays are also helpful in the diagnosis. Neuroimaging reveals agenesis of the cerebellar vermis and hypoplasia of the temporal lobes.

Management. Treatment consists of a high-carbohydrate, low-fat, low-protein diet. Carnitine supplements and riboflavin supplements may be of benefit.

Box 23-5. Glutaric Aciduria Type II

Common Name: Glutaric aciduria type II
Inheritance: Autosomal recessive
Metabolic Defect: Multiple acyl-CoA dehydrogenase deficiency
Clinical Pattern: Neonatal: severe metabolic acidosis, cardiomyopathy, hypoglycemia, macrocephaly, high forehead, flat nasal bridge, and malformed ears.

Table 23-2.		
Inheritance Patterns for Phenylketonuria		
Disease	Inheritance Pattern	Chromosome
PKU	AR	12
Malignant PKU	AR	4

Phenylketonuria

Biochemistry and clinical characteristics

Phenylketonuria (PKU) is an autosomal recessive disorder (Table 23-2, Box 23-6) that results in decreased phenylalanine hydroxylase (conversion of phenylalanine to tyrosine). Patients born with phenylketonuria appear normal at birth, but symptoms begin shortly after birth and after exposure to phenylalanine.[18,19] Vomiting is one of the first symptoms. By several months of age, the patients have developmental delay, with seizures in the more severely affected. In untreated patients, a variety of physical signs are noted, including fair skin, blue eyes, blonde hair, hyperreflexia, hyperkinetic activity, photosensitivity, eczema-like rash, and a musty body odor. Malignant PKU, the stiff baby variant, results from dihydropterin reductase (biopterin) deficiency.

Evaluation and pathology

The phenylalanine screen is positive if phenylalanine level is more than 20 mg/dL. The level should be checked at birth and at 2 weeks of age. If phenylalanine levels are high, a biopterin screen should be obtained. Tyrosine levels are low.

In the untreated, the EEG often reveals paroxysmal activity and hysarrhythmia. The EEG may be normal in the treated patients. Imaging findings remain abnormal even when treated. The MRI reveals atrophy and increased T-2 signal intensity in the posterior deep white matter. There is also decreased metabolism in the caudate and putamen.[20]

Management

Treatment consists of a low-phenylalanine diet for PKU. Infants with malignant PKU require treatment with supplemental biopterin. Even with treatment, malignant PKU has a poor prognosis.[21-23]

Nonketotic Hyperglycinemia

Biochemistry and clinical characteristics

The nonketotic hyperglycinemias (Box 23-7) are a relatively common group of disorders with widely variable genetics, phenotypes, and severities.[24] There are five reported forms of the disease, with four arising during infancy or childhood. The neonatal form is the most common. This form consists of initial hypotonia progressing to hypertonia. Seizures are a common complication. The condition typically progresses to coma, respiratory arrest, and death. Survivors have severe developmental delay and mental retardation.[24,25]

A rare, transient form appears to occur in some patients who are heterozygous for the disease. These patients have a brief, self-limited syndrome that is clinically similar to the more common neonatal form. The late infantile form typically arises toward the end of the first year, with cognitive decline, decerebrate posturing, and extrapyramidal findings. The juvenile form is associated with mild mental retardation and language dysfunction.

Evaluation and pathology

Nonketotic hyperglycinemia is rarely identified on newborn screening.[26] Laboratory evaluation requires spinal fluid evaluation. Elevation of the CSF glycine/serum glycine ratio (ratio > 0.10) is diagnostic. The EEG can reveal burst suppression, hypsarrhythmia, or focal epileptiform discharges. Neuroimaging reveals atrophy and hypomyelination.[27]

Management

The principle treatment is supportive care and treatment of the seizures with antiepileptic medication.

Table 23-3.

Disorders of the Urea Cycle

Disorder	Inheritance	Chromosome
Ornithine transcarbamylase deficiency	X-linked	Xp
Carbamoyl phosphate synthetase deficiency	AR	2q
Argininosuccinate synthetase deficiency (citrullinemia)	AR	9q
N-acetylglutamate sythetase	AR	17q
Argininosuccinic aciduria	AR	7
Arginase deficiency	AR	6q

Urea Cycle Defects

Biochemistry and clinical characteristics

The disorders of the urea cycle all result in hyperammonemia and therefore have similar symptom complexes (Table 23-3).[28-30] Symptoms usually arise during the neonatal period. These conditions should always be considered when an infant's ammonia level is elevated. Carbamoyl phosphate synthetase deficiency is the most severe of the urea cycle defects. When the enzyme is completely absent, it is usually fatal. Partial absence or dysfunction of the enzyme results in variable degrees of severity. The clinical presentation includes coma, seizures, hypotonia, respiratory arrest, occasional intracranial hemorrhages, vomiting, and death without treatment. Some patients, especially with milder forms of the disease, may be normal with early treatment.

Evaluation and pathology

Disorders of the urea cycle are usually associated with dramatic elevations of serum ammonia, often more than 500 mg/dL.[31] Increased glutamine levels are found on serum amino acid testing. Hepatic function studies typically reveal elevated AST and ALT levels. Neuroimaging studies reveal cerebral edema with occasional intracranial hemorrhage. A number of findings are common on microscopic pathologic evaluation including cerebral edema, Alzheimer type II cells, decreased myelination, and neuronal loss. Alzheimer type II cells are not common in carbamoyl phosphate synthetase deficiency, most likely because it is often rapidly fatal.

Management

Treatment consists primarily of hemodialysis to decrease ammonia and dietary restriction of nitrogen (low-protein diet). Valproate should be avoided for seizures since this drug increases ammonia production.[32]

Box 23-8. Hartnup Disease

Common Name: Hartnup disease
Incidence: 1:33,000
Inheritance: Familial
Metabolic Defect: Defect in Na-dependent neutral amino acid transport
Clinical Pattern: Failure to thrive, photosensitive scaly rash, intermittent ataxia, personality changes, nystagmus, and tremor.

Renal Amino Acid Transport

Hartnup disease

Biochemistry and clinical characteristics. Hartnup disease (Box 23-8) is a familial disorder of renal amino acid transport caused by defective Na-dependent neutral amino acid transport in the small intestine and renal tubules, leading to increased fecal and urinary amino acid excretion.[33] The symptoms begin during infancy. The clinical presentation is highly variable, with failure to thrive, a photosensitive scaly rash, intermittent ataxia, personality changes, nystagmus, and a tremor.[34] The symptoms tend to improve with age; in some cases there is slow progression.

Evaluation and pathology. Intermittent cerebral symptoms should suggest the diagnosis. Laboratory studies may reveal low serum tryptophan on neutral amino acid screening.

Management. Treatment includes a high-protein diet with nicotinic acid supplements (niacin). Tryptophan ethylester can also be of benefit. There is, however, a general improvement with increasing age.

Lowe syndrome (oculocerebrorenal syndrome)

Lowe syndrome (Box 23-9), a disorder of renal amino acid transport, is thought to be caused by a membrane transport defect. It is transmitted in an X-linked recessive pattern.[35] The symptoms typically begin during the neonatal period. The clinical presentation includes

---

Box 23-9. Lowe Syndrome

Common Name: Lowe syndrome
Inheritance: X-linked recessive
Metabolic Defect: Membrane transport defect
Clinical Pattern: Oculocerebrorenal syndrome—The symptoms typically begin during the neonatal period with mental retardation, developmental delay, glaucoma, cataracts, myopathy, and pendular nystagmus. Punctate cortical lens opacities may be the only sign in heterozygote female carriers. Death usually occurs secondary to renal failure.

Box 23-10. Maple Syrup Urine Disease

Common Name: Maple syrup urine disease
Incidence: 1:150,000
Inheritance: Autosomal recessive
Metabolic Defect: Alpha-ketoacid dehydrogenase deficiency
Clinical Pattern: Symptoms typically begin during the neonatal period with hypertonia, opisthotonos, fluctuating ophthalmoplegia, generalized seizures, and developmental delay. The patient eventually becomes flaccid and areflexic. Coma ensues without treatment. The prognosis is good if treatment is instituted within 5 days.

Box 23-11. Homocystinuria

Common Name: Homocystinuria
Inheritance: Autosomal recessive
Metabolic Defect: Cystathionine beta synthase deficiency
Clinical Pattern: Marfanoid habitus, codfish vertebra (biconcave), ocular anomalies include ectopia lentis, myopia, glaucoma, and optic atrophy. Central nervous system complications include mental retardation, seizures, behavioral disorders, and stroke.

---

mental retardation and developmental delay, glaucoma, cataracts, myopathy, and pendular nystagmus.[36] In addition, punctate cortical lens opacities may be the only sign in heterozygote female carriers. Death usually occurs secondary to renal failure. Pathology reveals loss of both central and peripheral myelinated fibers.

Maple syrup urine disease

Biochemistry and clinical characteristics. Maple syrup urine disease (Box 23-10) is a disorder of branched-chain amino acid metabolism secondary to a defect of alpha-ketoacid dehydrogenase deficiency resulting in abnormal oxidative decarboxylation.[37] It is inherited in an autosomal recessive pattern. The symptoms typically begin during the neonatal period. The clinical presentation includes hypertonia, opisthotonos, fluctuating ophthalmoplegia that correlates with serum leucine levels, clonus, generalized seizures, and developmental delay.[38] The patient eventually becomes flaccid and areflexic. Coma ensues without treatment. Conversely, the prognosis is good and the patient may have a normal IQ if treatment is instituted within 5 days.

Evaluation and pathology. Laboratory evaluation reveals elevated branched-chain amino acids (leucine, isoleucine, and valine) on serum amino acid screening. Approximately 50% of patients develop severe hypoglycemia. The urine has a characteristic odor and tests positive for 2,4-dinitrophenylhydrazine (DNPH).[39] Imaging during the acute phase reveals cerebral edema greatest in cerebellar deep white matter and brainstem. Pathologic specimens reveal white matter cystic degeneration and gliosis.

Management. Treatment consists of thiamine supplementation and dietary restriction of branched-chain amino acids.[40]

Homocystinuria

Biochemistry and clinical characteristics. Homocystinuria (Box 23-11) is a genetic disorder of homocysteine metabolism with AR inheritance (chromosome 21).

Cystathionine beta synthase deficiency results in accumulation of homocysteine and methionine.[41] There is also impaired methylation of homocysteine to methionine from enzyme deficiency or cofactor B_{12} deficiency. The onset and severity of symptoms are variable. The clinical presentation includes marfanoid habitus and codfish vertebra (biconcave). Ocular anomalies include ectopia lentis (lens displaced downward) in 90% of patients, myopia, glaucoma, and optic atrophy. Central nervous system complications include mental retardation, seizures, behavioral disorders, and stroke (beginning at age 5 to 9 months).[42]

Evaluation and pathology. Laboratory evaluation reveals increased homocysteine on serum and urine amino acids, and a positive methionine challenge test. Pathologic evaluation reveals intimal thickening and fibrosis of blood vessels leading to arterial and venous thrombosis.

Management. Treatment consists of dietary restriction of methionine, pyridoxine supplements, vitamin B_{12} supplements, and cysteine supplements.

PURINE METABOLISM

Lesch-Nyhan Syndrome

Biochemistry and clinical characteristics

Lesch-Nyhan syndrome (Box 23-12) is a rare disorder of purine metabolism secondary to hypoxanthine-guanine

---

Box 23-12. Lesch-Nyhan Syndrome

Common Name: Lesch-Nyhan syndrome
Incidence: 1:400,000 in males
Inheritance: X-linked recessive
Metabolic Defect: Hypoxanthine-guanine phosphoribosyl transferase deficiency
Clinical Pattern: Symptoms typically begin about age 6 months with developmental delay, choreoathetosis, dystonia, opisthotonos, hyperreflexia, mental retardation, and self-mutilating behavior.

phosphoribosyl transferase deficiency. It is inherited in an X-linked recessive pattern. Symptoms typically begin about age 6 months. The clinical presentation includes developmental delay, choreoathetosis, dystonia, opisthotonos, hyperreflexia, mental retardation, and self-mutilating behavior.[43]

Evaluation and pathology

Laboratory evaluation reveals crystalluria and hyperuricemia.[44]

Management

Treatment includes allopurinol 20 mg/kg/d (blocks uric acid synthesis). L-5-hydroxytryptophan plus L-dopa can help with symptomatic management. Physical restraint may be necessary given the risk of self-mutilating behavior. Fluphenazine may also help decrease self-mutilating behavior.[45]

LIPOPROTEIN METABOLISM

Abetalipoproteinemia (Bassen-Kornzweig Disease)

Biochemistry and clinical characteristics

Abetalipoproteinemia, or Bassen-Kornzweig disease (Box 23-13), is an AR disorder of lipoprotein metabolism resulting from a decreased posttranslational processing of apolipoprotein B.[46] Abetalipoproteinemia typically manifests neurological symptoms by age 12 years. The clinical manifestations include fat malabsorption with diarrhea and steatorrhea; acanthocytosis; retinopathy; vitamins A, D, E, and K deficiency; neuropathy with decreased reflexes, proprioception, and sensation; progressive ataxia; positive Romberg sign; decreased night vision (retinitis pigmentosa); and weakness.[47]

Evaluation and pathology

The laboratory evaluation of abetalipoproteinemia reveals acanthocytosis (Figure 23-3); absent beta-lipoproteins

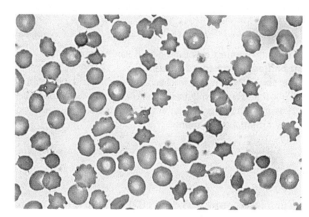

FIGURE 23-3 ■ Blood smear showing acanthocytosis. (*Reproduced with permission from Lichtman M, Beutler E, Kipps T, Seligohn U, Kaushansky K, Prchal J, eds. Williams Hematology. 7th ed. New York: McGraw-Hill; 2006:color plate III-11.*)

(chylomicrons, LDL, VLDL); decreased triglycerides and cholesterol; low vitamin A, D, E, and K levels (fat-soluble vitamins); and increased PT. Nerve conduction velocities are slow. Pathologic findings include loss of large myelinated fibers and spinocerebellar and posterior column degeneration.

Management

Treatment includes dietary restriction of triglycerides. Vitamin E supplements may also be of some benefit.[48]

Tangier Disease

Biochemistry and clinical characteristics

Tangier disease (Box 23-14) is an AR disorder of lipoprotein metabolism resulting from a deficiency of alpha-lipoprotein. The clinical manifestations include large orange tonsils, lymphadenopathy, splenomegaly, corneal infiltrates, relapsing multiple mononeuropathies, and loss of pain and temperature sensation. Peripheral neuropathy occurs in 50% of patients with demyelinating sensory, sensorimotor, or motor neuropathy.

Evaluation and pathology

The laboratory evaluation of Tangier disease reveals decreased total cholesterol and LDL, triglycerides normal

---

Box 23-13. Bassen-Kornzweig Disease

Common Name: Bassen–Kornzweig disease
Inheritance: Autosomal recessive
Metabolic Defect: Decreased posttranslational processing of apolipoprotein B
Clinical Pattern: Fat malabsorption with diarrhea and steatorrhea; acanthocytosis; retinopathy; vitamin A, D, E, and K deficiency; neuropathy with decreased reflexes, proprioception, and sensation; progressive ataxia; positive Romberg sign; decreased night vision (retinitis pigmentosa); and weakness.

Box 23-14. Tangier Disease

Common Name: Tangier disease
Inheritance: Autosomal recessive
Metabolic Defect: Deficiency of alpha-lipoprotein
Clinical Pattern: Large orange tonsils, lymphadenopathy, splenomegaly, corneal infiltrates, relapsing multiple mononeuropathies, loss of pain and temperature sensation (peripheral neuropathy).

Box 23-15. Cerebrotendinous Xanthomatosis

Common Name: Cerebrotendinous xanthomatosis
Inheritance: Autosomal recessive
Metabolic Defect: Absent chenodeoxycholic acid (bile acid)
Clinical Pattern: Dementia, ataxia, seizures, paresis, peripheral neuropathy, juvenile cataracts, xanthoma, atherosclerosis, and mental retardation.

---

or increased, and very low HDL. Nerve conduction velocities are typically slow in the demeylinating range. Pathologic findings include lipid droplets in Schwann cells and in reticular endothelial system (RES) of other cells, evidence of neuropathy with demyelination/remyelination, and a syringomyelia-like syndrome with axonal degeneration.

Management

There is no reliable treatment.

Cerebrotendinous Xanthomatosis

Biochemistry and clinical characteristics

Cerebrotendinous xanthomatosis (Box 23-15) is an AR disorder of lipoprotein metabolism resulting from absent chenodeoxycholic acid (bile acid).[49] The clinical manifestations include dementia, ataxia, seizures, paresis, peripheral neuropathy, juvenile cataracts, xanthoma, atherosclerosis, and mental retardation.

Evaluation and pathology

The laboratory evaluation of cerebrotendinous xanthomatosis reveals increased cholestanol.[50] Nerve conduction velocities are typically slow. Neuroimaging reveals diffuse hypomyelination on MRI and diffuse hypomyelination with hyperdensities in the cerebellum on CT. Pathologic findings include extensive demyelination greatest in the cerebellum and brainstem.

Management

Treatment consists of chenodeoxycholic acid 750 mg/d.[50]

PORPHYRIA

Biochemistry and Clinical Characteristics

Porphyria occurs in several subtypes, including acute intermittent porphyria (AIP), hereditary coproporphyria, and variegate porphyria.[51] The general characteristics of porphyria are outlined in Table 23-4.

Table 23-4.

Porphyria: Symptoms, Signs, and Medications

Symptom	Frequency (%)	Sign	Frequency (%)
Abdominal pain	95	Tachycardia	80
Extremity pain	50	Dark urine	74
Back pain	29	Motor deficit	60
Chest pain	12	Proximal limbs	48
Nausea and	43	Generalized	42
vomiting	48	Distal limbs	10
Constipation	43	Altered mentation	40
Diarrhea		Hypertension	36
		Sensory deficit	26
		Seizure	20

Medications in Porphyria	Dangerous	Probably Safe
Anticonvulsants	Barbiturates	Bromides
	Carbamazepine	Diazepam
	Clonazepam	Magnesium sulfate
	Ethosuximide	
	Phenytoin	
	Primidone	
	Valproic acid	
Hypnotics	Barbiturates	Chloral hydrate
	Chlordiazepoxide	Chlorpromazine
	Ethchlorvynol	Diphenhydramine
	Glutethimide	Lithium
	Meprobamate	Lorazepam
	Methyprylon	Meclizine
	Trifluoperazine	
Other	Alpha-methyldopa	ACTH
	Danazol	Allopurinol
	Ergots	Aminoglycosides
	Estrogens	Aspirin
	Griseofulvin	Codeine
	Imipramine	Colchicine
	Pentazocine	Furosemide
	Pyrazinamide	Ibuprofen
	Insulin	
	Meperidine	
	Morphine	
	Naproxen	
	Penicillin	
	Warfarin	

Adapted with permission from Geyer J, Keating J, Potts D, Carney P, eds. Neurology for the Boards. 3rd ed. Philadelphia, PA: Lippincott Williams & Wilkins; 2006.

Porphyria can be challenging to diagnose, especially early in the syndrome. The differential diagnosis includes Guillain–Barré syndrome, lead intoxication, and hereditary tyrosinemia.

Evaluation and Pathology

The laboratory evaluation includes elevated porphobilinogen (PBG) in urine, quantitative aminolevulinic acid (ALA), PBG, and porphyrins in urine and feces.[52] There is patchy demyelination and axonal degeneration.

Management

It is of utmost importance to avoid medications and other potential exacerbating factors. Treatment also includes hematin 1.5 to 3 mg/kg IV.[52] Symptomatic treatment is very important, but must be administered with care given the risk of some medications exacerbating the porphyria. Pain should be managed with analgesics, morphine, and chlorpromazine. Hyponatremia should be treated with normal saline (NS) + diuretics. Many seizure medications exacerbate porphyria. Valium is usually well tolerated in the patient with porphyria. Several of the newer antiepileptic agents are relatively safe in this population as well.

METAL METABOLISM

Wilson Disease (Hepatolenticular Degeneration)

Biochemistry and clinical characteristics

Wilson disease, or hepatolenticular degeneration (Box 23-16), is an AR disorder (chromosome 13) of metal metabolism resulting from ATPase deficiency.[53] Wilson disease typically manifests itself between ages 11 and 25 years. The clinical manifestations include cirrhosis, tremor (wing-beating), rigidity, dystonia, chorea, Kayser–Fleischer rings (present in 100% of neurological Wilson disease patients; Figure 23-4), seizures, and psychosis.[54]

Evaluation and pathology

The laboratory evaluation of Wilson disease reveals low or absent ceruloplasmin (low or absent in 96% of cases).[54,55] Aminoaciduria is also common. Kayser–Fleischer rings are present in 100% of neurologic Wilson cases.

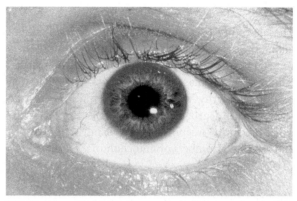

FIGURE 23-4 ■ A Kayser–Fleischer ring. Although in this case the brownish ring rimming the cornea is clearly visible to the naked eye, confirmation is usually by slit-lamp examination. (*Reproduced with permission from Kasper DL, Braunwald E, Hauser SL, Longo DL, Jameson JL, Loscalzo J, eds.* Harrison's Principles of Internal Medicine. *17th ed. New York: McGraw-Hill; 2008:2450, Figure 354-1.*)

Neuroimaging reveals caudate and putamen atrophy (lenticular degeneration). Pathologic findings include brick-red basal ganglia, spongy degeneration of the putamen, Alzheimer astrocytes, and neuronal dropout with axonal degeneration.

Management

Treatment includes a copper-poor diet. Sulfide 20 mg tid and penicillamine 500 to 1000 mg tid can also be of some benefit. L-dopa may be effective for the dystonia.

Kinky Hair Disease (Menkes Disease)

Biochemistry and clinical characteristics

Kinky hair disease, or Menkes disease (Box 23-17), is disorder of metal metabolism resulting from copper ATPase deficiency.[56] The incidence is approximately 1 in 250,000 live births. Kinky hair disease usually becomes clinically apparent during infancy. The clinical manifestations include hypothermia, poor feeding, seizures, hypotonia, a cherubic face, colorless friable kinky hair, and hydronephrosis.

Box 23-16. Wilson Disease

Common Name: Wilson disease
Inheritance: Autosomal recessive
Metabolic Defect: ATPase deficiency
Clinical Pattern: Hepatolenticular degeneration—cirrhosis; tremor (wing-beating); rigidity; dystonia; chorea; Kayser–Fleischer rings; seizures; and psychosis.

Box 23-17. Kinky Hair Disease

Common Name: Kinky hair disease
Incidence: 1:250,000 live births
Inheritance: Autosomal recessive
Metabolic Defect: Copper ATPase deficiency
Clinical Pattern: Hypothermia, poor feeding, seizures, hypotonia, a cherubic face, colorless friable kinky hair, and hydronephrosis.

Evaluation and pathology

The laboratory evaluation of kinky hair disease reveals a falling ceruloplasmin on serial measurements.[56,57] Neuroimaging reveals atrophy and focal encephalomalacia. Subdural hematomas are also common. The EEG often reveals hypsarrhythmia. Pathologic findings include focal cortical degeneration, prominent cerebellar neuronal dropout, "weeping willow" dendritic processes, and increased numbers of mitochondria.

Management

The primary treatment is copper histidine.

REFERENCES

1. Kemper AR, Hwu WL, Lloyd-Puryear M, Kishnani PS. Newborn screening for Pompe disease: synthesis of the evidence and development of screening recommendations. *Pediatrics.* 2007;120:e1327-1334.
2. Di Rocco M, Buzzi D, Tarò M. Glycogen storage disease type II: clinical overview. *Acta Myol.* 2007;26:42-44.
3. Koeberl DD, Kishnani PS, Chen YT. Glycogen storage disease types I and II: treatment updates. *J Inherit Metab Dis.* 2007;30:159-164.
4. Kishnani PS, Corzo D, Nicolino M, et al. Recombinant human acid [alpha]-glucosidase: major clinical benefits in infantile-onset Pompe disease. *Neurology.* 2007;68:99-109.
5. Shin YS. Glycogen storage disease: clinical, biochemical, and molecular heterogeneity. *Semin Pediatr Neurol.* 2006; 13:115-120.
6. Nogales-Gadea G, Arenas J, Andreu AL. Molecular genetics of McArdle's disease. *Curr Neurol Neurosci Rep.* 2007;7:84-92. Review.
7. Pillarisetti J, Ahmed A. McArdle disease presenting as acute renal failure. *South Med J.* 2007;100:313-316.
8. Haller RG. Treatment of McArdle disease. *Arch Neurol.* 2000;57:923-924.
9. Ronquist G. Glycogenosis type VII (Tarui's disease): diagnostic considerations and late sequelae. *South Med J.* 2002; 95:1361-1362.
10. Nakajima H, Raben N, Hamaguchi T, Yamasaki T. Phosphofructokinase deficiency; past, present and future. *Curr Mol Med.* 2002;2:197-212.
11. Massa R, Sancesario G, Bernardi G. Muscle phosphofructokinase deficiency. *Neurology.* 1997;49:899.
12. Auray-Blais C, Cyr D, Drouin R. Quebec neonatal mass urinary screening programme: from micromolecules to macromolecules. *J Inherit Metab Dis.* 2007;30:515-521.
13. Dionisi-Vici C, Deodato F, Röschinger W, Rhead W, Wilcken B. "Classical" organic acidurias, propionic aciduria, methylmalonic aciduria and isovaleric aciduria: long-term outcome and effects of expanded newborn screening using tandem mass spectrometry. *J Inherit Metab Dis.* 2006;29:383-389.
14. Sperl W. Diagnosis and therapy of organic acidurias. *Pediatr Pathol.* 1993;28:3-8.
15. Chaves-Carballo E. Detection of inherited neurometabolic disorders. A practical clinical approach. *Pediatr Clin North Am.* 1992;39:801-820.
16. Ozand PT, Gascon GG. Organic acidurias: a review. Part 1. *J Child Neurol.* 1991;6:196-219.
17. Ozand PT, Gascon GG. Organic acidurias: a review. Part 2. *J Child Neurol.* 1991;6:288-303.
18. Committee on Genetics, Kaye CI, Accurso F, La Franchi S, et al. Introduction to the newborn screening fact sheets. *Pediatrics.* 2006;118:1304-1312.
19. Kerruish NJ, Robertson SP. Newborn screening: new developments, new dilemmas. *J Med Ethics.* 2005; 31:393–398.
20. Laule C, Vavasour IM, Mädler B, et al. MR evidence of long T2 water in pathological white matter. *J Magn Reson Imaging.* 2007;26:1117-1121.
21. Giovannini M, Verduci E, Salvatici E, Fiori L, Riva E. Phenylketonuria: dietary and therapeutic challenges. *J Inherit Metab Dis.* 2007;30:145-152.
22. Böhles H. Possibilities and limitations of dietary therapy for inborn errors of metabolism. *Forum Nutr.* 2003; 56:225–226.
23. Giovannini M, Riva E, Salvatici E, et al. Treating phenylketonuria: a single centre experience. *J Int Med Res.* 2007;35:742-752.
24. Korman SH. Diagnosis of nonketotic hyperglycinemia in patients treated with valproic acid. *Pediatr Neurol.* 2007; 37:77.
25. Tan ES, Wiley V, Carpenter K, Wilcken B. Non-ketotic hyperglycinemia is usually not detectable by tandem mass spectrometry newborn screening. *Mol Genet Metab.* 2007;90:446-448.
26. Applegarth DA, Toone JR. Glycine encephalopathy (nonketotic hyperglycinemia): comments and speculations. *Am J Med Genet A.* 2006;140:186-188.
27. Shah DK, Tingay DG, Fink AM, Hunt RW, Dargaville PA. Magnetic resonance imaging in neonatal nonketotic hyperglycinemia. *Pediatr Neurol.* 2005;33:50-52.
28. Saudubray JM, Sedel F, Walter JH. Clinical approach to treatable inborn metabolic diseases: an introduction. *J Inherit Metab Dis.* 2006;29:261-274.
29. Endo F, Matsuura T, Yanagita K, Matsuda I. Clinical manifestations of inborn errors of the urea cycle and related metabolic disorders during childhood. *J Nutr.* 2004;134 (suppl): 1605S–1609S; discussion 1630S-1632S, 1667S-1672S.
30. Gropman AL, Batshaw ML. Cognitive outcome in urea cycle disorders. *Mol Genet Metab.* 2004;81(suppl):S58-S62.
31. Häberle J, Koch HG. Genetic approach to prenatal diagnosis in urea cycle defects. *Prenat Diagn.* 2004;24:378-383.
32. Nassogne MC, Héron B, Touati G, Rabier D, Saudubray JM. Urea cycle defects: management and outcome. *J Inherit Metab Dis.* 2005;28:407-414.
33. Buehler BA. Inherited disorders of amino acid transport in relation to the kidney. *Ann Clin Lab Sci.* 1981;11:274-278.
34. Irons M, Levy HL. Metabolic syndromes with dermatologic manifestations. *Clin Rev Allergy.* 1986;4:101-124.
35. Lavin CW, McKeown CA. The oculocerebrorenal syndrome of Lowe. *Int Ophthalmol Clin.* 1993;33:179-191.
36. Charnas LR, Gahl WA. The oculocerebrorenal syndrome of Lowe. *Adv Pediatr.* 1991;38:75-107.

37. Fernstrom JD. Branched-chain amino acids and brain function. *J Nutr.* 2005;135(suppl):1539S-1546S.

38. Schadewaldt P, Wendel U. Metabolism of branched-chain amino acids in maple syrup urine disease. *Eur J Pediatr.* 1997;156(suppl):S62-S66.

39. Velázquez A, Vela-Amieva M, Cicerón-Arellano I, et al. Diagnosis of inborn errors of metabolism. *Arch Med Res.* 2000;31:145-150.

40. Saudubray JM, Nassogne MC, de Lonlay P, Touati G. Clinical approach to inherited metabolic disorders in neonates: an overview. *Semin Neonatol.* 2002;7:3-15.

41. Miles EW, Kraus JP. Cystathionine beta-synthase: structure, function, regulation, and location of homocystinuria-causing mutations. *J Biol Chem.* 2004;279:29871-29874.

42. Finkelstein JD. Inborn errors of sulfur-containing amino acid metabolism. *J Nutr.* 2006;136(suppl):1750S-1754S.

43. Jinnah HA, Visser JE, Harris JC, et al.; Lesch-Nyhan Disease International Study Group. Delineation of the motor disorder of Lesch-Nyhan disease. *Brain.* 2006;129:1201-1217.

44. McCarthy G. Medical diagnosis, management and treatment of Lesch Nyhan disease. *Nucleosides Nucleotides Nucleic Acids.* 2004;23:1147-1152.

45. Cusumano FJ, Penna KJ, Panossian G. Prevention of self-mutilation in patients with Lesch-Nyhan syndrome: review of literature. *ASDC J Dent Child.* 2001;68:175-178.

46. Rampoldi L, Danek A, Monaco AP. Clinical features and molecular bases of neuroacanthocytosis. *J Mol Med.* 2002;80:475-491.

47. Stevenson VL, Hardie RJ. Acanthocytosis and neurological disorders. *J Neurol.* 2001;248:87-94.

48. Grant CA, Berson EL. Treatable forms of retinitis pigmentosa associated with systemic neurological disorders. *Int Ophthalmol Clin.* 2001;41:103-110.

49. Moghadasian MH. Cerebrotendinous xanthomatosis: clinical course, genotypes and metabolic backgrounds. *Clin Invest Med.* 2004;27:42-50.

50. Federico A, Dotti MT. Cerebrotendinous xanthomatosis: clinical manifestations, diagnostic criteria, pathogenesis, and therapy. *J Child Neurol.* 2003;18:633-638.

51. Sassa S. Modern diagnosis and management of the porphyrias. *Br J Haematol.* 2006;135:281-292.

52. Poblete-Gutiérrez P, Wiederholt T, Merk HF, Frank J. The porphyrias: clinical presentation, diagnosis and treatment. *Eur J Dermatol.* 2006;16:230-240.

53. Pfeiffer RF. Wilson's disease. *Semin Neurol.* 2007;27:123-132.

54. Madsen E, Gitlin JD. Copper and iron disorders of the brain. *Annu Rev Neurosci.* 2007;30:317-337.

55. Ala A, Walker AP, Ashkan K, Dooley JS, Schilsky ML. Wilson's disease. *Lancet.* 2007;369:397-408.

56. de Bie P, Muller P, Wijmenga C, Klomp LW. Molecular pathogenesis of Wilson and Menkes disease: correlation of mutations with molecular defects and disease phenotypes. *J Med Genet.* 2007;44:673-688.

57. Madsen E, Gitlin JD. Copper and iron disorders of the brain. *Annu Rev Neurosci.* 2007;30:317-337.

CHAPTER 24

Inherited Neurodegenerative Disorders

Alan K. Percy

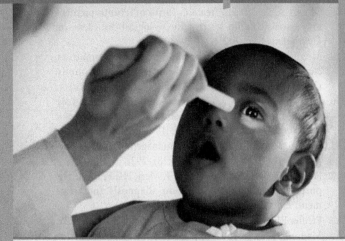

Understanding the inherited neurodegenerative diseases of childhood has evolved dramatically in the past 40 years. Fundamental discoveries in biochemistry uncovered the metabolic basis for many of these diseases. The subsequent identification of variant forms created additional challenges for the clinician. These variant forms share similar, if not identical, biochemical defects, but exhibit widely differing clinical expressions. Recent progress followed the rapid development and application of molecular-genetic strategies and the close linkage between clinical observations and basic science advances. The successes of molecular genetics have provided significant clarifications, but have also generated further examples of the marked heterogeneity within these disorders. These advances explain how disorders with clearly different phenotypic expression can result from different mutations within the same gene and, conversely, how disorders with similar clinical features result from mutations in different genes. Examples of the former include GM2-gangliosidosis variants and examples of the latter include the neuronal ceroid lipofuscinoses. Thus, at the clinical, biochemical, and molecular level, the clinician is faced with an increasingly complex knowledge base, the unraveling of which may present major diagnostic hurdles.

Inherited neurodegenerative diseases represent a significant proportion of referrals to tertiary care centers, especially those specializing in the care of children. For all inherited neurometabolic diseases as a group, the overall incidence is about 1 in 3700 births, and for those neurodegenerative disorders considered here, incidence may approach 1 in 5000 births. Technological advancements have in no way diminished the need for careful characterization of the clinical phenotype. Rather, enhanced diagnostic capabilities raise important public health policy issues including development of the necessary infrastructure to monitor outcome of diagnosis and treatment and to analyze the overall impact on society.

Regardless of the biochemical and molecular mechanisms, common patterns of disease expression emerge according to age at onset. Disorders presenting in infancy and early childhood are characterized by delayed development or loss of acquired developmental milestones that follows a period of delay or plateau in development. Onset in school-aged children or adolescents is characterized by declining school performance and behavioral or personality changes. In adulthood, faltering personal or work habits suggest declining cognitive abilities, movement disorder, or gait difficulties. As such, clinical assessment should include historical information regarding changes in development or behavior, evidence of cognitive difficulties, and altered motor control and a careful family history including consanguinity, previous deaths in childhood or adolescence, early-onset dementia, or a diagnosis of *progressive* cerebral palsy. Progressive neurological manifestations fall outside the established pathogenesis for cerebral palsy. A thorough clinical examination should incorporate assessment for dysmorphic features, hepatosplenomegaly, or skeletal deformities, and careful neurological and ophthalmologic evaluations, the latter for abnormalities of voluntary eye movement, corneal clouding, lens opacities, and retinal abnormalities such as retinitis pigmentosa, macular degeneration, cherry-red spot maculae, and optic atrophy.

Neurodegenerative disease may be explained by a number of processes that should be excluded including other metabolic conditions such as diabetes mellitus or porphyria, toxic encephalopathies (heavy metal poisoning, antiepileptic or neuroleptic preparations, or drugs of abuse), chronic viral infections (subacute sclerosing panencephalitis and the AIDS complex group), immunopathic disorders (systemic lupus erythematosis and related conditions), intracranial neoplasms, and psychiatric or behavioral disorders including autistic spectrum disorder and environmental deprivation.

Laboratory diagnosis involves a variety of biochemical, enzymatic, and molecular methodologies as well as clinical neurophysiology, neuroimaging, and histopathology. Careful clinical assessment should allow a quite precise tailored approach. However, for this to occur, a high index of suspicion for an inherited neurodegenerative process is essential.

In sum, the inherited neurodegenerative diseases represent important opportunities for advancement of knowledge, but at the same time present significant challenges to the neurologist in providing timely diagnosis, appropriate family counseling, and the consideration of new therapeutic strategies.

This chapter explores four groups of inherited neurodegenerative diseases presenting in childhood: the sphingolipidoses, the adrenoleukodystrophy complex, the neuronal ceroid lipofuscinoses, and the sialidosis/sialuria complex.[1,2] Clinical heterogeneity is summarized and current approaches to diagnosis and treatment examined. In the past, these disorders have been classified in discrete forms according to age at onset and clinical severity. We now recognize that age at onset and clinical severity fall along a clinical continuum. Detailed descriptions of these diseases can be found elsewhere.

SPECIFIC DISEASE ENTITIES

The sphingolipidoses, adrenoleukodystrophy complex, neuronal ceroid lipofuscinoses, and sialidosis/sialuria complex include disorders affecting both neuronal and glial function.[1,2] Within each group, the principal clinical variants will be discussed in terms of age at onset, clinical features, prognosis, mode of inheritance, stored material when relevant, and enzyme defects when known. Variant forms that may begin in adolescence or adulthood are included for comparison.

Sphingolipidoses

The sphingolipidoses (Table 24-1) represent a model for understanding the inherited neurodegenerative diseases of children, encompassing within the respective disorders both neuronal storage and white matter involvement.[3-11] The sphingolipids are normal lipid constituents of biological membranes. The sphingolipidoses reflect accumulation of the disease-related sphingolipid within the affected organ(s) as the result of defective catabolism.

Catabolism of sphingolipids occurs within lysosomes by specific acid hydrolases (lysosomal hydrolases). With the exception of galactosylceramide lipidosis (Krabbe disease), the disease-related sphingolipid accumulates up to 100-fold that seen in normal tissue. Accumulation of the sphingolipid, galactosylceramide, does not occur in Krabbe disease, except within globoid bodies, the neuropathologic hallmark of this disease. In contrast, galactosylsphingosine (psychosine), the deacylated form of galactosylceramide and the principal cytotoxic component of Krabbe disease does accumulate.

GM2 GANGLIOSIDOSES

The GM2 gangliosidoses (Box 24-1) are generally classified as acute (infantile), subacute (juvenile), and chronic (adult) types according to age at onset (Table 24-1). The majority manifest the acute-onset form, that is, classic Tay-Sachs disease. At least 10 clinical phenotypes are recognized,[12] each caused by deficiency of hexosaminidase A, except in the case of Sandhoff disease and its variant forms that feature deficiencies of both hexosaminidase A and B (Hex A and Hex B), or the very rare form caused by deficiency of the GM2 activator protein. Tay-Sachs disease has been recognized in several population isolates, including Ashkenazi Jews, French-Canadians, Pennsylvania Dutch, and Cajuns (from Acadia). The incidence of Tay-Sachs disease is approximately 1 in 4000 among Ashkenazi Jews and about 1 in 200,000 in the general population. Only Hex A metabolizes GM2 ganglioside. Hex B metabolizes the neutral sphingolipid, globoside, in addition to the other compounds noted above. Children with GM2 activator deficiency resemble Tay-Sachs disease clinically. They have normal Hex A and Hex B activity, but lack the activator protein required for metabolism of GM2 ganglioside.

Box 24-1. Tay-Sachs Disease

Common Name: Tay-Sachs disease; Sandhoff disease
Incidence: 1:4000 in Ashkenazi Jews; 1:220,000 otherwise
Inheritance: Autosomal recessive
Relevant Metabolite: GM2 ganglioside, asialo-GM2, lyso-GM2
Metabolic Defects: Hexosaminidase A, hexosaminidase B, GM2 activator
Mutation: *HEXA*-chromosome 15q23-24, *HEXB*-chromosome 5q13, *GM2A*-chromosome 5q31.3-33.1
Clinical Pattern: Multiple phenotypes reflecting different mutations

Table 24-1.

Inherited Neurodegenerative Disorders of Childhood: Clinical Features

Disease	Onset Age	Clinical Features	Longevity	Inheritance
Sphingolipidoses				
GM2-Gangliosidosis	6-12 mo	Psychomotor decline Seizures Cherry-red maculae	Death by age 5	AR
Juvenile type	2-5 y	Seizures Gait difficulty Psychomotor decline	Death by age 15	AR
Adult type	Adolescence to adulthood	Spinocerebellar degeneration Distal muscle wasting Dystonia Intact mentation	Slow progression usual	AR
Sandhoff type	6-12 mo	Hepatosplenomegaly Psychomotor decline Seizures Cherry-red maculae	Death by age 5	AR
GM1-Gangliosidosis (Generalized gangliosidosis)				
Type I—Infantile	Infancy	Hurler-like appearance Hepatomegaly Psychomotor decline	Death by age 2	AR
Type II—Late infantile	6-12 mo	Psychomotor decline	Death in 3-10 y	AR
Type III—Juvenile	5 y	Ataxia Dysarthria Mild dementia	Prolonged survival	AR
Type IV—Adult	Adolescence to adulthood Gait difficulty Variable dementia	Dystonia Bradykinesia	Prolonged survival	AR
Globotriaosylceramide *lipidosis* (Fabry disease)	Adolescence to adulthood	Cutaneous angiokeratoma Painful neuropathy Heat intolerance Renal disease Cardiac/CNS disease	Middle age	XLR
Sphingomyelin Lipidosis (Niemann-Pick Disease)				
Type A–Infantile (85% of total)	Infancy	Hepatosplenomegaly Failure to thrive Psychomotor decline	Death by age 4	AR
Type B—Adult (10%-15% of total)	Childhood	Hepatomegaly Pulmonary infections	Prolonged survival	AR
Type C—Late infantile	1-6 y	Initial hepatosplenomegaly, then gait difficulty Psychomotor decline	Death in teens	AR
Type D—Nova Scotia	1-6 y	Similar to type III	Death in teens	AR
Glucosylceramide Lipidosis (Gaucher Disease)				
Type I—Adult (80% of total)	By teens	Hepatosplenomegaly	Prolonged survival	AR

(Continued)

Table 24-1. (*Continued*)

Inherited Neurodegenerative Disorders of Childhood: Clinical Features

Disease	Onset Age	Clinical Features	Longevity	Inheritance
Type II—Infantile (15% of total)	Infancy	Hepatosplenomegaly Laryngospasm Extensor posturing Psychomotor decline	Death by age 2	AR
Type III—Juvenile (Norrbotten type)	4-8 y	Initial hepatosplenomegaly Seizures Dementia Motor difficulties	Death by age 10-15 with some prolonged	AR
Galactosylceramide Lipidosis (Krabbe Disease)				
Type I—Infantile	Infancy	Irritability Extensor posturing Optic atrophy Cortical blindness Psychomotor deterioration	Death by age 12 mo	AR
Type II—Late infantile	1-3 y	Gait difficulty Psychomotor decline Visual failure	Death by age 10-12	AR
Sulfatide Lipidosis (Metachromatic Leukodystrophy)				
Type I—Late infantile	6-24 mo	Gait difficulty Ataxia Hypotonia	Death in 5-6 y	AR
Type II—Juvenile	4-8 y	Gait difficulty Ataxia prominent Psychomotor decline	Death in 10-15 y	AR
Type III—Adult	15 y or older	Dementia Depression Psychotic behavior Motor difficulty	Slow progression usual	AR
Type IV—Mucosulfatidosis	6–18 mo	Hepatosplenomegaly Skeletal deformity, Psychomotor decline	Death by age 10-12	AR
Ceramide Lipidosis (Farber Disease)	Early infancy	Subcutaneous granuloma Painful, fixed joints Failure to thrive Hypotonia	Death by age 2	AR
Adrenoleukodystrophy Complex				
Adrenoleukodystrophy	4-15 y	Behavioral difficulty Poor school performance Quadriparesis Seizures Visual decline Hypoadrenalism in ~50%	Death in 6-10 y from onset	XLR
Adrenomyeloneuropathy	20-40 y	Spastic paraparesis Urinary retention Impotence Distal neuropathy Hypoadrenalism from childhood	Prolonged survival	XLR

(*Continued*)

Table 24-1. (*Continued*)

Inherited Neurodegenerative Disorders of Childhood: Clinical Features

Disease	Onset Age	Clinical Features	Longevity	Inheritance
Adrenoleukomyelo-neuropathy	10-20 y	Behavioral difficulty Pyramidal tract and cerebellar difficulty Pseudobulbar palsy Mild dementia Hypoadrenalism	Death in 10 y	XLR
Neonatal adrenoleukodystrophy	Infancy	Severe hypotonia Seizures Profound psychomotor decline Ultimately blind and deaf Normal adrenal function Hypoplastic adrenals Optic atrophy or dysplasia	Death in 1-5 y	AR
Neuronal Ceroid Lipofuscinoses				
Infantile type (Haltia-Santavuori)	6 mo-2 y	Myoclonus Seizures Blindness Profound psychomotor decline	Death by age 10	AR
Late-infantile type (Jansky-Bielschowsky)	2-4 y	Seizures Dementia Visual disturbance later	Death by age 10-20	AR
Juvenile type (Spielmeyer-Vogt)	5-10 y	Early visual loss Seizures and dementia later	Death by age 20	AR
Sialidosis/Sialuria Complex				
Sialidosis I	Adolescence	Cherry-red maculae Myoclonus Gait difficulties and ataxia Normal intellect common Visual acuity decline	Prolonged survival	AR
Sialidosis II				
Infantile type (Mucolipidosis I)	Infancy	Seizures Myoclonus Hurler-like coarse features Corneal clouding Cherry-red maculate Hepatosplenomegaly Growth failure Profound psychomotor delay	Death by age 5	AR
Juvenile type	5–15 y	Myoclonus Ataxia Coarse features Psychomotor delay Cherry-red maculae Visual acuity decline	Death in adolescence to young adulthood	AR
Sialuria Complex				
Infantile type	At birth	Profound psychomotor delay Coarse features Hepatosplenomegaly Sparse white hair Diarrhea Anemia	Death by age 2	AR

(*Continued*)

Table 24-1. (*Continued*)				
Inherited Neurodegenerative Disorders of Childhood: Clinical Features				
Disease	Onset Age	Clinical Features	Longevity	Inheritance
Salla type	1 y	Psychomotor delay Coarse features Ataxia Athetosis Quadriparesis	Prolonged survival	AR

AR, autosomal recessive; XLR, X-linked recessive.

Clinical Characteristics

Acute GM2 gangliosidosis

Acute GM2 gangliosidosis type I (Tay-Sachs disease) has its onset in infancy, following uneventful early development, marked by increasing irritability, seizures, exaggerated startle response, and rapidly progressive psychomotor deterioration. Weakness, hypotonia, and hyporeflexia appear initially and are gradually replaced by spasticity and extensor posturing. Seizures include repetitive generalized myoclonic jerks of the trunk and extremities. EEG may reveal hypsarrhythmia or multifocal cortical spike discharges and may be associated with laughter (gelastic seizures). Neuroimaging techniques demonstrate hyperdense cerebral cortical zones, decreased white matter, ventricular dilatation, and small cerebellum and brainstem. Electroretinography (ERG) is normal, but VERs are delayed. Death occurs by age 5. Cherry-red maculae, reflecting storage material within retinal ganglion cells and obscuring the choroidal vessels, were once considered a hallmark of the disease. They may also appear in other storage diseases, including GM1 gangliosidosis, metachromatic leukodystrophy, sphingomyelin lipidosis, and sialidase deficiency. Cherry-red maculae are easily detected at the onset, but may be obscured during later stages, so their absence does not rule out the diagnosis. Macrocephaly, if present, is due to gliosis and not GM2-ganglioside storage.

GM2 gangliosidosis type II (Sandhoff disease) differs clinically from type I by the presence of hepatosplenomegaly and biochemically by deficiency of both hexosaminidase A and B. GM2 ganglioside accumulates within the central nervous system and globoside, the principal glycosphingolipid of red cells, accumulates in visceral organs. The clinical onset, pattern, and progression of type II GM2 gangliosidosis are similar to Tay-Sachs disease. Death occurs by age 5.

Subacute GM2 gangliosidosis

Subacute (Juvenile) forms of Tay-Sachs and Sandhoff diseases present between 2 and 5 years as gait disturbance with ataxia and psychomotor deterioration.[13] Neither cherry-red maculae nor hepatosplenomegaly are noted. Progression is relentless, with death occurring by adolescence.

Chronic GM2 gangliosidosis

Chronic forms of GM2 gangliosidosis present a variety of neurological manifestations, typically appearing in adolescents and adults, reflecting dysfunction of specific neuronal populations including anterior horn cells, brainstem, basal ganglia, thalamus, and cerebellum.[14,15] These include spinal muscular atrophy, motor neuron disease, spinocerebellar degeneration, and progressive dystonia. Neurological involvement of one system often dominates, but significant overlap may occur. Mentation is generally preserved although progressive dementia or significant psychiatric manifestations ranging from depression to schizophrenia may occur.[16,17] Most chronic forms of GM2 gangliosidosis appear to be due to deficiency of Hex A.

Pathology

Brain weight and volume increase markedly secondary to gliosis during the second year of life, often exceeding 2000 g (normal = 1000 g). Cystic degeneration of the cerebral white matter, along with atrophy of the cerebellar hemispheres, is frequently present. Neurons, including anterior horn cells, and glia store GM2 ganglioside. Myenteric plexus ganglion cells are also ballooned and distorted. Historically, rectal biopsy was performed as a diagnostic procedure for the storage diseases, but is obsolete due to the availability of biochemical and molecular diagnostic methodologies. Electron microscopy reveals lipid profiles within neuronal cytoplasm (most likely within lysosomes) referred to as membranous cytoplasmic bodies. In late-onset GM2 gangliosidosis, storage is preferentially localized to thalamus, substantia nigra, brainstem nuclei, and cerebellum.

Biochemistry

GM2 ganglioside accumulates in this group of disorders in neurons in the central, peripheral, and autonomic nervous systems (Table 24-2). Asialo-GM2-ganglioside (GM2 ganglioside minus sialic acid) and lyso-GM2 (GM2 ganglioside minus the fatty acid) also accumulate. The lyso-compound may be cytotoxic. Hex A activity is deficient in tissues of patients with Tay-Sachs disease and its variant forms, although total hexosaminidase activity may be increased. Hex A and B activities are deficient in Sandhoff disease and its variants. Diagnosis of each form of GM2 gangliosidosis can be made in leukocytes or cultured skin fibroblasts. In GM2 activator deficiency, Hex A and B activities are normal versus synthetic substrate, but GM2 metabolism is deficient in the absence of the activator. Multiple mutations in the respective genes have been identified.[18]

Management

Definitive therapy is not available. Carrier detection and prenatal diagnosis are feasible. Ashkenazi Jewish individuals are at high risk for transmitting the type I disorder. A population-based screening program has substantially reduced its incidence in this group.[19,20]

GM1 GANGLIOSIDOSES

Clinical Characteristics

Acute GM1 gangliosidosis

Type I GM1 gangliosidosis, the most common form, is a rapidly progressive disorder of early infancy manifesting as profound psychomotor deterioration and hepatosplenomegaly as well as the dysmorphic and radiologic features of Hurler disease (Table 24-1, Box 24-2). The last consist of multiple bone deformities (skull, vertebral bodies, ribs, and extremities) called dysostosis multiplex, hence the former name of Hurler variant or Tay-Sachs disease with Hurler features.

Onset occurs within the first weeks of life with evident psychomotor delay marked by apathy, exaggerated startle, generalized seizures, and hypotonia that progresses to spasticity. Cherry-red maculae are found in about 50% of cases. Systemic features include corneal clouding, gingival hyperplasia, macroglossia, kyphoscoliosis, broad hands, and flexion contractures, particularly of fingers, elbows, and knees. Death occurs by age 2.

Neuroimaging reveals prominent atrophy, increased density of thalami and reduced density of basal ganglia by CT, and hyperintensity of thalami and basal ganglia on T_1 and hypointensity on T_2, along with evidence of delayed myelination by MRI.[21] Electroretinography is normal whereas VERs are delayed. EEG findings generally consist of nonspecific slowing.

Subacute GM1 gangliosidosis

Type II GM1 gangliosidosis presents at 6 to 12 months with psychomotor regression after normal early development. Neurological features are dominated by spasticity, ataxia, dystonia, and prominent myoclonic and generalized seizures. Corneal clouding, cherry-red maculae, dysmorphic facies, and hepatosplenomegaly are not seen. Bony changes are typically limited to moderate beaking of vertebral bodies and hypoplasia of the hips. EEG and neuroimaging findings are similar to type I. Progression is relentless leading to death by age 3 to 10 years.

Chronic GM1 gangliosidosis

Type III begins in early childhood with slowly progressive ataxia and mild cognitive impairment followed by slurred speech and progressive extrapyramidal signs (dystonia and rigidity) in adulthood.[22] Dysmorphic features, cherry-red maculae, corneal clouding, and hepatosplenomegaly are absent. Bony abnormalities of the vertebral bodies and hips are mild. MRI may show increased intensity of the putamen on T_2. Longevity appears normal.

Pathology

Pathologic findings are described best for type I. Neurons, including those in Meissner plexus, and glia are involved diffusely, their cytoplasm stuffed with PAS-positive storage material. Bone pathology is similar to that for Hurler disease. Diffuse neuronal involvement is less evident in later onset forms. Neuronal involvement in type III is most prominent in caudate and putamen.

Biochemistry

GM1 ganglioside comprises 80% to 90% (normal = 20%) of total gray matter gangliosides (Table 24-2). Asialo-GM1 (GM1 minus sialic acid) also accumulates, exceeding normal values by up to 20 times. In the acute form, GM1 also accumulates in liver and spleen. In the chronic form, GM1 accumulation is generally limited to caudate and putamen. Deficient β-galactosidase activity in leukocytes or cultured skin fibroblasts establishes the diagnosis. Multiple mutations have been identified in *GBL1*, although five common mutations account for the majority.

A separate transcript of *GBL1* encodes a β-galactosidase-like protein without enzyme activity and identical to the elastin-binding protein (EBP). Six infants with GM1 gangliosidosis and prominent cardiac involvement had *GBL1* mutations in the region common to both enzyme and EBP proteins.

Table 24-2.

Inherited Neurodegenerative Disorders of Childhood: Biochemical and Diagnostic Features

Disease	Stored Material	Enzyme Defect	Tissue for Diagnosis
Sphingolipidoses			
GM2-Gangliosidosis	GM2-ganglioside Asialo GM2-analogue	Hexosaminidase A	Leucocytes Cultured skin fibroblasts
GM2-Gangliosidosis Sandhoff Type	GM2-ganglioside Asialo GM2-analogue Globoside in non-neural organs	Hexosaminidase A and B	Leucocytes Cultured skin fibroblasts
GM1-Gangliosidosis	GM1-ganglioside Asialo GM2-ganglioside Keratan sulfate	GM1-ganglioside beta-galactosidase	Leucocytes Cultured skin fibroblasts
Globotriaosylceramide lipidosis	Globotriaosylceramide	Alpha-galactosidase	Leucocytes Cultured skin fibroblasts
Sphingomyelin Lipidosis Types I/II	Sphingomyelin	Sphingomyelinase (phospholipase C)	Leucocytes Cultured skin fibroblasts
Glucosylceramide Lipidosis	Glucosylceramide Glucosylsphingosine	Glucosylceramide beta-glucosidase	Leucocytes Cultured skin fibroblasts
Galactosylceramide Lipidosis	Galactosylceramide Galactosylsphingosine	Galactosylceramide beta-galactosidase	Leucocytes Cultured skin fibroblasts
Sulfatide Lipidosis	Sulfatide	Sulfatide sulfatase (arylsulfatase a)	Leucocytes Cultured skin fibroblasts
Mucosulfatidosis	Sulfatide Cholesterol sulfate Mucopolysaccharide sulfate	Multiple sulfatases	Leucocytes Cultured skin fibroblasts
Ceramide Lipidosis (Farber Disease)	Ceramide	Ceramidase	Leucocytes Cultured skin fibroblasts

Adrenoleukodystrophy
  Group Neuronal Ceroid
  Lipofuscinoses
	Very-long-chain fatty acids	Defective peroxisomal
		  fatty acid oxidation
			Plasma
			Cultured skin fibroblasts

CLN1	Saposins A and D	Palmitoylprotein thioesterase	Leucocytes Cultured skin fibroblasts Plasma Cerebrospinal fluid
CLN2	ATP synthase subunit c Saposins A and D	Pepstatin-insensitive peptidase	Leucocytes Cultured skin fibroblasts
CLN3	ATP synthase subunit c Saposins A and D	None known	*CLN3* mutations
CLN5	ATP synthase subunit c Saposins A and D	None known	*CLN5* mutations
CLN6	Unknown	None known	*CLN6* mutations
CLN8	ATP synthase subunit c	None known	*CLN8* mutations
Sialidosis			

Type I and II	Sialic acid-containing oligo-
	  saccharides/glycoproteins
		Oligosaccharide alpha-
		  sialidase
			Culture skin fibroblasts

Sialic Acid Storage Disorders			
Infantile Type	Sialic acid in urine and tissues	Unknown	Increased sialic acid in urine

Salla Type	Sialic acid in urine and
	  fibroblasts
		Unknown	Increased sialic acid in
			  urine

Box 24-2. Generalized Gangliosidosis

Common Name: Generalized gangliosidosis; Hurler variant
Incidence: 1:400,000
Inheritance: Autosomal recessive
Relevant Metabolite: GM1 ganglioside, asialo-GM1, keratan sulfate, oligosaccharides
Metabolic Defect: GM1 β-galactosidase
Mutation: GLB1-chromosome 3p21.33
Clinical Pattern: Variable phenotypes reflecting different mutations; allelic with Morquio B

A unique feature of the acute-onset form is increased keratan sulfate levels in various tissues and excessive urinary excretion accounting for the Hurler-like appearance. Both GM1 ganglioside and keratan sulfate have a terminal β-galactose. Morquio disease, a mucopolysaccharidosis, is characterized by keratan sulfate accumulation and deficient β-galactosidase activity. As such, Morquio B disease is allelic with GM1 gangliosidosis, that is, both diseases are due to mutations in the same gene.

A number of children with mild to moderate reduction of β-galactosidase activity were once considered as variants of GM1 gangliosidosis. This disorder, galactosialidosis, is due to deficiency of a protective protein for sialidase deficiency and β-galactosidase (see p. 295).

Management

Effective treatment for GM1 gangliosidosis is lacking.

GLOBOTRIAOSYLCERAMIDE LIPIDOSIS (FABRY DISEASE)

Box 24-3 gives an overview of Fabry disease.

Box 24-3. Fabry Disease

Common Name: Fabry disease; angiokeratoma corporis diffusum universale
Incidence: 1:40,000 males
Inheritance: X-linked recessive
Relevant Metabolite: Globotriaosylceramide, digalactosyl-ceramide
Metabolic Defect: α-galactosidase
Mutation: *GLA*-chromosome Xq22.1
Clinical Pattern: Males—cutaneous, vascular, and renal disease, ocular changes and peripheral neuropathy
Atypical males—cardiac disease
Carrier females—rare renal, cardiac, or neurological disease; ocular changes common

Clinical Characteristics

Globotriaosylceramide lipidosis (angiokeratoma corporis diffusum universale, Fabry disease) is the lone X-linked sphingolipid storage disease (Table 24-1). The principal clinical manifestations involve skin, heart, and kidney. The cutaneous features (angiokeratoma) consist of violaceous angiectatic lesions over the genitalia, thighs, buttock, back, and lower abdomen. These are not unique to Fabry disease, occurring in fucosidosis, β-mannosidosis, galactosialidosis, and Schindler disease. Difficulties with sweating (hypohidrosis) result in temperature intolerance. Lymphedema and episodic diarrhea are also common. Fabry disease has its onset in adolescence or early adulthood,[23-25] but despite major clinical issues, survival is often quite prolonged with death from renal or cardiac involvement in the fourth or fifth decades. Later-onset variants are now recognized.[26] Cardiac involvement includes left ventricular hypertrophy, valvular dysfunction (especially mitral insufficiency), and conduction abnormalities.[27] Obstructive pulmonary disease occurs in about one-third, usually after age 25. Interestingly, subclinical hypothyroidism appears to be more frequent as well.[28]

The principal neurological problem is painful peripheral neuropathy, generally involving the distal extremities (acroparesthesias). Both severe crises of lancinating pain precipitated by exercise, fatigue, stress, or exposure to sunshine or hot weather, and chronic, unremitting pain, may occur. Corneal and lenticular opacifications and retinal vasculopathies are common. CNS vaso-occlusive events, especially in the posterior circulation and periventricular white matter supply, should place Fabry disease in the differential diagnosis of cerebrovascular accidents in the young male.[29] Cranial imaging may suggest prior vaso-occlusive events even without clinical accompaniment.[30]

Female carriers may develop signs similar to affected males, but usually in middle life. Corneal opacifications occur in approximately 75% of carriers. Other manifestations, while less common, may be as severe as in males, especially the painful peripheral neuropathy.

Natural history studies demonstrate cerebral lesions in some males in their mid-twenties but involvement is found in all males by age 55, whereas chronic renal insufficiency and end-stage renal disease are noted by age 40 to 50. Overall survival in males is age 50 and in carrier females age 70.

Cardiac variant

A variant form is limited to cardiac involvement. The specific gene defect in this form results in more residual enzyme activity. Onset of cardiac disease is typically at age 40 or older but without the other features of Fabry disease except for mild proteinuria.

Pathology

Lipid accumulation occurs in vascular smooth muscle and endothelium, kidney, cornea, peripheral nerves, and in neurons of the autonomic nervous system, both central and peripheral. Electron microscopy of peripheral nerves reveals lamellar inclusions in perineurial cells. Peripheral nerve involvement can be easily assessed by analysis of skin biopsy.

Biochemistry

Globotriaosylceramide is a quantitatively significant sphingolipid in kidney and is also the first intermediate in the degradation of globoside, the prominent sphingolipid of red cell membranes (Table 24-2). Accumulation occurs in kidney, liver, and lung ranging from 30 to 300 times normal. Alpha-glactosidase (globotriaosylceramide α-galactosidase) activity is deficient. Diagnosis can be made in leukocytes and cultured skin fibroblasts. Numerous mutations have been described.[31] A more benign mutation is associated with the cardiac variant.

Management

Renal transplantation may be required for renal failure, but may not result in overall improvement. Enzyme replacement therapy can reduce lipid storage and neuropathic pain and improve renal function and cerebral perfusion.[32-38] Replacement therapy has also been safe and effective in symptomatic females.[39] Individuals with the cardiac variant may benefit from infusion of galactose, which acts as a molecular chaperone to stabilize mutant enzyme activity. Carbamazepine, phenytoin, or gabapentin may be effective therapy for neuropathic pain or dysesthesias.

SPHINGOMYELIN LIPIDOSIS (NIEMANN-PICK DISEASE)

Box 24-4 gives an overview of Niemann-Pick disease.

Box 24-4. Niemann-Pick Disease

Common Name: Niemann-Pick disease
Incidence: Acute form 1:20,000-40,000, chronic form 1:80,000, both in Ashkenazi Jews; much lower in general population
Inheritance: Autosomal recessive
Relevant Metabolite: Sphingomyelin, bis(monoacylglycero)phosphate, sphingosylphosphorylcholine
Metabolic Defect: Acid sphingo-myelinase (phospholipase C)
Mutation: *ASM*-chromosome 11p15-15.4
Clinical Pattern: Different clinical phenotypes featuring hepatospleno megaly; chronic form spares CNS; acute form rapidly progressive CNS dysfunction

---

Clinical Characteristics

Sphingomyelin lipidosis is characterized by storage of sphingomyelin (Table 24-1). Acute (type A) and chronic (type B) forms are clinically distinct. Two variants (types C and D), previously thought to have similar etiologies, are not disorders of sphingomyelin catabolism.

Acute sphingomyelin lipidosis

Type A is the predominant form, occurring prominently in Ashkenazi Jews and accounting for 85% of the total. Onset occurs in infancy, characterized by severe failure to thrive, hepatosplenomegaly, psychomotor retardation, and frequent respiratory infections. Persistent neonatal jaundice and ascites in later stages may be noted. Neurological abnormalities include hypotonia and weakness initially with progression to spasticity and rigidity. Seizures are rare. Cherry-red maculae are seen in approximately 50% and the ERG response may be diminished. EEG findings consist of nonspecific slowing and voltage attenuation. ABRs may be abnormal and nerve conduction velocities reduced. Death occurs by age 4.

Chronic sphingomyelin lipidosis

Type B sphingomyelin lipidosis typically spares the central nervous system. Onset occurs in childhood marked by hepatosplenomegaly and respiratory infections. Progression is remarkably indolent, the principal problems arising from the hepatosplenomegaly, cirrhosis, and chronic pulmonary disease. Survival into middle adulthood is usual.

Pathology

Neuropathologic findings are derived from type A. Brain weight is approximately 75% of normal. Light microscopy reveals large, distended neurons lacking their pyramidal shape. Neuronal storage is prominent, but lipid accumulation also occurs in liver, spleen, lymph nodes, bone marrow, and lung. Peripheral nerves are abnormal with segmental demyelination and cytoplasmic inclusions within axoplasm and Schwann cells.

Biochemistry

Sphingomyelin accumulation in brain and other tissues is characteristic of type A (Table 24-2). Sphingomyelin in brain is increased up to 50 times and may represent two-thirds of total phospholipid (normal = 20%). Tissue cholesterol levels are also increased up to 10-fold. Another phospholipid, bis(monoacylglycero)phosphate, is increased nearly 100-fold, and lyso-sphingomyelin or sphingosylphosphorylcholine is also increased in brain, liver, and spleen in type A, but only in liver and spleen in type B. Their role in the pathogenesis of neurological abnormalities is unknown. Brain content of sphingomyelin is normal in type B. Deficient sphingomyelinase activity in leucocytes and cultured skin fibroblasts is profound in both types. Sparing of the central nervous system and prolonged survival in type B patients reflects greater residual enzyme activity and possibly other factors. Multiple mutations have been defined in *ASM*, but three account for most of type A in the Ashkenazi population. A separate and less severe mutation is found in the majority of type B.

Niemann-Pick C (formerly types C and D) has its onset in early childhood (ages 1-6) with hepatosplenomegaly and hepatic dysfunction, gait difficulties, ataxia, vertical gaze deficit, and cognitive decline. Progression is relentless with death usually in adolescence. Lipid storage consists mainly of cholesterol but also both sphingomyelin and glucosylceramide. Sphingomyelin catabolism is normal in cultured skin fibroblasts. Deficient cholesterol esterification is the hallmark of Nieman-Pick C.

Management

Effective treatment is lacking for type A. Enzyme replacement should be effective in type B, but systematic trials have not been initiated.[40]

GLUCOSYLCERAMIDE LIPIDOSIS (GAUCHER DISEASE)

Glucosylceramide lipidosis (Gaucher disease; Box 24-5) has three principal forms (Table 24-1). Type I is prominent in Ashkenazi Jews with an incidence of 1:1600, the general incidence being 1:80,000-160,000. The variant forms are explained by different mutations in the gene for glucosylceramide β-glucosidase.[41]

Clinical Characteristics

Chronic glucosylceramide lipidosis

Type I, the chronic non-neuronopathic form, is the most common, representing approximately 85% of the

---

total.[42] The CNS is generally spared, although oculomotor apraxia, seen in acute and subacute forms, has been described. Onset occurs in childhood or adolescence with progressive hepatosplenomegaly.[43] It may begin in early adulthood or later. Significant intrafamilial variability has been noted.[44] Survival is typically prolonged, although early death from severe pancytopenia or other complications is possible. The principal clinical problems are hypersplenism, bony abnormalities including infarction, osteomyelitis, pathologic fractures, arthritis, chronic pulmonary hypertension, and growth retardation. Secondary neurological problems have been described.[45] An association exists between Gaucher disease and Parkinson disease in the Ashkenazi population, but has not been noted in Norway.[46-49] With the exception of multiple myeloma, cancer rates are not elevated.[50]

Acute glucosylceramide lipidosis

Type II (neuronopathic) or infantile glucosylceramide lipidosis is a fulminant disorder. Prominent features are failure to thrive, extensor posturing, laryngospasm, profound psychomotor retardation, and hepato-splenomegaly. Weakness and hypotonia quickly progress to rigidity. Oculomotor apraxia or strabismus is typical. Seizures may occur in later stages. Onset occurs in early infancy with survival rare beyond age 2. Fetal hydrops, also seen in other lysosomal disorders (ceramide lipidosis, sialidosis type II, galactosialidosis, β-glucuronidase deficiency, and infantile sialic acid storage disease) may be the presenting sign.[51]

Subacute glucosylceramide lipidosis

Type III (Norrbottnian form; subacute neuronopathic) is an intermediate form. Particularly prevalent in Sweden, this form occurs in childhood (4-8 years) with hepatosplenomegaly, horizontal gaze apraxia, motor dysfunction, seizures, and progressive cognitive impairment. In particular, progressive myoclonic epilepsy may be noted.[52] Significant intrafamilial variability occurs, some presenting in early childhood, others with a more indolent course. Death often occurs during adolescence, whereas survival into middle age is possible.

Pathology

Lipid-laden cells are seen in liver, spleen, and bone marrow. The Gaucher cell, a derivative of the reticuloendothelial system, is characterized by wrinkled blue cytoplasm and easily distinguished from cells with foamy cytoplasm in Niemann-Pick disease. Neuronal loss and perivascular accumulation of glucosylceramide are noted in CNS.[47] Neuronal loss (type III in particular) is most pronounced in the bulbar nuclei. Typical Gaucher cells are found in pyramidal cell layers of cerebral cortex.

Box 24-5. Gaucher Disease

Common Name: Gaucher disease
Incidence: Chronic form: 1:1,600 in Ashkenazi Jews; all forms: 1:80,000-160,000 in general population
Inheritance: Autosomal recessive
Relevant Metabolite: Glucosylceramide, glucosylsphingosine
Metabolic Defect: Glucosylceramide β-glucosidase
Mutation: *GBA*-chromosome 1q21
Clinical Pattern: Variable phenotypes; chronic form, sparing CNS, most common; acute and subacute forms involve CNS progressively

Biochemistry

Glucosylceramide levels in liver and spleen may reach 100 times normal (Table 24-2). In types II and III, glucosylceramide content is increased by 80-fold in cerebral cortex and 40-fold in cerebellar cortex. Levels of glucosylsphingosine (lyso-glucosylceramide) are increased up to 1000-fold. Glycosphingosine accumulation, a potential cytotoxin, is prominent already in early fetal life.

Glucosylceramide β-glucosidase activity in leukocytes and cultured skin fibroblasts is markedly deficient. Variable levels of residual enzyme activity within the broad range of *GBA* mutations are responsible for the clinical variants. However, other biological or epigenetic factors could explain intrafamilial variability in type III (Norrbottnian).

Multiple mutations in *GBA* have been identified although five mutations account for more than 95% of those in the Ashkenazi population, but only about 50% of those in non-Jewish individuals.[53] Different mutations are most common in neuronopathic forms.[54] In the African-American population, the most common type I mutations are not seen, and seven other mutations are noted.

Deficiency of an activator protein that is essential for normal glucosylceramide β-glucosidase activity underlies a variant form of Gaucher disease similar to the subacute form. In this variant, glucosylceramide content is elevated in liver, spleen, and brain as in types II and III, while glucosylceramide β-glucosidase activity is normal.

Management

Replacement therapy using recombinant enzyme (glucosylceramide β-glucosidase) results in decreased accumulation of lipid in juvenile and adult forms of Gaucher disease.[55–61] In chronic Gaucher disease, complete reversal of systemic involvement is possible. In type III, high-dose enzyme replacement ameliorates systemic involvement and stabilizes neurological involvement in the majority although pulmonary involvement is not improved.

Bone marrow transplantation has led to significant improvement, particularly in type III. Inhibitors of glycosphingolipid synthesis have provided modest benefit and may be adjunctive, especially in individuals who may not tolerate enzyme replacement therapy.[62,63]

In some individuals, splenectomy may be required. In type I Gaucher disease, it may be followed by increased bone pathology, and in type III may accelerate decline in cognitive function and increase glucosylceramide accumulation in other organs. Partial splenectomy may be a more prudent approach, allowing accumulation of glucosylceramide in the remaining splenic tissue.

GALACTOSYLCERAMIDE LIPIDOSIS (KRABBE DISEASE, GLOBOID CELL LEUKODYSTROPHY)

Globoid cell leukodystrophy (Box 24-6) occurs in three principal forms: infantile (the more common) and two with later onset (Table 24-1). The incidence is 1 per 50,000 in Sweden but less than 1:100,000 outside Scandinavia. Both central and peripheral nervous systems are affected.

Clinical Characteristics

Acute galactosylceramide lipidosis

Infantile globoid cell leukodystrophy usually appears by 6 months of age characterized by developmental stagnation, marked irritability, hypertonia, increased muscle stretch reflexes, psychomotor regression, and unexplained fever. Subsequently, extensor posturing, rigidity, exaggerated startle response, optic atrophy, and cortical blindness are noted. Hypotonia then replaces hypertonia and muscle stretch reflexes are lost, reflecting peripheral nerve involvement. Microcephaly may be seen. Death usually occurs by age 12 months. Nerve conduction velocities are reduced and CSF protein is increased significantly, occasionally exceeding 300 mg/dL. Cranial CT reveals diminished white matter and increased density of internal capsule, thalamus, and basal ganglia as noted for GM1-gangliosidosis. Cranial MRI confirms the failure of myelination.

Subacute galactosylceramide lipidosis

Late-onset globoid cell leukodystrophy occurs from 1 to 10 years of age after a period of normal development.[64] Gait abnormalities and ataxia progressing to spasticity, visual loss with optic atrophy and cortical blindness, and mild to profound psychomotor retardation may be seen. CSF protein and nerve conduction velocities may be normal. Cranial MRI demonstrates diffuse central white matter and pyramidal tract loss. Death may occur within 3 years or not until 20 years after onset.

Box 24-6. Krabbe Disease

Common Name: Krabbe disease; globoid cell leukodystrophy
Incidence: 1:50,000 in Sweden; 1:100,000-200,000 generally
Inheritance: Autosomal recessive
Relevant Metabolite: Galactosylceramide, galactosylsphingosine
Metabolic Defect: Galactosylceramide β-galactosidase
Mutation: *GALC*-chromosome 14q24.3-32.1
Clinical Pattern: Progressive psychomotor deterioration; delayed onset/adult-onset forms: later onset and slower progression of motor impairment; mentation is often spared

Chronic galactosylceramide lipidosis

Adult onset features slowly progressive gait difficulties leading to spastic paraparesis.[65] Dysmetria, brisk muscle stretch reflexes with clonus and extensor plantar responses, and optic disc pallor may be seen. Mentation is generally preserved. Nerve conduction velocities and CSF protein are typically normal. Cranial MRI and MRS reveal symmetrical subcortical white matter and pyramidal tract lesions.[66] Periventricular and cerebellar white matter appears uninvolved.

Pathology

In the acute form, cerebral atrophy is prominent with marked gliosis and diminished white matter. Oligodendroglia are markedly reduced or absent. Globoid cells (multinucleate giant cells), apparently elicited by galactosylceramide, are numerous. Segmental demyelination is seen in peripheral nerves.

Biochemistry

Brain galactosylceramide levels are reduced, but globoid cells accumulate this lipid (Table 24-2). Galactosylsphingosine, or psychosine (lyso-galactosylceramide), accumulates up to 100 times normal. The loss of oligodendroglia is due to psychosine cytotoxicity. Psychosine promotes cytokine and inducible nitric oxide synthase production.

Galactosylceramide β-galactosidase activity in peripheral leucocytes or cultured skin fibroblasts is markedly deficient. Multiple mutations have been described, some associated with the late-onset forms.

Management

Effective therapy for globoid cell leukodystrophy is lacking, although recent hematopoietic stem-cell transplantation results are somewhat encouraging.[67,68]

SULFATIDE LIPIDOSIS (METACHROMATIC LEUKODYSTROPHY)

Metachromatic leukodystrophy (MLD; Box 24-7), due to deficient arylsulfatase activity,[69] occurs in three principal forms: late infantile (the most common), juvenile, and adult (Table 24-1). The juvenile form includes varying phenotypes. Children with sulfatide activator deficiency and normal arylsulfatase A activity display the juvenile pattern. MLD has an incidence of 1 in 40,000 except in the Navajo (1 in 2520 births). A separate entity due to deficiency of multiple sulfatase enzymes has the

---

Box 24-7. Metachromatic Leukodystrophy

Common Name: Metachromatic leukodystrophy
Incidence: 1:40,000
Inheritance: Autosomal recessive
Relevant Metabolite: Galactosyl-3-sulfate ceramide (sulfatide),lyso-sulfatide, lactosylsulfate ceramide
Metabolic Defect: Sulfatide sulfatase (arylsulfatase A)
Mutation: *ARSA*-22q13.31-ter
Clinical Pattern: Multiple phenotypes of varying age of onset and rate of progression. Acute form: rapidly progressive psychomotor deterioration; Subacute form: somewhat rapidly progressive motor and cognitive difficulties; Chronic form: slowly progressive motor and severe cognitive impairments or psychosis

---

clinical appearance of a mucopolysaccharidosis, but follows the late infantile MLD course.

Clinical Characteristics

Acute sulfatide lipidosis

Late infantile MLD presents at 6 months to 2 years of age after normal early development. Regression includes gait difficulties, ataxia, optic atrophy, hypotonia, and extensor plantar responses. Muscle stretch reflexes are diminished or absent due to peripheral nerve involvement. Progression to a vegetative state is rapid. Nerve conduction velocities are markedly reduced and CSF protein is increased up to 300 mg/dL. Cranial CT and MRI reveal symmetric white matter abnormalities. Death occurs by age 6 years.

Subacute sulfatide lipidosis

Juvenile metachromatic leukodystrophy may exhibit different patterns. An early form, noted between 4 and 8 years of age, features gait disturbance, intellectual decline, ataxia, and upper motor neuron signs. Extrapyramidal signs and seizures may appear subsequently. Muscle stretch reflexes are increased initially but lost eventually. Progression is slower than in late infantile MLD, but death within 6 years of onset is typical.

A second juvenile form appears between 6 and 16 years of age. Personality and behavior changes and declining school performance are prominent, as well as seizures. Motor dysfunction occurs later. Progression is even slower, with survival into late adolescence or early adulthood. In both forms, nerve conduction velocities are reduced and CSF protein is elevated, but less than in the late infantile form. Cranial MRI demonstrates diminution of white matter and cortical atrophy.

Chronic sulfatide lipidosis

Adult-onset metachromatic leukodystrophy presents as decline in cognitive function or psychosis with onset ranging from 16 to 60 years. Declining school or work performance often is the first sign. Motor dysfunction progresses very slowly to spastic quadriparesis and signs of basal ganglia involvement, especially dystonia. Nerve conduction velocities and CSF protein may be normal. Cranial MRI demonstrates significant cortical atrophy and moderate white matter involvement as compared to other forms.

Multiple sulfatase deficiency disease

Multiple sulfatase deficiency disease combines features of the late infantile form of metachromatic leukodystrophy, steroid sulfatase deficiency, and mucopolysaccharidoses. The clinical features of multiple sulfatase deficiencies deviate from MLD in that development is abnormal from birth with regression by age 1 year. Ichthyosis is apparent at birth. By 1 year of age, coarse facial features, hepatosplenomegaly, skeletal abnormalities, peripheral lens opacities, and retinal degeneration appear.

Pathology

MLD affects not only the central and peripheral nervous systems, but kidney, pancreas, adrenal, liver, and gallbladder. Neuropathology consists of widespread loss of central myelin, loss of oligodendroglia, and segmental demyelination of peripheral nerves. Light microscopy reveals PAS-positive metachromatic, birefringent material throughout cerebral white matter and peripheral nerve. Metachromatic material accumulates within glia and neurons.

Pathologic findings in multiple sulfatase deficiency reflect storage of both sulfatides and mucopolysaccharides.

Biochemistry

In the acute form, white matter sulfatide levels are 4 to 8 times normal (Table 24-2). White matter sulfatide levels in adult MLD are increased only 1.2- to 2.5-fold. Unlike the acute form, significant sulfatide storage is noted in gray matter. Lyso-sulfatide is also markedly increased (up to 100 times normal). Sulfatide, along with the lactosylsulfate analogue, is increased in kidney and liver. Excretion of sulfatide in urine served as the diagnostic marker prior to enzyme diagnosis. Markedly decreased arylsulfatase A activity in leukocytes or cultured skin fibroblasts occurs in each type of MLD except those with activator protein deficiency.[69] Peripheral nerve biopsy for the detection of metachromatic material is no longer required.

Several mutations have been identified in the arylsulfatase gene, but two major alleles are known, one detected exclusively in the late infantile form and the other in the juvenile and adult forms, providing a molecular basis for the phenotypic heterogeneity.[70-72]

Some individuals with the juvenile-onset phenotype have normal levels of arylsulfatase A, but lack the activator protein necessary for sulfatide degradation. Demonstrating abnormal sulfatide catabolism in cultured skin fibroblasts and absence of activator in leukocytes or cultured fibroblasts using specific antibodies will establish the diagnosis.

Multiple sulfatase deficiency disease is characterized by abnormal activity of several different enzymes comprising the known sulfatases. Mutations have not been found in the respective sulfatase genes. Rather, abnormal posttranslational processing of these sulfatases is responsible for abnormal enzyme catalytic activity.

Management

No effective treatment is available. Enzyme replacement by bone marrow transplantation may provide possible benefit in terms of improved arylsulfatase A activity and slowed disease progression, but beneficial response has not been seen uniformly.

CERAMIDE LIPIDOSIS (FARBER DISEASE; LIPOGRANULOMATOSIS)

Ceramide lipidosis (Farber disease; Box 24-8), initially called lipogranulomatosis, is a very rare disorder of early infancy leading to death by age 2 (Table 24-1).[73] The principal clinical features are subcutaneous granulomas, most prominent over the interphalangeal and metacarpophalangeal joints and wrists and over the trunk and scalp, skeletal deformities including painful, swollen, and fixed joints, pulmonary infiltrates and frequent respiratory difficulties, hoarseness, cutaneous lesions, and psychomotor deterioration. Fetal hydrops may be the presenting feature. Feeding difficulties are significant leading to failure to thrive. Neurological involvement is not prominent, although hypotonia is common and cherry red maculae have been described. CSF protein is often increased. Cranial imaging reveals diffuse cortical atrophy.

Box 24-8. Farber Disease

Common Name: Farber disease; lipogranulomatosis
Incidence: Unknown—very rare
Inheritance: Autosomal recessive
Relevant Metabolite: Ceramide
Metabolic Defect: Ceramidase
Mutation: AC-chromosome 8p21.3-22
Clinical Pattern: Progressive skeletal deformities, subcutaneous granulomas, joint contractures, and respiratory difficulties with early death; milder variants described with preserved mentation

Milder variants have been described with delayed onset and slower progression.

An additional variant with a phenotype more closely resembling acute glucosylceramide lipidosis (type II) is the result of a combined activator deficiency producing marked reduction in activity of three sphingolipid hydrolases: ceramidase, glucosylceramide β-glucosidase, and galactosylceramide β-galactosidase.

Pathology

Farber disease is a systemic disorder with firm, yellowish, periarticular and subcutaneous nodules, enlarged lymph nodes, and foam cells in lung, liver, spleen, and bone marrow. Neurons including anterior horn cells are involved throughout the CNS.

Biochemistry

Ceramide is increased up to 60-fold and may comprise one-fifth of total lipid within the granulomas and in lung, liver, kidney, lymph nodes, and neurons (Table 24-2). Ceramidase activity in leucocytes and cultured skin fibroblasts is significantly reduced. Several mutations have been identified in the ceramidase gene.[74]

Management

Effective treatment is lacking.

ADRENOLEUKODYSTROPHY/ADRENOMYELONEUROPATHY COMPLEX

Clinical Characteristics

X-linked adrenoleukodystrophy (X-ALD) has a variable onset age, although typically appearing at age 6-10 years (Table 24-1, Box 24-9). The phenotypic expression of X-linked ALD can be quite variable also. Of more than 1000 individuals noted to have elevated VLCFA

Box 24-9. X-Linked Adrenoleukodystrophy

Incidence: 1:20,000-40,000 males
Inheritance: X-linked recessive
Relevant Metabolite: Very-long-chain fatty acids (VLCFAs)
Metabolic Defect: VLCFA acyl-CoA synthetase, adrenoleukodystrophy protein
Mutation: *ALDP*-chromosome Xq28
Clinical Pattern: Childhood (most common), juvenile and adult onset; cognitive and behavioral decline, vision and hearing impaired, motor difficulties

---

(very-long-chain fatty acids), 45% have the X-ALD phenotype with 38% beginning in childhood, 27% have X-AMN (adrenomyeloneuropathy), 10% have Addison disease, and 9% are asymptomatic.[75] The most common presentation is in the early school age (Table 24-1), featuring behavioral disturbance and cognitive impairment, resulting in declining school performance. Impaired hearing and vision, motor difficulties, and seizures develop later. Visual and auditory evoked responses are reduced. Seizures are noted in 20% of children, often as the presenting feature. CSF protein is elevated. Cerebral progression occurs in 50% of those who are asymptomatic in childhood. Death usually occurs within 6 to 10 years of onset.

X-AMN, a variant of X-ALD, presents in young adulthood as slowly progressive spastic paraparesis. Sexual and urinary dysfunction and posterior column sensory difficulties usually present later. Reduced motor and sensory nerve conduction velocities and auditory and visual evoked responses are seen.[76] Survival is typically prolonged. Both X-ALD and X-AMN may occur in the same kindred. More than 25% of individuals with X-AMN will develop cerebral demyelination.

Cranial imaging in X-ALD reveals progressive, symmetrical (occasionally unilateral) cerebral demyelination beginning occipitally and progressing rostrally with enhancing margins suggesting an inflammatory process. In AMN, cranial imaging is typically normal, although central abnormalities may occur. Prediction of disease progression is often difficult on clinical grounds. Contrast-enhanced cranial MRI may distinguish individuals likely to progress.[77] Proton magnetic resonance spectroscopy (MRS) may predict disease progression more effectively.[78]

More than 90% with X-ALD and two-thirds with X-AMN have adrenal insufficiency.[79] Occasionally, Addison disease is the only manifestation. Measurement of VLCFA is indicated in all males, including children, with Addison disease.

Female carriers may be symptomatic, almost all with signs of spastic paraparesis.[80,81] About 10% to 15% of female heterozygotes have significant neurological problems and 50% have mild abnormalities.[82] Adrenal function is normal. Typical X-ALD has been noted in some females.

Pathology

Neuropathology reveals cerebral demyelination with caudal-rostral progression and relative sparing of cortex. Perivascular inflammation is prominent. In X-AMN, the major abnormality is in spinal cord. Axonal changes are noted in corticospinal tracts and posterior columns. Peripheral neuropathic findings that may occur in both forms include loss of myelinated fibers.

Adrenocortical cells and Schwann cells contain characteristic lamellar inclusions representing VLCFA cholesterol esters.

Biochemistry

Both X-ALD and X-AMN display elevated levels of saturated VLCFA (Table 24-2). These can be readily measured in plasma, cultured skin fibroblasts, and amniocytes. No correlation exists between VLCFA levels and type or severity of disease. The gene responsible for X-ALD encodes the X-ALD protein (ALDP), a peroxisomal membrane protein.[83] ALDP is required for localization of VLCFA CoA synthetase within the peroxisome. It is unclear how mutations in the ALDP produce the glial responses and inflammatory changes.[84,85] Numerous mutations in *ALDP* have been identified.

Plasma VLCFA levels are elevated in approximately 90% of obligate female carriers. Prenatal diagnosis of X-ALD is highly accurate, but cannot predict age of onset or severity of disease.

Management

Treatment is generally supportive. Dietary modification with restricted VLCFA intake and added erucic acid may normalize plasma VLCFA levels, but neurological improvement does not occur. Bone marrow transplantation retards disease progression when initiated before onset or with mild involvement.[86] Presymptomatic treatment is confounded by the fact that some individuals with elevated plasma VLCFA will remain asymptomatic.

NEONATAL ADRENOLEUKODYSTROPHY

Clinical Characteristics

Neonatal adrenoleukodystrophy (NALD) is quite different from X-ALD (Table 24-1). Profound hypotonia is apparent at birth and developmental delay and seizures are noted in early infancy. Later neurological signs include tremor, ataxia, hyperreflexia, sensory deficits, and progressive visual and auditory dysfunction. Mid-facial hypoplasia is also noted. Developmental progress occurs in the first year of life such as walking, but cognitive function is severely impaired and speech is limited. Thereafter regression ensues. Mild cranial MRI reveals severe white matter deficiency. Adrenal insufficiency is rarely apparent, although response to ACTH is reduced. Most die within the first 5 years with occasional survival into adolescence.

Pathology

Neuropathologic findings include heterotopias, polymicrogyria, and demyelination similar to, but milder than in the related peroxisomal disorder, Zellweger syndrome. Adrenal cortical atrophy and lipid inclusions are prominent.

Conclusion

Each adrenoleukodystrophy disorder features elevated plasma and tissue very-long-chain fatty acids levels due to defective oxidation in peroxisomes (Table 24-2). The neonatal form is distinctly different, reflecting a pervasive defect in peroxisomal function due to the absence of recognizable peroxisomes.

NEURONAL CEROID LIPOFUSCINOSES

The neuronal ceroid lipofuscinoses are autosomal recessive lysosomal storage disorders characterized by accumulation of autofluorescent material in neurons throughout the nervous system (Table 24-1), and as a group represent the most common inherited neurodegenerative storage disease of children with an overall incidence of 1 in 10,000.[87-90] They have been referred to collectively as Batten disease, although this term should be reserved for the juvenile form. They result from abnormalities in lysosomal proteolysis or membrane function. The stored material in INCL, LINCL, and JNCL has a characteristic ultrastructural appearance, that is, granular osmiophilic deposits (GRODs) in INCL, curvilinear bodies in LINCL, and fingerprint bodies in JNCL. However, some children do not follow this pattern, such that definitive diagnosis cannot be based on biopsy findings alone. With the establishment of the molecular basis for these diseases, this discrepancy has been clarified.

Eight general categories have been described based on age at onset and clinical pattern: infantile, late infantile (LINCL), a Finnish LINCL (vLINCL), juvenile (JNCL), early JNCL (EJNCL), progressive epilepsy with mental retardation (EPMR), and adult (ANCL). A ninth category involving congenital onset has also been described in a small number of neonates and has now been associated with deficiency of cathepsin D activity and a specific mutation in this gene.[91] In the United States, JNCL represents about one-half, LINCL one-third, and INCL one-tenth. ANCL or Kufs disease accounts for about 1%. In Newfoundland, LINCL predominates. The childhood forms are relentlessly progressive whereas ANCL (Kufs disease) is much more indolent.[92]

INFANTILE NEURONAL CEROID LIPOFUSCINOSIS

Clinical Characteristics

INCL is the most rapidly progressive form, presenting from 6 to 24 months, characterized by severe psychomotor deterioration, blindness with macular degeneration, microcephaly, hypotonia, ataxia, and myoclonic epilepsy (Table 24-1, Box 24-10). Hand stereotypies, which progress to choreoathetosis, may be noted early. Hand stereotypies, microcephaly, and visual inattentiveness may suggest the diagnosis of Rett syndrome, but the rapid progression of INCL leads to the correct diagnosis as spasticity and extensor posturing replace hypotonia. The EEG reveals generalized spike and wave activity and prominent amplitude reduction becoming isoelectric by age 2 to 3 years. Both ERG and VER are absent. This differs from Tay-Sachs disease in which the ERG is normal. Cranial CT and MRI reveal profound cerebral and cerebellar atrophy. Death occurs by age 10.

Pathology

Granular osmiophilic deposits (GRODs) are noted in epithelial cells of multiple organs and in neurons throughout the central and peripheral nervous systems. The brain is extremely firm, neuronal loss is profound, and white matter is minimal.

Biochemistry

The stored material includes specific lysosomal activator proteins required for sphingolipid catabolism, saposins A for glucosylceramide and galactosylceramide and D for ceramide (Table 24-2). The defective enzyme, lysosomal palmitoyl protein thioesterase, can be measured in leucocytes, cultured skin fibroblasts, plasma, CSF, amniotic fluid cells, and chorionic villi. Saposins A and D appear to be substrates for this enzyme. GRODs can be identified in skin or conjunctival biopsy, although the yield is often low, requiring multiple samples. A variant form with the clinical pattern of LINCL or JNCL and GRODs on biopsy was found to be allelic with INCL, representing different mutations within the same gene. More recently, adult onset has been described in association with mutations in the *CLN1* gene.[93]

LATE INFANTILE NEURONAL CEROID LIPOFUSCINOSIS

Clinical Characteristics

LINCL has its onset from age 2 to 4 years. The initial features are seizures and psychomotor deterioration followed by loss of vision (Table 24-1, Box 24-11). Myoclonus and ataxia are prominent. Death by age 15 is usual. EEG reveals exaggerated occipital response to photic stimulation. ERG is reduced and ultimately extinguished. VERs and SSEPs are exaggerated initially and then lost. Cranial imaging reveals cerebral and cerebellar atrophy and hyperintense periventricular white matter.

Pathology

Brain atrophy is evident, particularly involving the cerebellum, with loss of neurons and white matter. Autofluorescent material is present within neurons, and curvilinear bodies are seen by electron microscopy within neurons, glia, endothelial cells, and Schwann cells.

Biochemistry

ATP synthase subunit c is the principal storage material along with saposins A and D (Table 24-2). LINCL results from deficient lysosomal pepstatin-insensitive tripeptidyl-peptidase that can be measured in leucocytes, cultured

---

Box 24-10. Santavuori-Haltia-Hagberg Disease

Common name: Santavuori-Haltia-Hagberg disease
Incidence: 1:13,000; mainly in Finnish
Inheritance: Autosomal recessive
Relevant Metabolite: Specific lysosomal activator proteins: saposins A and D
Metabolic Defect: Lysosomal palmitoyl protein thioesterase
Mutation: *CLN1/PPT*-chromosome 1p32
Clinical Pattern: Onset in infancy, rapid psychomotor deterioration, blindness, myoclonic epilepsy, death by age 10

Box 24-11. Jansky-Bielschowsky Disease

Common Name: Jansky-Bielschowsky disease
Incidence: 1:45,000 in British Columbia
Inheritance: Autosomal recessive
Relevant Metabolite: ATP synthase subunit c, saposins A and D
Metabolic Defect: Lysosomal pepstatin-insensitive peptidase
Mutation: *CLN2/TPP1*-chromosome 11p15
Clinical Pattern: Onset age 2-4, seizures, psychomotor deterioration, later visual loss and macular degeneration, death by age 15

20

skin fibroblasts, amniotic cells, and chorionic villi. This enzyme appears to be required for degradation of ATP synthase subunit c. Curvilinear bodies are present in skin or conjunctival biopsies, but again the yield may be low. Significant molecular heterogeneity has been described in individuals with the clinical picture of LINCL with some having mutations in the genes for INCL or JNCL whereas others with clinical features of JNCL had mutations in the LINCL gene. Mutations in this gene (*CLN2*) appear to impede transport of the enzyme into lysosomes.[94]

JUVENILE NEURONAL CEROID LIPOFUSCINOSIS

Clinical Characteristics

JNCL, the most common form of NCL appears at age 5 to 10 years, characterized by visual loss, declining school performance, and seizures (Table 24-1, Box 24-12). Dysarthria, ataxia, and extrapyramidal signs (rigidity and athetosis) follow the onset of seizures. Blindness is inevitable. Macular degeneration is noted with diminished ERGs and VERs. Agitation, restlessness, and psychotic or delusional behavior may occur. Efforts to codify behavior and adaptive function have led to development of a standardized rating scale.[95,96] Cranial MRI reveals mild to moderate cerebral and cerebellar atrophy and increased intensity of periventricular white matter. EEG shows prominent slow spike-and-wave activity and background slowing. Death typically occurs by age 20.

Pathology

Brain atrophy is moderate. Neuronal storage of autofluorescent material is prominent but neuronal loss is minimal. Fingerprint bodies are noted both in neurons and axons as well as in skin and conjunctival biopsies.

Biochemistry

The stored materials are ATP synthase subunit c and, to a lesser extent, saposins A and D (Table 24-2). The JNCL gene encodes a lysosomal transmembrane protein called battenin, which appears to function as a palmitoyl-protein Δ-9 desaturase critical for proteolipid protein processing.[97] Diagnosis is suggested by detection of fingerprint bodies in skin or conjunctival biopsy, but detection of specific mutations in the *CLN3* gene is definitive.

ADULT NEURONAL CEROID LIPOFUSCINOSIS

Clinical Characteristics

Kufs disease is the least common NCL. Both dominant and recessive forms have been described, the latter being more common. Onset occurs by age 30 leading to death in 10 to 15 years (Table 24-1, Box 24-13). Variable clinical manifestations presenting in two principal forms are noted. The more common form begins as progressive myoclonic epilepsy. Dementia and ataxia soon follow. The second features dementia, dysarthria, ataxia, and a prominent movement disorders (especially facial dyskinesia). Vision is spared in each form. EEG shows background slowing and generalized spike-and-wave activity. ERG and VER are normal.

Pathology

Mild cerebral and prominent cerebellar atrophy is noted. Granular autofluorescent material is noted within neurons. Electron microscopy reveals curvilinear, fingerprint, and granular inclusion bodies within neurons.

Biochemistry

The biochemical and molecular bases of Kufs disease are unknown.

Box 24-12. Spielmeyer-Vogt-Sjögren Disease

Common Name: SpielmeyerVogt-Sjögren disease; Batten disease
Incidence: 1:20,000-25,000 in Finland and northern Europe; most common U form
Inheritance: Autosomal recessive
Relevant Metabolite: ATP synthase subunit c, saposins A and D
Metabolic Defect: Lysosomal transmembrane CLN3 protein—battenin
Mutation: *CLN3*-chromosome 16p12
Clinical Pattern: Onset age 5-10, early visual loss and psychomotor delay, seizures later, death by age 20

Box 24-13. Kufs Disease

Common Name: Kufs disease
Incidence: Unknown—very rare
Inheritance: Autosomal dominant and recessive
Relevant Metabolite: Unknown
Metabolic Defect: Unknown
Mutation: *CLN4*-Unknown
Clinical Pattern: Onset about age 30, variable pattern: progressive myoclonic epilepsy, then dementia and ataxia or only dementia and ataxia, death in 10-15 years

Neuronal Ceroid Lipofuscinosis Variants

vLINCL

vLINCL, also called CLN5, has been mapped to chromosome 13q22. This form has a phenotype with features of both LINCL and JNCL, that is, later onset and slower progression of LINCL pattern. Onset occurs from age 4 to 7 with psychomotor regression followed by seizures, myoclonus, ataxia, and visual decline. Macular degeneration and loss of ERG are noted. Death occurs within 10 to 20 years. Cerebral atrophy and neuronal loss are prominent. Electron microscopy reveals fingerprint and curvilinear (more rectilinear) profiles. ATP synthase subunit c and small amounts of saposins A and D are stored. *CLN5* encodes lysosomal transmembrane protein CLN5, whose function remains to be determined. Mutations are uniformly severe.[98]

EJNCL

EJNCL or CLN6 has been linked to chromosome 15q21-23. This form follows the clinical pattern of JNCL with early visual loss followed by seizures, myoclonus, and psychomotor deterioration. Onset is noted at 4 to 5 years, earlier than JNCL, and death occurs from age 10 to 30. ERG is absent. Both curvilinear and fingerprint bodies are noted. The stored material has not been identified, but mutations in a novel transmembrane protein gene have been identified.

EPMR

EPMR or CLN8 is localized to the Finnish population. Onset occurs between age 5 and 10 years, characterized by progressive generalized or complex partial epilepsy and progressive cognitive and motor impairments. Storage material, comprised of ATP synthase subunit c, has curvilinear profiles. The gene encodes a transmembrane protein of unknown function with localization to the endoplasmic reticulum. Its role in the pathogenesis of CLN8 remains to be established. A single mutation has been identified with a carrier frequency of 1 in 135 in this population. It also appears that a variant LINCL form (*CLN7*) occurring in the Turkish population shares mutations with *CLN8*.[99]

SIALIDOSES

The sialidoses are characterized by deficient α-neuraminidase (sialidase) activity or by abnormal lysosomal transport of sialic acid. Two forms of sialidase deficiency are allelic representing different mutations in the same gene: type I, the cherry-red spot-myoclonus syndrome; and type II, the infantile form (also called mucolipidosis I). A third disorder, galactosialidosis,

---

> **Box 24-14. Sialidose Deficiency**
>
> **Common Name:** Type I: cherry-red spot-myoclonus syndrome; Type II: mucolipidosis I
> **Incidence:** Unknown—very rare
> **Inheritance:** Autosomal recessive
> **Relevant Metabolite:** Sialic acid-containing oligosaccharides
> **Metabolic Defect:** Sialidase
> **Mutation:** *NEU*-chromosome 6p21.3
> **Clinical Pattern:** Type I: progressive myoclonus, ataxia, and visual loss; Type II: severe physical and neurological impairment

---

results from deficient activity of both sialidase and GM1 β-galactosidase due to an abnormal protective protein required for stabilizing each enzyme. Two disorders of lysosomal sialic acid storage, infantile sialic acid storage disease (ISSD) and Salla disease, are allelic. A third type of sialic acid storage in cytoplasm, sialuria, unlike the other sialidoses is an autosomal dominant disorder involving the cyptoplasmic enzyme UDP-N-acetylglucosamine 2-epimerase/N-acetylmannosamine kinase (Box 24-14).

Clinical Characteristics

Type I presents in adolescence with visual impairment, generalized myoclonus, or gait difficulty (Table 24-1). Visual loss is progressive involving disproportionate night blindness or loss of color vision. The cherry-red spot is uniformly present, and punctate lenticular opacities may occur. Myoclonus may be stimulus-sensitive or increased by stress, excitement, smoking, or menses and responds poorly to treatment. Intelligence is normal initially, but cognitive decline follows with abilities falling into the educable range. Generalized tonic-clonic seizures and worsening ataxia are noted. EEG reveals progressive background slowing and bilateral, photosensitive fast spike-and-wave activity. Cranial CT and MRI reveal progressive cerebral and cerebellar atrophy. Survival into the thirties is typical.

Type II sialidosis is much more devastating, closely resembling GM1 gangliosidosis. Onset is in infancy characterized by major joint contractures, mild dysostosis multiplex, coarse, puffy facies, hypertrophic gums, inguinal herniae, and hepatosplenomegaly. Severe nephropathy may develop. Type II may also present at birth as hydrops fetalis as in other lysosomal storage diseases. Neurological findings include progressive cognitive decline, cherry-red maculae, ataxia, hypotonia, reduced muscle mass, and peripheral neuropathy. Death in the infantile form occurs in the first or second decade. Survival is brief with neonatal onset. A juvenile form may have a more protracted course.

Pathology

Type I features diffuse cortical atrophy with neuronal storage as well as vacuolar inclusions in liver. Type II neuropathology is much more extensive with diffuse neuronal storage including brainstem nuclei, sympathetic neurons, and peripheral nerves.

Biochemistry

Glycoprotein sialidase and ganglioside sialidase are distinct enzymes (Table 24-2). Sialidosis I and II represent deficiency of glycoprotein sialidase activity. Ganglioside sialidase activity is normal. Tissue and urine sialic acid-containing oligosaccharide levels are elevated. Deficient sialidase (α-neuraminidase) activity should be measured in cultured skin fibroblasts. Several mutations have been identified in *NEU* with clinical severity correlating with mutation type.[100-103]

GALACTOSIALIDOSIS

Clinical Characteristics

Galactosialidosis results from deficiencies of glycoprotein-specific α-neuraminidase and GM1 β-galactosidase activities secondary to mutations in a protective protein gene (Box 24-15). This protective protein is necessary for post-translational stabilization of the two enzymes and is identical with the serine protease, cathepsin A. The protective and protease functions appear distinct.

Three different phenotypic expressions have been described. Cherry-red maculae are noted uniformly along with coarse facies, skeletal abnormalities, inguinal herniae, and visceromegaly. The early infantile form resembles early infantile type II sialidosis. Onset is at birth with coarse facies and fetal hydrops. Death occurs in infancy. The infantile form occurs in the first months of life featuring coarse facies, severe skeletal dysplasia, hepatosplenomegaly, inguinal herniae, hearing loss, and valvular heart disease. Neurological involvement is mild, if any, and survival is prolonged. The juvenile/adult onset form, described almost exclusively in the Japanese, occurs in adolescence or later, with coarse facies, mild skeletal changes (mainly vertebrae), angiokeratoma as in Fabry disease, fucosidosis, and β-mannosidosis. Corneal clouding and punctate lens opacities but not hepatosplenomegaly have been described. Neurological involvement resembles type I sialidosis with progressive myoclonus and cognitive decline, ataxia, and generalized seizures leading to death within 20 to 30 years.

Pathology

Cerebral atrophy and neuronal storage are prominent. Involvement is most severe in the early infantile form.

Biochemistry

Urinary excretion of sialic acid–containing oligosaccharides is markedly increased. GM1-ganglioside is mildly elevated, GM3-ganglioside is increased 10-fold, and sialylglycoproteins are increased significantly in cerebral cortex. GM1 β-galactosidase and glycoprotein-specific α-neuraminidase activities are deficient in leukocytes and cultured skin fibroblasts. Several mutations in the protective protein gene have been identified.

SIALIC ACID STORAGE DISEASES

Clinical Characteristics

Salla disease, prevalent in Finland, and infantile sialic acid storage disease are due to abnormal sialic acid transport (Table 24-1, Box 24-16). Free sialic acid is markedly increased in tissues, serum, urine, and cultured skin fibroblasts. In Salla disease, clinical features include cognitive decline, hypotonia, nystagmus, ataxia,

---

Box 24-15. Galactosialidosis

Incidence: Unknown—(<100 described)
Inheritance: Autosomal recessive
Relevant Metabolite: Sialic acid-containing oligosaccharides
Metabolic Defect: Protective protein/cathepsin A
Mutation: *PPCA*-chromosome 20q13.1
Clinical Pattern: Very similar to type II sialidosis; variable onset from infancy to adulthood; juvenile form mainly in Japanese

---

Box 24-16. Infantile Sialic Acid Storage Disease

Common Name: Infantile sialic acid storage disease (ISSD); Salla disease
Incidence: ISSD: Unknown—very rare; Salla disease: 1:7000; mainly seen in Finland
Inheritance: Autosomal recessive
Relevant Metabolite: Sialic acid
Metabolic Defect: Sialic acid lysosomal transport
Mutation: *ASD*-chromosome 6q14-15
Clinical Pattern: ISSD: onset near birth, severe psychomotor decline, coarse features, early death; Salla: onset in infancy, milder features; psychomotor delay, slow progression, and near normal survival

and extrapyramidal (mainly athetosis) movements. Onset occurs in infancy with coarse facies and somatic growth retardation.[104] One-fourth to one-third do not walk. By adulthood, intelligence is moderately to severely impaired. Absence-type seizures appear in later years. Cranial MRI reveals an arrest of myelination at the infantile level with hypoplasia of the corpus callosum and increased T_2-weighted signal in white matter. Peripheral nerve myelin is abnormal with reduced nerve conduction velocities and prolonged distal latencies. Survival is prolonged, if not normal.

Infantile sialic acid storage disease has its onset prior to or at birth. Fetal hydrops may be seen. Severe failure to thrive, coarse facies, dysostosis multiplex, hepatosplenomegaly, and severe psychomotor deterioration are uniform. Death occurs by age 2. Cranial MRI reveals severely reduced white matter.

Pathology

In ISSD, brain atrophy is severe, mainly from reduced white matter. Neuronal storage is diffuse. In Salla disease, storage is less extensive. Cytoplasmic inclusions are present in lymphocytes and cultured skin fibroblasts.

Biochemistry

The basic defect is blockade of sialic acid transport[105] from lysosomes resulting in tissue sialic acid storage and increased excretion in urine (Table 24-2). In ISSD, the increase is 100-fold over normal whereas in Salla disease it is approximately10-fold. Glucuronic acid, which utilizes the same transport system, is also stored. Increased sialic acid excretion in urine establishes the diagnosis, disease severity correlating with the level of sialic acid excretion. ISSD and Salla disease are allelic, due to different mutations in the sialic acid transporter gene.[106,107]

SIALURIA

Sialuria is an autosomal dominant disorder described in only a handful of individuals characterized by developmental delay, coarse features, hepatosplenomegaly, and mild to moderate impairment of cognitive and fine-motor functions.[108] Sialic acid levels in urine are increased 100-fold, confirming the diagnosis. Failure of feedback inhibition of UDP-N-acetylglucosamine 2-epimerase by CMP-neuraminic acid is responsible. Mutations have been identified in the gene, *GNE*.

Distinctly different mutations in *GNE* are associated with the autosomal recessive disorder, hereditary inclusion body myopathy, another example of different disorders arising from mutations in the same gene.[109-112] This disorder has been described in multiple ethnic groups, but predominantly in Jewish individuals of Persian descent. The principal clinical features occur in adulthood as a slowly progressive lower extremity myopathy with sparing of the quadriceps accompanied by vacuolar, filamentous inclusions in muscle.

Neuroimaging Assessment

Neuroimaging is particularly useful in the assessment of the leukodystrophies (Table 24-3).[1,2] The principal CT finding is a decrease in density of white matter with later appearance of atrophy. In general, the later-onset forms have milder abnormalities. For example, the decrease in density is diffuse and symmetrical in the late infantile and juvenile types of sulfatide lipidosis, whereas the adult form may mainly show central and cortical atrophy, with variable and focal decrease in white matter density. Galactosylceramide lipidosis (Krabbe disease) may be distinguished from the others by the appearance of increased density in the cerebellum, thalami, caudate nuclei, brainstem, and corona radiata. These areas show markedly shortened T_1 and T_2 values by MRI, whereas the areas of decreased density in white matter show increased T_1 and T_2 values and appear similar to plaques in multiple sclerosis. This finding is particularly relevant in light of the proposed cytotoxic effect of psychosine.

Cranial CT is also helpful in the diagnosis of adrenoleukodystrophy, revealing attenuation in the periventricular white matter posteriorly with contrast enhancement at the periphery of the low-density lesions and a pattern of posterior-to-anterior progression. Enhancement decreases or disappears as the disease process progresses. Atypical findings noted on CT include low-density, non-enhancing frontal lesions and unilateral lesions with suggestion of mass effect. Adrenomyeloneuropathy, by contrast, has either normal findings or mild ventricular dilatation. MRI readily demonstrates demyelination in X-ALD and detects abnormal white matter in the cerebrum, pons, and spinal cord of adrenomyeloneuropathy despite a normal pattern by CT. The neonatal form, in comparison, demonstrates diffuse and symmetrical white matter lucencies with central contrast enhancement.

Cranial imaging is not of particular help in the diagnosis or differentiation of the neuronal storage disorders, including the sphingolipidoses, GM1- and GM2-gangliosidoses, the neuronal ceroid lipofuscinosis, and the sialidoses/sialuria complex.

Clinical Neurophysiologic Assessment

Clinical neurophysiologic assessments of the peripheral and central pathways in the inherited neurodegenerative

Table 24-3.

Inherited Neurodegenerative Disorders of Childhood: Neuroimaging

Disorder	Computed Tomography	Magnetic Resonance Imaging
Sphingolipidoses		
GM2-Gangliosidosis	Hyperdense cortical zones	Hyperdense cortical zones
Acute types including Sandhoff	Decreased white matter	Decreased white matter
	Dilated ventricles	Dilated ventricles
	Small cerebellum and brainstem	Small cerebellum and brainstem
Juvenile and adult types	Normal to cerebellar atrophy and mild cerebral cortical atrophy	Marked cerebellar atrophy
GM1-Gangliosidosis		
Acute type	Prominent atrophy	Prominent atrophy
	Increased density of thalami	Thalami and basal ganglia hyperintense on T_1 and hypointense on T_2
	Reduced density of basal ganglia	
Adult type	Normal to moderate ventricular dilatation and cortical atrophy; possible caudate atrophy	Normal to moderate ventricular dilatation and cortical atrophy; possible caudate atrophy
Globotriaosylceramide lipidosis	Normal to evidence of stroke	Normal to evidence of stroke
Galactosylceramide lipidosis		
Infantile type	Symmetrical attenuation decrease in white matter and increase in cerebellum, thalami, caudate, brainstem, and corona radiata	Markedly shortened T_1 and T_2 in areas of increased density on CT
	No contrast enhancement	Increased T_1 and T_2 in centrum semiovale
	Severe atrophy later	
Late infantile type	Mild ventricular dilatation	Diffuse myelin loss in central white matter and pyramidal tracts
	Decreased density of anterior periventricular white matter	
Sulfatide Lipidosis		
Late infantile and juvenile types	Diffuse, symmetrical attenuation in cerebral and cerebellar white matter progressing anterior to posterior with gradual appearance of atrophy	Symmetrical white matter loss
		Cortical atrophy
	No contrast enhancement	
Adult type	Central and cortical atrophy	Central and cortical atrophy
	Variable focal (frontal and parietal) decrease in white matter density	Variable focal (frontal and parietal) decrease in white matter density
Adrenoleukodystrophy Complex		
Adrenoleukodystrophy		
Typical pattern	Attenuation in periventricular cerebral white matter near trigone with contrast enhancement in butterfly pattern	Loss of gray-white contrast in occipital region, increased T_2 in periventricular region posteriorly
	Posterior to anterior progression	
	Enhancement disappears or diminishes as disease progresses	
	No mass effect	
Atypical pattern	(a) Low density non-enhancing frontal lesion	(a) Low density non-enhancing frontal lesion
	(b) Unilateral lesions and suggestion of mass effect	(b) Unilateral lesions and suggestion of mass effect
Adrenomyeloneuropathy	No abnormality to mild ventricular dilatation	Often normal
Adrenoleukomyeloneuropathy	Mild ventricular dilation	May see central white matter loss
	Atrophy of pons and cerebellum	Increased T_1/T_2 in corpus callosum, cerebral white matter, internal capsule, pons, and cord

(Continued)

Table 24-3. (Continued)

Inherited Neurodegenerative Disorders of Childhood: Neuroimaging

Disorder	Computed Tomography	Magnetic Resonance Imaging
Neonatal Type	Normal early	NI
	Then diffuse, symmetrical white matter lucencies with central contrast enhancement	NI
Neuronal Ceroid Lipofuscinoses		
CLN1	Normal early; then profound cerebral and cerebellar atrophy	Profound cerebral and cerebellar atrophy
CLN2	Profound cerebral and cerebellar atrophy Hyperintense periventricular white matter	Profound cerebral and cerebellar atrophy Hyperintense periventricular white matter
CLN3	At age greater than 13, 1/6 normal	Mild to moderate cerebral and cerebellar atrophy
	At age less than 23, 6/8 normal	Hyperintense periventricular white matter
Sialic Acid Disorders		
Sialidosis I	Progressive cerebral and cerebellar atrophy	Progressive cerebral and cerebellar atrophy
Sialidosis II		
Infantile type	Severe cortical atrophy	Severe cortical atrophy
Juvenile type	Normal	NI
Sialuria		
Infantile type	NI	Arrested myelination at infantile level Hypoplastic corpus callosum Increased T_2 in white matter
Salla type	Marked cerebral atrophy	Markedly reduced white matter Thin corpus callosum Cerebellar atrophy

NI, no information found.

disorders provide powerful tools. The information in Table 24-4 represents the collation of individual cases as well as in-depth studies of specific disorders.[1,2]

The electroretinogram (ERG) is particularly useful in the diagnosis of the neuronal ceroid lipofuscinosis, as responses range from small amplitude to absent. In few of the other entities is the response sufficiently reduced to confuse the diagnosis. Although ERG and VER responses may be markedly diminished in neonatal adrenoleukodystrophy, this disorder should be differentiated on clinical findings (see Table 24-1).

Visual evoked responses (VER) may also be extremely helpful. In Tay-Sachs disease, the VERs are lost in a progressive fashion. The VER is also abnormal in the neuronal ceroid lipofuscinoses, but the difference in the ERG response should be differentiating. Within the NCL group, the late infantile type demonstrates enlarged or exaggerated VERs, whereas the infantile and juvenile types display small to absent responses.

It is possible to discriminate between the leukodystrophies based on auditory brainstem responses (ABR) and nerve conduction velocities. Nerve conduction velocities are markedly reduced in both the early forms of galactosylceramide lipidosis and sulfatide lipidosis, whereas such studies are generally normal in disorders of the adrenoleukodystrophy complex, at least during the beginning stages of the disorder.

ABRs reveal abnormalities in disorders of white matter that range from prolonged interwave intervals to an absence of response after wave 1. White matter diseases have abnormal ABRs together with high-amplitude irregular delta activity on EEG, whereas gray matter disease is characterized by normal to minimally abnormal ABRs and EEGs that consist of paroxysmal sharp waves and spike-and-wave activity, in addition to diffuse slowing and progressive voltage reduction. Freeman and McKhann[113] promulgated the concept of gray versus white matter differentiation in the expression of the inherited neurodegenerative diseases to direct strategies for clinical diagnosis. Clinical neurophysiology assessments provide support for this concept.

Table 24-4.

Inherited Neurodegenerative Disorders of Childhood: Clinical Neurophysiologic Assessment

Disorder	ERG	VER	ABR	SSEP	EEG	NCV
Sphingolipidoses						
GM2-Gangliosidosis						
Infantile type	Normal to slight decrease in amplitude	Normal early; abnormal to absent later with loss of definition of early components initially	Prolonged latencies	Peripheral components normal	Progressive slowing initially High then decreasing voltage Paroxysmal spike events may be infrequent	NI
Late infantile type	Normal	Variable loss	Abnormal in 1/2 tested Prolonged I-V interval	NI	Similar to infantile type	Normal
Juvenile type	Normal	Normal high-voltage response	Normal	NI	Normal to progressive diffuse slowing	Normal
Adult type	Normal	NI	NI	NI	Normal to diffuse slowing	Normal
Sandhoff type	Similar to infantile	Similar to infantile	Similar to infantile	NI	Similar to infantile	Normal
GM1-Gangliosidosis						
Infantile/juvenile types	Normal	Abnormal	Normal in 1/1 tested	NI	Generalized slowing Occasionally with spike/wave	Normal
Adult type	NI	NI	NI	NI	Normal	Normal
Sphingomyelin Lipidosis						
Infantile type	Normal to reduced	Progressive decrease in amplitude	Normal to delayed	NI	Normal early May be epileptiform with slowing late	Normal to reduced
Glucosylceramide Lipidosis						
Infantile type	NI	NI	Lengthening of peak latencies Progressive loss of waves III-V Associated with loss of neurons in cochlear nuclei and hypoplastic superior olivary complex	NI	Diffuse slow waves and spike-wave discharges Abnormal sharp waves on photic stimulation	NI

(Continued)

Table 24-4. (Continued)

Inherited Neurodegenerative Disorders of Childhood: Clinical Neurophysiologic Assessment

Disorder	ERG	VER	ABR	SSEP	EEG	NCV
Galactosylceramide Lipidosis						
Infantile type	Normal	Progressive decrease to no response in late stage	Only waves I and II noted rest absent	Delayed major component (P 100)	Normal early Moderate to severe generalized high-voltage slowing	Markedly reduced
Sulfatide Lipidosis						
Late infantile type	Normal	Normal early; then prolonged latencies No response late	Prolonged latencies for waves I and V and I-V interval Absent waves III-V Delayed Wave I	Low amplitude Prolonged latencies to absent response	Normal early Progressive diffuse slowing Occasionally spike-and-wave paroxysms late	Markedly reduced
Juvenile type	Normal	Same as late infantile	Prolonged latencies	Prolonged latencies	Same as late infantile	Markedly reduced
Adult type	NI	Normal to prolonged latencies	Normal	NI	Low voltage Diffusely slow	Normal to reduced
Adrenoleukodystrophies						
Adrenoleukodystrophy	Normal	Normal early Prolonged latency later	Normal at onset Prolonged interwave intervals to absent response after wave I Prolonged in obligate heterozygotes	Prolonged latency Abnormal in 4/7 female relatives	Normal early Irregular high voltage delta More prominent posteriorly Loss of normal arousal response	Normal early Reduced later
Adrenomyeloneuropathy	Normal	Normal	No waves after I or prolonged interwave intervals	Prolonged latency	Normal	Normal to mildly reduced

Adrenoleukomyelo-neuropathy	Normal	Normal	Prolonged I-III and III-V intervals	Prolonged latency	Normal to mild diffuse slowing	Normal early Reduced later Worse in lower extremities
Neonatal adrenoleukodystrophy	Absent	Absent—info from one infant	Marked central pathway dysfunction	NI	Diffusely epileptiform Marked frontally Progresses from focal to multifocal spikes to burst suppression	Normal to reduced
Neuronal Ceroid Lipofuscinoses						
Infantile type	Small to absent	Small to absent by age 3-4	NI	NI	Slowing initially (normal 12-15 mo) with progressive decrease in amplitude, especially central, frontal, and temporal regions); no response to photic stimulation before 2 y; after age 3, isoelectric	Normal
Late infantile type	Small to absent	Grossly enlarged response early Absent late	NI	Exaggerated response early with normal latency Later, little response within and rostral to brainstem	Loss of background rhythm Diffusely slow with temporal spike and wave spikes Exaggerated photic response	Usually normal
Juvenile type	Small to absent Early	Small amplitude early Then absent	NI	Markedly reduced Amplitudes	Early diffuse slowing Increased amplitude Spike/wave discharges	Slight decrease especially in sensory fibers

(Continued)

Table 24-4. (Continued)

Inherited Neurodegenerative Disorders of Childhood: Clinical Neurophysiologic Assessment

Disorder	ERG	VER	ABR	SSEP	EEG	NCV
Sialidosis/Sialuria Complex						
Sialidosis I	Normal	Normal to decreased amplitude	Normal	NI	Normal early Decreased voltage with fast background Occasional generalized spike/wave	NI
Sialidosis II						
Infantile type	NI	NI	NI	NI	Marked epileptiform activity	NI
Juvenile type	Normal	Normal early Decreased amplitude later	NI	NI	Normal to diffuse fast activity early Irregular background with spike discharges later	Normal
Sialuria						
Infantile type	Normal	Normal	Normal	NI	Multifocal spike discharges	Normal
Salla type	Normal	Normal	Normal	NI	Progressive voltage decrease With voltage decrease, no response to eye-opening or photic stimulation	Normal

NI, no information found.

Chemical and Biochemical Assays

The clinical presentation of neurodegenerative disorders and the results of cranial imaging and clinical neurophysiology should allow the clinician to tailor specific diagnostic laboratory studies, in many instances focusing the diagnostic approach to a specific entity (Table 24-2).

For the sphingolipidoses and sialidoses, specific enzyme assays will confirm the diagnosis. For the adrenoleukodystrophy complex, measurements of very-long-chain fatty acids must be made in plasma or cultured skin fibroblasts. For the sialuria group, sialic acid can be measured in urine or in cultured skin fibroblasts. For the neuronal ceroid lipofuscinoses, specific enzymatic or molecular testing is possible. The use of conjunctival, skin, or nerve biopsies for ultrastructural analysis is less often employed because of its low yield and, more importantly, the availability of more precise and specific biochemical and molecular testing.

Carrier Identification and Prenatal Diagnosis

Carrier identification and prenatal diagnosis are now feasible for many of the inherited neurodegenerative diseases.[114,115] Despite recent advances in molecular genetic diagnosis, analysis of the specific enzyme deficiency or detection of the relevant metabolite remains the gold standard in most instances. The number of different mutations in most of these disorders makes DNA analysis impractical on a broad scale. In families with known mutations, molecular testing should offer the most specific information.

Careful consideration should be given to medical, social, and ethical consequences of carrier identification and prenatal diagnosis including the outcome analysis of these programs. One must be aware of the possibility of revealing non-paternity with carrier identification.

Therapy

For most inherited neurodegenerative and neurometabolic diseases, treatment remains problematic (Table 24-5).[116] Established strategies for some have been effective including dietary (PKU) and enzyme replacement (storage diseases).[117-122] Enzyme replacement in Gaucher disease and Fabry disease has proved effective but costly. Bone marrow transplantation has also been beneficial in neuronopathic (type III) Gaucher disease, but of uncertain benefit in many other storage diseases involving the CNS.[123]

Molecular advances offer the opportunity to replace specific genes. Alternatively, multipotent neural progenitor cells (stem cells) have been engineered to express specific genes whose products would then supply deficient cells.

Table 24-5.

Inherited Neurodegenerative Disorders of Childhood: Enzyme Replacement Therapy

Modality	Result
Substrate reduction	Erucic acid appears to delay or block onset of X-ALD
	Miglustat may be beneficial in Gaucher disease
Specific enzyme	Limited efficacy in neurodegenerative types
	Effective in non-neuronal types of Gaucher and Fabry disease
Organ transplant	Limited efficacy except in Gaucher and Fabry disease
Bone marrow transplant	In general, no benefit in altering involvement of central nervous system
	Disease progression slowed in type I Krabbe disease and juvenile sulfatide lipidosis

Alternative strategies have also been considered involving manipulation of substrate load through the use of chemical inhibitors or through the use of molecular chaperones designed to protect or stabilize enzyme function.[124-129] This approach has been applied specifically to the sphingolipidoses. To date, the results have been relatively modest in terms of reducing substrate load; however, in combination with enzyme replacement therapy, this remains an approach warranting further study.

Evaluation of effective therapies requires the development of objective outcome data. This includes measurable motor, cognitive, and behavioral endpoints. Aiding this process is the implementation of quantitative measures of specific metabolites using techniques such as magnetic resonance spectroscopy.

REFERENCES

1. Scriver C, Sly W, Childs B, et al. *The Metabolic and Molecular Bases of Human Disease.* 8th ed. New York: McGraw-Hill; 2005.
2. Percy A. Inherited neurometabolic diseases. In: Griggs R, Joynt R, eds. *Baker's Clincial Neurology on CD ROM.* Philadelphia: Lippincott-Wliiams & Wilkins; 2004.
3. Risch N, Tang H, Katzenstein H, Ekstein J. Geographic distribution of disease mutations in the Ashkenazi Jewish population supports genetic drift over selection. *Am J Hum Genet.* 2003;72:812-822.
4. Sillence DJ, Platt FM. Storage diseases: new insights into sphingolipid functions. *Trends Cell Biol.* 2003;13:195-203.
5. Buccoliero R, Futerman AH. The roles of ceramide and complex sphingolipids in neuronal cell function. *Pharmacol Res.* 2003;47:409-419.

6. Lukacs Z, Keil A, Peters V, et al. Towards quality assurance in the determination of lysosomal enzymes: a two-centre study. *J Inherit Metab Dis.* 2003;26:571-581.

7. Zhang X, Kiechle FL. Review: Glycosphingolipids in health and disease. *Ann Clin Lab Sci.* 2004;34:3-13.

8. Ginzburg L, Kacher Y, Futerman AH. The pathogenesis of glycosphingolipid storage disorders. *Semin Cell Dev Biol.* 2004;15:417-431.

9. Walkley SU. Secondary accumulation of gangliosides in lysosomal storage disorders. *Semin Cell Dev Biol.* 2004;15:433-444.

10. Ozkara HA. Recent advances in the biochemistry and genetics of sphingolipidoses. *Brain Dev.* 2004;26:497-505.

11. Kolter T, Sandhoff K. Sphingolipid metabolism diseases. *Biochim Biophys Acta.* 2006;1758:2057-2079.

12. Shapiro BE, Hatters-Friedman S, Fernandes-Filho JA, et al. Late-onset Tay-Sachs disease: adverse effects of medications and implications for treatment. *Neurology.* 2006;67:875-877.

13. Nassogne MC, Commare MC, Lellouch-Tubiana A, et al. Unusual presentation of GM2 gangliosidosis mimicking a brainstem tumor in a 3-year-old girl. *AJNR Am J Neuroradiol.* 2003;24:840-842.

14. Inglese M, Nusbaum AO, Pastores GM, et al. MR imaging and proton spectroscopy of neuronal injury in late-onset GM2 gangliosidosis. *AJNR Am J Neuroradiol.* 2005;26:2037-2042.

15. Rucker JC, Shapiro BE, Han YH, et al. Neuro-ophthalmology of late-onset Tay-Sachs disease (LOTS). *Neurology.* 2004;63:1918-1926.

16. Frey LC, Ringel SP, Filley CM. The natural history of cognitive dysfunction in late-onset GM2 gangliosidosis. *Arch Neurol.* 2005;62:989-994.

17. Zaroff CM, Neudorfer O, Morrison C, et al. Neuropsychological assessment of patients with late onset GM2 gangliosidosis. *Neurology.* 2004;62:2283-2286.

18. Branda KJ, Tomczak J, Natowicz MR. Heterozygosity for Tay-Sachs and Sandhoff diseases in non-Jewish Americans with ancestry from Ireland, Great Britain, or Italy. *Genet Test.* 2004;8:174-180.

19. Gason AA, Sheffield E, Bankier A, et al. Evaluation of a Tay-Sachs disease screening program. *Clin Genet.* 2003;63:386-392.

20. Gason AA, Metcalfe SA, Delatycki MB, et al. Tay Sachs disease carrier screening in schools: educational alternatives and cheekbrush sampling. *Genet Med.* 2005;7:626-632.

21. Gururaj A, Sztriha L, Hertecant J, et al. Magnetic resonance imaging findings and novel mutations in GM1 gangliosidosis. *J Child Neurol.* 2005;20:57-60.

22. Muthane U, Chickabasaviah Y, Kaneski C, et al. Clinical features of adult GM1 gangliosidosis: report of three Indian patients and review of 40 cases. *Mov Disord.* 2004;19:1334-1341.

23. Ries M, Gupta S, Moore DF, et al. Pediatric Fabry disease. *Pediatrics.* 2005;115:e344-e355.

24. Ramaswami U, Whybra C, Parini R, et al. Clinical manifestations of Fabry disease in children: data from the Fabry Outcome Survey. *Acta Paediatr.* 2006;95:86-92.

25. Desnick RJ, Brady RO. Fabry disease in childhood. *J Pediatr.* 2004;144:S20-S26.

26. Spada M, Pagliardini S, Yasuda M, et al. High incidence of later-onset Fabry disease revealed by newborn screening. *Am J Hum Genet.* 2006;79:31-40.

27. Senechal M, Germain DP. Fabry disease: a functional and anatomical study of cardiac manifestations in 20 hemizygous male patients. *Clin Genet.* 2003;63:46-52.

28. Hauser AC, Gessl A, Lorenz M, et al. High prevalence of subclinical hypothyroidism in patients with Anderson-Fabry disease. *J Inherit Metab Dis.* 2005;28:715-722.

29. Altarescu G, Moore DF, Schiffmann R. Effect of genetic modifiers on cerebral lesions in Fabry disease. *Neurology.* 2005;64:2148-2150.

30. Marino S, Borsini W, Buchner S, et al. Diffuse structural and metabolic brain changes in Fabry disease. *J Neurol.* 2006;253:434-440.

31. Schaefer E, Mehta A, Gal A. Genotype and phenotype in Fabry disease: analysis of the Fabry Outcome Survey. *Acta Paediatr Suppl.* 2005;94:87-92.

32. Kleinert J, Lorenz M, Hauser AC, et al. Measurement of renal function in patients with Fabry disease. *Acta Paediatr Suppl.* 2005;94:19-23.

33. Eto Y, Ohashi T, Utsunomiya Y, et al. Enzyme replacement therapy in Japanese Fabry disease patients: the results of a phase 2 bridging study. *J Inherit Metab Dis.* 2005;28:575-583.

34. Shah JS, Elliott PM. Fabry disease and the heart: an overview of the natural history and the effect of enzyme replacement therapy. *Acta Paediatr Suppl.* 2005;94:11-14.

35. Hughes DA, Mehta AB. Vascular complications of Fabry disease: enzyme replacement and other therapies. *Acta Paediatr Suppl.* 2005;94:28-33.

36. Hilz MJ, Brys M, Marthol H, et al. Enzyme replacement therapy improves function of C-, A-delta-, and A-beta-nerve fibers in Fabry neuropathy. *Neurology.* 2004;62:1066-1072.

37. Wilcox WR, Banikazemi M, Guffon N, et al. Long-term safety and efficacy of enzyme replacement therapy for Fabry disease. *Am J Hum Genet.* 2004;75:65-74.

38. Hajioff D, Enever Y, Quiney R, et al. Hearing loss in Fabry disease: the effect of agalsidase alfa replacement therapy. *J Inherit Metab Dis.* 2003;26:787-794.

39. Baehner F, Kampmann C, Whybra C, et al. Enzyme replacement therapy in heterozygous females with Fabry disease: results of a phase IIIB study. *J Inherit Metab Dis.* 2003;26:617-627.

40. McGovern MM, Aron A, Brodie SE, et al. Natural history of Type A Niemann-Pick disease: possible endpoints for therapeutic trials. *Neurology.* 2006;66:228-232.

41. Sidransky E. Gaucher disease: complexity in a "simple" disorder. *Mol Genet Metab.* 2004;83:6-15.

42. Kaplan P, Andersson HC, Kacena KA, Yee JD. The clinical and demographic characteristics of nonneuronopathic Gaucher disease in 887 children at diagnosis. *Arch Pediatr Adolesc Med.* 2006;160:603-608.

43. Grabowski GA, Andria G, Baldellou A, et al. Pediatric non-neuronopathic Gaucher disease: presentation, diagnosis and assessment. Consensus statements. *Eur J Pediatr.* 2004;163:58-66.

44. Amato D, Stachiw T, Clarke JT, Rivard GE. Gaucher disease: variability in phenotype among siblings. *J Inherit Metab Dis.* 2004;27:659-669.

45. Pastores GM, Barnett NL, Bathan P, Kolodny EH. A neurological symptom survey of patients with type I Gaucher disease. *J Inherit Metab Dis.* 2003;26:641-645.

46. Toft M, Pielsticker L, Ross OA, et al. Glucocerebrosidase gene mutations and Parkinson disease in the Norwegian population. *Neurology.* 2006;66:415-417.

47. Wong K, Sidransky E, Verma A, et al. Neuropathology provides clues to the pathophysiology of Gaucher disease. *Mol Genet Metab.* 2004;82:192-207.

48. Aharon-Peretz J, Rosenbaum H, Gershoni-Baruch R. Mutations in the glucocerebrosidase gene and Parkinson's disease in Ashkenazi Jews. *N Engl J Med.* 2004; 351:1972-1977.

49. Bembi B, Zambito Marsala S, Sidransky E, et al. Gaucher's disease with Parkinson's disease: clinical and pathological aspects. *Neurology.* 2003;61:99-101.

50. Rosenbloom BE, Weinreb NJ, Zimran A, et al. Gaucher disease and cancer incidence: a study from the Gaucher Registry. *Blood.* 2005;105:4569-4572.

51. Mignot C, Gelot A, Bessieres B, et al. Perinatal-lethal Gaucher disease. *Am J Med Genet A.* 2003; 120:338-344.

52. Park JK, Orvisky E, Tayebi N, et al. Myoclonic epilepsy in Gaucher disease: genotype-phenotype insights from a rare patient subgroup. *Pediatr Res.* 2003;53:387-395.

53. Diaz-Font A, Cormand B, Blanco M, et al. Gene rearrangements in the glucocerebrosidase-metaxin region giving rise to disease-causing mutations and polymorphisms. Analysis of 25 Rec NciI alleles in Gaucher disease patients. *Hum Genet.* 2003;112:426-429.

54. Zhao H, Bailey LA, Elsas LJ 2nd, et al. Gaucher disease: in vivo evidence for allele dose leading to neuronopathic and nonneuronopathic phenotypes. *Am J Med Genet A.* 2003;116:52-56.

55. El-Beshlawy A, Ragab L, Youssry I, et al. Enzyme replacement therapy and bony changes in Egyptian paediatric Gaucher disease patients. *J Inherit Metab Dis.* 2006; 29:92-98.

56. Aerts JM, Hollak CE, van Breemen M, et al. Identification and use of biomarkers in Gaucher disease and other lysosomal storage diseases. *Acta Paediatr Suppl.* 2005; 94:43-46; discussion 37-48.

57. Deegan PB, Cox TM. Clinical evaluation of biomarkers in Gaucher disease. *Acta Paediatr Suppl.* 2005;94:47-50; discussion 37-48.

58. Baldellou A, Andria G, Campbell PE, et al. Paediatric non-neuronopathic Gaucher disease: recommendations for treatment and monitoring. *Eur J Pediatr.* 2004; 163:67-75.

59. Charrow J, Andersson HC, Kaplan P, et al. Enzyme replacement therapy and monitoring for children with type 1 Gaucher disease: consensus recommendations. *J Pediatr.* 2004;144:112-120.

60. Burrow TA, Cohen MB, Bokulic R, et al. Gaucher disease: progressive mesenteric and mediastinal lymphadenopathy despite enzyme therapy. *J Pediatr.* 2007; 150:202-206.

61. Charrow J, Dulisse B, Grabowski GA, Weinreb NJ. The effect of enzyme replacement therapy on bone crisis and bone pain in patients with type 1 Gaucher disease. *Clin Genet.* 2007;71:205-211.

62. Elstein D, Hollak C, Aerts JM, et al. Sustained therapeutic effects of oral miglustat (Zavesca, N-butyldeoxynojirimycin, OGT 918) in type I Gaucher disease. *J Inherit Metab Dis.* 2004;27:757-766.

63. Germain DP. Gaucher's disease: a paradigm for interventional genetics. *Clin Genet.* 2004;65:77-86.

64. Del Bigio MR, Chudley AE, Booth FA, Pacin S. Late infantile onset krabbe disease in siblings with cortical degeneration and absence of cerebral globoid cells. *Neuropediatrics.* 2004;35:297-301.

65. Arenson NE, Heydemann PT. Late-onset Krabbe's disease mimicking acute disseminated encephalomyelitis. *Pediatr Neurol.* 2005;33:208-210.

66. Brockmann K, Dechent P, Wilken B, et al. Proton MRS profile of cerebral metabolic abnormalities in Krabbe disease. *Neurology.* 2003;60:819-825.

67. Siddiqi ZA, Sanders DB, Massey JM. Peripheral neuropathy in Krabbe disease: effect of hematopoietic stem cell transplantation. *Neurology.* 2006;67:268-272.

68. Escolar ML, Poe MD, Provenzale JM, et al. Transplantation of umbilical-cord blood in babies with infantile Krabbe's disease. *N Engl J Med.* 2005;352:2069-2081.

69. Diez-Roux G, Ballabio A. Sulfatases and human disease. *Annu Rev Genomics Hum Genet.* 2005;6:355-379.

70. Rauschka H, Colsch B, Baumann N, et al. Late-onset metachromatic leukodystrophy: genotype strongly influences phenotype. *Neurology.* 2006;67:859-863.

71. Anlar B, Waye JS, Eng B, Oguz KK. Atypical clinical course in juvenile metachromatic leukodystrophy involving novel arylsulfatase A gene mutations. *Dev Med Child Neurol.* 2006;48:383-387.

72. Marcao AM, Wiest R, Schindler K, et al. Adult onset metachromatic leukodystrophy without electroclinical peripheral nervous system involvement: a new mutation in the ARSA gene. *Arch Neurol.* 2005;62:309-313.

73. Park JH, Schuchman EH. Acid ceramidase and human disease. *Biochim Biophys Acta.* 2006;1758:2133-2138.

74. Muramatsu T, Sakai N, Yanagihara I, et al. Mutation analysis of the acid ceramidase gene in Japanese patients with Farber disease. *J Inherit Metab Dis.* 2002;25:585-592.

75. Cox CS, Dubey P, Raymond GV, et al. Cognitive evaluation of neurologically asymptomatic boys with X-linked adrenoleukodystrophy. *Arch Neurol.* 2006;63:69-73.

76. Zackowski KM, Dubey P, Raymond GV, et al. Sensorimotor function and axonal integrity in adrenomyeloneuropathy. *Arch Neurol.* 2006;63:74-80.

77. Loes DJ, Fatemi A, Melhem ER, et al. Analysis of MRI patterns aids prediction of progression in X-linked adrenoleukodystrophy. *Neurology.* 2003;61:369-374.

78. Eichler F, Mahmood A, Loes D, et al. Magnetic resonance imaging detection of lesion progression in adult patients with X-linked adrenoleukodystrophy. *Arch Neurol.* 2007;64:659-664.

79. Wichers-Rother M, Grigull A, Sokolowski P, et al. Adrenal steroids in adrenomyeloneuropathy. Dehydroepiandrosterone sulfate, androstenedione and 17alpha-hydroxyprogesterone. *J Neurol.* 2005;252:1525-1529.

80. Maier EM, Kammerer S, Muntau AC, et al. Symptoms in carriers of adrenoleukodystrophy relate to skewed X inactivation. *Ann Neurol.* 2002;52:683-688.

81. Jung HH, Wimplinger I, Jung S, et al. Phenotypes of female adrenoleukodystrophy. *Neurology.* 2007;68:960-961.

82. Fatemi A, Barker PB, Ulug AM, et al. MRI and proton MRSI in women heterozygous for X-linked adrenoleukodystrophy. *Neurology.* 2003;60:1301-1307.

83. Wanders RJ. Metabolic and molecular basis of peroxisomal disorders: a review. *Am J Med Genet A.* 2004; 126:355-375.

84. Paintlia AS, Gilg AG, Khan M, et al. Correlation of very long chain fatty acid accumulation and inflammatory disease progression in childhood X-ALD: implications for potential therapies. *Neurobiol Dis.* 2003;14:425-439.

85. Linnebank M, Kemp S, Wanders RJ, et al. Methionine metabolism and phenotypic variability in X-linked adrenoleukodystrophy. *Neurology.* 2006;66:442-443.

86. Schonberger S, Roerig P, Schneider DT, et al. Genotype and protein expression after bone marrow transplantation for adrenoleukodystrophy. *Arch Neurol.* 2007; 64:651-657.

87. Williams RE, Aberg L, Autti T, et al. Diagnosis of the neuronal ceroid lipofuscinoses: an update. *Biochim Biophys Acta.* 2006;1762:865-872.

88. Siintola E, Lehesjoki AE, Mole SE. Molecular genetics of the NCLs—status and perspectives. *Biochim Biophys Acta.* 2006;1762:857-864.

89. Mole SE. Neuronal ceroid lipofuscinoses. *Eur J Paediatr Neurol.* 2006;10:255-257.

90. Haltia M. The neuronal ceroid-lipofuscinoses. *J Neuropathol Exp Neurol.* 2003;62:1-13.

91. Siintola E, Partanen S, Stromme P, et al. Cathepsin D deficiency underlies congenital human neuronal ceroid-lipofuscinosis. *Brain.* 2006;129:1438-1445.

92. Hobert JA, Dawson G. Neuronal ceroid lipofuscinoses therapeutic strategies: past, present and future. *Biochim Biophys Acta.* 2006;1762:945-953.

93. Ramadan H, Al-Din AS, Ismail A, et al. Adult neuronal ceroid lipofuscinosis caused by deficiency in palmitoyl protein thioesterase 1. *Neurology.* 2007;68:387-388.

94. Steinfeld R, Steinke HB, Isbrandt D, et al. Mutations in classical late infantile neuronal ceroid lipofuscinosis disrupt transport of tripeptidyl-peptidase I to lysosomes. *Hum Mol Genet.* 2004;13:2483-2491.

95. Adams H, de Blieck EA, Mink JW, et al. Standardized assessment of behavior and adaptive living skills in juvenile neuronal ceroid lipofuscinosis. *Dev Med Child Neurol.* 2006;48:259-264.

96. Marshall FJ, de Blieck EA, Mink JW, et al. A clinical rating scale for Batten disease: reliable and relevant for clinical trials. *Neurology.* 2005;65:275-279.

97. Narayan SB, Rakheja D, Tan L, et al. CLN3P, the Batten's disease protein, is a novel palmitoyl-protein delta-9 desaturase. *Ann Neurol.* 2006;60:570-577.

98. Pineda-Trujillo N, Cornejo W, Carrizosa J, et al. A CLN5 mutation causing an atypical neuronal ceroid lipofuscinosis of juvenile onset. *Neurology.* 2005;64:740-742.

99. Ranta S, Topcu M, Tegelberg S, et al. Variant late infantile neuronal ceroid lipofuscinosis in a subset of Turkish patients is allelic to Northern epilepsy. *Hum Mutat.* 2004;23:300-305.

100. Seyrantepe V, Landry K, Trudel S, et al. Neu4, a novel human lysosomal lumen sialidase, confers normal phenotype to sialidosis and galactosialidosis cells. *J Biol Chem.* 2004;279:37021-37029.

101. Seyrantepe V, Poupetova H, Froissart R, et al. Molecular pathology of NEU1 gene in sialidosis. *Hum Mutat.* 2003;22:343-352.

102. Pattison S, Pankarican M, Rupar CA, et al. Five novel mutations in the lysosomal sialidase gene (NEU1) in type II sialidosis patients and assessment of their impact on enzyme activity and intracellular targeting using adenovirus-mediated expression. *Hum Mutat.* 2004;23:32-39.

103. Rodriguez Criado G, Pshezhetsky AV, Rodriguez Becerra A, Gomez de Terreros I. Clinical variability of type II sialidosis by C808T mutation. *Am J Med Genet A.* 2003;116:368-371.

104. Martin RA, Slaugh R, Natowicz M, et al. Sialic acid storage disease of the Salla phenotype in American monozygous twin female sibs. *Am J Med Genet A.* 2003;120:23-27.

105. Yarovaya N, Schot R, Fodero L, et al. Sialin, an anion transporter defective in sialic acid storage diseases, shows highly variable expression in adult mouse brain, and is developmentally regulated. *Neurobiol Dis.* 2005;19:351-365.

106. Biancheri R, Verbeek E, Rossi A, et al. An Italian severe Salla disease variant associated with a SLC17A5 mutation earlier described in infantile sialic acid storage disease. *Clin Genet.* 2002;61:443-447.

107. Kleta R, Aughton DJ, Rivkin MJ, et al. Biochemical and molecular analyses of infantile free sialic acid storage disease in North American children. *Am J Med Genet A.* 2003;120:28-33.

108. Leroy JG, Seppala R, Huizing M, et al. Dominant inheritance of sialuria, an inborn error of feedback inhibition. *Am J Hum Genet.* 2001;68:1419-1427.

109. Eisenberg I, Avidan N, Potikha T, et al. The UDP-N-acetylglucosamine 2-epimerase/N-acetylmannosamine kinase gene is mutated in recessive hereditary inclusion body myopathy. *Nat Genet.* 2001;29:83-87.

110. Broccolini A, Pescatori M, D'Amico A, et al. An Italian family with autosomal recessive inclusion-body myopathy and mutations in the GNE gene. *Neurology.* 2002;59: 1808-1809.

111. Vasconcelos OM, Raju R, Dalakas MC. GNE mutations in an American family with quadriceps-sparing IBM and lack of mutations in s-IBM. *Neurology.* 2002;59: 1776-1779.

112. Arai A, Tanaka K, Ikeuchi T, et al. A novel mutation in the GNE gene and a linkage disequilibrium in Japanese pedigrees. *Ann Neurol.* 2002;52:516-519.

113. Freeman JM, and McKhann GM. Degenerative disease of the central nervous system. *Adv Pediatr.* 1969;16:121-175.

114. Meikle PJ, Grasby DJ, Dean CJ, et al. Newborn screening for lysosomal storage disorders. *Mol Genet Metab.* 2006;88:307-314.

115. Meikle PJ, Ranieri E, Simonsen H, et al. Newborn screening for lysosomal storage disorders: clinical evaluation of a two-tier strategy. *Pediatrics.* 2004;114:909-916.

116. Beutler E. Lysosomal storage diseases: natural history and ethical and economic aspects. *Mol Genet Metab.* 2006;88:208-215.

117. Beck M. New therapeutic options for lysosomal storage disorders: enzyme replacement, small molecules and gene therapy. *Hum Genet.* 2007;121:1-22.

118. Fox TE, Finnegan CM, Blumenthal R, Kester M. The clinical potential of sphingolipid-based therapeutics. *Cell Mol Life Sci.* 2006;63:1017-1023.

119. Desnick RJ. Enzyme replacement therapy for Fabry disease: lessons from two alpha-galactosidase A orphan products and one FDA approval. *Expert Opin Biol Ther.* 2004;4:1167-1176.

120. Eto Y, Shen JS, Meng XL, Ohashi T. Treatment of lysosomal storage disorders: cell therapy and gene therapy. *J Inherit Metab Dis.* 2004;27:411-415.

121. Wenger DA, Coppola S, Liu SL. Insights into the diagnosis and treatment of lysosomal storage diseases. *Arch Neurol.* 2003;60:322-328.

122. Grabowski GA, Hopkin RJ. Enzyme therapy for lysosomal storage disease: principles, practice, and prospects. *Annu Rev Genomics Hum Genet.* 2003;4:403-436.

123. Peters C, Steward CG. Hematopoietic cell transplantation for inherited metabolic diseases: an overview of outcomes and practice guidelines. *Bone Marrow Transplant.* 2003;31:229-239.

124. Suzuki Y. Beta-galactosidase deficiency: an approach to chaperone therapy. *J Inherit Metab Dis.* 2006;29:471-476.

125. Iwasaki H, Watanabe H, Iida M, et al. Fibroblast screening for chaperone therapy in beta-galactosidosis. *Brain Dev.* 2006;28:482-486.

126. Platt FM, Jeyakumar M, Andersson U, et al. Substrate reduction therapy in mouse models of the glycosphingolipidoses. *Philos Trans R Soc Lond B Biol Sci.* 2003;358:947-954.

127. Ellinwood NM, Vite CH, Haskins ME. Gene therapy for lysosomal storage diseases: the lessons and promise of animal models. *J Gene Med.* 2004;6:481-506.

128. Kacher Y, Futerman AH. Genetic diseases of sphingolipid metabolism: pathological mechanisms and therapeutic options. *FEBS Lett.* 2006;580:5510-5517.

129. Cox TM. Substrate reduction therapy for lysosomal storage diseases. *Acta Paediatr Suppl.* 2005;94:69-75; discussion 57.

ACKNOWLEDGMENTS

This work was supported in part by the Civitan International Research Center and National Institutes of Health grant HD38985 (Mental Retardation Research Center).

DISCLOSURES

The author has nothing to disclose beyond that noted above.

CHAPTER 25

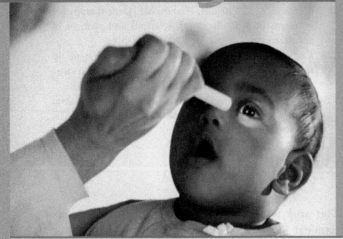

Brain Tumors

Gregory A. Murad, Michael Lynn,
Amy A. Smith, David V. Smullen,
Sharatchandra S. Bidari, Anna Co,
and David W. Pincus

DEFINITIONS AND EPIDEMIOLOGY

Pediatric brain tumors represent the second most common form of pediatric cancer and the most common solid malignancy. The most recent statistics available report findings from 2004, and they show that the incidence of pediatric brain tumors is approximately 1100 per year, representing 20% of all childhood cancers. These neoplasms also represent the second leading cause of cancer death in US children, and the sixth leading cause of death in US children overall.[1,2] Survival for children with central nervous system (CNS) neoplasms, however, has dramatically risen over the past 30 years,

with 5-year survival rates of 74%, up from 57% in 1977. Most of these results are due to a combination of improved chemotherapeutic regimens, more accurately targeted and dosed radiation, and safer, more accurate surgical resection techniques.[1,3]

The location of childhood tumors differs from those in adults. Most pediatric tumors occur in the posterior fossa, with medulloblastoma, juvenile pilocytic astrocytoma (JPA), and ependymoma making up the majority of these lesions.[1-4]

The etiology of childhood tumors is poorly understood. Although certain genetic syndromes are responsible for an increased risk of tumorigenesis (Table 25-1),

Table 25-1.

Imaging Characteristics of Pediatric Tumors in the Posterior Fossa

	Medulloblastoma	Juvenile Pilocytic Astrocytoma	Ependymoma
Location	Vermis	Cerebellar hemisphere	4th ventricle with spread through foramina of Luschka and Magendie
Noncontrast CT	Hyperdense	Hypodense	Iso- to hypodense
Enhancement	Avid homogeneous	Mural nodule—avid Homogeneous Cyst—no enhancement	Minimal to moderate More heterogeneous
Calcification	15%-20% Speckled	< 10%	40%-50% Typically punctate
Cyst formation	10%-20%	60%-80%	10%-15%
Hemorrhage	3%	< 5%	10%
T1WI	Iso- to hypointense	Hypointense	Iso- to hypointense
T2WI/FLAIR	Iso- to hyperintense	Hyperintense	Iso- to hyperintense
Gadolinium	Enhances	Mural nodule enhances avidly	Variable enhancement
DWI	Restricted diffusion	Nonrestricted diffusion	Nonrestricted diffusion

From Grossman RI and Yousem DM, Neuroradiology. 2nd ed. St. Louis, MO: Mosby; 2003:123.

the majority of tumors arise de novo. Certain environmental exposures have also been implicated in the development of tumors, including toxic chemicals, cigarette smoke, radiation, medications, home microwave ovens, cellular telephones, and electromagnetic fields. Of these, the only exposure that has a proven link to tumorigenesis is ionizing therapeutic radiation.[5]

Brain tumors arise from multiple different cell lineages, and thus are a heterogeneous population of tumors. In this review, we will examine the following lesions: low-grade glioma, high-grade glioma, medulloblastoma, ependymoma, juvenile pilocytic astrocytoma, brainstem glioma, craniopharyngioma, and pineal region tumors (usually germ cell).

Pediatric brain tumors appear to arise from a different set of circumstances than do similar adult lesions. Craniopharyngiomas represent remains of embryonic cells that slowly differentiate over time, leading to growth of large lesions. Medulloblastomas are primitive neuroectodermal tumors (PNETs) that arise from similar but more aggressive embryonic rests. High- and low-grade gliomas are derived from newly differentiated glial cells that undergo multiple different genetic mutations, leading to malignant transformation.[6]

CLINICAL PRESENTATION

Presentation of pediatric brain tumors can differ depending on location and vary from subtle changes to fulminant coma with the need for emergent neurosurgical treatment (Table 25-2). The most common symptom of mass lesions is headache. This can be difficult to localize, and headache in the absence of other neurological signs is not an indication for neuroimaging. Other signs and symptoms include seizures, nausea/vomiting, ataxia/dysmetria, visual disturbances, macrocephaly/hydrocephalus, weakness (focal deficit), altered level of consciousness, and endocrine disturbances (including weight loss/gain, precocious

puberty, amenorrhea, hypothyroidism, and diabetes insipidus).[7]

DIAGNOSIS

History and Physical Examinations

Diagnosis of pediatric brain tumors starts with a detailed clinical history and physical examinations. A combination of findings from the list of symptoms described in the earlier section will often lead to an imaging study.[7] In the vast majority of cases, neuroimaging will lead to discovery and, often, diagnosis of a lesion. For emergency situations, computed tomography (CT) scanning is the study of choice. CT scanning, however, has low soft-tissue resolution, which can limit its ability to identify intrinsic brain lesions. CT also has the disadvantage of using ionizing radiation. Thus, if there is appropriate clinical suspicion, magnetic resonance imaging (MRI) is indicated. MRI allows for multiplanar imaging and much more sensitive and subtle differentiation of normal and abnormal tissues. MRI is especially suited for posterior fossa imaging, where beam hardening artifact from CT often makes accurate diagnosis of a lesion difficult or impossible. Enhanced MRI with the administration of gadolinium increases sensitivity and reveals areas of breakdown of the blood-brain barrier. This accurately depicts the tumor nidus, although this does not necessarily imply tumor grade.[8]

Postoperatively, enhanced MRI is the gold standard for evaluation of residual tumor. Other more specialized imaging techniques, including MR-spectroscopy and positron-emission tomography (PET) scanning, may give additional information regarding brain lesions. These technologies, however, are currently reserved for monitoring tumor response to therapy and differentiating tumor regrowth versus treatment effects such as radiation necrosis.[9] The specific imaging characteristics of

Table 25-2.

Imaging Characteristics of Pediatric Tumors in the Pineal Region

	Germinoma	Teratoma	Pineoblastoma/Pineocytoma	Astrocytoma
Noncontrast CT	Slightly hyperdense	Variable density	Hyperdense	Slightly hypodense
Enhancement	Avid homogeneous	Irregular heterogeneous	Moderate homogeneous	Variable Less homogeneous
Calcification	Within pineal gland	Common; intratumoral	Uncommon; intratumoral	Rare; intratumoral
T1WI	Isointense	Variable	Hypo- to isointense	Hypointense
T2WI	Iso- to hypointense	Variable	Hyperintense	Hyperintense
Gadolinium	Avid enhancement	Mild enhancement	Moderate enhancement	Variable enhancement
DWI	Nonrestricted diffusion	Nonrestricted diffusion	Nonrestricted diffusion	Nonrestricted diffusion

From Grossman RI and Yousem DM, Neuroradiology. 2nd ed. St. Louis, MO: Mosby; 2003:158.

different types of tumors will be discussed with each separate lesion.

TUMOR TYPES

Medulloblastoma

Medulloblastoma is a highly aggressive form of childhood brain tumor and is the most common malignant central nervous system tumor in children. The term "medulloblastoma" is actually a misnomer, derived from the idea that these tumors arose from multipotential cells known as medulloblasts. These tumors have since been reclassified as PNETs and thus can be referred to interchangeably as PNET-MB, medulloblastoma, or infratentorial PNET. MB represents about 20% of all pediatric brain tumors and 30% of posterior fossa tumors. There is a 2 to 1 male predominance. These tumors present with a classic posterior fossa syndrome, including headache that is worse in the morning, nausea, vomiting, and a fairly rapid decline over 1 to 2 months. Occasionally presentation can be related to spinal pathology from drop metastases, including back pain, leg pain, or paraparesis. Physical examination findings include papilledema, sixth-nerve palsies, lethargy, or ataxia. The diagnostic evaluation of these lesions begins with imaging. CT can be used for emergent symptoms, but contrasted MRI is the study of choice. CT shows hyperdensity in the area of the vermis, often with speckled calcifications, ± cyst formation (Figure 25-1). MRI will show T_1 iso- to

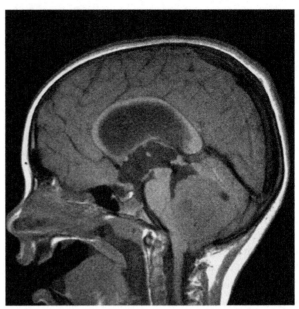

FIGURE 25-2 ■ T_1 sagittal image in a 6-year-old boy with medulloblastoma shows a large isointense fourth ventricle-based mass causing obstructive hydrocephalus.

hypodensity and T_2 hyperintensity, as well as avid enhancement with contrast (Figures 25-2 to 25-4). Diffusion-weighted imaging can also help differentiate these tumors from others, as it will often reveal restricted diffusion as a consequence of the lesions' hypercellularity (Figures 25-5 and 25-6). Due to the propensity of these

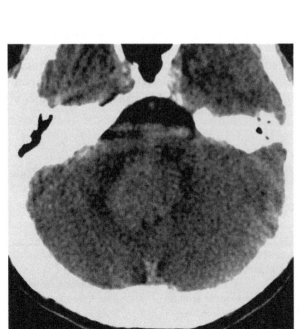

FIGURE 25-1 ■ Noncontrast axial CT image of a medulloblastoma shows that the mass is slightly more dense that the adjacent cerebellum due to the high nuclear to cytoplasmic ratio of the tumor cells.

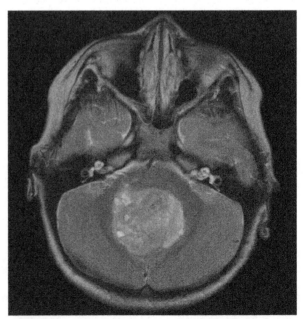

FIGURE 25-3 ■ T_2 axial image shows the mass is heterogeneously hyperintense. The mass completely occupies and expands the fourth ventricle with mass effect on the pons, middle cerebellar peduncles, and cerebellum.

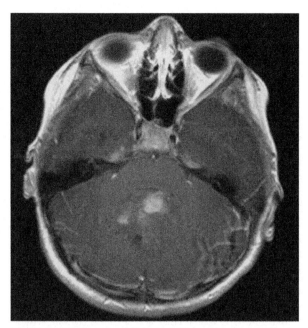

FIGURE 25-4 ■ T$_1$ postgadolinium axial image shows areas of nodular enhancement with the mass.

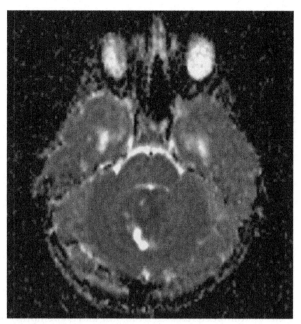

FIGURE 25-6 ■ ADC map shows that the corresponding regions of mass have darkening confirming the water restriction. Restriction on DWI is thought to be due to high nuclear to cytoplasmic ratio seen in medulloblastoma and other PNET.

tumors to spread through the neural axis, MR imaging of the entire neuraxis to assess for drop metastases is also indicated (Figure 25-7).[10,11]

Initial treatment is aimed at stabilizing the patient, often with the administration of steroids. Occasionally, emergent cerebrospinal fluid diversion such as external ventricular drain placement or endoscopic third ventriculostomy is performed. This should be followed by surgical

evaluation. Tumor resection is the treatment of choice and allows for relief of mass effect, cerebrospinal fluid (CSF) diversion/drainage, and tissue diagnosis. Due to the location of these tumors and their adherence to critical brain

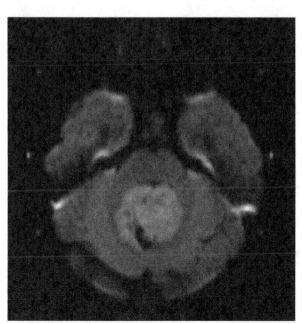

FIGURE 25-5 ■ Diffusion-weighted image shows water restriction with the mass.

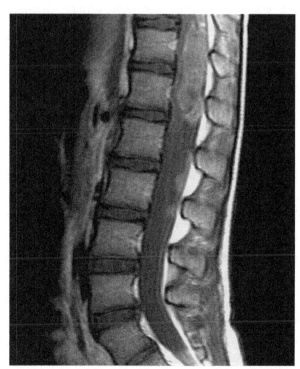

FIGURE 25-7 ■ Postgadolinium T$_1$ sagittal image of lumbar spine shows drop metastasis of medulloblastoma as enhancing mass in the conus region and two enhancing nodules along the dorsal margin of thecal sac.

structures, morbidity is fairly high, on the order of 25% to 40%. Complications include cranial nerve deficits, swallowing/breathing difficulties, cerebellar mutism, gaze abnormalities, hydrocephalus, and infection.[12]

After surgical resection, the next step in treatment is adjuvant, in the form of chemotherapy and radiation. For children older than 3 years, radiation to the tumor bed and the craniospinal axis, followed by chemotherapy alone, is the current standard.[13,14] For those considered to be high risk (age less than 3 years, >1.5 mL of residual tumor, tumor dissemination) are offered chemotherapy alone if younger than 3 years, and either concurrent chemotherapy/irradiation followed by chemotherapy, or induction chemotherapy with stem cell rescue if the patient is older than 3 years. Five-year survival for low-risk tumors is as high as 80%, and recent data for recurrent and progressive disease indicates 5-year survival of almost 70% with a stem cell rescue strategy.[15] Overall, however, continued research is ongoing and is attempting to focus not only on survival, but also on the morbidity, especially neurocognitive, of these treatments.

Ependymoma

Ependymomas represent about 10% of pediatric brain tumors and 15% of posterior fossa tumors.[2,16] They are the third most common pediatric brain tumor behind medulloblastoma and cerebellar astrocytoma. These tumors arise from ependymal cells that line the ventricular system. The presentation of posterior fossa ependymoma is similar to that of medulloblastoma, although rarely as rapid. Signs and symptoms of hydrocephalus, compression of the brainstem, and cranial neuropathies are the most common. Classically, it is not uncommon for these patients to have gastrointestinal (GI) problems including nausea, vomiting, and poor appetite that have gone on for a prolonged period, resulting in a prolonged gastrointestinal workup prior to eventual neuroimaging that reveals a brain tumor.[16-20] The best diagnostic study is contrasted MRI. These tumors will be iso- to hypointense on T_1 and T_2 and show heterogeneous enhancement (Figures 25-8 to 25-10). The tumor can often be seen arising from the floor of the fourth ventricle and also exiting through the foramina of the fourth ventricle, including Luschka and Magendie (Figures 25-10 and 25-11). The extrusion of ependymomas out of the fourth ventricle is often referred to as plastic ependymoma. Imaging of the entire spinal axis is also indicated due to the rare (<10 %) occurrence of drop metastases. This imaging preoperatively is also important to distinguishing between new tumor spread and expected postoperative changes.[8,9]

Surgical treatment of these tumors is the first option. This allows for pathologic diagnosis, tumor gross total resection if possible, and reestablishment of CSF flow channels. Following diagnosis, the current

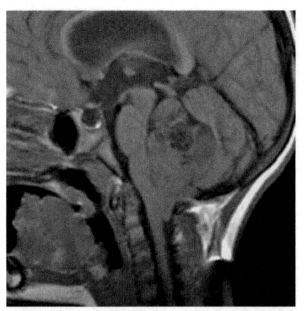

FIGURE 25-8 ■ T_1 sagittal image in a 5-year-old boy with ependymoma shows a large fourth ventricle-based mass that has predominantly isointense signal, but with some areas of hypointensity that correspond to cystic portion of the tumor. Note the tumor extension into cisterna magna and inferiorly into the spinal canal dorsal to the cord.

mainstay of adjuvant therapy is conformal local radiation therapy. This currently includes conformal radiotherapy to the tumor bed in a variety of fractions and total doses ranging from 54 to 59.4 Gy.[21-24] Chemotherapy also has a role in this disease, and multiple different

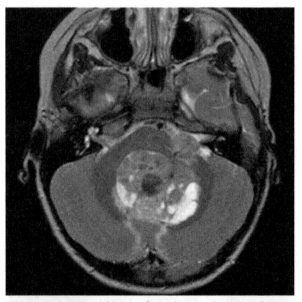

FIGURE 25-9 ■ T_2 axial image of ependymoma shows that the mass is heterogeneously hyperintense with few cystic areas causing mass effect on brainstem, middle cerebellar peduncles, and cerebellum. The T_2 dark areas in the center of mass are hemorrhagic foci. See the tumor extension into left CP angle cistern through foramen of Lushka (plastic ependymoma).

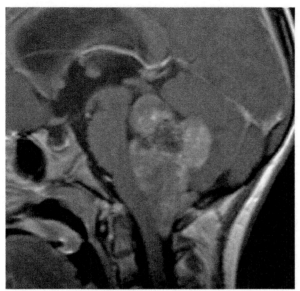

FIGURE 25-10 ■ Postgadolinium T$_1$ sagittal image shows enhancement of the mass, expect the central hemorrhagic area. The dorsal extension into cisterna magna is much better seen on postcontrast study.

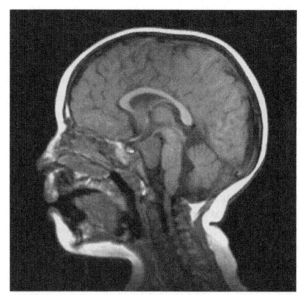

FIGURE 25-12 ■ T$_1$ sagittal image of a large hypothalamic JPA that extended into the prepontine cistern.

regimens have been used, with cisplatin appearing to be the most effective agent, with approximately a 40% response rate.[25-28] Overall, 5-year survival for patients with ependymoma is approximately 55% in historical studies, with some improvement recently to as high as 70% with gross total resection followed by adjuvant local involved field radiation.

Juvenile Pilocytic Astrocytoma

Juvenile pilocytic astrocytoma (JPA) is another of the most common pediatric brain tumors and is most often located in the posterior fossa. It is the second most common posterior fossa tumor, representing approximately 20% to 35% of these lesions.[1,2] These tumors can also be found in the hypothalamus (Figure 25-12), optic nerves (Figure 25-13), thalamus, and the cerebral hemispheres.

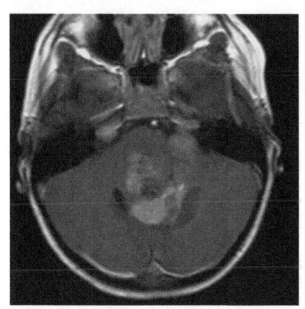

FIGURE 25-11 ■ Post-gadolinium T$_1$ axial image shows enhancement of the mass except the central hemorrhagic and cystic areas. The enhancing mass within the left CP angle cistern confirms the tumor extension through the foramen of Lushka.

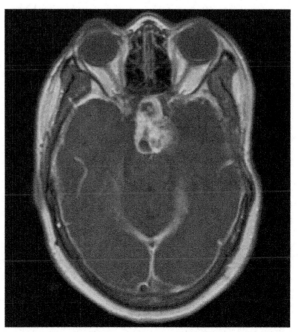

FIGURE 25-13 ■ Postgadolinium T$_1$ axial image of enhancing chaismatic JPA.

Pilocytic tumors are also associated with neurofibromatosis type I, and the optic nerve and hypothalamic lesions are more common in this setting. Pathologically, the classic finding with JPA is fibrillar astrocytes against a microcystic background and the presence of eosinophilic intracytoplasmic inclusions called Rosenthal fibers. Signs and symptoms of these tumors are similar to other posterior fossa lesions, including headaches, ataxia, and hydrocephalus. Optic nerve lesions can lead to visual loss.[29] The diagnostic workup for these tumors is contrasted MRI. Often, these tumors have a cystic appearance with an enhancing mural nodule. Solid lesions can also have varying degrees of contrast enhancement. In spite of this enhancement, however, these tumors are often benign in their course.[8] Surgical removal, when possible, is the treatment of choice.[29-31] For WHO grade I tumors, survival exceeds 90% at 10 years with gross total resection. Adjuvant therapy for JPA is usually reserved for subtotally resected lesions that show signs of continued growth or for recurrent lesions after gross total resection. Radiotherapy has not been shown to affect overall survival in the nonrecurrent setting, although it has shown some efficacy in preventing disease progression.[32] Chemotherapy has also not been greatly effective for these lesions in the posterior fossa, although multiple trial regimens are available.[29]

Craniopharyngioma

Craniopharyngiomas represent 3% to 5% of pediatric brain tumors. These tumors also occur in a bimodal distribution and are also represented in the sixth decade of life (Table 25-3). The greatest incidence in children is in the ages of 6 to 10 years.[2] These tumors are benign histologically, but can cause severe morbidity due to their location. The two histologic subtypes are adamantinomatous

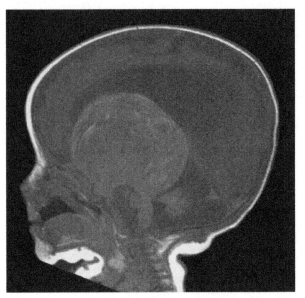

FIGURE 25-14 ■ T$_1$ sagittal image in new born baby with craniopharyngioma shows a large mass in the sella and suprasellar region that is extending superiorly and completely compressing the third ventricle.

and squamous papillary. The adamantinomatous variety is that which occurs in childhood. These tumors arise from embryologic remnants of Rathke pouch, located in the region stretching from the sella turcica through the pituitary and hypothalamus up to the third ventricle (Figures 25-14 and 25-15). They often contain epithelial

Table 25-3.

Imaging Characteristics of Craniopharyngioma

	Craniopharyngioma
Location	Typically suprasellar ± sellar extension
Noncontrast CT	Predominantly hypodense cystic mass with slightly hyperdense solid component
Enhancement	Nodular heterogeneous
Calcification	80%-90%; commonly peripheral and nodular
Cyst formation	85%
T1WI	Variable; often hyperintense
T2WI	Solid component—iso- to hypointense
	Cystic areas—hyperintense
Gadolinium	Solid component enhances avidly
DWI	May have restricted diffusion

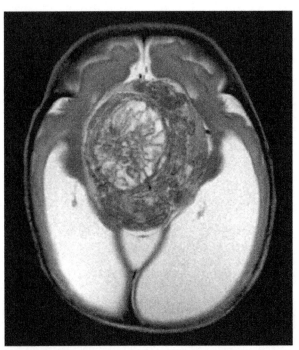

FIGURE 25-15 ■ T$_2$ axial image of a large craniopharyngioma shows heterogeneous high signal within the mass. Obstruction of third ventricle causes marked hydrocephalus.

remnants, and have large amounts of epithelial cells and keratin, and have associated oily cysts that can calcify. Craniopharyngiomas present with headaches in 60% to 75% of cases. Other symptoms include visual loss, hormonal changes including delayed sexual maturation, weight gain, diabetes insipidus, or growth failure; and for larger lesions, problems with cognition or seizures. Radiologically, craniopharyngiomas appear as cystic lesions arising from the sella with variable amounts of calcification. CT scanning can also show erosion or remodeling of the skull base and sella. MR imaging will also show a cystic lesion with the solid portions being hypointense on T_1 and avidly enhancing with contrast (Figures 25-16 and 25-17). Cyst fluid will usually be hyperintense on T_2 and have variable intensity on T_1 due to the heterogeneity of the cyst contents. Sagittal MRI can also be used to distinguish these lesions from pituitary adenoma by visualizing the normal pituitary gland (Fig. 25-18).[33,34] Treatment of craniopharyngioma has evolved over the years due to the nature of these tumors. As stated previously, the benign nature and location make the gross total resection of these tumors possible. However, the proximity and involvement of the hypothalamus may make gross total resection a highly morbid procedure in many instances. Complete resection of tumors with significant hypothalamic and third ventricular extension may result in severe disturbance of thirst and hunger inhibition as well as cognitive impairment. Virtually all patients have panhypopituitarism following aggressive resection. Complete resection, however, does result in 10-year

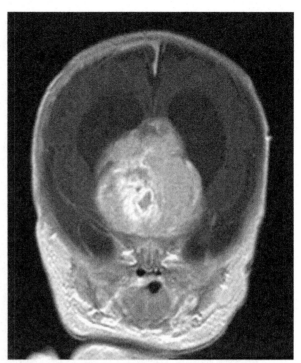

FIGURE 25-17 ■ Postgadolinium T_1 coronal image shows avid enhancement of the craniopharyngioma. Note the complete obstruction of third ventricle.

progression-free survival rates around 80%. Thus, this area remains an area of considerable dispute among pediatric neurosurgeons. Surgery remains necessary to remove mass effect, treat hydrocephalus, establish a diagnosis, and decompress the optic apparatus. Alternative treatment strategies have moved toward a less aggressive surgical technique, sparing the hypothalamus and using adjuvant therapies such as intracystic or external beam radiotherapy. Morbidity of treatment is still significant, but overall survival for craniopharyngioma is 70% to 100% at 5 years, and 60% to 90% at 10 years.[35-40]

Supratentorial Low-Grade Glioma

Supretentorial low-grade glioma (SLGG) is a heterogeneous group of glial tumors that can include astrocytoma, oligdendroglioma, dysembryoplastic neuroepithelial tumors (DNT), ganglioglioma, and pleomorphic xanthoastrocytoma (PXA). These tumors are located anywhere in the supratentorial space and represent about 10% to 15% of pediatric tumors (Figures 25-19 to 25-30).[1] Focal neurological findings can be seen, depending on tumor location, but headaches and seizure are the most common presenting complaints.[41] The lesion types also appear different on imaging. Plain head CT is often nondiagnostic, so contrasted MRI is

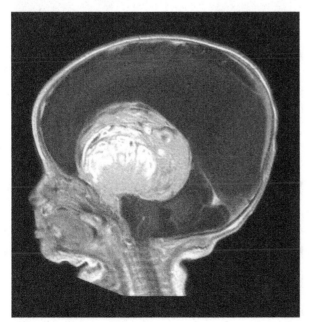

FIGURE 25-16 ■ Postgadolinium T_1 sagittal image shows avid enhancement of the craniopharyngioma.

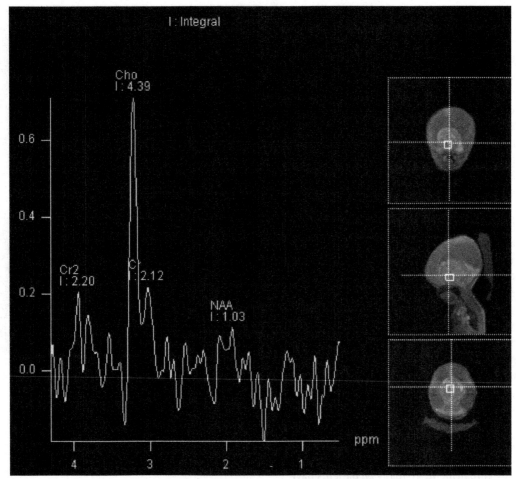

FIGURE 25-18 ■ MRS of the craniopharyngioma shows loss of NAA peak with markedly elevated choline peak.

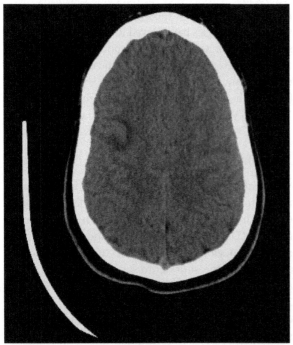

FIGURE 25-19 ■ Noncontrast CT in 17-year-old male with seizures shows a low-density lesion in the right high frontal convexity.

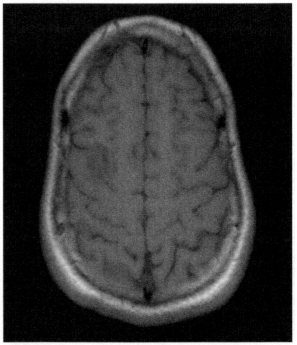

FIGURE 25-20 ■ T₁ axial image shows that this lesion is slightly hypointense to the gray and white matter.

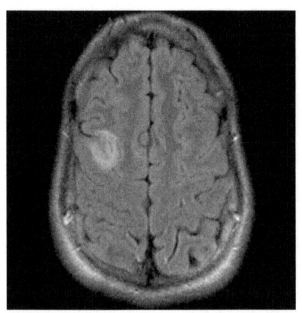

FIGURE 25-21 ■ FLAIR axial image shows that the lesion is hyperintense to gray and white matter.

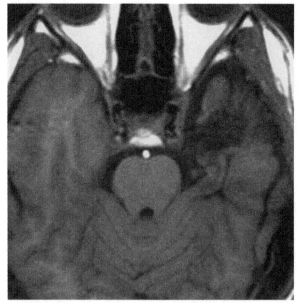

FIGURE 25-23 ■ T$_1$ axial image of a pathologically proven ganglioglioma in the left medial temporal lobe with associated cortical dysplasia.

again the primary diagnostic modality. This will show a variety of findings, including hypo- to isointensity on T$_1$, very minimal contrast enhancement, and iso- to hyperintensity on T$_2$. FLAIR imaging is often better able to differentiate between normal and pathologic brain. Ganglioglioma, DNT, and PXA can also be associated with cyst formation.[8] Treatment for these tumors

is variable. Initially, if symptoms are nonspecific, they can be followed with neuroimaging. Surgery offers the option for tissue sampling, removal of mass effect, therapeutic treatment of seizures, and in many cases, cure. For astrocytoma and oligodendrogliomas in accessible locations, gross total resection offers increased progression-free survival.[41,42]

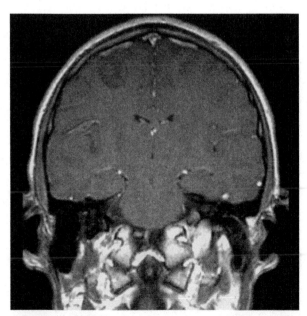

FIGURE 25-22 ■ Postgadolinium T$_1$ coronal image shows no enhancement of the lesion. Pathologically proven dysembryoplastic neuroepithelial tumor (DNT).

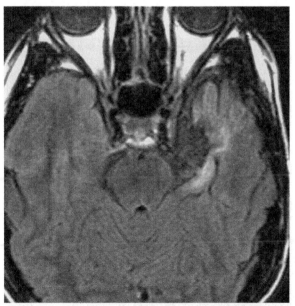

FIGURE 25-24 ■ FLAIR axial image of a pathologically proven ganglioglioma in the left medial temporal lobe with associated cortical dysplasia.

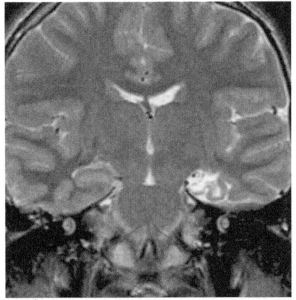

FIGURE 25-25 ■ T$_2$ coronal image of a pathologically proven ganglioglioma in the left medial temporal lobe with associated cortical dysplasia.

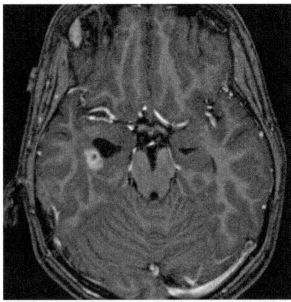

FIGURE 25-27 ■ Postgadolinium T$_1$ axial image shows an enhancing nodule adjacent to right temporal horn obstructing it—PXA.

Adjuvant treatment of SLGG is variable, depending on the pathology and extent of surgical resection. For tumors that are nonresectable, especially in the hypothalamus or optic nerves/pathways, chemotherapy and radiotherapy, either separately or in combination, allow for slowed time to progression and 5- and 10-year survival rates in the range of 60% to 80% and 55% to 70%, respectively.[43-45] Ganglioma and DNT typically present with seizures and are commonly cured with complete excision.

Supratentorial High-Grade Glioma

Supratentorial high-grade glioma (SHGG) tumors are similar histologically to those found in adult patients and are represented by anaplastic astrocytoma, anaplastic oligodendroglioma, and glioblastoma multiforme. SHGG are relatively rare in the pediatric population, representing about 20% of all supratentorial gliomas and 5% to 10% of all pediatric tumors.[2-5,46] Their

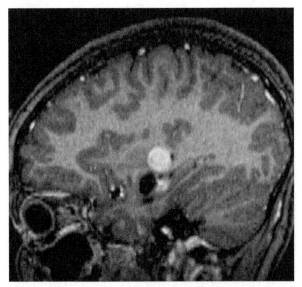

FIGURE 25-26 ■ Postgadolinium T$_1$ sagittal image shows an enhancing nodule adjacent to temporal horn—PXA.

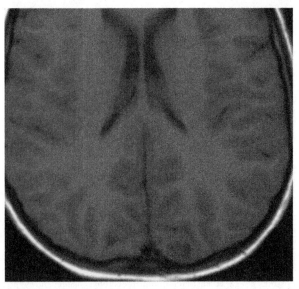

FIGURE 25-28 ■ T$_1$ axial image shows a isointense lesion in the left occipital cortex—PXA.

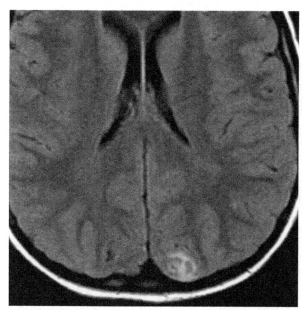

FIGURE 25-29 ■ FLAIR axial image shows a hyperintense lesion in the left occipital cortex—PXA.

presentation varies, but includes similar symptoms such as headache, seizure, or focal neurological deficit, depending on tumor location. On imaging, these tumors are more likely to show surrounding edema, central necrosis, and ring enhancement on T_1 MR with contrast. Treatment begins with diagnosis via tissue sampling. For lesions that are easily accessible, gross total resection has been shown to improve outcome and

overall survival.[46-51] However, for more deep-seated lesions and those in eloquent cortex, resection may not be feasible. For these lesions, as well as postoperatively, chemotherapy and radiation are indicated to slow progression of the disease. Multiple different chemotherapeutic and radiation delivery methods have been used and newer methods of targeted chemotherapy for specific genetic markers are in development. Survival rates for these more aggressive lesions, however, remain low, with 5-year survivals from 6% to 40%.[49-53]

Brainstem Glioma

Brainstem gliomas represent about 10% of pediatric brain tumors. These tumors can be divided into diffuse intrinsic tumors (also known as diffuse pontine tumors) representing 75% to 80% of brainstem tumors and the remaining heterogeneous group of lesions, which include tectal lesions, cystic tumors, and exophytic cervicomedullary tumors (Figure 25-31 to 25-37).[3,54] Brainstem gliomas present with symptoms of cranial neuropathies, long-tract signs such as spasticity and ataxia, and occasionally with headache or hydrocephalus.[54] These symptoms are usually rapid in onset for diffuse tumors. Diagnosis of these tumors is usually by imaging only, as radical resection of diffuse brainstem tumors is not an option, and biopsy is often not indicated, unless imaging is not classic or there has been a prolonged clinical course with some question as to the nature of the lesion.[55,56] MR imaging will show diffuse pontine enlargement with T_1 hypointensity, T_2 hyperintentsity,

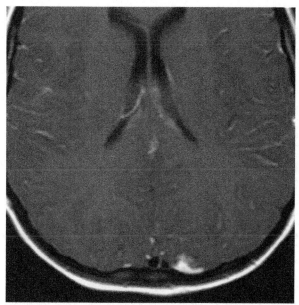

FIGURE 25-30 ■ Postgadolinium T_1 axial image shows avid enhancement in the left occipital cortex—PXA.

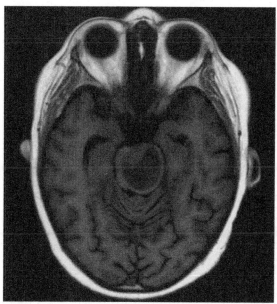

FIGURE 25-31 ■ T_1 axial image of a low-grade pontine glioma in an 8-year-old boy shows that the mass is of low intensity.

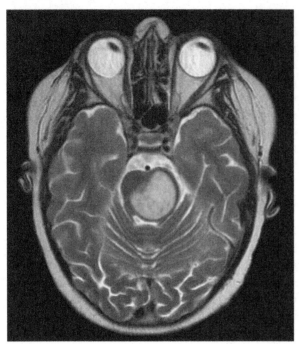

FIGURE 25-32 ■ T$_2$ axial image of a low-grade pontine glioma in an 8-year-old boy shows high signal.

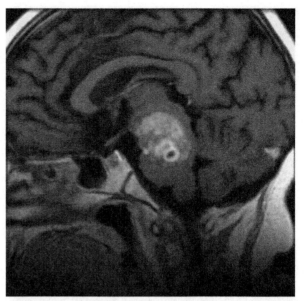

FIGURE 25-34 ■ Postgadolinium T$_1$ axial image of a low-grade pontine glioma in an 8-year-old boy shows heterogeneous enhancement, atypical for low-grade tumors.

and little contrast enhancement. Treatment for diffuse tumors is usually supportive or with radiation therapy. Chemotherapy trials have had little success.[57] The subset of tumors that are not diffuse can have some benefit from surgical resection, although morbidity rates for these types of procedures remain high.[58] Overall, survival for diffuse lesions is poor, with less than 25%

at 2 years. The remaining lesions have different survival rates depending on extent of resection and tumor histology.[54,55,59,60]

Pineal Region Tumors

The pineal region is home to multiple different types of tumors, including germ cell tumors (germinoma,

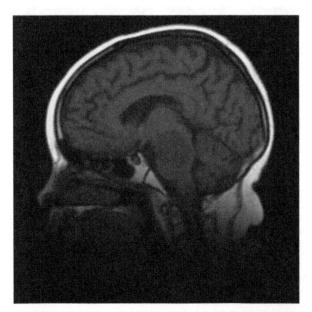

FIGURE 25-33 ■ T$_1$ sagittal image of a low-grade pontine glioma in an 8–year-old boy shows the craniocaudal extent of the mass.

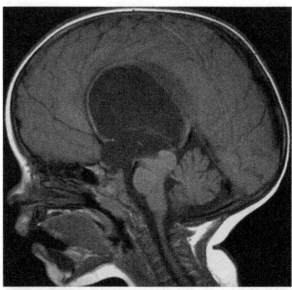

FIGURE 25-35 ■ T$_1$ sagittal image of a tectal glioma in a 2-year-old girl. Tectal mass is seen to cause aqueduct stenosis and obstructive hydrocephalus.

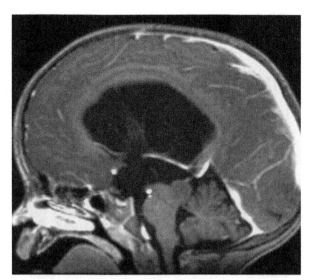

FIGURE 25-36 ■ Postgadolinium T₁ sagittal image of a tectal glioma in a 2-year-old girl. Tectal mass is seen to cause aqueduct stenosis and obstructive hydrocephalus. The mass shows no enhancement.

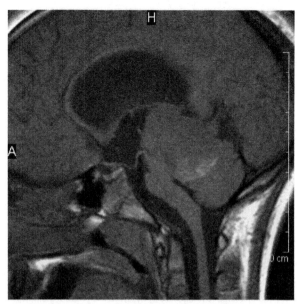

FIGURE 25-38 ■ T₁ sagittal image in an 8-year-old boy with pineal PNET shows a large predominantly isointense pineal region mass.

embryonal cell carcinoma, endodermal sinus tumors, choriocarcinoma, teratoma), astrocytomas, pineoblastoma, and pineocytomas (Figures 25-38 to 25-45). They make up 5% to 8% of pediatric brain tumors. The majority of germ cell tumors are germinomas (~70%).[61]

Pineal tumors present with signs of mass effect, including hydrocephalus, headaches, and nausea and vomiting. A classic finding is that of Parinaud syndrome, which is upgaze palsy, light-near dissociation on pupillary examination, convergence retraction nystagmus, and eyelid retraction. This is all due to compression of the superior colliculus and tectal plate.[7] Germinomas may be associated with endocrinopathies, specifically

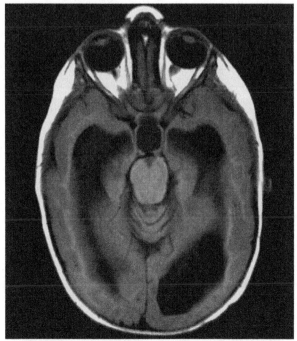

FIGURE 25-37 ■ T₁ axial image of a tectal glioma in a 2-year-old girl. Mass is isointense in signal. Dilated ventricles due to aqueduct obstruction.

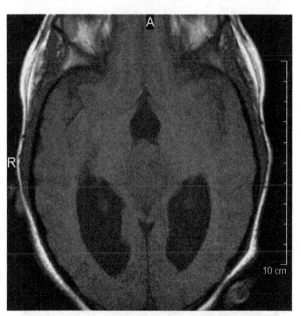

FIGURE 25-39 ■ T₁ axial image in an 8-year-old boy with pineal PNET shows a large isointense pineal region mass that completely occupies the superior cerebellar cistern.

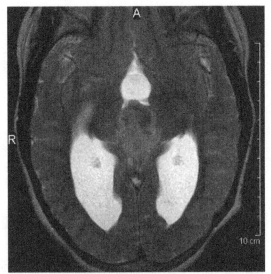

FIGURE 25-40 ■ T₂ axial image in an 8-year-old boy with pineal PNET shows a large heterogeneously hyperintense pineal region mass.

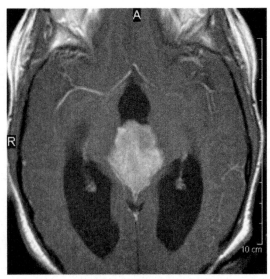

FIGURE 25-42 ■ Postgadolinium T₁ axial image in an 8-year-old boy with pineal PNET shows a large isointense pineal region mass that completely occupies the superior cerebellar cistern.

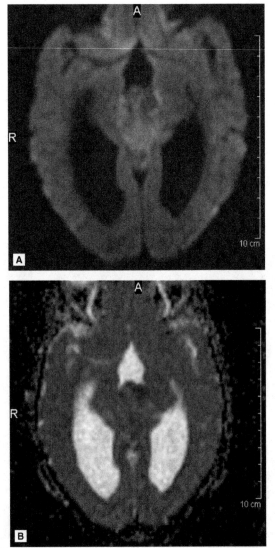

FIGURE 25-41 A AND B ■ Diffusion-weighted images and ADC maps show fluid restriction, again due to the high nuclear to cytoplasmic ratio seen in PNET's.

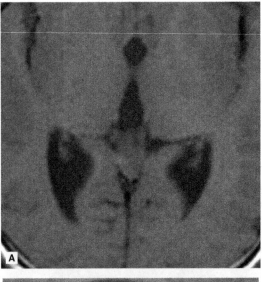

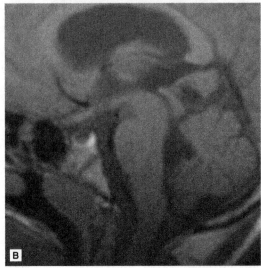

FIGURE 25-43 A AND B ■ T₁ axial and sagittal images show an isointense pineal mass with a small cyst—pineoblastoma.

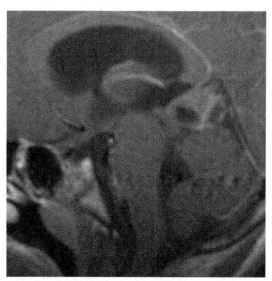

FIGURE 25-44 ■ Postgadolinium T₁ sagittal image shows enhancement of the pineal mass—pineoblastoma.

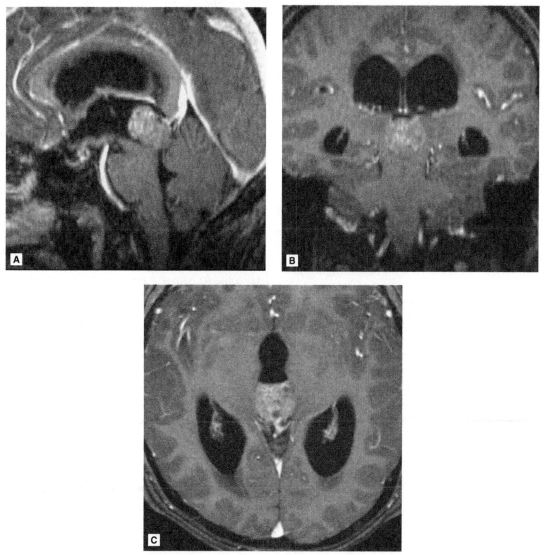

FIGURE 25-45, A, B, AND C ■ Postgadolinium T₁ sagittal, coronal, and axial images show an enhancing pineal mass that causes significant mass effect on the tectal plate causing obstruction to CSF flow at the cerebral aqueduct. This represents a case of pineal germinoma presenting clinically with headaches and Parinaud syndrome.

diabetes insipidus primary or metastatic lesions occur in the pituitary stalk. The diagnostic workup for these lesions begins with neuroimaging. Any tumor found in the pineal region should initiate MRI with and without contrast of the entire craniospinal axis. MRI characteristics of germinoma are usually hypointense on T_1 with iso- to hyperintensity on T_2 and avid contrast enhancement. Non-germinomatous lesions are more likely to be irregular in shape and enhancement, and may have evidence of calcification or cyst formation.[8] Blood and cerebrospinal fluid sampling for tumor markers (alpha-fetoprotein, beta-hCG, and placental alkaline phosphatase [PLAP]) are also helpful in the diagnosis of germ cell tumors. At this time, biopsy of the lesion, either endoscopically or stereotactically, can be carried out. Once a diagnosis is made, the mainstay of treatment for germinoma is chemotherapy and radiotherapy.[61-64] A variety of chemotherapeutic and radiotherapeutic options are available for non-germinomatous tumors, and for non–germ-cell tumors. Surgical resection is usually reserved for those tumors that recur or are nonresponsive to medical treatment.[65] Other treatment strategies designed to limit the total dose of radiation with the use of adjuvant chemotherapeutic regimens have been examined, with the goal to limit treatment-related morbidity.[66,67] Overall survival for germinomas is greater than 90% at 5 years. The other tumors in this location, however, are much more difficult to control, with average survival lesser than 50% overall.

In conclusion, tumors of the pediatric CNS are relatively common, although each particular subtype is rare. The most common presenting signs and symptoms of these lesions are headache, seizure, or focal neurological deficit. Increasing head circumference or failure to meet developmental milestones are also important indications of CNS pathology. Prompt referral for neuroimaging, in most cases MRI scanning, and referral to a neurosurgeon are of paramount importance. With aggressive treatment, the majority of children with CNS neoplasms can survive into adulthood. Rates of treatment-related morbidity and long-term cognitive and developmental side effects, however, remain high. Newer therapies, imaging modalities, surgical techniques, radiation and chemotherapy, as well as molecular and genetic diagnostic methods, will likely only improve not only survival but quality of life for future patients.[3,4,6,46,68]

REFERENCES

1. Jemal A, Siegel R, Ward E, et al. Cancer statistics 2007. *CA Cancer J Clin.* 2007;57:43.
2. Rickert CH, Paulus W. Epidemiology of central nervous system tumors in childhood and adolescence based on the new WHO classification. *Childs Nerv Syst.* 2001;17:503.
3. Packer RJ. Progress and challenges in childhood brain tumors. *J Neurooncol.* 2005;75:239.
4. Robertson PL. Advances in treatment of pediatric brain tumors. *NeuroRx.* 2006;3:276.
5. Bestak M. Epidemiology of brain tumors. In: Keating RF, Goodrich JT, Packer RJ, eds. *Tumors of the Pediatric Central Nervous System.* New York: Thieme; 2001:14-22.
6. Tamber MS, Bansal K, Liang M, et al. Current concepts in the molecular genetics of pediatric brain tumors: implications for emerging therapies. *Childs Nerv Syst.* 2006; 22:1379.
7. Duchatelier S, Wolf SM. Diagnostic principles. In: Keating RF, Goodrich JT, Packer RJ, eds. *Tumors of the Pediatric Central Nervous System.* New York: Thieme; 2001:22-27.
8. Vezina G, Booth TN. Neuroradiology. In: Keating RF, Goodrich JT, Packer RJ, eds. *Tumors of the Pediatric Central Nervous System.* New York: Thieme; 2001:27-44.
9. Vezina LG. Neuroradiology of childhood brain tumors: new challenges. *J Neurooncol.* 2005;75:243.
10. Packer RJ, Cogen P, Vezina G, et al. Medulloblastoma: clinical and biologic aspects. *Neurooncol.* 1999;1:232.
11. Packer RJ. Medulloblastoma. *J Neurosurg.* 2005;103(suppl): 299.
12. Robertson PL, Muraszko KM, Holmes EJ, et al. Incidence and severity of postoperative cerebellar mutism syndrome in children with medulloblastoma: a prospective study by the Children's Oncology Group. *J Neurosurg.* 2006;105(suppl): 444.
13. Packer RJ, Goldwein J, Nicholson HS, et al. Treatment of children with medulloblastomas with reduced-dose craniospinal radiation therapy and adjuvant chemotherapy: a Children's Cancer Group Study. *J Clin Oncol.* 1999; 17:2127.
14. Packer RJ. Standard-risk medulloblastoma treated by adjuvant chemotherapy followed by reduced-dose craniospinal radiation therapy. *Curr Neurol Neurosci Rep.* 2007;7:129.
15. Packer RJ. Risk-adapted craniospinal radiotherapy followed by high-dose chemotherapy and stem-cell rescue in children with newly diagnosed medulloblastoma. *Curr Neurol Neurosci Rep.* 2007;7:130.
16. Allen JC, Siffert J, Hukin J. Clinical manifestations of childhood ependymoma: a multitude of syndromes. *Pediatr Neurosurg.* 1998;28:49.
17. Foreman NK, Love S, Thorne R. Intracranial ependymomas: analysis of prognostic factors in a population-based series. *Pediatr Neurosurg.* 1996;24:119.
18. Perilongo G, Massimino M, Sotti G, et al. Analyses of prognostic factors in a retrospective review of 92 children with ependymoma: Italian Pediatric Neuro-Oncology Group. *Med Pediatr Oncol.* 1997;29:79.
19. Pollack IF, Gerszten PC, Martinez AJ, et al. Intracranial ependymomas of childhood: long-term outcome and prognostic factors. *Neurosurgery.* 1995;37:655.
20. Horn B, Heideman R, Geyer R, et al. A multi-institutional retrospective study of intracranial ependymoma in children: identification of risk factors. *J Pediatr Hematol Oncol.* 1999;21:203.
21. Robertson PL, Zeltzer PM, Boyett JM, et al. Survival and prognostic factors following radiation therapy and chemotherapy for ependymomas in children: a report of the Children's Cancer Group. *J Neurosurg.* 1998;88:695.

22. Jaing TH, Wang HS, Tsay PK, et al. Multivariate analysis of clinical prognostic factors in children with intracranial ependymomas. *J Neurooncol.* 2004;68:255.

23. Rousseau P, Habrand J, Sarrazin D, et al. Treatment of intracranial ependymomas of children: review of a 15-year experience. *Int J Radiat Biol Phys.* 1994;28:381.

24. Merchant TM, Mulhern RK, Krasin MJ, et al. Preliminary results from a phase II trial of conformal radiation therapy and evaluation of radiation-related CNS effects for pediatric patients with localized ependymoma. *J Clin Oncol.* 2004;22:3156.

25. Grill J, Le Deley MC, Gambarelli D, et al. Postoperative chemotherapy without irradiation for ependymoma in children under 5 years of age: a multicenter trial of the French Society of Pediatric Oncology. *J Clin Oncol.* 2001; 19:1288.

26. Duffner PK, Horowitz ME, Krischer JP, et al. Postoperative chemotherapy and delayed radiation in children less than three years of age with malignant brain tumors. *N Engl J Med.* 1993;328:1725.

27. Needle MN, Goldwein JW, Grass J, et al. Adjuvant chemotherapy for the treatment of intracranial ependymoma of childhood. *Cancer.* 1997;80:341.

28. Evans AE, Anderson JR, Lefkowitz-Boudreaux IB, et al. Adjuvant chemotherapy of childhood posterior fossa ependymomas: cranial-spinal irradiation with or without adjuvant CCNU, vincristine, and presnisone: a Children's Cancer Group Study. *Med Pediatr Oncol.* 1996;27:8.

29. Koeller KK, Rushing EJ. From the archives of the AFIP: pilocytic astrocytoma: radiologic-pathologic correlation. *Radiographics.* 2004;24:1693.

30. Benesch M, Eder HG, Sovinz P, et al. Residual or recurrent cerebellar low-grade glioma in children after tumor resection: is re-treatment needed? A single center experience from 1983 to 2003. *Pediatr Neurosurg.* 2006; 42:159.

31. Akay KM, Izci Y, Baysefer A, et al. Surgical outcomes of cerebellar tumors in children. *Pediatr Neurosurg.* 2004; 40:220.

32. Marcus KJ, Goumnerova L, Billett AL, et al. Stereotactic radiotherapy for localized low-grade gliomas in children: final results of a prospective trial. *Int J Radiat Oncol Biol Phys.* 2005;61:374.

33. Harwood-Nash DC. Neuroimaging of childhood craniopharyngioma. *Pediatr Neurosurg.* 1994;21:2.

34. Tsuda M, Takahashi S, Higano S, et al. CT and MR imaging of craniopharyngioma. *Eur Radiol.* 1997;7:464.

35. Fahlbusch R, Honegger J, Paulus W, et al. Surgical treatment of craniopharyngiomas: experience with 168 patients. *J Neurosurg.* 1999;90:237.

36. Tomita T, McLone DG. Radical resections of childhood craniopharyngiomas. *Pediatr Neurosurg.* 1993;19:6.

37. Hoffman HJ, De Silva M, Humphreys RP, et al. Aggressive surgical management of craniopharyngiomas in children. *J Neurosurg.* 1992;76:47.

38. Yasargil MG, Curcic M, Kis M, et al. Total removal of craniopharyngiomas. Approaches and longterm results in 144 patients. *J Neurosurg.* 1990;73:3.

39. Van Effenterre R, Boch AL. Craniopharyngioma in adults and children: a study of 122 surgical cases. *J Neurosurg.* 2002;97:3.

40. Puget S, Garnett M, Wray A, et al. Pediatric craniopharyngiomas: classification and treatment according to the degree of hypothalamic involvement. *J Neurosurg.* 2007; 106(suppl):3.

41. Rilliet B, Vernet O. Gliomas in children: a review. *Childs Nerv Syst.* 2000;16:735.

42. Burzynski SR. Treatments for astrocytic tumors in children: current and emerging strategies. *Paediatr Drugs.* 2006;8:167.

43. Reddy AT, Packer RJ. Chemotherapy for low-grade gliomas. *Childs Nerv Syst.* 1999;15:506.

44. Perilongo G. Considerations on the role of chemotherapy and modern radiotherapy in the treatment of childhood low grade glioma. *J Neurooncol.* 2005;75:301.

45. Combs SE, Schulz-Ertner D, Moschos D, et al. Fractionated stereotactic radiotherapy of optic pathway gliomas: tolerance and long-term outcome. *Int J Radiat Oncol Biol Phys.* 2005;62:814.

46. Rood BR, MacDonald TJ. Pediatric high-grade glioma: molecular genetic clues for innovative therapeutic approaches. *J Neurooncol.* 2005;75:267.

47. Tamber MS, Rutka JT. Pediatric supratentorial high-grade gliomas. *Neurosurg Focus.* 2003;14:e1.

48. Campbell JW, Pollack IF, Martinez AJ, et al. High grade astrocytomas in children: radiologically complete resection is associated with an excellent long-term prognosis. *Neurosurgery.* 1996;38:258.

49. Finlay JL, Wisoff JH. The impact of extent of resection in the management of malignant gliomas of childhood. *Childs Nerv Syst.* 1999;15:786.

50. Wisoff JH, Boyett JM, Berger MS, et al. Current neurosurgical management and the impact of the extent of resection in the treatment of malignant gliomas of childhood: a report of the Children's Cancer Group trial no. CCG-945. *J Neurosurg.* 1998;89:52.

51. Kramm CM, Wagner S, Van Gool S, et al. Improved survival after gross total resection of malignant gliomas in pediatric patients from the HIT-GBM studies. *Anticancer Res.* 2006;26:3773-3779.

52. Finlay JL, Boyett JM, Yates AJ, et al. Randomized phase III trial in childhood high-grade astrocytoma comparing vincristine, lomustine, and prednisone with the eight-drugs-in-1-day regimen. Childrens Cancer Group. *J Clin Oncol.* 1995;13:112.

53. Wolff JE, Gnekow AK, Kortmann RD, et al. Preradiation chemotherapy for pediatric patients with high-grade glioma. *Cancer.* 2002;94:264.

54. Freeman CR, Farmer JP. Pediatric brain stem gliomas: a review. *Int J Radiat Oncol Biol Phys.* 1998;40:265.

55. Wagner S, Warmuth-Metz M, Emser A, et al. Treatment options in childhood pontine gliomas. *J Neurooncol.* 2006;79:281.

56. Epstein F, Constantini S. Practical decisions in the treatment of pediatric brain stem tumors. *Pediatr Neurosurg.* 1996;24:24.

57. Packer RJ, Krailo M, Mehta M, et al. A phase I study of concurrent RMP-7 and carboplatin with radiation therapy for children with newly diagnosed brainstem gliomas. *Cancer.* 2005;104:1968.

58. Jallo GI, Shiminski-Maher T, Velazquez L, et al. Recovery of lower cranial nerve function after surgery for medullary brainstem tumors. *Neurosurgery.* 2005;56:74.

59. Mauffrey C. Paediatric brainstem gliomas: prognostic factors and management. *J Clin Neurosci.* 2006;13:431.

60. Finlay JL, Zacharoulis S. The treatment of high grade gliomas and diffuse intrinsic pontine tumors of childhood and adolescence: a historical—and futuristic—perspective. *J Neurooncol.* 2005;75:253.

61. Blakely JO, Grossman SA. Management of pineal region tumors. *Curr Treat Options Oncol.* 2006;7:505.

62. Weiner HL, Lichtenbaum RA, Wisoff JH, et al. Delayed surgical resection of central nervous system germ cell tumors. *Neurosurgery.* 2002;50:727.

63. Jaing TH, Wang HS, Tung IJ, et al. Intracranial germ cell tumors: a retrospective study of 44 children. *Pediatr Neurol.* 2002;26:369.

64. Ausman JI, Nicholson JC, Takakura K, et al. Clinical controversy: how do you manage germ cell tumors of the CNS? *Surg Neurol.* 2003;60:5.

65. Shim KW, Kim TG, Suh CO, et al. Treatment failure in intracranial primary germinomas. *Childs Nerv Syst.* 2007 Oct;23(10):1155-1161.

66. Douglas JG, Rockhill JK, Olson JM, et al. Cisplatin-based chemotherapy followed by focal, reduced-dose irradiation for pediatric primary central nervous system germinomas. *J Pediatr Hematol Oncol.* 2006;28:36.

67. Kellie SJ, Boyce H, Dunkel IJ, et al. Primary chemotherapy for intracranial nongerminomatous germ cell tumors: results of the second international CNS germ cell study group protocol. *J Clin Oncol.* 2004;22:846.

68. Ullrich NJ, Pomeroy SL. Molecular genetics of pediatric central nervous system tumors. *Curr Oncol Rep.* 2006; 8:423.

CHAPTER 26

Malformations of the Nervous System in Relation to Ontogenesis

Harvey B. Sarnat and
Laura Flores-Sarnat

Embryonic development of the nervous system is a series of overlapping processes.[1] To understand neural development, a traditional view of morphogenesis must be integrated with what we know about molecular genetic programming of the neural tube and fetal brain. Understanding these normal ontogenetic processes is necessary to comprehend neural malformations, which arise as disturbances in one or more of these processes. Malformations of the brain and spinal cord may be caused by genetic mutations or by environmental or acquired influences. Examples of acquired and environmental causes are teratogenic toxins and drugs, fetal ischemia and infarcts, intrauterine trauma from maternal trauma or invasive procedures, cerebral hemorrhages, and infections affecting the fetal brain.

Knowledge of neuroembryology provides insight into the pathogenesis and mechanisms of neural malformations and how the brain determines dysgeneses of many non-neurological structures, such as developmental craniofacial disorders. Molecular genetics has profoundly changed our understanding of the mechanisms of both normal and abnormal development of the nervous system. These advances, combined with medical advances in neuroimaging, clinical neurophysiology, and neuropathologic tissue examination, provide a way to understand malformations of the nervous system. Thus, this chapter is not presented as a traditional list of various known neural malformations, each with their clinical, radiologic, and pathologic findings; nor is it intended as a tabulation of known genetic mutations and deletions associated with specific dysgeneses. It is presented as a modern approach to better understand malformations in the context of development, a new neuroembryology that integrates descriptive morphogenesis and genetic programming.

DEFINITIONS AND PRINCIPLES OF NERVOUS SYSTEM DEVELOPMENT

Neural development is better thought of as a set of simultaneously occurring processes than as a set of sequential steps.

Traditional classifications list a series of developmental processes as a linear sequence of events, one following another. Some processes are indeed step-wise, each dependent upon the preceding one. Among these are:

- Gastrulation
- Establishment of the body axes
- Curling of the primitive neuroepithelium or neural plate to form the neural tube

All of these processes occur before maturation of individual cells and structural organization of the neural tube.

Other neurodevelopmental processes occur late in embryonic development. Synaptogenesis can only occur after the formation of dendrites and dendritic spines, maturation of the neuronal membrane to form synapses, and the synthesis of neurotransmitters and their release at axonal terminals. Myelination of axons does not occur during the projection phase of axonal growth before the axon has reached its target and initiated synapse formation.

However, most processes occur simultaneously, such that they must be considered in relation to one another. Among these are:

- Neuroblast migration
- Maturation of the neuroblast membrane capable of developing a resting membrane potential
- Projection of the axonal growth cone from the migratory neuroblast

▪ Vascular perfusion of the brain
▪ The formation of glial cells in relation to capillaries to form a blood–brain barrier

Nevertheless, it is useful both for classification and understanding to list the developmental processes and then consider them individually. This classification must integrate traditional morphogenesis with an understanding of molecular genetic programming of nervous system development. Finally, the relation of nervous system development to the development of non-neural tissues, or neural induction, must also be considered along with development of non-neural cells and tissue within the brain, such as the vascular system for cerebral perfusion, microglia (resident macrophages), and the development of the immune system. Table 26-1 lists the developmental processes considered in the next sections.

The (Perhaps) Outdated Concept of Germ Layers

The concept of germ layers, which give origin to various tissues, as primitive ectoderm, mesoderm, and endoderm, is a traditional and long-accepted basic concept in embryology, conceived in the 19th century and based upon the best embryologic morphologic observations of that time. This concept continued to be accepted until the advent of molecular genetics in the late 1980s and early 1990s, when this deeply ingrained idea began to seem artificial and arbitrary. Gene families are expressed in all three layers, both in initial stages of tissue differentiation and also in maturing and mature tissues. For example, the *HOX* gene family programs segmentation of the neural tube but also is essential in the development of mesodermal structures of the extremities, endochondral long bones and muscle, and some endocrine organs of endodermal derivation. Neural crest cells of ectodermal origin form many mesodermal structures.

Ganglia: Not Small, Simple Brains

Understanding the development of the brain requires a basic knowledge of ganglia, which are not simple brains, and the components of a simple brain. The differences between brains and ganglia are listed in Table 26-2. A scientific definition of a brain must exclude functional criteria, especially those involving intellect, language, problem-solving, and reasoning. To introduce unique human qualities, or even those of more complex animals, as criteria, removes the definition from the realm of objective science and misrepresents it as philosophy or religion.

Acute Functional Changes to Nervous System Not Invoked by Birth

In many systems of the body, such as the cardiovascular and pulmonary, the abrupt transition from an intrauterine to the extrauterine environment involves profound physiologic changes. The nervous system is not in this category, *and the programmed rate of maturation of the central nervous system is not influenced by the time of birth, whether preterm or at term, in the healthy infant.* An infant born at 28 weeks gestation (3 months early) has the same neurological examination and EEG

Table 26-1.

Sequential/Simultaneous Developmental Process in the Ontogenesis of the Nervous System

1. Gastrulation (16 d): establishment of body symmetry and axes; birth of the nervous system
2. Gradients of genetic expression in the axes of the neural plate and neural tube
3. Neurulation (24-28 d) and neural crest separation
4. Neural induction: notochordal induction of neural tube and neural crest induction of craniofacial development and of formation of the peripheral nervous system and associated tissues
5. Segmentation of the neural tube
6. Cellular proliferation
7. Apoptosis
8. Cellular lineage: differentiation of neurons, glial, and epenydmal cells
9. Neuroblast migration
10. Neuronal maturation: establishment of an ATPase energy pump, resting membrane potential, and membrane receptors
11. Axonal projection and pathfinding; retraction of excessive or redundant axonal collaterals
12. Dendritic arborization
13. Neurotransmitter synthesis
14. Synaptogenesis; remodeling of synaptic circuits
15. Myelination

Table 26-2.

Comparison of Brain and Ganglion

Brain	Ganglion
Cephalic site only	Variable sites in body
Serves entire body	Serves limited regions or segments
Bilobar with commissures	Alobar without commissures
Neurons form surface, axons form core	Homogeneous mixture of neurons and axons
Interneurons predominate	Interneurons sparse
Multisynaptic intrinsic circuits	Monosynaptic relays
Specialized local functions	No localized specialization of function

From Sarnat HB, Netsky MG. When does a ganglion become a brain? Evolutionary origin of the central nervous system. Semin Pediatr Neurol. 2002;9:240-253.

maturation and myelination pattern at postnatal age 3 months as a full-term neonate just born, unless hypoxemia or other pathologic conditions cause a delay in maturation. In assessing neurological maturation of preterm infants, *conceptional age* (gestational age at birth + chronological age since birth) always must be considered, including head circumference and size of the fontanelles. This is clinically important and makes it crucial that the developmental age of a child be considered when assessing his or her neurological function.

Gradients of Genetic Expression Along the Axes of the Neural Tube

Various developmental genes of the nervous system are expressed as early as gastrulation, the stage of the primitive streak and the Henson node. Others appear later during neural plate development and especially after the neural tube is formed. With the establishment of bilateral symmetry and the formation of the neural tube, three major axes are identified: longitudinal, vertical, and horizontal (Figure 26-1). Genes that are expressed this early are expressed in a gradient along one or more of the three neural axes, with strongest expression at one site and progressively diminishing expression distal to that site. In each of the axes, one of two gradients is possible: in the longitudinal axis, the gradient may either be rostrocaudal or caudorostral; in the vertical axis, the gradient is either dorsoventral or ventrodorsal; in the horizontal axis, it is mediolateral or lateromedial. The bending of the neural tube with the formation of flexures does not alter the axes, which bend with the tube and follow its contour.

Nearly all developmental processes of the neural tube are genetically programmed. Many of the genes that appear at various stages to mediate specific processes are known[2-4] and many more remain to be discovered.

A majority of cerebral malformations may be understood in the context of these axes and gradients. In general, up-regulation of a gene results in hypertrophy or duplication of structures at its strongest site of expression; down-regulation results in hypoplasia or noncleavage or midline "fusion" of structures. Many genes are antagonistic to others, and the down-regulation of one may lead to an appearance of up-regulation of the other, but this overexpression of one gene function is not due to increased synthesis of that gene's product mRNA or protein. This relatively recent molecular genetic insight may be integrated with traditional descriptive morphogenesis to provide a new means of classifying CNS malformations.[5]

Neural Tube Development: Concentric Zones

At 6 weeks gestation, the neural tube is fully closed, but the concentric zones of internal architecture are not yet fully developed. At the level of the telencephalon, only

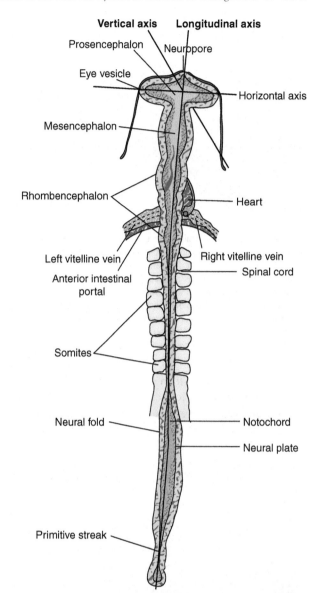

FIGURE 26-1 ■ Drawing of early neural tube showing the three fundamental cerebral vesicles and the three axes: longitudinal, vertical, and horizontal, along which genetic gradients are expressed during development.

two zones are found: a (peri-) *ventricular zone* of undifferentiated neuroepithelium with cells still in the mitotic/proliferative stage and a *marginal zone* as a peripheral rim that has relatively few cells (Figure 26-2). The neuroepithelium is densely cellular, with most tightly packed with large nuclei and sparse cytoplasm and very little intercellular neuropil. No ependymal differentiation is present at the ventricular surface.[6]

By 8 weeks gestation, four concentric zones can be distinguished histologically (Figure 26-3):

1. The *ventricular zone* is still prominent, forming the ventricular wall and surface.
2. The *subventricular zone*, also known as the *germinal matrix* is peripheral to the ventricular zone. It should be noted that this is an imprecise

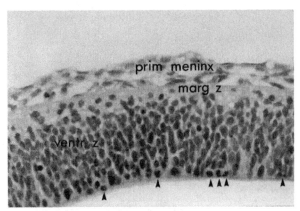

FIGURE 26-2 ■ Section of primitive human telencephalon at 6 weeks gestation. The ventricular surface is formed by undifferentiated neuroepithelium still in the mitotic phase, with most mitoses occurring at the margin of the ventricle (arrows). Ependyma is not yet differentiated. Peripheral to this neuroepithelial "ventricular zone" is a cell-sparse "marginal zone" in which future Cajal-Retzius and subplate neurons and a preplate plexus of neurites are found, but the first wave of radial migration has not yet occurred and the cortical plate is not yet formed. The primitive meninx (primordium of the leptomeninges) is at the surface of the telencephalon. Haematoxylin-eosin. X100.

but traditional term used by neuropathologists but not by strict neuroembryologists. Radial glial cells differentiate within the subventricular zone and send their long, slender process centrifugally to the pial surface, but do not have attachments to the ventricular surface as do neuroepithelial cells of the ventricular zone.

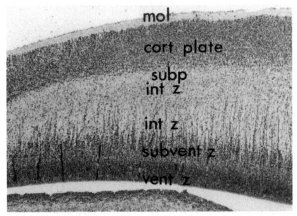

FIGURE 26-3 ■ Section of human telencephalon at 8 weeks gestation. Four layers of the parenchyma are now defined. The innermost periventricular layer is the "ventricular zone" (**vent z**). Just distal to it is the "subventricular zone" (**subvent z**), consisting of postmitotic, premigratory neuroblasts and glioblasts and the site of the radial glial cell bodies. The middle layer is called the "intermediate zone" (**int z**), through which radial glial fibres and migratory neuroblasts and glioblasts pass; it is the future subcortical white matter. The previous marginal zone is now divided into thirds by the formation of the cortical plate (cort plate) in the middle of this zone by neuroblasts that have completed their radial migration. The peripheral part of the original marginal zone becomes the "molecular layer" (mol) or layer 1 of the mature, laminated neocortex. The area deep to the cortical plate from the original marginal zone becomes the "subplate layer" (subp), a transitory fetal layer that later becomes incorporated into the deep cortical laminae and loses its distinction.

3. The *intermediate zone* lies peripheral to the subventricular zone and is the future white matter of the centrum semiovale.
4. The *cortical plate* forms from the migratory neuroblasts in the middle of the marginal zone, thus dividing the marginal zone into three layers:
   - A superficial part that persists as the *molecular layer*, which will be layer 1 of the mature cortex
   - A middle layer that is the cortical plate proper
   - A deep layer between the cortical plate and the intermediate zone that is called the *subplate zone*
5. With maturation of the cortical plate, the subplate zone becomes incorporated into layer 6; hence it is a transitory lamina.

Elimination of Redundancies

A fundamental principle of development is the overproduction and subsequent reduction of excessive cells, axonal collaterals, dendritic spines, and synapses. Redundancy of neuroblasts in every part of the brain and spinal cord, mediated by apoptosis, may be modulated by the need for, and provides for the potential repair or replacement of, cells lost early in gestation by physical, metabolic, or toxic injury to the developing brain.

Two Fundamental CNS Plans of Architecture: Nuclear and Cortical

During development, two cellular arrangements are present throughout the neuraxis. A nucleus is a cluster of the same type of neurons for a common, though not necessarily identical, purpose. Cranial nerve nuclei are a good example. Most of the thalamus and the basal telencephalic nuclei (ie, "basal ganglia") are organized with nuclear architecture. Also, more than one type of neuron may be included in nuclei. Many nuclei include interneurons as well as primary sensory or motor neurons. Cortical architecture is a laminar arrangement of neurons of the same type in each layer, with synaptic connections between layers. Examples of cortical architecture are the cerebral neocortex, hippocampus (paleocortex), lateral geniculate body of the thalamus, superior colliculus (optic tectum of the rostral midbrain), cerebellar cortex, olfactory bulb, and retina. The cerebral cortical plate at mid-gestation is not yet a laminated structure, and has a fetal architecture that is more columnar than laminar, corresponding to the recently completed phase of neuroblast radial migration (Figure 26-4). In one type of focal cortical dysplasia, this columnar architecture persists (Figure 26-5).

Gyration

Because the mammalian brain has cortices with laminar architecture, but a limited cranium in which the

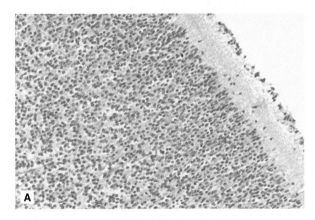

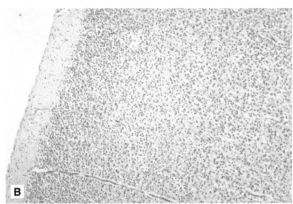

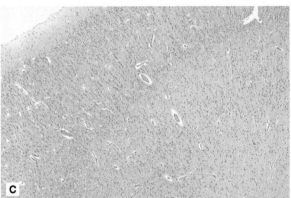

FIGURE 26-4 ■ Sections of cerebral cortex of human fetuses at **(A)** 20 weeks gestation, **(B)** 28 weeks, and **(C)** 38 weeks. The arrangement of cells within the cortical plate at 20 weeks is radial columnar more than horizontal laminar, and the immature neurons are tightly packed because they have little cytoplasm and the neuropil is very sparse. By 28 weeks there is distinctive histological layering of the cortex superimposed on the earlier fetal columnar architecture, but the distinctive six layers of the mature cortex are not evident until near-term. Note the prominent thin layer of cells at the surface of the brain at 20 weeks and more disperse at 28 weeks and only occasional persistent cells at 38 weeks; this is the subpial granular glial layer of Brun that is transitory and disappears with maturation. Haemotoxylin-eosin X100.

brain must fit, an increase in surface area without a corresponding volume increase is necessary. This is accomplished in the mammalian brain with folding of the cortex to form gyri and sulci in the cerebrum and folia in the cerebellum. Fissures and sulci of the cerebral cortex are similar but not identical because they form differently (see section "Fissures, Sulci, and Gyri of the Cortex").

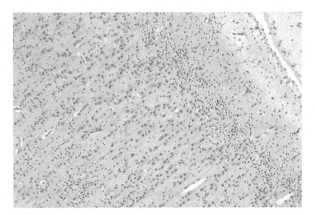

FIGURE 26-5 ■ Cerebral cortex with abnormal persistent radial columnar architecture in a 6-week-old male infant born at 29 weeks gestation (conceptional age 35 weeks at death) with DiGeorge syndrome, genetically confirmed. This cortex is an example of maturational arrest. He also had absence of the anterior commissure and hypoplasia of the corpus callosum. Haematoxylin-eosin. X100.

Thalamic Modulation of Ascending Sensory Information to Forebrain

Almost all primary sensory systems—somatosensory, proprioceptive, auditory, vestibular, visual, and taste—have synapses in the thalamus for modulation before relay to the sensory cortices. The notable exception is the olfactory system, in which olfactory nerve impulses are received in the olfactory bulbs and relayed via mitral and tufted neurons directly to neocortex, the entorhinal cortex (parahippocampal gyrus); local circuitry within the olfactory bulb functions as its own thalamus.[7]

SPECIFIC DEVELOPMENTAL PROCESSES

Gastrulation

Gastrulation occurs at 16 days postconception. The formation of the Henson node and primitive streak establish bilateral symmetry as the basic body plan of all vertebrates, and the three axes of the body and of the CNS:

1. *Longitudinal* (cephalic and caudal ends
2. *Vertical* (dorsal and ventral surfaces)
3. *Horizontal* (medial and lateral in relation to the midline of the longitudinal axis)

Gastrulation also is the "birthday" of the nervous system, as it is the earliest time when neuroepithelium can be distinguished from other tissues.

Neurulation

Neurulation is the bending of the neural plate to form a tube and changes the orientation of surfaces and edges of the neural plate. The dorsal surface becomes the inner surface facing the lumen of the central canal and ventricles; it is lined by neuroepithelium and later by ependyma. The lateral margin of the neural plate closes the tube in the dorsal midline and neural crest arises from most of this edge.

Closure of the neural tube begins in the cervical region and progresses rostrally and caudally. The anterior neuropore closes at 24 days, and the posterior at 28 days. There are multiple sites of closure in the position of the anterior and posterior neuropore.

Secondary neurulation is the formation of the most caudal sacral segments of spinal cord, posterior to the site of closure of the posterior neuropore. This part of the spinal cord does not develop as a folding of the neural plate, but rather is a solid cone of neuroepithelium with an ependymal central canal forming within its core.

Induction

Induction is the influence of one embryonic tissue upon another, each of which differentiates into different mature tissues. Neural crest cells separate from the dorsal midline of the neural tube at the time of its closure. The incipient neural crest or progenitor cells develop at the lateral margin of the neural plate. Neural crest arises from three sites of the neural tube and each migrates to give rise to specific structures (Table 26-3):

1. *Prosencephalic neural crest* is generated in the dorsal part of the lamina terminalis, the same place that gives origin to the bridge for the corpus callosum. It migrates rostrally as a thin vertical sheet of cells in the midline to the nose and forehead, and forms the intercanthal ligament between the embryonic orbit.

2. *Mesencephalic neural crest* arises from the dorsal midline of the mesencephalic neuromere and rhombomeres r1 and r2. It migrates as streams of cells in the horizontal plane to form most of the craniofacial structure, including the orbits, all cartilage and membranous bone of the face and cranial vault (but not endochondral bone of the cranial base, basioccipital, exoccipital and supraoccipital bones), dura mater including falx and tentorium, leptomeninges over the brain (but not over the spinal cord), the globe of the eye (except the retina, optic nerve, choroid, lens, and cornea), blood vessels, nerve sheaths (including Schwann cells, but not axons), and melanocytes.

3. *Rhombencephalic neural crest* arises from rhombomeres r3 through r8 including the spinal cord. It migrates as blocks of cells in streams and forms most of the peripheral autonomic nervous system (including sympathetic chain and parasympathetic ganglia in GI tract), chromaffin tissue (adrenal medulla; carotid body), nerve sheaths, dorsal root ganglia, stria vasculosa over the hair cells of the cochlea, melanocytes, and adipocytes.

Migratory neural crest cells do not differentiate into their mature identity until they reach their terminal site. Abnormalities of neural crest, known in human medicine as "neurocristopathies," include many neurocutaneous syndromes and aganglionic megacolon

Table 26-3.

Types of Neural Crest

Type of Neural Crest	Origin	Migration	Structures Generated
Prosencephalic	Dorsal part of lamina terminalis	Rostrally as thin sheet of cells to midline of face	Intercanthal ligament
Mesencephalic	Dorsal midline of mesencephalic neuromere and rhombomeres 1 and 2	As a stream of cells in the horizontal plane	Most of craniofacial structures: orbits, cartilage, and bone of face; dura mater, leptomeninges over brain; parts of the eye globe; blood vessels and nerve sheaths
Rhomboencephalic	Rhombomeres 3-8	As blocks of cells in streams	Most of the peripheral and autonomic nervous system, nerve sheaths, dorsal root ganglia, stria vasculosa over the hair cells of the cochlea; melanocytes adipocytes

(Hirschsprung disease). The mesencephalic origin of craniofacial structures also explains hereditary neurosensory deafness and craniofacial dysmorphisms also associated with many cerebral malformations.[8]

Segmentation

Segmentation of the neural tube or the formation of transitory physical compartments (neuromeres) restricts the longitudinal movement of cells during development.[9] Segmentation is mediated by a group of genes called *homeoboxes*, which are restricted DNA sequences composed of exactly 183 DNA base pairs. Homeobox genes encode a class of proteins that share a common or very similar 60-amino acid motif, the *homeodomain*.[10] Mammalian homeoboxes are identical to the segment polarity genes of invertebrates, and program the embryonic segmentation of the vertebrate neural tube.[11] For example, *HOX* genes are essential for limb development and the anterior and posterior orientation of the arms and legs. The human *EGR2* (*Krox-20* in the mouse) is expressed only in rhombomeres r3 and r5 in the neural tube, and is an essential gene for myelination in the peripheral nervous system (PNS).[12]

Cellular Proliferation and Apoptosis

Neural development is redundant and generates more neurons than are needed. There is a subsequent reduction of this abundance via the mechanism of apoptosis (programmed cell death). Most mitoses occur in the neuroepithelium at the ventricular wall (m-phase).[13,14] Neuroepithelial cells have long radial processes that span the neural tube, with end feet at the ventricular surface and the pial surface; nuclei travel to and fro within this thin cytoplasmic extension. When distal to the ventricular wall, the s-phase enables replication of DNA in preparation for the next mitosis.

If the mitotic spindle is oriented perpendicular to the ventricular surface (symmetrical mitosis), the two daughter cells each reenter the mitotic cycle. If the mitotic spindle is parallel to the ventricular wall, the cell next to the ventricle reenters the mitotic cycle and the other has completed its last mitosis and prepares for migration as a neuroblast. In the human, 33 mitotic cycles produce all the neurons of the cerebral cortex.[15]

There are 50% more motor neuroblasts produced in the spinal cord than needed, and this number is later reduced through apoptosis.[16] The Bcl-2 family of proteins plays an integral role in regulating the time and rate of apoptosis,[17] which usually occurs in undifferentiated or only incipiently differentiated neuroblasts. However, a second phase of apoptosis may involve more mature neurons during late development. Hormones and growth factors may influence the rate of apoptosis.

This process is more complex than most developmental processes because there is no single gene or gene combination that intiates the cascade of events comprising apoptosis, which is programmed into every cell, but only expressed when trophic factors secreted by nearby cells remove the inhibitors of this process that normally preserve metabolic integrity.

Until recently, it was thought that the mature brain has no capacity to generate new neurons; however, potentially neurogenic stem cells within the brain have now been identified in the periventricular regions. These are most numerous in the region of the dentate gyrus of the hippocampus and in the olfactory bulb. In fact, there is a constant turnover of some neurons in both locations. Primary olfactory receptor neurons are continuously renewed, but interneurons (granule cells) in the olfactory bulb are also regenerated.[18,19]

Cellular Lineage and Differentiation

The origin and migration, or lineage, of any neural cell determines not only whether it will be as a neuron, glial cell, or ependymal cell within the neural tube, but also which type of neuron, which neurotransmitter it will synthesize, which receptors will form in its plasma membranes, and where it will project its axon. Glial cells similarly must differentiate as astrocytes, oligodendrocytes, and specialized astrocytes such as the transitory radial glial cells of the cerebrum or the permanent Bergmann glial cells of the cerebellar cortex. Lineage in general is genetically programmed, but may be induced to change if pathologic conditions ensue in the fetal brain.

The development of a stable resting membrane potential depends upon the formation of the ATPase energy pump. Associated with that are other maturational features of the neuron and its plasma membrane: membrane channels and receptors, neurotransmitter biosynthesis, neuron-specific proteins, and intermediate filaments.

Regulator genes are important factors not only in whether a progenitor cell will become a neuron, a glial or ependymal cell, but also in which type of cell within these categories it becomes. Some developmental disorders of the brain are due to mixed cellular lineage, as in tuberous sclerosis and hemimegalencephaly, in which cells not only express a mixture of neuronal and glial proteins but show morphologic and growth aberrations, sometimes even leading to neoplastic transformation.

Neuronal differentiation

A neuron is a secretory cell with an electrically polarized membrane. Neuroblasts, however, are postmitotic cells with a committed neuronal lineage, but not yet mature enough to be neurons. The features of maturation that define neurons are:

1. Synthesis and expression of neuronal proteins and filaments, such as neuronal nuclear antigen (NeuN) and neurofilament proteins (NFP)
2. An energy-producing pump for maintaining a resting membrane potential, generally the Na/K adenosine triphosphatase (ATPase) pump
3. Development of specialized membrane receptors and ion channels
4. Neurosecretory functions to enable the biosynthesis of a neurotransmitter, and to transport it and package it in vesicles; ribosomes and rough endoplasmic reticulum and a Golgi apparatus are required.

It should be noted that the presence of neurites is is not sufficient to define a cell as a neuron. For example, chromaffin cells of the adrenal medulla and carotid body are not neurons without dendrites or axons.

Ependymal differentiation

The fetal ependyma provides unique functions not required in the adult. Differentiation of the ependyma from the neuroepithelium at the ventricular surface arrests all mitotic activity at that site.[20] Ependyma does not completely cover the lateral ventricular surface until 22 weeks gestation.[21-23] Genetic and environmental influences, such as toxins, teratogens, and viral infections, can cause precocious differentiation of the ependyma. Early ependymal formation decreases the number of neurons and may result in microencephaly and other malformations with later functional correlates, such as mental retardation and epilepsy.

Fetal ependymal cells have basal processes that radiate into the parenchyma, but do not extend to the pial surface and do not guide migratory neuroblasts. They secrete molecules that help guide the intermediate trajectory of growing axons by either repelling them or attracting them. Both the neuronal targets of the roof plate and floor plate are ependymal, and the floor plate is the first cellular differentiation in the neural tube, even before closure. Figure 26-6 shows the normal relations of the sclerotome with the notochord in its centre to the neural tube overlying it, in the spinal cord of a 6-week human embryo; the notochord produces the gene Sonic hedgehog (SHH), which induces the floor plate of the neural tube and the first motor neuroblasts. Figure 26-7 shows the spinal cord roof plate ependymal processes in an 8-week fetus that extend dorsally in the midline to separate the developing dorsal columns of the two sides of the spinal cord by both acting as a physical barrier and by secreting glycosaminoglycans that repel growing axons, so that right-left orientation is not confused in the brain by aberrant decussations of these axons in the spinal cord. Figure 26-8 shows the growing axons in the dorsal columns in a longitudinal (frontal) section of the dorsal part of the spinal cord in a 6-week human embryo, impregnated with silver stain.

Disorders related to disturbances in cell lineage and differentiation

Disturbances in neural cell lineage and differentiation are the cause of several human neural malformations. In these malformations, cells often show a mixed lineage with expression of both neuronal and glial proteins. Tuberous sclerosis is the prototype example.[24] Another good example is hemimegalencephaly, with many cells of mixed lineage and abnormal architecture resulting from disturbed migration due both to abnormal radial glial cells and abnormalities in the migratory neuroblasts.[25] Other examples include cerebellar dysplastic gangliocytoma (Lhermitte-Duclos disease), dysembryoplastic neuroepithelial tumour (borderland between dysplasia and neoplasia), and the Taylor-type of focal cortical dysplasia.

Neuroblast and Glioblast Migrations

Almost all mature neurons migrate from their point of cellular origin to where they are in the mature nervous system. Cells migrate mainly centrifugally, to a distant site before completing their cellular maturation. Migration may proceed along radial glial processes or along axons.

Radial migration to the cerebral cortical plate is guided by a scaffold of slender radial processes of specialized astrocytes that differentiate in the subventricular zone and project their processes centrifugally to the pial surface (Figure 26-8). Neuroblasts and glioblasts are guided to their destination along the outside of these radial glial fibers, as if riding a monorail. The continued proliferation of radial glial cells in the subvenricular zone stops at midgestation.[26] After migration is complete, the radial process retracts and most radial glial cells become fibrillary astrocytes of the white matter. In the cerebellar cortex, the specialized radial glial cells are called Bergmann cells; their soma is in the Purkinje cell layer, and their processes extend radially through the molecular zone to guide external granule cells to their mature site in the internal granular layer, beneath the row of Purkinje cells. Radial glia are also found in the early brainstem and spinal cord to guide neuroepithelial cells, but they are mixed with basal processes of ependymal cells, which extend for longer distances in the brainstem than in the telencephalon (Figure 26-9).

In addition to radial migration to the cerebral cortical plate, there also is tangential migration along several pathways from the ganglionic eminence of the embryonic forebrain that is part of the germinal matrix, along axons into the developing cortical plate. These neurons that arrive by tangential migration are GABAergic inhibitory interneurons of the cortex and they comprise about 18% to 20% of total cortical neurons. A subset of these neurons is identified by reactivity to calretinin in both the fetal and adult brain (Figure 26-10).

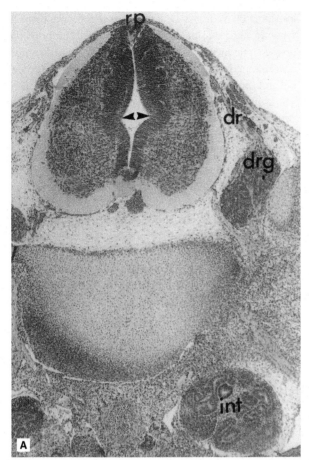

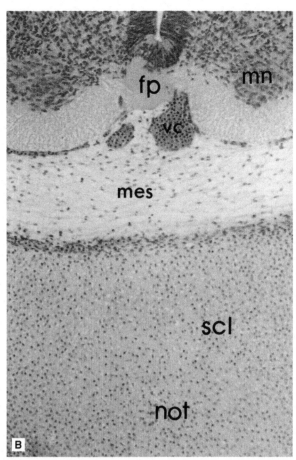

FIGURE 26-6 ■ Transverse section of 6-week human fetal spinal region at **(A)** low and **(B)** higher magnifications, to show the relation of the sclerotome (scl) or primordial vertebral body with its enclosed notochord (not) to the overlying mesenchyma (mes) separating it from the neural tube. The notochord strongly expresses the gene Sonic hedgehog (SHH) and induces the floor plate (fp) of the midline ventral ependyma and also induces the differentiation of motor neuroblasts (mn). The roof plate (rp) in the dorsal midline of the spinal cord is at the surface because the dorsal columns are not yet formed. The central canal is much larger, relative to the spinal cord parenchyma than at older ages and is a narrow vertical space. Arrows indicate the sulcus limitans in the central canal that demarcates the basal and alar plates, ventral and dorsal to this sulcus, respectively. Dorsal roots (dr) extend farther ventrally than at more mature stages and the dorsal root ganglia (drg) lie opposite the basal, rather than the more dorsal alar, plate of the spinal cord. The intestine (int) is seen ventral to the sclerotome. Vacular channels (vc) are not yet mature capillaries or other vessels and contain mainly nucleated erythrocytes. Haematoxylin-eosin. A. X40; B. X250.

Migration depends upon characteristics of the migratory cells, the cells and molecules they secrete, as well as proteins in the extracelluar matrix that guide the migration. Many genes that mediate the migratory process have been identified, not only in the CNS but also in the migration of neural crest cells to the periphery. Mutation, down-regulation, or lack of expression of each produces characteristic malformations.[4,5,27-29]

Fissures, Sulci, and Gyri of the Cortex

Fissures and sulci are grooves that form in the smooth external surface of the cortex to facilitate folding, which increases the surface area without a concomitant augmentation of volume or mass of the brain tissue. Fissures form earlier than sulci and generally are deeper, but the principal difference is the forces that mediate their formation: fissures are a reaction to external physical stresses and bending of the brain, whereas sulci result from internal stresses due to an increased and growing volume of the parenchyma from growth of cells and especially the production of neurites and glial processes that form the neuropil between neurons. The development of the ventricular system influences the formation of fissures but not sulci because the ventricles act as an external force; even through they are enclosed within the brain, they are not part of the parenchyma.

Four fissures form in the forebrain: (1) the interhemispheric fissure that creates two telencephalic hemispheres from a single prosencephalon at 4 to 5 weeks gestation; (2) the hippocampal fissure that develops with rotation of the hippocampus ventrally from its initial dorsal position; (3) the sylvian fissure that results from telencephalic flexure or ventral bending of the caudal third of the primitive telencephalon, beginning at about 9 weeks

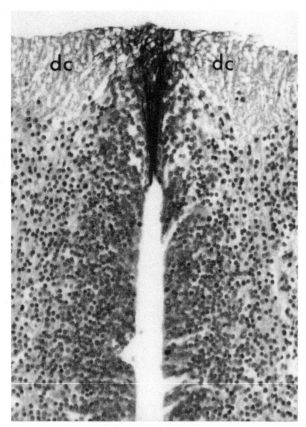

FIGURE 26-7 ■ Transverse section of dorsal third of spinal cord of an 8-week human fetus. The central canal is mainly still lined by primitive neuroepithelium without ependyma, but the roof plate is formed in the dorsal midline and projects basal extensions to the pial surface to form the dorsal median septum. The dorsal columns (dc) are now forming on either side of this septum, and the septum prevents axonal growth cones from aberrant decussations, both by forming a physical barrier and also a chemical barrier by its secretion of keratin sulfate, a glycosaminoglycan that strongly repels growing axons. Vimentin immunoreactivity. X250.

and completed when the operculum completely covers the insula at 36 weeks; and (4) the calcarine fissure on the medial side of the occipital lobe, developing at about 12 weeks.[30] More than 30 sulci form, beginning at about 22 weeks gestation. They follow a precise temporal and spatial pattern and create predictable identifiable gyri of the mature cerebral cortex. Fissures of the brainstem include the sagittal and transverse intercollicular fissures of the tectum of the midbrain and the fissure that forms at the pontomedullary junction to demarcate the caudal end of the basis pontis. The folia of the cerebellum, by contrast, correspond to gyri and sulci and develop in the vermis sooner than in the lateral hemispheres, but the parasagittal grooves that demarcate the vermis from the medial side of the lateral hemispheres are fissures.

Synaptogenesis

The formation of synapses depends not only upon axonal trajectories to reach the target neurons with which they form contact, but also the ability of the presynaptic neurons to synthesize secretory products (neurotransmitters) and to transport them distally within the axon and store them in synaptic vesicles at the axonal terminal. Furthermore, the postsynaptic membrane of the recipient neuron also must have matured to have developed a resting membrane potential and specialized receptors and membrane ion channels. The sequence of synaptogenesis in the brain is as precisely time-linked and spatially sequential as other developmental processes and may be demonstrated in tissue sections of human fetal and neonatal brain by immunocytochemical markers for synaptic vesicle proteins, such as synaptophysin.[31] Figure 26-11 shows the hippocampus of (A) a midgestational fetus, with strong synaptophysin reactivity limited to the molecular zone of the dentate gyrus and the CA2 sector of Ammon's horn, with weaker activity in CA3 and none in CA4, and (B) a full-term neonate with uniformly strong reactivity thoughout all grey matter structures of the dentate gyrus and Ammon's horn. Figure 26-12 shows synaptophysin in the frontal neocortex of (A) a 26-week fetus with reactivity limited to the molecular layer and the deep part of the cortical plate, and in ascending thalamocortical axons; (B) a full-term neonate with uniformly strong reactivity throughout the cortex. These may be combined with more specific tissue markers identifying specific neurotransmitters. Heterotopic neurons in the white matter are not "isolated" as they appear histologically, but are synaptically connected with each other and with the overlying cortex, and may contribute to epileptic circuitry.

Myelination

Myelination is dependent upon the cellular lineage of oligodendrocyte precursors and also by expression of genes directing the mature oligodendroglial cell to synthesize myelin lipoproteins.[32-34] The wrapping of individual axons by oligodendroglial processes that synthesize myelin is a late process in neural development. It is not initiated until the growing axonal growth cone has passed through its intermediate trajectory and made synaptic contact with a target neuron. In most longitudinal pathways of the central nervous system, the entire axon acquires its myelin sheath at the same time; for example, the spinothalamic tracts. Some pathways myelinate along a proximal (near to the neuronal soma) to distal gradient. The corticospinal tract is an example of this pattern. In the full-term neonate, corticospinal axons possess myelin in the corona radiata, internal capsule, and middle third of the cerebral peduncle; minimal myelin is present in the basis pontis; and none is seen by conventional myelin stains in the pyramids or spinal cord.

Many normal axons never become myelinated. In the peripheral nervous system, the sympathetic nerves are an example. In the central nervous system, only 40% of axons of the corpus callosum are myelinated in the adult. These axons still function well. Myelination increases the speed of conduction along an axon by saltatory conduction between nodes of Ranvier, but this has no effect on the speed of thinking or movement.

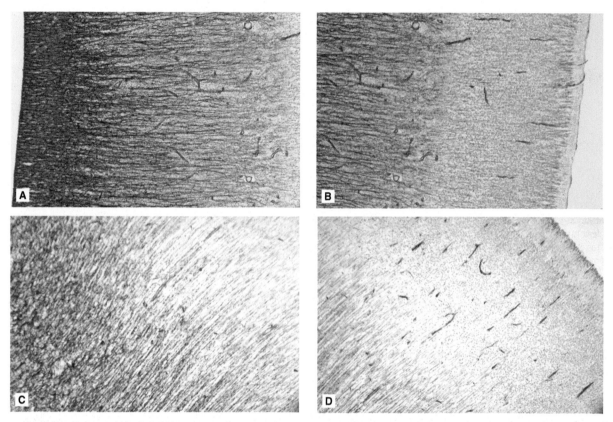

FIGURE 26-8 ■ Fetal cortex at **(A, B)** 18 weeks gestation and **(C, D)** 28 weeks. Vimentin demonstrates strong reactivity of radial glial fibres that are not seen with haematoxylin-eosin, (A,C) from their origin in the subventricular zone to (B,D) extension through the cortical plate to the pial surface. These fibres serve as monorail guides for migratory neuroblasts and glioblasts to the cortex. Vimentin immunoreactivity. X100.

The earliest axons to myelinate are the ventral roots of the spinal cord, at about 16 weeks gestation. As with other aspects of neural development, temporal and spatial sequences of myelination are precisely timed and predictable. Some pathways complete their "myelination cycle" early, within days or a couple of fetal weeks. Other are slower, even over years. The corpus callosum does not begin to myelinate until 4 months of age by MRI criteria, though myelin stains show early myelination in tissue sections at about 2 months. Myelination is not complete in the corpus callosum until adolescence. The last pathway to acquire myelin in normal development is the ipsilateral frontotemporal and frontoparietal association bundles, delayed to 32 years of age.[35] Table 26-4 lists major and some minor CNS pathways with the initiation and termination of their myelination cycles.

FIGURE 26-9 ■ Horizontal section of dorsal columns of spinal cord in a 7-week human fetus to show the growing axons (ax) of the incipient dorsal columns and the dorsal median septum between the two sides. Bielschowsky silver impregnation. X100.

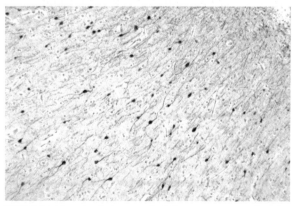

FIGURE 26-10 ■ Cerebral cortex of a full-term neonate to show distribution of an important subgroup of GABAergic inhibitory interneurons within the cortex, that arrive by tangential rather than radial migration. These neurons are distributed in all layers of the cortex but more prominently in the sensory layers 2 and 4. Axons and proximal dendrites are demonstrated, as well as the cytoplasm of the soma. Calretinin immunoreactivity. X100.

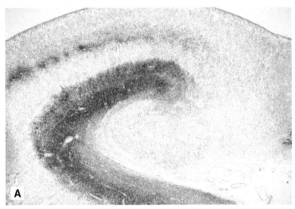
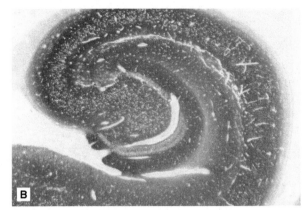

FIGURE 26-11 ■ Hippocampi of a **(A)** 20-week fetus and **(B)** full-term neonate to show the distribution of synaptic vesicle reactivity, a means of demonstrating synaptogenesis. In the midgestational fetus strong reactivity is limited to the molecular zone of the dentate gyrus and the CA2 sector of Ammon's horn, with weaker reactivity seen in CA3. In the term infant, all grey matter structures are uniformly strongly reactive. Synaptophysin immunoreactivity. A. X100; B. X40.

VASCULAR DEVELOPMENT

The development of major blood vessels, both arteries and venous sinuses and veins, is equally precise in its timing and coordination with neural development. The basilar artery initially is a pair of vessels at the base of the rostral neural tube, the longitudinal neural arteries. At about 4 weeks gestation, they undergo a true fusion to form the single midline basilar artery. At that time, the direction of blood flow is rostrocaudal because the early basilar artery is connected with the internal carotid arteries by a series of segmental communicating arteries, the most constant of which are named the trigeminal, otic, and hypoglossal arteries. The vertebral arteries form from a plexus of vessels. When these connect with the basilar artery and there is atrophy and disappearance of the transitory connections between the carotid and basilar artery, the direction of blood flow is reversed and becomes caudorostral. The anterior and middle cerebral arteries are formed separately from the internal carotid and only later fuse on each side with the carotid. The anterior cerebral artery arises in the first pharyngeal (brachial) pouch associated with rhombomere 1, and the middle cerebral artery arises from the second pharyngeal pouch and rhombomere 2. The posterior cerebral arteries arise from pharyngeal pouch 3 and fuse with the rostral end of the basilar artery. The circle of Willis, including the anterior and posterior communicating arteries, is the last major arterial element to form.

NEURAL REGENERATION, REPAIR, AND PLASTICITY

Stem cells persist in the human brain and are capable of proliferation and then differentiation as neurons. This is a relatively new finding and has challenged the long-held dogma that the brain had all the neurons it would ever have at birth, and that nerve cells were too specialized to regenerate or repair injuries. Stem cells in the adult human brain are localized mainly to the olfactory bulb and the hippocampus, around the dentate gyrus,

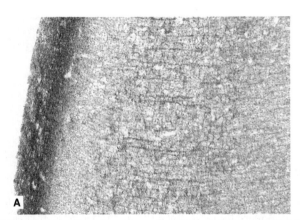
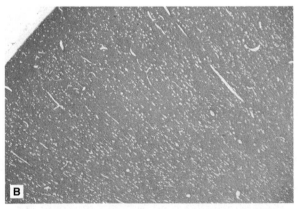

FIGURE 26-12 ■ Frontal neocortex of a **(A)** 26-week fetus and **(B)** full-term neonate to show the distribution of synaptic vesicle reactivity as a reflection of synaptogenesis. In the fetus there is reactivity in the molecular zone, in deep, but not superficial parts of the cortical plate, and in ascending thalamocortical axons that appear as lines within the cortical plate, perpendicular to the pial surface. The term infant shows uniformly strong reactivity in all layers of the cerebral cortex. Synaptophysin immunoreactivity. A. X100; B. X40.

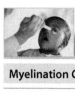

Table 26-4.

Myelination Cycles in the Human Nervous System, Based Upon Myelin Tissue Stains

Pathway	Begins (weeks gestation)	Completed (weeks gestation, or postnatal months or years)
Prenatal Onset		
Spinal motor roots	16	42 wk
Cranial motor nerves III, IV, V, VI, VII, X, XI, XII	20	28 wk
Spinal sensory roots	20	5 mo
Medial longitudinal fasciculus	24	28 wk
Acoustic nerve (cranial nerve VIII)	24	36 wk
Ventral commissure, spinal cord	24	4 mo
Trapezoid body and lateral lemniscus	25	36 wk
Inferior cerebellar peduncle (inner part)	26	36 wk
Inferior cerebellar peduncle (outer part)	32	4 mo
Superior cerebellar peduncle	28	6 mo
Middle cerebellar peduncle	42	3 y
Habenulopeduncular tract	28	34 wk
Dorsal columns, spinal cord	28	36 wk
Ansa reticularis	28	8 mo
Medial lemniscus	32	12 mo
Optic nerve	38	6 mo
Corticospinal tract	38	2 y
Geniculocalcarine tract (optic radiations)	40	6 mo
Thalamocortical acoustic radiations	40	3 y
Postnatal Onset		
Tornix	2 mo	2 y
Corpus callosum	2 mo	14 y
Mamillothalamic tract	8 mo	6 y
Ipsilateral frontotemporal and frontoparietal association axons	3 mo	32 y

Reproduced with permission from Sarnat HB. Cerebral Dysgenesis. Embryology and Clinical Expression. New York: Oxford University Press; 1992:61.

but periventricular sites in the telencephalon also may contribute new neurons. Primary olfactory neurons are continually regenerated.

The term *neural plasticity* is used to describe many processes, but fundamentally involves all the processes of neural development. Proliferation of stem cells is only one aspect; others include the formation of new dendritic spines, synapses, and synaptic circuits. For example, in the hippocampus, synaptic remodeling is used to form new memories. This is also the basis of learning and problem-solving in the neocortex.

Plasticity is much greater in the fetal and postnatal immature brain, than in the adult mature brain. The result is that damage, such as early fetal infarcts, may not necessarily cause a permanent deficit because some functions can be transferred to other healthy parts of the brain. For example, language functions can sometimes develop in the right cerebral hemisphere if the left hemisphere is damaged early in gestation.

Hemimegalencephaly is an asymmetrical malformation that develops early in fetal life, yet some children have no asymmetry of motor or sensory function because of the other side of the brain subserves both sides of the body. Similarly, hemicerebellar hemispheric infarcts early in gestation may not necessarily be expressed as ipsilateral tremor and dyssynergia because of the "rewiring" that enables the other preserved cerebellar hemisphere to provide motor coordination on both sides of the body.

Cysts form more readily in the fetal and postnatal brain than in the adult brain, which is more likely to form dense gliosis unless the infarct is very large. This is because the neonatal brain has about 6 times fewer astrocytes per unit volume of white matter than mature brain, and so is less able to mobilize glia. Thus, the neonatal brain tends to have larger infarcts because of the poor collateral circulation within the microvascular network of immature brain.

CNS MALFORMATIONS IN RELATION TO ONTOGENESIS

Historical Context

Until the era of molecular genetics of neural development, little was known about the pathogenesis of neural malformations, and thus they were classified in broad categories based upon descriptive morphology, such as disorders of neural tube closure, midline disorders, migratory disorders, and disturbances of cellular growth and differentiation. After it became clear that there is a precise spatial and temporal pattern of genetic expression in development, not only in the nervous system but in all other organs as well, classifications shifted to the opposite extreme, often ignoring morphogenesis and focusing on lists of gene defects. Morphology has been reintroduced by advances and refinements in neuroimaging, particularly magnetic resonance imaging (MRI), but these imaging techniques all have the inherent limitation of demonstrating only structural changes large enough to visualize with the naked eye. Microscopic differences in cells and protein and gene expression cannot be seen, even with the best imaging techniques available today. Thus the next frontier is to correlate anatomic findings in living patients with modern molecular genetics and modern neuropathology from postmortem studies of the same disorders.[36] An additional frontier that is only in incipient stages of correlation is of neurophysiologic alterations, in EEG in particular, among the various malformations, with aberrations of developmental processes such as synaptogenesis.[37]

Dysgeneses As Disorders of Gradients of Genetic Expression in Axes of the Neural Tube

As discussed earlier, genetic up-regulation, in the vertical axis in particular, results in hypertrophy and/or duplication of structures; down-regulation results in hypoplasia and/or noncleavage or fusion of structures.

Holoprosencephaly

Holoprosencephaly (HPE) is a prototype malformation that well illustrates the genetic gradients in all three major axes of the neural tube, as well as disturbances in neural induction of craniofacial development (Figure 26-9).[38,39] The strictly morphologic concept of holoprosencephaly is that it is a disorder of midline cleavage with several variants of uncertain relation to each other: alobar, semilobar, and lobar.[40] In addition to identifying many additional details of abnormal macroscopic and microscopic structure in HPE, Golden presented this malformation as an abnormality of genetic programming with the variants being degrees of severity.[40]

We attempted to further recognize the variants of the malformation as an overall problem of down-regulation of genes, with the length of their gradients in each of the axes explaining the degrees of morphologic and clinical expression, as well as the midfacial hypoplasia in some, but not all, cases. It is now recognized that there are six, and perhaps eight, distinctive genes in which mutations may cause the same forms of HPE, and that these only represent about 20% of total cases examined genetically; undoubtedly there will be many more genes discovered in the future. HPE is thus not a single disease with one etiology, but rather a syndrome that can be associated with many different genetic defects, but that all have a common mechanism to produce a similar or identical end result.

The variations of the mediolateral gradient of gene expression may explain many clinical features of HPE, such as the extent of mental retardation and cognitive deficiencies and the presence and severity of epilepsy. Only 41% of children with HPE have epilepsy,[42,43] by contrast with lissencephalic disorders, in which nearly 100% of patients are epileptic. Endocrine disorders also are complications of HPE,[43,44] another aspect of the rostrocaudal gradient of the longitudinal axis reaching the diencephalon. A related disorder, septo-optic-pituitary dysplasia (de Morsier syndrome), shares many embryologic aspects with HPE.[45]

Neural tube disorders

In addition to HPE, many other disorders of embryonic development of the neural tube can also be explained by gradients of genetic expression (Figure 26-10). In the spinal cord, duplication of the dorsal horns is an expression of up-regulation of a dorsalizing gene in the vertical axis; duplication of the central canal and, in more extreme form, complete diplomyelia, are due to up-regulation of a ventralizing gene.[38] Severe dysplasia of the spinal cord and a single midline ventral horn in the caudal regions of the spinal cord may occur in some cases of lumbosacral agenesis. This is explained by down-regulation of a ventralizing gene, *Sonic hedgehog*, but simultaneous disturbance in the caudorostral gradient of the longitudinal axis also is evident.[38] In the cerebellum, up-regulation in the dorsoventral gradient is associated with cerebellar vermal hypertrophy, whereas down-regulation in this gradient may result in rhombencephalosynapsis or agenesis of the vermis with fusion of the two lateral cerebellar hemispheres and the dentate nuclei. In the forebrain (telencephalon and diencephalon), up-regulation in the dorsoventral gradient may produce an abnormally thick corpus callosum and duplication of the hippocampus on one or both sides (the hippocampus begins its development as a dorsal structure in humans, but later rotates to a more ventral position; in rodents it remains a dorsal structure even in adult life). Down-regulation of the dorsoventral gradient in the forebrain produces agenesis of the corpus callosum, hypoplasia of the hippocampus, and hypotelorism because of a defective intercanthal ligament arising from the prosencephalic neural crest. These examples serve to emphasize a general principle that many CNS malformations can be understood in the context of gradients of genetic expression.

Dysgeneses As Disorders of Segmentation of the Neural Tube

Compartmentalization of the neural tube into neuromeres was discussed earlier. As with the gradients, both up-regulation and down-regulation of segmentation homeobox genes may be the basis of some malformations. In general, up-regulation may cause *ectopic expression* of a gene in neuromeres where it is not normally expressed. Down-regulation, by contrast, results in hypoplasia or even aplasia of the particular neuromeres that rely upon that gene for their integrity. A good example is the rare malformation, congenital agenesis of the mesencephalon and metencephalon (midbrain and rostral pons), which corresponds to the embryonic mesencephalic neuromere and rhombomere 1 and part of r2.

Up-regulation of segmental homeobox genes in murine models causes ectopic expression, so that more rostral structures might form in more caudal segments than normal. The most likely and most common human dysgenesis that might be attributed to such up-regulation is the Chiari II and Chiari III malformations.[46] This might also account for at least some cases of Chiari I malformations, but other mechanisms might also be involved. Chiari II malformations are nearly always associated with lumbosacral meningomyeloceles, and Chiari III also involves a posterior encephalocele. A molecular genetic segmental hypothesis of Chiari II malformation has been presented that can explain these other features, as well as the meningomyelocele.[46,47] The candidate gene is one of the *HOX* family. This particular homeobox gene family is primordial in embryonic hindbrain segmentation, but they also are essential for the formation of endochrondral, but not membranous, bone. Most of the cranial vault and facial skeleton is membranous bone, derived from neural crest. The basioccipital, exoccipital, and supraoccipital bones, however, are endochondral. These bones are hypoplastic in Chiari II malformation, explaining the low insertion of the convergence of venous sinuses at the torcula, which reduces the volume of the infratentorial space of the posterior fossa. HOX gene mutations can cause this and also can cause multiple primary brainstem dysgenesis, including aqueductal stenosis, dysplasias of the inferior olivary nuclei, and "tectal beaking" of the inferior colliculi. Because the whole spinal cord is derived from rhombomere 8, posterior neural tube defects also might result, and would not necessarily be expressed at all levels

of the spinal cord. Indeed, the meningomyelocele sometimes occurs at more rostral spinal levels.

Congenital Absence of Specific Types of Neurons

Regulator genes program late developmental events such as synaptogenesis and myelin formation. These genes are also are responsible for the differentiation of cell types, not only cellular lineage but the specific type of neuron or glial cell that develops, as discussed earlier.

In Dandy-Walker malformation and related disorders, a part of the cerebellum may be deficient, such as the posterior vermis, even though similar neurons with the same morphologic and metabolic profiles[48] are normal. This may be explained not as a genetic program of individual neurons but as a defect in gradients. A difference between the partial vermal agenesis in Dandy–Walker and Joubert syndromes from rhombencephalosynapsis is that the medial sides of the two cerebellar hemispheres remain separated by an extension of the subarachnoid space to replace the vermis, rather than fusing.

Defects in genetic regulation of cellular differentiation and growth result not only in malformations in which the architecture of neural tissue is disrupted, but also cause abnormalities in individual cells. Regions of both abnormal tissue organization and abnormal cells are called *hamartomas* (Figure 26-11). The most prominent examples of these diseases are tuberous sclerosis,[24] hemimegalencephaly,[25] and dysplastic gangliocytoma of the cerebellum (Lhermitte-Duclos disease).[1]

Disorders of Neuroblast Migration

This group of cerebral malformations is one of the best understood, because many genes responsible for specific malformations are now known, and because many features can be recognized macroscopically, allowing establishment of the diagnosis with neuroimaging and confirmation with specific genetic studies. Many of these disorders have distinctive facial dysmorphisms and clinical neurological features that enable them to be suspected from the initial history and physical examination, before any laboratory investigations are even carried out.

Neurons do not and cannot migrate. Migratory cells of neuronal lineage are neuroblasts; hence the term "neuronal migration" is a misnomer and, despite its widespread use, is more properly designated *neuroblast migration*. Axons may form during migration, but dendritic arborization awaits final positioning of the neuroblast. Heterotopia are embryologically defined as cells displaced within their organ of origin, and ectopia are cells displaced outside their organ of origin. Considering the brain as an organ or origin, a neuron abnormally displaced in the deep white matter is heterotopic, and a neuron isolated in the leptomeninges is ectopic. Heterotopia may be single cells or may be groups of cells to form nodules large enough to visualize by imaging.

Disorders of neuroblast migration are often readily diagnosed by neuroimaging because abnormal migration is associated with heterotopia and abnormal gyration, or lack of gyration, of the cerebral cortex. These heterotopia and convolutional abnormalities are so characteristic that the diagnosis frequently can be diagnosed from the MRI even without confirmation by genetic studies or postmortem neuropathologic examination. Such disorders can be divided into groups based upon where the migratory arrest has occurred, that is, how far the neurons were able to migrate before stopping.

In some malformations, there is little or no migration radially from the subventricular zone, and *periventricular nodular heterotopia* results. Another group is characterized by partial migration with arrest of migratory neuroblasts in the subcortical white matter to form a sheet of gray matter, *subcortical laminar heterotopia* or *band heterotopia* (also called "double cortex"), but this term is a poor one because the heterotopia are not organized as laminar cortex. One of the known genes that is defective in periventricular nodular heterotopia is called *Filamin-A* (*FLM-A*); the best known gene causing subcortical laminar heterotopia is *Doublecortin* (*DCX*). Both of these genes are essential for building microtubles that allow cellular motility. A third group consists of abnormal positioning of neurons within the cortical plate so that the cerebral cortex itself is abnormally laminated and has disoriented and displaced neurons in the wrong layers. *Reelin* (*RELN*) is an essential gene and its protein product signals the correct organization of the cortical plate. Reelin is secreted by Cajal-Retzius neurons of the molecular zone present in the preplate plexus before the first wave of migratory neurons arrives. Defective *RELN* results in abnormal lamination and orientation of neurons in the cortex (Figure 26-12).[6,27] The genes that cause Walker-Warburg syndrome or lissencephaly type II, *POM-T1*(locus 9q34.2) and *POM-T2* (locus 14q24.3), are important for the glycolysation of the cytoskeletal protein α-dystroglycan, which connects the neuronal cytoskeleton to extracellular matrix proteins, which is required for cell movements.[28,29] Striated muscle membranes also are affected, hence the coexpression of congenital muscular dystrophy. Overmigration beyond the pia mater into the leptomeninges, called *glioneuronal heterotopia*, also may occur. The breach in the glial limiting membrane and pia mater may be associated with a defect in the subpial granular glial layer of Brun. This feature is common to many neuroblast migratory disorders, but also is very common in holoprosencephaly, in which one of the more constant defects is a paucity or total absence of subpial granular glial cells of Brun.[1]

Appendix
James D. Geyer and Paul R. Carney

DISORDERS OF PRIMARY NEURULATION

Anencephaly

Anencephaly occurs because of a failure of anterior neuropore closure. Since the anterior neuropore closes at less than 24 days, this disorder occurs within the first month of fetal development. Anencephaly affects the forebrain and variable portions of brainstem but several different subtypes may occur depending on the level of the defect. Holoacrania occurs with a defect to the foramen magnum. Meroacrania occurs with the defects slightly higher than the foramen magnum.

Approximately 75% of these children are stillborn. It is most common in whites, Irish, females, and children born to either very old or very young mothers. The risk of anencephaly in subsequent pregnancies is 5% to 7%.

Myeloschisis

Myeloschisis develops with failure of *posterior* neuropore closure. It is associated with iniencephaly, or a malformation of skull base. Most of these children are stillborn.

Encephalocele

An encephalocele is a restricted defect in *anterior* neural tube closure. These defects consist of a protrusion of brain and intracranial structures through a skull defect. These are typically migration defects or heterotopia involving these patients. Approximately 75% occur in the occipital region and 50% are associated with hydrocephalus.

Myelomeningocele

A myelomeningocele develops secondary to a restricted defect in *posterior* neural tube closure. There is a herniation of the spinal cord or meninges through a vertebral defect. Most of these defects occur in the lumbar region. Approximately 90% of the cases with lumbar defects have associated hydrocephalus. If the defect occurs in some other region, only 60% of the patients have hydrocephalus. The symptoms include motor, sensory, and sphincter dysfunction. Spina bifida occulta occurs with a defect in the vertebral arch but no abnormalities of the spinal cord or meninges.

Chiari Malformations

Type I Chiari malformation is an isolated displacement of the cerebellar tonsils into the cervical canal. This may be either congenital or acquired in patients with low intracranial pressure. The type I malformation can be associated with a syrinx, a kinked cervical spinal cord, and hydrocephalus. Most of the type I patients have no associated symptoms. In rare cases, the patient may have headaches, tinnitus, or ataxia. In severe cases, surgical decompression is the primary treatment.

Type II Chiari malformation occurs with displacement of the cerebellum into cervical canal, displacement of the medulla and fourth ventricle into the cervical canal, a long, thin medulla and pons, tectum deformity, and skull base and upper cervical spine defects. Hydrocephalus is a common complication secondary to fourth ventricle obstruction or aqueductal stenosis. Myelomeningocele occurs in all patients and 96% have cortex malformations (heterotopia, polymicrogyria, etc.). Brainstem malformations are less common but occur in three-quarters of patients. Other common findings include cerebellar dysplasia, thoracolumbar kyphoscoliosis, diastematomyelia (bifid cord), and syringomyelia. The patient usually presents as a neonate with neurological deterioration including respiratory failure, stridor, and hydrocephalus. Treatment includes surgical decompression and shunting. Severe neurological sequelae typically persist.

Type III Chiari malformation includes all of the features of the type II malformation with herniation of the occipital lobes, cerebellum, and brainstem into an associated low occipital or high cervical encephalocele. The neurological consequences are severe and the outcome is poor.

Meckel syndrome occurs in some patients following *maternal hyperthermia* or fever on days 20 to 26 following conception. The features includes encephalocele, microcephaly, microphthalmia, cleft lip, polydactyly, polycystic kidneys, and ambiguous genitalia.

Neural Tube Defects

Neural tube defects occur in association with a number of disorders including chromosomal abnormalities (trisomy 13, trisomy 18), teratogens (thalidomide, valproate, phenytoin), single mutant gene (Meckel syndrome), and as a multifactorial syndrome. Diagnosis is made by increased alpha-fetoprotein, increased acetylcholinesterase, and by ultrasound. These defects can in some cases be prevented by maternal supplemental folate. The recurrence rate in subsequent children is 2% to 3%.

DISORDERS OF SECONDARY NEURULATION—OCCULT DYSRAPHIC STATES

The disorders of secondary neurulation have an intact dermal layer over the lesion but 80% have an overlying dermal lesion (dimple, hairy tuft, lipoma, or hemangioma). The spinal cord is frequently tethered. All patients have an abnormal conus and filum terminale. Most patients have vertebral defects. Siblings have a 4% chance of a disorder of primary neurulation.

1. Caudal regression syndrome—dysraphic sacrum and coccyx with atrophic muscle and bone
2. Myelocystocele—cystic central canal
3. Diastematomyelia—bifid cord
4. Meningocele—rare with no associated hydrocephalus
5. Lipomeningocele
6. Subcutaneous lipoma/teratoma
7. Dermal sinus

DISORDERS OF PROSENCEPHALIC DEVELOPMENT

Aprosencephaly is the absence of the telencephalon and diencephalon. Atelencephaly is the absence of the telencephalon but a normal diencephalon. The skull and skin are intact. These disorders are frequently associated with cyclopia, absent eyes, and abnormal limbs and genitalia.

Holoprosencephaly

Holoprosencephaly occurs with a defect in prosencephalic cleavage resulting in defective division of the hemispheres. All patients have anosmia because of absent olfactory bulbs and tracts. A single-lobed cerebrum and single ventricle are common. The optic nerve is either hypoplastic or single. There is agenesis of the corpus callosum. Neuronal migration defects are common. A number of caial defects can occur, including ethmocephaly (hypertelorism with proboscis between eyes), cebocephaly (single nostril), cyclopia (single eye with or without proboscis), and a cleft lip. Patients typically present with or develop seizures, apnea, decreased hypothalamic function, developmental delay, anosmia, and a single maxillary incisor. Several chromosomal abnormalities can lead to holoprosencephaly including trisomy 13, ring 13, and the SHH gene on chromosome 7. The recurrence rate for siblings is approximately 6%, and 2% are infants of diabetic mothers.

Disorders Associated with Agenesis of the Corpus Callosum
Holoprosencephaly
Absent septum pellucidum
Neuronal migration disorders, schizencephaly
Chiari II malformation
Septo-optic dysplasia/septo-opto-hypothalamic dysplasia
Aicardi syndrome

Disorders Associated with Congenital Hydrocephalus
Aqueductal stenosis—33%
Chiari malformation—28%
Communicating hydrocephalus—22%
Dandy-Walker Malformation—7%
Tumor
Vein of Galen obstruction
X-linked aqueductal stenosis

Dandy-Walker Malformation

The Dandy-Walker malformation occurs secondary to failed or delayed development of the foramen of Magendie. There is systic dilation of the fourth ventricle and cerebellar agenesis with maldevelopment of the cerebellar vermis. Hydrocephalus is a common complication. Many patients have agenesis of the corpus callosum, neuronal migration disorders (70%), a large inion, a large posterior fossa, cardiac anomalies, and urinary tract abnormalities. Seizures are a common complication.

NEURONAL PROLIFERATION AND MIGRATION DISORDERS

Disorders of Proliferation
Microcephaly—decreased *size* of proliferative units
Radial microbrain—decreased *number* of proliferative units
Macrencephaly—well-formed but large
Unilateral macrencephaly (hemimegencephaly)

Disorders of Migration

Schizencephaly occurs with a cleft or space connecting the ventricle and the subarachnoid space. There is no associated gliosis. Heterotopia frequently occur in the wall of the cleft. In type I, the lips of the cleft are closed or in contact with each other. In type II, the lips of the cleft are open and do not touch. Schizencephaly may be genetic or related to a sporadic ischemic insult early in gestation.

Porencephaly is a variable communication between the ventricles and the subarachnoid space. Unlike schizencephaly, there is gliosis in the cleft wall. Porencephaly is felt to be secondary to ischemia later in gestation.

Lissencephaly is a disorder of migration with the development of few or no gyri. This results in a "smooth brain." Heterotopia occur frequently in lissencephaly. Type I lissencephaly is associated with a partial deletion of chromosome 17 (the LIS1 gene). Type II lissencephaly is associated with a disorganized cortex, neuronal overmigration, and a thickened, somewhat cobblestone-appearing cortex. Pachygyria is a subtype of lissencephaly with a few broad thick gyri. Seizures, mental retardation, and death at an early age are common.

Miller–Dieker syndrome is associated with lissencephaly. There is a large chromosome 17 deletion in 90% of cases. The clinical presentation includes microcephaly, seizures, hypotonia, poor feeding, craniofacial defects, cardiac defects, and genital abnormalities.

Polymicrogyria occurs with too many small gyri, giving the brain the appearance of a wrinkled chestnut. This disorder usually occurs secondary to an ischemic injury or infection resulting in poor migration. Polymicrogyia occurs in X-linked dominant Aicardi syndrome. Inherited peroxisomal disorders such as Zellweger syndrome (cerebro-hepato-renal syndrome) may also result in polymicrogyria.

Heterotopia or remains of neurons in the white matter occur secondary to arrested radial migration. These heterotopia are frequently associated with seizures. There are several subtypes: periventricular, laminar (in deep white matter), and band-like (between cortex and ventricular surface).

REFERENCES

1. Sarnat HB. *Cerebral dysgenesis. Embryology and Clinical Expression.* New York: Oxford University Press; 1992.
2. Sarnat HB, Menkes JH. How to construct a neural tube. *J Child Neurol.* 2000;15:110-124.
3. Pinter JD, Sarnat HB. Neuroembryology. In: Winn HR, ed. *Youman's Neurological Surgery.* 5th ed. Philadelphia: Saunders; 2004;1:45-69.
4. Sarnat HB. CNS malformations. Gene locations of known human mutations. *Eur J Paediatr Neurol.* 2005;9: 427-431.
5. Sarnat HB, Flores-Sarnat L. Integrated morphological and molecular genetic classification of malformations of the CNS. *Am J Med Genet.* 2004;126A:386-392.
6. Sarnat HB, Flores-Sarnat L. Cajal-Retzius and subplate neurons: their role in cortical development. *Eur J Paediatr Neurol.* 2002;6:91-97.
7. Kay LM, Sherman SM. An argument for an olfactory thalamus. *Trends Neurosci.* 2007;30:49-53.
8. Sarnat HB, Flores-Sarnat L. Embryology of the neural crest: its inductive role in the neurocutaneous syndromes. *J Child Neurol.* 2005;20:637-643.
9. Lumsden A. The cellular basis of segmentation in the developing hindbrain. *Trends Neurosci.* 1990;13: 329-335.

10. McGinnis W, Krumlauf R. Homeobox genes and axial patterning. *Cell.* 1992;68:283-302.

11. De Pomerai D. *From Gene to Animal: An Introduction to the Molecular Biology of Animal Development.* 2nd ed. Cambridge, UK: Cambridge University Press; 1990.

12. Topilko P, Schneider-Maunoury S, Levi G, et al. *Krox-20* controls myelination in the peripheral nervous sytem. *Nature.* 1994;371:796-799.

13. Sauer FC. Mitosis in the neural tube. *J Comp Neurol.* 1935;62:377-405.

14. Smart IHM. Proliferative characteristics of the ependymal layer during the early development of the spinal cord in the mouse. *J Anat.* 1972;111:365-380.

15. Caviness VS Jr., Williams RS. Cellular pathology of developing human cortex. In: Katzman R, ed. *Congenital and Acquired Cognitive Disorders.* NY: Raven; 1979:669-689.

16. Okado N, Oppenheim RW. Cell death of motoneurons in the chick embryo spinal cord. *J Neurosci.* 1984;4:1639-1652.

17. LeGrand JN, Vanderluit J, Arbour N, et al. MCL-1 is required for neuronal survival. *Can J Neurol Sci.* 2007;34(suppl):S30. Abstract.

18. Crews L, Hunter D. Neurogenesis in the olfactory epithelium. *Perspect Dev Neurobiol.* 1994;2:151-161.

19. Pierre-Olivier BD, Parent A, Saghatelyan A. Role of sensory activity in the fate specification of newly generated cells in the adult olfactory bulb. *Can J Neurol Sci.* 2007;34(suppl):S24. Abstract.

20. Sarnat HB. Role of human fetal ependyma. *Pediatr Neurol.* 1992;8:163-178.

21. Dooling EC, Chi JG, Gilles FH. Ependymal changes in the human fetal brain. *Ann Neurol.* 1977;1:535-541.

22. Sarnat HB. Regional differentiation of the human fetal ependyma: immunocytochemical markers. *J Neuropathol Exp Neurol.* 1992;51:58-75.

23. Sarnat HB. Histochemistry and immunocytochemistry of the developing ependyma and choroid plexus. *Microsc Res Tech.* 1998;41:14-28.

24. Curatolo P, ed. *Tuberous Sclerosis Complex. From Basic Science to Clinical Phenotypes.* London, UK: MacKeith Press; 2003.

25. Flores-Sarnat L, Sarnat HB, Dávila-Gutiérrez G, Álvarez A. Hemimegalencephaly: part 2. Neuropathology suggests a disorder of cellular lineage. *J Child Neurol.* 2003;18:776-785.

26. Schmechel DE, Rakic P. Arrested proliferation of radial glial cells during midgestation in rhesus monkey. *Nature.* 1979;277:303-305.

27. Greesens P. Pathogenesis of migration disorders. *Curr Opin Neurol.* 2006;19:135-140.

28. Van Reeuwijk J, Janssen M, van den Elzen C, et al. *POMT2* mutations cause alpha-dystroglycan hypoglycosylation and Walker-Warburg syndrome. *J Med Genet.* 2005; 42:907-912.

29. Mendell JR, Boue DR, Martin PT. The congenital muscular dystrophies: recent advances and molecular insights. *Pediatr Devel Pathol.* 2006;9:427-443.

30. Sarnat HB, Flores-Sarnat L. Telencephalic flexures and schizencephaly. Submitted.

31. Sarnat HB, Flores-Sarnat L. Synaptogenesis of the developing human brain: hippocampus and neocortex. Synaptophysin reactivity in 162 fetuses and neonates from 6 to 41 weeks gestation. *J Neuropathol Exp Neurol.* 2009; in press.

32. Lemke G. The molecular genetics of myelination. An update. *Glia.* 1993;7:263-271.

33. Yu WP, Collarini EJ, Pringle NP, et al. Embryonic expression of myelin genes: evidence for a focal source of oligodendrocyte precursors in the ventricular zone of the neural tube. *Neuron.* 1994;12:1353-1362.

34. Noll E, Miller RH. Regulation of oligodendrocyte differentiation: a role for retinoic acid in the spinal cord. *Development.* 1994;120:649-660.

35. Yakovlev PI, Lecours AR. The myelination cycles of regional maturation of the brain. In: Minkowski A, ed. *Regional Development of the Brain in Early Life.* Philadelphia: Davis; 1967:3-70.

36. Barkovich AJ. *Pediatric Neuroimaging.* 4th ed. Philadelphia, PA: Lippincott Williams & Wilkins; 2005:30-41.

37. Sarnat HB, Flores-Sarnat L, Trevenen CL. Synaptogenesis in the human fetal hippocampus and neocortex. *J Neuropathol Exp Neurol.* 2009:in press.

38. Sarnat HB. Molecular genetic classification of central nervous system malformations. *J Child Neurol.* 2000; 15:675-687.

39. Sarnat HB, Flores-Sarnat L. Neuropathologic research strategies in holoprosencephaly. *J Child Neurol.* 2001;16:918-931.

40. Golden JA. Holoprosencephaly: a defect in brain patterning. *J Neuropathol Exp Neurol.* 1998;57:991-999.

41. Friede RI. *Developmental Neuropathology.* 2nd ed. Berlin: Springer-Verlag; 1989.

42. Hahn, JS, Pinter JD. Holoprosencephaly: genetic, neuroradiological and clinical advances. *Semin Pediatr Neurol.* 2002;9:309-319.

43. Hahn JS. Holoprosencephaly. In: Sarnat HB, Curatolo P, eds. *Elsevier Handbook of Clinical Neurology.* Vol. 87, 3rd series. New York: Elsevier. 2008;13-38.

44. Hahn JS, Hahn SM, Kammann H, et al. Endocrine disorders associated with holoprosencephaly. *J Pediatr Endocrinol Metab.* 2005;18:935-941.

45. Humphreys P. Septo-optic-pituitary dysplasia. In: Sarnat HB, Curatolo P, eds. *Elsevier Handbook of Clinical Neurology.* Vol. 87, 3rd series. New York: Elsevier. 2008;39-52.

46. Sarnat HB. Regional ependymal upregulation of vimentin in Chiari II malformation, aqueductal stenosis and hydromyelia. *Pediatr Dev Pathol.* 2004;7:48-60.

47. Sarnat HB. Disorders of segmentation of the neural tube: Chiari malformations. In: Sarnat HB, Curatolo P, eds. *Elsevier Handbook of Clinical Neurology.* 2007;82: in press.

48. Russo R, Fallet-Bianco C. Isolated posterior cerebellar vermal defect: a morphological study of midsagittal cerebellar vermis in 4 fetuses—early stage of Dandy-Walker continuum or new vermal dysgenesis? *J Child Neurol.* 2007;22:492-500.

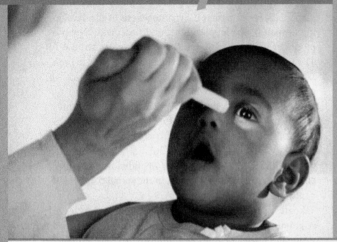

CHAPTER 27

Autism

Richard E. Frye

DEFINITIONS AND EPIDEMIOLOGY

Autism spectrum disorder (ASD) is a behaviorally defined neurologically-based developmental disorder with an onset before 3 years of age. ASD encompasses three diagnoses: autism, Asperger disorder (AD), and pervasive developmental disorders not otherwise specified (PDD-NOS). Autism is defined by abnormal development and/or regression in social interaction and communication along with repetitive and stereotyped interests and behaviors.[1] Although the DSM-IV-TR also lists disintegrative and Rett disorder as subtypes of ASD, the former is rarely diagnosed and the latter is recognized as a distinct neurodegenerative disorder. Diagnosis of autism is usually made around the age of 18 to 24 months, although, upon reflection, parents typically report concerns in the first year of life. This gap between parents' early concerns and the relatively late diagnosis, along with the importance of early intervention, highlights the necessity to find reliable tools for early diagnosis. Recent studies have suggested that symptoms of autism may be detectable as early as 14 months of age using standardized assessments.[2] ASD associated with developmental regression accounts for approximately one-third of the cases and usually occurs between the first and second years of life. Late-onset developmental regression, particularly after 3 years of age, highly suggests an underlying neurological disorder.

The prognosis of ASD is variable. It has been estimated that 40% to 70% of children with ASD will manifest subnormal intellectual function with higher early levels of intellectual, adaptive, language, and social function predictive of later autism symptoms and acquisition of cognitive skills.[3-5] Data collected through the Autism and Developmental Disabilities Monitoring Network from 14 surveillance areas in the United States suggest that the average prevalence of ASD as 6.6 per 1000 children (approximately 1:150), with this prevalence ranging from 3.3 to 10.6 per 1000 children.[6] These data also suggested that the previously noted increase in the prevalence of ASD has recently stabilized and confirmed previous reports that ASD is more prevalent in males than females with a ratio ranging from 3.4:1 to 6.5:1.[6]

The etiology of ASD is unknown, but it is becoming clear that ASD probably results from a genetically vulnerable individual being exposed to an environmental agent or endogenous stressor during a critical period in development. This so-called *triple hit hypothesis* attempts to account for both the complex nature of this disorder and lack of simple associations found between ASD and genetic markers.[7] Investigation of environmental pollutants has been facilitated by modern information technology. Studies have linked clinical databases coordinated by the Centers for Disease Control and Prevention with monitoring databases from the Environmental Protection Agency.[8,9] Such studies have suggested that environmental toxins, particularly mercury, may be related to an increased risk of ASD.[8-10] The role of immunizations containing thimerosal, a mercury-containing preservative, is still unclear. While recent large-scale studies have demonstrated little influence of thimerosal on neuropsychological outcomes in childhood,[11] meta-analysis of epidemiologic studies and a comparison of outcomes of children receiving vaccines containing different amounts of thimerosal have indicated the possibility of a link between thimerosol and ASD.[12,13] Regardless of the safety of thimerosal-containing vaccines, it is clear that the public perception of vaccine safety could significantly affect the health of children.[14-16]

Known genetic syndromes associated with ASD are discussed later in this chapter, but these probably account for less than 10% of individuals diagnosed with ASD.[17] Twin studies suggest a strong genetic component, but genetic studies that have evaluated candidate genes or whole genome screens have failed to find one genetic cause. Researchers have focused on several schemes to increase the sensitivity of their analysis, including examining the genetic basis of endophenotypes,[18,19] using large samples derived from the Autism Genetic Resource Exchange,[20] and examining the shared genetic pathways between known genetic syndromes associated with ASD.[21] Most researchers have concluded that multiple genes interact to predispose an individual to developing ASD.[17]

PATHOGENESIS

Table 27-1 lists the reported anatomic brain abnormalities found in ASD. Abnormalities in cortical white[22-25] and gray[24,26,27] matter, the limbic system,[28-31] particularly the hippocampus and amygdala,[32,33] as well as in the cerebellum,[24,26,28,34] have been reported. The functional and developmental significance of these neuropathologic abnormalities has led to speculation regarding pathogenic mechanisms underlying ASD. The reduced number of Purkinje cells in the cerebellum with few significant changes in the inferior olive may point to a prenatal onset.[28] The abnormally increased white matter volume has been proposed to be the result of an increase in the short association fibers in the frontal and temporal lobes due to an increased number of microcolumns.[22] This, in turn, has been proposed to result in too much intracortical communication, an imbalance between local and distant cortical communication, and a deficit in large-scale cortical integration that is required for

high-order cognitive processes such as language, behavioral regulation, and context-based social interactions. Abnormalities of the amygdala have been linked to abnormal fear conditioning in animal models.[35] Clearly ASD is associated with widespread abnormalities of brain development, but the timing, localization, and links between these abnormalities are still not known. In addition, the connection between these neuropathologic findings and the derailment of cognitive development is a matter of intense debate. As discussed next, these abnormalities may be related to abnormal brain growth, maturation, and/or immune system dysregulation.

Brain growth appears to be dysregulated in ASD. Several lines of evidence point to an acceleration in brain growth during the first years of life followed by premature cessation of further brain growth by early childhood.[36,37] A retrospective examination of head circumference (HC) measurements during the first 2 years of life demonstrated that HC growth was greater in every child with autism as compared to children with PDD-NOS and typically developing children.[26] More recent prospective studies suggest that the accelerated growth is not isolated to the cranium, but may be a part of a more general dysregulation in growth[38] related to higher levels of growth-related hormones.[39] While reports have linked an early acceleration in HC to brain volume[23,40] other studies suggest that the increase in HC is better correlated with increases in non-neural tissue volume.[41]

Several lines of evidence point to abnormalities of the immune system. Investigators have identified autoantibodies to neural tissue, including neuron-axon filament proteins, cerebellar neurofilaments, myelin basic protein, caudate, serotonin receptors and endothelial cells, abnormal cytokine levels in the CSF and blood, and alterations in the number and activity of T cells, monocytes, and natural killer cells.[42] The important role of the immune system in nervous system development is being increasingly realized. For example, major histocompatibility complex-deficient mouse models demonstrate abnormal synaptic pruning[43] and an absence of long-term depression.[44] A link between immune system dysfunction and autism would help explain the association of autism with prenatal and postnatal infections, familial autoimmunity, gastrointestinal inflammation, animal models, and findings of immune system dysregulation.[42]

CLINICAL PRESENTATION

Medical History

Gestational and neonatal

In utero exposure to several agents is associated with an increased incidence of ASD (Table 27-2). Fetal anticonvulsant syndrome associated autistic disorder was

Table 27-1.

Neuropathology of Autism

Head Circumference	Abnormal Growth and Size[36]
White matter	Increased volume on MRI[23,24]
Gray matter	Increased volume on MRI[24,26]
	Smaller, more compact and numerous minicolumns in frontotemporal areas[27]
Corpus callosum	Small compared to brain size[25]
Limbic system	Reduced neuronal size and increased packing density[28,29]
Amygdala	Abnormal volume on MRI[32,33]
Hippocampi	Decreased CA1 and CA4 dendritic branching[30]
	Smaller CA4 neurons[30]
	Increased volume on MRI[31]
Cerebellum	Increased volume on MRI[24,26]
	Vermis agenesis[34]
	Reduced Purkinje and granule cells[28]

Table 27-2.

Medical History Associated with Autism

Gestational	*Medications:* Anticonvulsants,[45,46] thalidomide,[47]
	Drugs: Alcohol,[48] cocaine[49]
	Viral Infections: CMV, rubella, and measles[50]
	Newly Diagnosis Medical Condition: Asthma, allergy[63]
Medical	*Sleep Disruption:* Behavioral sleep problem,[55] circadian sleep–wake problems,[55] anxiety-associated sleep disorder[55]
	Early Brain Injury: Amygdala,[53] cerebellum,[51] neonatal encephalopathy[52]
	Gastrointestinal: Ileo-colonic lymphoid nodular hyperplasia,[57] inflammation of the colorectum, small bowel and stomach[57]
Development	Regression in language, motor or social skills
	Speech, motor, or social delay
	Reciprocal interactions
Family	Twin or sibling with autism[59,68]
	Relatives with PDD,[61] anxiety,[61] OCD,[61] autoimmune thyroid disease,[64,65] rheumatic fever[65]
	Father with type 1 diabetes[66]
	Mother with ulcerative colitis,[66] psychiatric disorders,[62] personality disorders,[62] psoriasis[63]
Social	Maternal and paternal age[69]
	Environmental pollutants[8–10]

described in 4.6% of children exposed to either sodium valproate or carbamazepine in utero.[45] In utero phenytoin and diazepam exposure in combination with sodium valproate or carbamazepine has also been associated with ASD.[46] Older studies have documented the link between thalidomide and maternal alcohol and cocaine intake, and in utero viral infections to an increased risk of ASD.[47-50] Nonfocal and focal brain damage early in life has also been associated with ASD.[51-53]

Medical

The prevalence of sleep disorders in children with autism ranges between 44% and 83%.[54] Behavioral sleep problems appear to be the most common, but circadian sleep–wake problems are also common. Many children manifest multiple sleep problems.[55] Sleep problems are important to address since sleep disturbance has been associated with impaired daytime function, appetite, and growth.[54,56]

Children with ASD have been documented to have a higher prevalence of ileo-colonic lymphoid nodular hyperplasia,[57] although the risk of gastrointestinal disorders in general may not be elevated.[58] It is

important to recognize gastrointestinal symptoms, since such symptoms can result in behavioral instability, and improvement of such symptoms may improve functional outcome.

Development

Children with ASD typically have a history of developmental delay or regression in early language and social development. Fine-motor milestones are also typically affected but gross motor milestones are usually intact.

Family

Monozygous twins have a very high concordance rate (approximately 80%) of ASD symptoms while dizygous twins demonstrate a much lower concordance rate (approximately 10%), suggesting a clear genetic component in the development of ASD.[59] Recurrence risk of idiopathic ASD in siblings is estimated to be approximately 5% to 10%.[59] A family history of psychiatric, but not neurological, disease has been associated with ASD.[60-62] While several studies have found increases in specific autoimmune diseases in family relatives of individuals with ASD (Table 27-2), others have not.[63-66] Interestingly, while one study did not find a major association between ASD and a specific autoimmune diseases, it did find that the risk of ASD increased as the numbers of family members with autoimmune disease increased, supporting the idea of an interaction between a general immune defect and the environment.[67]

Social

Both advanced maternal and paternal age are independently associated with an increase risk of ASD.[68,69] As described in the previous section, environmental pollutants, particularly mercury, appear to be associated with a higher risk of ASD.[8-10]

Symptoms

Delay or regression of early language and social development constitute the core symptoms of ASD (Table 27-3). Regression of skills may be subtle, especially if early, representing a minor loss in attained skills with a static developmental course. Some children will also present with fluctuations in language development, with parents noting both gain and loss of language skill. Some children lose or never attain typical early language, such as "mama" or "dada," and instead gain rather idiosyncratic words or phrases. When ASD children start to speak in more than one word, the phrases used are atypical, usually being very stereotypical "scripted" phrases without pronouns. In addition, once recognizable speech develops, the intonation and volume is rather inconsistent and odd and may even have a sing-song type quality.

Table 27-3.

Symptoms Associated with Autism

Language	Immediate and delayed echolalia, scripted and/or stereotyped phases and language, poor modulation of volume, odd intonation
Behavior	Aloof, alone
	Hyperfocused, hyperactive, staring episodes
	Poor eye contract
	Does not point for wants
	Poor initiation and maintenance of friendships
	Poor temperament, upset by change in routine
	Stereotype and/or repetitive movements
Neurological	Poor fine motor skills, seizures
Gastroenterologic	Constipation, diarrhea

Children with ASD lack well-modulated social interactions. It is important to differentiate between a child who does not interact because of a severe speech delay from one who truly has an underlying abnormality in social development. It is not the quantity of eye contact per se that suggests ASD, but the ability of the child to use eye contact to initiate, terminate, and regulate social interactions. Children with ASD are usually aloof and alone, choosing to play by themselves rather than seeking social interactions. They do not indicate their wants by pointing and may lead their parent by the hand to the item they want. Attention is dysregulated rather than purely increased or decreased. For example, sometimes children will be hyperfocused whereas other times attention will appear absent, sometimes accompanied by hyperactivity. While alone and hyperfocused, a child with ASD may line up small cars or other objects. As the ASD child becomes older and enters school, he or she has difficulties both initiating and maintaining friendships and typically requires significant assistance with social interactions.

Behavior is typically tenuous in children with ASD and can change very easily. Behavioral outbursts and tantrums are not unusual and can be a daily occurrence even in the high-functioning school-aged ASD child. Children with ASD can become very upset by change in routine or even on a daily basis due to the change from one classroom to another. One of the core components of ASD is stereotypical repetitive movements or interests. Motor stereotypies may arise during times of excitement or frustration and may be manifested by typical hand-flapping or spinning or, sometimes, more idiosyncratic complex movements.

Physical and Neurological Examination

There are limited, but key, examination findings in children with ASD (Table 27-4). Children should be monitored for unusual growth patterns and the physical examination should concentrate on dysmorphology and neurocutaneous stigmata in order to identify

Table 27-4.

Physical and Neurological Findings Associated with Autism

Physical Examination	
Growth	Weight and head circumference
Dysmorphic features ·	Associated with syndromes listed in Table 27-5
Skin with Woods lamp	Neurocutaneous stigmata associated with tuberous sclerosis
Neurological Examination	
Language	Echolalaia
	Scripted and/or stereotyped phases and language
	Poor modulation of volume and/or odd intonation
Behavior	Hyperfocused, hyperactive, uninhibited
	Poor use of eye contact to regulate social interaction
	Poor initiation and maintenance of social interaction
	Motor impersistence, imitative behavior
Motor	Hypotonia, complex stereotyped movements
Gait	Asymmetric gait with running

Table 27-5.

Genetic Disorders Associated with ASD

Disorder	Prevalence in Disorder (%)
Angelman syndrome[70]	2
Cornelia Down de Lange[71]	53
Fragile X syndrome[72-74]	2
Möbius sequence[76]	40
Prader-Willi syndrome[70]	25
Smith-Lemli-Opitz syndrome[75]	50
Velocardiofacial syndrome[77]	50

Table 27-6.

Medical Disorders Presenting as ASD

Metabolic	Mitochondrial disorders
	■ Respiratory chain complex deficiencies[78–82]
	■ Coenzyme Q10[79]
	■ Aspartate-glutamate carrier SLC25A12[83,84]
	■ mtDNA mutation and depletion[82,85,86]
	■ HEADD[82]
	■ Long-chain acyl-CoA dehydrogenase[87]
	■ X-linked creatine transporter deficiency[88]
	Urea cycle disorder[92]
	Organic acidemia[93]
	Partial biotinidase deficiency[94,95]
	Cerebral folate deficiency[96]
Neurological	Tuberous sclerosis complex[87,98–100]
	Rett disorder[101]
	Migrational anomalies[107]
	Epileptic
	■ Epileptiform aphasia/encephalopathy[105]
	■ Nonspecific epileptiform abnormalities[103,104]
	■ Landau-Kleffner syndrome[103–106]
	■ Electrical status epilepticus during slow-wave sleep[106]

underlying genetic syndromes (Table 27-5) or tuberous sclerosis complex (TSC). Neurological examination should initially concentrate on cognitive factors, looking for symptoms described earlier and listed in Table 27-3. It is very difficult to perform a formal examination on many patients, but those who will cooperate may demonstrate "frontal" signs such as motor impersistence and may even imitate and mirror the examiner's movements. Hypotonia is not an uncommon finding on motor examination, and reflexes are sometimes generally depressed. Findings of hypertonia, dystonia, weakness, spasticity, or brisk reflexes would suggest a primary underlying neurological disease. Complex stereotyped mannerisms are not uncommon, but dyskinesia or choreoathetoid movements are abnormal for ASD. Gait tends to be asymmetric, with the child leading with one side of the body, particularly during running.

DIFFERENTIAL DIAGNOSIS

Genetic Disorders

Genetic disorders commonly associated with ASD and the prevalence of ASD in these disorders are given in Table 27-5.[70-77]

Metabolic Disorders

Although mitochondrial dysfunction has been associated with ASD (Table 27-6), it remains unclear whether such dysfunction is secondary to other underlying conditions or the primary biochemical abnormality leading to ASD.[78-89] Mitochondrial abnormalities underlie hypotonia, epilepsy, autism, and developmental delay (HEADD) syndrome.[82] Association and linkage studies have associated ASD with aspartate-glutamate carrier SLC25A12

gene single-nucleotide polymorphisms,[83,84] although some have not been able to confirm this finding[90] and such polymorphisms are not associated with biochemical abnormalities.[91] Several isolated cases of other metabolic disorders have also been associated with ASD.[92-96] Most of these reported cases manifested abnormal EEGs and seizures. CSF organic acids may have abnormal levels of ethanolamine.[97]

Neurological Disorders

ASD is found in 25% to 50% of individuals with TSC, but this only represents between 1% and 4% of patients with ASD.[98] The total number of TSC lesions appears to be associated with autistic features, and studies have suggested that lesions in the right frontal and temporal lobes are more common in ASD patients who also have TSC.[87,99,100] Rett syndrome should be considered in any female with language regression, characteristic hand-wringing, and acquired microcephaly. Such girls should undergo genetic testing for the MeCP2 mutation.[101]

The relationship between epilepsy and autism is complicated. Children with ASD associated with a known genetic syndrome have a particularly high rate of clinical motor seizures. However, epileptic aphasia with subclinical seizures may also be particularly prevalent in ASD.[102] The prevalence of EEG abnormalities was found to range from 30%[103] to 60%[104] using 24-hour EEG monitoring, while a prevalence of epileptiform abnormalities was approximately 82% using MEG.[105] The significance and prevalence of subclinical epileptiform activity in ASD is unknown. Language regression and autistic-like behavior can be observed in epileptiform aphasias, such as Landau–Kleffner syndrome (LKS) and electrical status-epilepticus during slow-wave sleep (ESES).[106] Brain lesions and migrational anomalies have also been associated with ASD.[51,53,73,107]

DIAGNOSIS

Behavioral Evaluation

Few reliable tools are available for screening children younger than 18 months, but the AAP recommends the Communication and Symbolic Behavior Scales Developmental Profile Infant/Toddler Checklist.[108] Screening tools for toddlers and children older than 18 months fall into two categories: level 1, shorter questionnaires used to screen for children at-risk for ASD; and level 2, longer questionnaires combined with clinical examination that require more experienced clinical acumen. Level 2 helps differentiate ASD from global developmental delay and specific language impairment.[109-113] The more reliable tools are outlined in Table 27-7. Verification of the diagnosis of ASD should involve more in-depth examination and caretaker interview. The Autism Diagnostic Observation Schedule (ADOS) combined with the Autism Diagnostic Interview (ADI) have become a standard, at least for research studies. These instruments require specialized training and their accuracy may be improved by an extended developmental examination that includes an evaluation of language and adaptive functioning.[114-117] If the neurologist believes that the child has any other developmental or behavioral disorders regardless of signs and symptoms of ASD, the patient should be referred to a psychologist, neuropsychologist, or physical or occupational therapist if appropriate.

Neurological Studies

The particularly high prevalence of epileptiform abnormalities in ASD children without clinical seizures suggests a screening EEG study should be conducted.[102] Although a routine EEG that includes sleep can be used, it is often difficult to obtain an adequate study, usually because the child needs to be sedated for lead placement. Thus, it is preferable to obtain a 24-hour overnight EEG in order to collect an adequate sample of sleep without medication effect and to determine the frequency and severity of epileptiform abnormalities.[103,104,106]

Table 27-7.

Diagnostic Tests

Behavioral Evaluations	
Level 1 screening tools	Autism: Checklist for Autism in Toddlers[109,110]
	Asperger: Childhood Asperger Syndrome Test[111]
Level 2 screening tools	Autism: Autism Diagnostic Rating Scale[112]
	Asperger: Krug Asperger's Disorder Index[113]
Autism diagnostic tools	Autism Diagnostic Interview[114–116]
	Autism Diagnostic Observation Schedule[114–116]
Neurological Studies	
Neurophysiological tests	24-hour EEG[103,104,106]
	Magnetoencephalography[105]
Neuroimaging tests	Magnetic resonance imaging[51,53,73,107,118]
	Magnetic resonance spectroscopy[88]
	Diffusion tensor imaging[119–121]
	Volumetric imaging[122,123]
	PET[107]
Other Medical Studies	
Metabolic	Ammonia, serum[124]
	Amino acids, serum: alanine[78,124]
	Aspartate aminotransferase, serum[78]
	Carnitine, serum[124]
	Creatine, urine, and serum[73,88]
	Creatine kinase[78]
	Folic acid (5-methyltetrahydrofolate), CSF[96]
	Folic acid transporter antibody, serum[125]
	Guanidinoacetic acid, urine, and serum[73,88]
	Lactate, serum[78,80,91,124]
	Organic acids, urine[73,80]
	Pyruvate, serum[91,124]
	Respiratory chain complex activities, muscle[80]
Genetic studies	Karyotype[73,74]
	Chromosomal microarray[131]
	PTEN tumor suppressor gene[74,126–130]
	Targeted genetic syndromes (Tables 27-5 and 27-6).

The location of the epilepsy focus may be related to ASD symptoms in children with epileptic aphasia. For example, although both LKS and ESES have manifestations of language regression, autistic type behavior is more common in ESES. The cortical distribution of epileptic discharges is different in these two groups.[106] MEG provides a superior ability to localize the focus of discharges and has been used to show a correspondence between behavior and location of epileptiform discharges. Indeed, MEG has demonstrated that the primary epileptiform activity may be limited to the left perisylvian region in children with LKS, while autistic children may manifest epileptiform abnormalities similar to the children with LKS plus independent epileptiform activity outside of the left perisylvian region, particularly in the right perisylvian and/or frontal regions.[105] Taken together, EEG and MEG studies appear to suggest that autistic symptoms are associated with more widespread epileptiform disturbance, with a possible implication of disturbances within the frontal cortex being related to autistic-type behavior, and suggest a pivotal role of neurophysiological studies in ASD.

Anatomic neuroimaging has uncovered lesions and migrational anomalies in children with ASD.[51,53,73,107] Lesions such as Chiari I malformation could explain unexplainable discomfort in ASD.[118] Magnetic resonance spectroscopy is essential for diagnosing a creatine deficiency.[88] One study suggests that PET may be useful after an initially unremarkable MRI scan since subtle neuronal migrational anomalies may be more obvious after knowledge of a regional metabolic abnormality.[107] PET may be particularly useful when EEG or MEG abnormalities are found and the anatomic MRI is normal. Other more advanced imaging methods may be well suited for diagnosing ASD, especially as these tools undergo rapid development and application to the clinical arena. For example, diffusion-weighted and tensor imaging demonstrates abnormalities in corpus callosum and cortical white matter anisotropy and diffusivity as well as white matter maturation,[119-121] and cortical volumetric changes have been associated with social and intellectual function in ASD.[122,123]

Metabolic Studies

Biochemical markers of mitochondrial dysfunction can be subtle. A combination of subtle abnormalities should raise the clinician's index of suspicion for a mitochondrial disorder. Some have suggested that mitochondrial disorders may be reflected by slight abnormalities in carnitine and lactate accompanied by more significant elevations in alanine and ammonia,[124] while others have suggested that slight elevations in creatine kinase and aspartate aminotransferase[78] can be associated with mitochondrial disorders. Case reports of creatine and cerebral folic acid deficiency suggest specific testing for these disorders. It should be noted that the child reported with cerebral folic acid deficiency demonstrated normal folic acid metabolite levels in non-nervous system tissues. The possibility of antibodies to the folate

transporter was not investigated in this reported case. Such a possibility could be ruled out with a serum test if lumbar puncture is contraindicated or difficult.[125]

Genetic Studies

Karyotype testing has been useful in identifying chromosomal abnormalities.[73,74] Dysmorphology, neurocutaneous stigmata, or a neurological course associated with Rett syndrome should suggest specific genetic testing. The *PTEN* tumor suppressor gene has been identified in significantly macrocephalic ASD patients.[74,126-130] A high frequency of cryptic chromosomal rearrangements has been identified by noncommercial chromosomal microarray in ASD patients.[131] Commercial chromosomal microarray products have not been evaluated in ASD, but the ability of these techniques to detect mutations associated with genetic syndromes associated with ASD as well as cryptic mutations make the cost-effectiveness of such products outstanding.

Workup

Although individually the various underlying abnormalities reported to underlie ASD may not seem to account for a substantial percentage of the ASD population, when added together, underlying medical abnormalities could account for a substantial percentage of the children with ASD. Most children with ASD do not receive a medical workup. With the large number of children diagnosed each year with ASD, identifying and treating an underlying etiology in even a small percentage of the population of children with ASD can have an incredible impact.

While Figures 27-1 and 27-2 outline the stepwise work up for the diagnosis of ASD and the investigation of underlying genetic abnormalities, Figure 27-3 provides an overview of the neurological workup. Any child with unexplained ASD should obtain a comprehensive workup including a 24-hour EEG, MRI, MRS, and complete metabolic testing as outlined in Table 27-7 (Figure 27-3). Further workup to determine the location of the focal abnormality using MEG or PET should be considered in children with focal or multifocal findings on EEG. Confirmed abnormal metabolic laboratory values, especially those that may represent mitochondrial dysfunction, should be investigated with pathologic and/or biochemical functional studies of the muscle, leukocytes, or skin.

TREATMENT

Treatment options are summarized in Tables 27-8 and 27-9 and Figure 27-2.

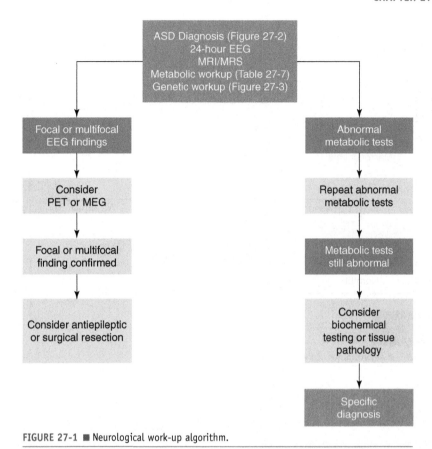

FIGURE 27-1 ■ Neurological work-up algorithm.

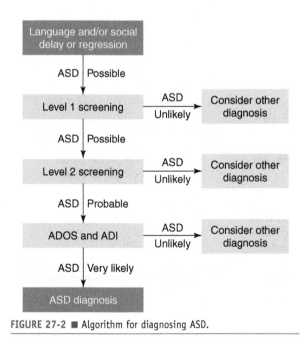

FIGURE 27-2 ■ Algorithm for diagnosing ASD.

Behavior

Stimulant medication such as methylphenidate, the selective norepinephrine reuptake inhibitor atomoxetine, alpha-adenergics such as clonidine, and antipsychotics such as risperidone, are useful for controlling behaviors such as hyperactivity, impulsivity, inattention, aggression, and explosive outbursts in children with ASD.[132-137] Several controlled trials have demonstrated the efficacy of selective serotonin reuptake inhibitors in improving anxiety, repetitive behaviors, and global functioning.[138-144]

Epilepsy

Common clinical epilepsy in ASD should be treated similarly to epilepsy in non-ASD patients, keeping in mind that side effects from anti-epileptic medications may manifest as severe behavioral dysregulation.[102] Many children with LKS or ESES respond to more specific anti-epileptic medications (high-dose sodium valproate with or without ethosuximide, benzodiazepines) and/or immunomodulatory treatment (steroids and intravenous immunoglobulin) in various treatment protocols.[145-148] Multiple subpial transections have been used in refractory cases with success.[146-148]

Metabolic Disorders

Children with underlying mitochondrial disorders should be provided with the standard mitochondrial

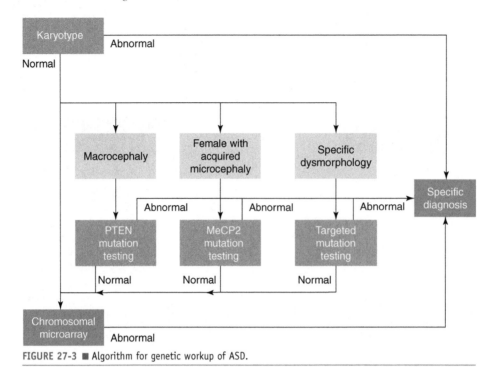

FIGURE 27-3 ■ Algorithm for genetic workup of ASD.

Table 27-8.

Treatments for Autism

Behavioral

Hyperactivity, impulsivity, inattention, aggression, and explosive outbursts	Atomoxetine[132]
	Clonidine[134]
	Methylphenidate[136]
	Risperidone[137]
Anxiety and repetitive behaviors	Citalopram[141]
	Escitalopram[139]
	Fluoxetine[142]
	Fluvoxamine[143]
	Sertraline[144]

Epilepsy

Clinical motor seizures	Standard antiepileptic therapy[102]
Epileptiform regression	Valproate[145–147]
	Valproate + ethosuxamide[145–147]
	Benzodiazepines[146,147]
	Multiple subpial transections[146–148]
	Steroids[146,147]
	Intravenous immunoglobulin[146,147]

Metabolic Disorders

Cerebral folate deficiency	Folinic acid [96]
Mitochondrial disorders	Mitochondrial cocktail

Sleep Disorders

Restless sleep and low ferritin insomnia	Iron supplementation[152]
	Ramelteon,[153] melatonin[154,155]

Table 27-9.

Medication Doses

Atomoxetine	20-100 mg/d[132]
Citalopram	5-40 mg/d[141]
Clonidine	0.1-0.3 mg/d[134]
Elemental iron	6 mg/kg/d[152]
Escitalopram	2.5-20 mg/d[139]
Ethosuxamide (ESM)	Combined with VPA: 13-37 mg/kg/d[145]
Fluoxetine	2.4-20 mg/d[142]
Fluvoxamine	1-3 mg/kg/d[143]
Folinic acid	0.5-1.0 mg/kg/d[96]
Melatonin	1-6 mg at bedtime Fast Release, 2 mg at bedtime Controlled Release[154,155]
Methylphenidate	10-50 mg/d[136]
Ramelteon	4-8 mg at bedtime[153]
Risperidone	0.5-3.5 mg/d[137]
Sertraline	25-200 mg/d[144]
Sodium valproate (VPA)	High-dose: 52-144 mg/kg/d[145] Combined with ESM: 18-36 mg/kg/d[145]

cocktail of the clinician's institution. This cocktail should be modified if a specific mitochondrial disorder is identified. Cerebral folic acid deficiency improves with folinic acid supplementation.[96] A trial of folinic acid may be appropriate while awaiting the results of metabolic and antibody testing. However, the clinician should be aware that the CSF levels of 5-methyltetrahydrofolate may normalize with folinic acid supplementation, making measurement of 5-methyltetrahydrofolate in the CSF prior to supplementation preferable. The development of two patients with X-linked creatine transporter disorder was not helped by creatine supplementation.[88] This is not unusual for this form of the disorder.[149] However, other forms of creatine deficiency have been reported to respond to supplementation.[150]

Sleep Disorders

The lack of treatment guidelines for sleep problems in ASD has been recognized by the American Academy of Pediatrics.[151] As with typically developing children, children with ASD who have restless sleep and low ferritin also respond to iron supplementation.[152] For insomnia, melatonin and the new melatonin agonist Ramelteon have both been shown to be successful,[153–155] as has behavioral management.[156] In practice, many children with ASD do not respond to behavioral treatment or melatonin and require medication such as clonidine for initiation of sleep.

REFERENCES

1. APA. *Diagnostic and Statistical Manual of Mental Disorders* (DSM-IV-TR). 4th ed. Washington, DC: American Psychiatric Association; 2000.
2. Landa RJ, Holman KC, Garrett-Mayer E. Social and communication development in toddlers with early and later diagnosis of autism spectrum disorders. *Arch Gen Psychiatry.* 2007;64:853-864.
3. Ben Itzchak E, Lahat E, Burgin R, Zachor AD. Cognitive, behavior and intervention outcome in young children with autism. *Res Dev Disabil.* 2008;5:447-58.
4. Ben-Itzchak E, Zachor DA. The effects of intellectual functioning and autism severity on outcome of early behavioral intervention for children with autism. *Res Dev Disabil.* 2007;28:287-303.
5. Baghdadli A, Picot MC, Michelon C, et al. What happens to children with PDD when they grow up? Prospective follow-up of 219 children from preschool age to midchildhood. *Acta Psychiatr Scand.* 2007;115:403-412.
6. Autism and Developmental Disabilities Monitoring Network Surveillance Year 2002 Principal Investigators; Centers for Disease Control and Prevention. Prevalence of autism spectrum disorders—autism and developmental disabilities monitoring network, 14 sites, United States, 2002. *MMWR Surveill Summ.* 2007;56:12-28.
7. Casanova MF. The neuropathology of autism. *Brain Pathol.* 2007;17:422-433.
8. Windham GC, Zhang L, Gunier R, Croen LA, Grether JK. Autism spectrum disorders in relation to distribution of hazardous air pollutants in the San Francisco bay area. *Environ Health Perspect.* 2006;114:1438-1444.
9. Palmer RF, Blanchard S, Stein Z, Mandell D, Miller C. Environmental mercury release, special education rates, and autism disorder: an ecological study of Texas. *Health Place.* 2006;12:203-209.
10. Zhang L, Wong MH. Environmental mercury contamination in China: sources and impacts. *Environ Int.* 2007; 33:108-121.
11. Thompson WW, Price C, Goodson B, et al. Early thimerosal exposure and neuropsychological outcomes at 7 to 10 years. *N Engl J Med.* 2007;357:1281-1292.
12. Geier DA, Geier MR. A meta-analysis epidemiological assessment of neurodevelopmental disorders following vaccines administered from 1994 through 2000 in the United States. *Neuro Endocrinol Lett.* 2006;27:401-413.
13. Geier DA, Geier MR. An evaluation of the effects of thimerosal on neurodevelopmental disorders reported following DTP and Hib vaccines in comparison to DTPH vaccine in the United States. *J Toxicol Environ Health* 2006;69:1481-1495.
14. Zimmerman RK, Wolfe RM, Fox DE, et al. Vaccine criticism on the World Wide Web. *J Med Internet Res.* 2005;7:e17.
15. Clements CJ, McIntyre PB. When science is not enough—a risk/benefit profile of thiomersal-containing vaccines. *Expert Opin Drug Saf.* 2006;5:17-29.
16. Hughes V. News feature: A shot of fear. *Nat Med.* 2006;12:1228-1229.
17. Muhle R, Trentacoste SV, Rapin I. The genetics of autism. *Pediatrics.* 2004;113:e472-e486.
18. Spence SJ, Cantor RM, Chung L, Kim S, Geschwind DH, Alarcón M. Stratification based on language-related endophenotypes in autism: attempt to replicate reported linkage. *Am J Med Genet B Neuropsychiatr Genet.* 2006;141:591-598.
19. Chen GK, Kono N, Geschwind DH, Cantor RM. Quantitative trait locus analysis of nonverbal communication in autism spectrum disorder. *Molec Psychiatry.* 2006;11: 214-220.
20. Ylisaukko-oja T, Alarcón M, Cantor RM, et al. Search for autism loci by combined analysis of Autism Genetic Resource Exchange and Finnish families. *Ann Neurol.* 2006;59:145-155.
21. Nishimura Y, Martin CL, Vazquez-Lopez A, et al. Genome-wide expression profiling of lymphoblastoid cell lines distinguishes different forms of autism and reveals shared pathways. *Hum Mol Genet.* 2007;16:1682-1698.
22. Casanova MF. White matter volume increase and minicolumns in autism. *Ann Neurol.* 2004;56:453.
23. Herbert MR. Large brains in autism: the challenge of pervasive abnormality. *Neuroscientist.* 2005;11:417-440.
24. Courchesne E, Karns CM, Davis HR, et al. Unusual brain growth patterns in early life in patients with autistic disorder: an MRI study. *Neurology.* 2001;57:245-254.
25. Stanfield AC, McIntosh AM, Spencer MD, Philip R, Gaur S, Lawrie SM. Towards a neuroanatomy of autism: a systematic review and meta-analysis of structural magnetic resonance imaging studies. *Eur J Psychiatry.* 2008;23: 289-99.
26. Courchesne E, Carper R, Akshoomoff N. Evidence of brain overgrowth in the first year of life in autism. *JAMA.* 2003;290:337-344.
27. Casanova MF, Buxhoeveden DP, Brown C. Clinical and macroscopic correlates of minicolumnar pathology in autism. *J Child Neurol.* 2002;17:692-695.
28. Bauman ML, Kemper TL. Neuroanatomic observations of the brain in autism: a review and future directions. *Int J Dev Neurosci.* 2005;23:183-187.

29. Bauman ML, Kemper TL. Neuroanatomic observations of the brain in autism. In: Bauman ML, Kemper TL, eds. *Neurobiology of Autism*. Baltimore: Johns Hopkins University Press; 1994:119-145.

30. Raymond GV, Bauman ML, Kemper TL. Hippocampus in autism: a Golgi analysis. *Acta Neuropathol*. 1996;91: 117-119.

31. Sparks BF, Friedman SD, Shaw DW, et al. Brain structural abnormalities in young children with autism spectrum disorder. *Neurology*. 2002;59:184-192.

32. Munson J, Dawson G, Abbott R, et al. Amygdalar volume and behavioral development in autism. *Arch Gen Psychiatry*. 2006;63:686-693.

33. Nacewicz BM, Dalton KM, Johnstone T, et al. Amygdala volume and nonverbal social impairment in adolescent and adult males with autism. *Arch Gen Psychiatry*. 2006;63:1417-1428.

34. Bobylova MY, Petrukhin AS, Dunaevskaya GN, Piliya SV, Il'ina ES. Clinical-psychological characteristics of children with dysgenesis of the cerebellar vermis. *Neurosci Behav Physiol*. 2007;37:755-759.

35. Markram K, Rinaldi T, La Mendola D, Sandi C, Markram H. Abnormal fear conditioning and amygdala processing in an animal model of autism. *Neuropsychopharmacology*. 2008; 33:901-12.

36. Courchesne E, Pierce K. Brain overgrowth in autism during a critical time in development: implications for frontal pyramidal neuron and interneuron development and connectivity. *Int J Dev Neurosci*. 2005;23:153-170.

37. Redcay E, Courchesne E. When is the brain enlarged in autism? A meta-analysis of all brain size reports. *Biol Psychiatry*. 2005;58:1-9.

38. van Daalen E, Swinkels SH, Dietz C, van Engeland H, Buitelaar JK. Body length and head growth in the first year of life in autism. *Pediatr Neurol*. 2007;37:324-330.

39. Mills JL, Hediger ML, Molloy CA, et al. Elevated levels of growth-related hormones in autism and autism spectrum disorder. *Clin Endocrinol*. 2007;67:230-237.

40. Courchesne E, Pierce K. Why the frontal cortex in autism might be talking only to itself: local over-connectivity but long-distance disconnection. *Curr Opin Neurobiol*. 2005;15:225-230.

41. Tate DF, Bigler ED, McMahon W, Lainhart J. The relative contributions of brain, cerebrospinal fluid-filled structures and non-neural tissue volumes to occipital-frontal head circumference in subjects with autism. *Neuropediatrics*. 2007;38:18-24.

42. Ashwood P, Wills S, Van de Water J. The immune response in autism: a new frontier for autism research. *J Leukoc Biol*. 2006;80:1-15.

43. Oliveira AL, Thams S, Lidman O, et al. A role for MHC class I molecules in synaptic plasticity and regeneration of neurons after axotomy. *Proc Natl Acad Sci U S A*. 2004; 101:17843-17848.

44. Boulanger LM, Shatz CJ. Immune signalling in neural development, synaptic plasticity and disease. *Nature Rev Neurosci*. 2004;5:521-531.

45. Rasalam AD, Hailey H, Williams JH, et al. Characteristics of fetal anticonvulsant syndrome associated autistic disorder. *Dev Med Child Neurol*. 2005;47:551-555.

46. Moore SJ, Turnpenny P, Quinn A, et al. A clinical study of 57 children with fetal anticonvulsant syndromes. *J Med Genet*. 2000;37:489-497.

47. Strömland K, Nordin V, Miller M, Akerström B, Gillberg C. Autism in thalidomide embryopathy: a population study. *Dev Med Child Neurol*. 1994;36:351-356.

48. Aronson M, Hagberg B, Gillberg C. Attention deficits and autistic spectrum problems in children exposed to alcohol during gestation: a follow-up study. *Dev Med Child Neurol*. 1997;39:583-587.

49. Davis E, Fennoy I, Laraque D, Kanem N, Brown G, Mitchell J. Autism and developmental abnormalities in children with perinatal cocaine exposure. *J Nat Med Assoc*. 1992;84:315-319.

50. Libbey JE, Coon HH, Kirkman NJ, et al. Are there altered antibody responses to measles, mumps, or rubella viruses in autism? *J Neurovirol*. 2007;13:252-259.

51. Limperopoulos C, Bassan H, Gauvreau K, et al. Does cerebellar injury in premature infants contribute to the high prevalence of long-term cognitive, learning, and behavioral disability in survivors? *Pediatrics*. 2007; 120:584-593.

52. Badawi N, Dixon G, Felix JF, et al. Autism following a history of newborn encephalopathy: more than a coincidence? *Dev Med Child Neurol*. 2006;48:85-89.

53. Shaw P, Lawrence EJ, Radbourne C, Bramham J, Polkey CE, David AS. The impact of early and late damage to the human amygdala on "theory of mind" reasoning. *Brain*. 2004;127:1535-1548.

54. Gail Williams P, Sears LL, Allard A. Sleep problems in children with autism. *J Sleep Res*. 2004;13:265-268.

55. Wiggs L, Stores G. Sleep patterns and sleep disorders in children with autistic spectrum disorders: insights using parent report and actigraphy. *Dev Med Child Neurol*. 2004;46:372-380.

56. Schreck KA, Mulick JA, Smith AF. Sleep problems as possible predictors of intensified symptoms of autism. *Res Dev Disabil*. 2004;25:57-66.

57. Wakefield AJ, Ashwood P, Limb K, Anthony A. The significance of ileo-colonic lymphoid nodular hyperplasia in children with autistic spectrum disorder. *Eur J Gastroenterol Hepatol*. 2005;17:827-836.

58. Black C, Kaye JA, Jick H. Relation of childhood gastrointestinal disorders to autism: nested case-control study using data from the UK General Practice Research Database. *BMJ*. 2002;325:419-421.

59. Chudley AE. Genetic landmarks through philately-autism spectrum disorders: a genetic update. *Clin Genet*. 2004;65:352-357.

60. Mouridsen SE, Rich B, Isager T. Epilepsy and other neurological diseases in the parents of children with infantile autism: a case control study. *Child Psychiatry Hum Dev*. 2008;39:1-8.

61. Micali N, Chakrabarti S, Fombonne E. The broad autism phenotype: findings from an epidemiological survey. *Autism*. 2004;8:21-37.

62. Mouridsen SE, Rich B, Isager T, Nedergaard NJ. Psychiatric disorders in the parents of individuals with infantile autism: a case-control study. *Psychopathology*. 2007; 40:166-171.

63. Croen LA, Grether JK, Yoshida CK, Odouli R, Van de Water J. Maternal autoimmune diseases, asthma and allergies, and childhood autism spectrum disorders: a case-control study. *Arch Pediatr Adolesc Med.* 2005; 159:151-157.

64. Molloy CA, Morrow AL, Meinzen-Derr J, et al. Familial autoimmune thyroid disease as a risk factor for regression in children with autism spectrum disorder: a CPEA study. *J Autism Dev Disord.* 2006;36:317-324.

65. Sweeten TL, Bowyer SL, Posey DJ, Halberstadt GM, McDougle CJ. Increased prevalence of familial autoimmunity in probands with pervasive developmental disorders. *Pediatrics* 2003;112:e420.

66. Mouridsen SE, Rich B, Isager T, Nedergaard NJ. Autoimmune diseases in parents of children with infantile autism: a case-control study. *Dev Med Child Neurol.* 2007; 49:429-432.

67. Comi AM, Zimmerman AW, Frye VH, Law PA, Peeden JN. Familial clustering of autoimmune disorders and evaluation of medical risk factors in autism. *J Child Neurol.* 1999;14:388-394.

68. Lauritsen MB, Pedersen CB, Mortensen PB. Effects of familial risk factors and place of birth on the risk of autism: a nationwide register-based study. *J Child Psychol Psychiatry.* 2005;46:963-971.

69. Croen LA, Najjar DV, Fireman B, Grether JK. Maternal and paternal age and risk of autism spectrum disorders. *Arch Pediatr Adolesc Med.* 2007;161:334-340.

70. Veltman MW, Craig EE, Bolton PF. Autism spectrum disorders in Prader-Willi and Angelman syndromes: a systematic review. *Psychiatr Genet.* 2005;15:243-254.

71. Berney TP, Ireland M, Burn J. Behavioural phenotype of Cornelia de Lange syndrome. *Arch Dis Child.* 1999;81: 333-336.

72. Brown W, Nolin SL, Dobkin CS, Spence SJ, Geschwind DH. Frequency of fragile X in multiplex autism: testing the AGRE families. In: *Society for Neuroscience.* San Diego: Society for Neuroscience; 2007.

73. Oliveira G, Ataíde A, Marques C, et al. Epidemiology of autism spectrum disorder in Portugal: prevalence, clinical characterization, and medical conditions. *Dev Med Child Neurol.* 2007;49:726-733.

74. Herman GE, Henninger N, Ratliff-Schaub K, Pastore M, Fitzgerald S, McBride KL. Genetic testing in autism: how much is enough? *Genet Med.* 2007;9:268-274.

75. Tierney E, Nwokoro NA, Porter FD, Freund LS, Ghuman JK, Kelley RI. Behavior phenotype in the RSH/Smith-Lemli-Opitz syndrome. *Am J Med Genet.* 2001;98:191-200.

76. Johansson M, Wentz E, Fernell E, Ströomland K, Miller MT, Gillberg C. Autistic spectrum disorders in Möbius sequence: a comprehensive study of 25 individuals. *Dev Med Child Neurol.* 2001;43:338–345.

77. Vorstman JA, Morcus ME, Duijff SN, et al. The 22q11.2 deletion in children: high rate of autistic disorders and early onset of psychotic symptoms. *J Am Acad Child Adolesc Psychiatry.* 2006;45:1104-1113.

78. Poling JS, Frye RE, Shoffner J, Zimmerman AW. Developmental regression and mitochondrial dysfunction in a child with autism. *J Child Neurol.* 2006;21:170-172.

79. Tsao CY, Mendell JR. Autistic disorder in 2 children with mitochondrial disorders. *J Child Neurol.* 2007;22: 1121-1123.

80. Oliveira G, Diogo L, Grazina M, et al. Mitochondrial dysfunction in autism spectrum disorders: a population-based study. *Dev Med Child Neurol.* 2005;47:185-189.

81. Filipek PA, Juranek J, Smith M, et al. Mitochondrial dysfunction in autistic patients with 15q inverted duplication. *Ann Neurol.* 2003;53:801-804.

82. Fillano JJ, Goldenthal MJ, Rhodes CH, Maríin-Garcia J. Mitochondrial dysfunction in patients with hypotonia, epilepsy, autism, and developmental delay: HEADD syndrome. *J Child Neurol.* 2002;17:435-439.

83. Segurado R, Conroy J, Meally E, Fitzgerald M, Gill M, Gallagher L. Confirmation of association between autism and the mitochondrial aspartate/glutamate carrier SLC25A12 gene on chromosome 2q31. *Am J Psychiatry.* 2005;162:2182-2184.

84. Ramoz N, Reichert JG, Smith CJ, et al. Linkage and association of the mitochondrial aspartate/glutamate carrier SLC25A12 gene with autism. *Am J Psychiatry.* 2004; 161:662-669.

85. Pons R, Andreu AL, Checcarelli N, et al. Mitochondrial DNA abnormalities and autistic spectrum disorders. *J Pediatr.* 2004;144:81-85.

86. Graf WD, Marin-Garcia J, Gao HG, et al. Autism associated with the mitochondrial DNA G8363A transfer RNA(Lys) mutation. *J Child Neurol.* 2000; 15:357-361.

87. Clark-Taylor T, Clark-Taylor BE. Is autism a disorder of fatty acid metabolism? Possible dysfunction of mitochondrial beta-oxidation by long chain acyl-CoA dehydrogenase. *Med Hypotheses.* 2004;62:970-975.

88. Póo-Argüelles P, Arias A, Vilaseca MA, et al. X-Linked creatine transporter deficiency in two patients with severe mental retardation and autism. *J Inherit Metab Dis.* 2006;29:220-223.

89. Lerman-Sagie T, Leshinsky-Silver E, Watemberg N, Lev D. Should autistic children be evaluated for mitochondrial disorders? *J Child Neurol.* 2004;19:379-381.

90. Rabionet R, McCauley JL, Jaworski JM, et al. Lack of association between autism and SLC25A12. *Am J Psychiatry.* 2006;163:929-931.

91. Correia C, Coutinho AM, Diogo L, et al. Brief report: High frequency of biochemical markers for mitochondrial dysfunction in autism: no association with the mitochondrial aspartate/glutamate carrier SLC25A12 gene. *J Autism Dev Disord.* 2006;36:1137-1140.

92. Görker I, Tüzün U. Autistic-like findings associated with a urea cycle disorder in a 4-year-old girl. *J Psychiatry Neurosci.* 2005;30:133-135.

93. Topcu M, Saatci I, Haliloglu G, Kesimer M, Coskun T. D-glyceric aciduria in a six-month-old boy presenting with West syndrome and autistic behaviour. *Neuropediatrics.* 2002;33:47-50.

94. Zaffanello M, Zamboni G, Fontana E, Zoccante L, Tatò L. A case of partial biotinidase deficiency associated with autism. *Child Neuropsychol.* 2003;9:184-188.

95. Colamaria V, Burlina AB, Gaburro D, et al. Biotin-responsive infantile encephalopathy: EEG-polygraphic study of a case. *Epilepsia.* 1989;30:573-578.

96. Moretti P, Sahoo T, Hyland K, et al. Cerebral folate deficiency with developmental delay, autism, and response to folinic acid. *Neurology.* 2005;64:1088-1090.

97. Perry TL, Hansen S, Christie RG. Amino compounds and organic acids in CSF, plasma, and urine of autistic children. *Biol Psychiatry*. 1978;13:575-586.

98. Wiznitzer M. Autism and tuberous sclerosis. *J Child Neurol* 2004;19:675-679.

99. Chou IJ, Lin KL, Wong AM, et al. Neuroimaging correlation with neurological severity in tuberous sclerosis complex. *Eur J Paediatr Neurol*. 2008;12:108-12.

100. Asano E, Chugani DC, Muzik O, et al. Autism in tuberous sclerosis complex is related to both cortical and subcortical dysfunction. *Neurology*. 2001;57:1269-1277.

101. Young DJ, Bebbington A, Anderson A, et al. The diagnosis of autism in a female: could it be Rett syndrome? *Eur J Pediatr*. 2008;167:661-9.

102. Canitano R. Epilepsy in autism spectrum disorders. *Eur Child Adolesc Psychiatry*. 2007;16:61-66.

103. McVicar KA, Ballaban-Gil K, Rapin I, Moshé SL, Shinnar S. Epileptiform EEG abnormalities in children with language regression. *Neurology*. 2005;65:129-131.

104. Chez MG, Chang M, Krasne V, Coughlan C, Kominsky M, Schwartz A. Frequency of epileptiform EEG abnormalities in a sequential screening of autistic patients with no known clinical epilepsy from 1996 to 2005. *Epilepsy Behav*. 2006;8:267-271.

105. Lewine JD, Andrews R, Chez M, et al. Magnetoencephalographic patterns of epileptiform activity in children with regressive autism spectrum disorders. *Pediatrics*. 1999;104:405-418.

106. Scholtes FB, Hendriks MP, Renier WO. Cognitive deterioration and electrical status epilepticus during slow sleep. *Epilepsy Behav*. 2005;6:167-173.

107. Schifter T, Hoffman JM, Hatten HP Jr., Hanson MW, Coleman RE, DeLong GR. Neuroimaging in infantile autism. *J Child Neurol*. 1994;9:155-161.

108. Johnson CP, Myers SM. Identification and evaluation of children with autism spectrum disorders. *Pediatrics*. 2007;120:1183-1215.

109. Wong V, Hui LH, Lee WC, et al. A modified screening tool for autism (Checklist for Autism in Toddlers [CHAT-23]) for Chinese children. *Pediatrics*. 2004;114:e166-e176.

110. Dumont-Mathieu T, Fein D. Screening for autism in young children: The Modified Checklist for Autism in Toddlers (M-CHAT) and other measures. *Ment Retard Dev Disabil Res Rev*. 2005;11:253-262.

111. Williams J, Allison C, Scott F, et al. The Childhood Asperger Syndrome Test (CAST): test-retest reliability. *Autism*. 2006;10:415-427.

112. Perry A, Condillac RA, Freeman NL, Dunn-Geier J, Belair J. Multi-site study of the Childhood Autism Rating Scale (CARS) in five clinical groups of young children. *J Autism Dev Disord*. 2005;35:625-634.

113. Campbell JM. Diagnostic assessment of Asperger's disorder: a review of five third-party rating scales. *J Autism Dev Disord*. 2005;35:25-35.

114. Gray KM, Tonge BJ, Sweeney DJ. Using the Autism Diagnostic Interview-Revised and the Autism Diagnostic Observation Schedule with young children with developmental delay: evaluating diagnostic validity. *J Autism Dev Disord*. 2008;38:657-67.

115. Le Couteur A, Haden G, Hammal D, McConachie H. Diagnosing autism spectrum disorders in pre-school children using two standardised assessment instruments: The ADI-R and the ADOS. *J Autism Dev Disord*. 2008; 38:362-72.

116. Lord C, Risi S, DiLavore PS, Shulman C, Thurm A, Pickles A. Autism from 2 to 9 years of age. *Arch Gen Psychiatry*. 2006;63:694-701.

117. Tomanik SS, Pearson DA, Loveland KA, Lane DM, Bryant Shaw J. Improving the reliability of autism diagnoses: examining the utility of adaptive behavior. *J Autism Dev Disord*. 2007;37:921-928.

118. Zeegers M, Van Der Grond J, Durston S, et al. Radiological findings in autistic and developmentally delayed children. *Brain Dev*. 2006;28:495-499.

119. Alexander AL, Lee JE, Lazar M, et al. Diffusion tensor imaging of the corpus callosum in Autism. *Neuroimage*. 2007;34:61-73.

120. Ben Bashat D, Kronfeld-Duenias V, Zachor DA, et al. Accelerated maturation of white matter in young children with autism: a high b value DWI study. *Neuroimage*. 2007;37:40-47.

121. Lee JE, Bigler ED, Alexander AL, et al. Diffusion tensor imaging of white matter in the superior temporal gyrus and temporal stem in autism. *Neurosci Lett*. 2007;424:127-132.

122. Rojas DC, Peterson E, Winterrowd E, Reite ML, Rogers SJ, Tregellas JR. Regional gray matter volumetric changes in autism associated with social and repetitive behavior symptoms. *BMC Psychiatry*. 2006;6:56.

123. Spencer MD, Moorhead TW, Lymer GK, et al. Structural correlates of intellectual impairment and autistic features in adolescents. *Neuroimage*. 2006;33:1136-1144.

124. Filipek PA, Juranek J, Nguyen MT, Cummings C, Gargus JJ. Relative carnitine deficiency in autism. *J Autism Dev Disord*. 2004;34:615-623.

125. Ramaekers VT, Rothenberg SP, Sequeira JM, et al. Autoantibodies to folate receptors in the cerebral folate deficiency syndrome. *N Engl J Med*. 2005;352:1985-1991.

126. Butler MG, Dasouki MJ, Zhou XP, et al. Subset of individuals with autism spectrum disorders and extreme macrocephaly associated with germline PTEN tumour suppressor gene mutations. *J Med Genet*. 2005;42:318-321.

127. Buxbaum JD, Cai G, Chaste P, et al. Mutation screening of the PTEN gene in patients with autism spectrum disorders and macrocephaly. *Am J Med Genet B Neuropsychiatr Genet*. 2007;144:484-491.

128. Greer JM, Wynshaw-Boris A. PTEN and the brain: sizing up social interaction. *Neuron*. 2006;50:343-345.

129. Herman GE, Butter E, Enrile B, Pastore M, Prior TW, Sommer A. Increasing knowledge of PTEN germline mutations: two additional patients with autism and macrocephaly. *Am J Med Genet A*. 2007;143:589-593.

130. Tan WH, Baris HN, Burrows PE, et al. The spectrum of vascular anomalies in patients with PTEN mutations: implications for diagnosis and management. *J Med Genet*. 2007;44:594-602.

131. Jacquemont ML, Sanlaville D, Redon R, et al. Array-based comparative genomic hybridisation identifies high frequency of cryptic chromosomal rearrangements in patients with syndromic autism spectrum disorders. *J Med Genet*. 2006;43:843-849.

132. Arnold LE, Aman MG, Cook AM, et al. Atomoxetine for hyperactivity in autism spectrum disorders: placebo-controlled crossover pilot trial. *J Am Acad Child Adolesc Psychiatry*. 2006;45:1196-1205.

133. Posey DJ, McDougle CJ. The pharmacotherapy of target symptoms associated with autistic disorder and other pervasive developmental disorders. *Harv Rev Psychiatry.* 2000;8:45-63.

134. Posey DJ, McDougle CJ. Pharmacotherapeutic management of autism. *Expert Opin Pharmacother.* 2001;2: 587-600.

135. Posey DJ, Wiegand RE, Wilkerson J, Maynard M, Stigler KA, McDougle CJ. Open-label atomoxetine for attention-deficit/ hyperactivity disorder symptoms associated with high-functioning pervasive developmental disorders. *J Child Adolesc Psychopharmacol.* 2006; 16:599-610.

136. Santosh PJ, Baird G, Pityaratstian N, Tavare E, Gringras P. Impact of comorbid autism spectrum disorders on stimulant response in children with attention deficit hyperactivity disorder: a retrospective and prospective effectiveness study. *Child Care Health Dev.* 2006;32: 575-583.

137. McCracken JT, McGough J, Shah B, et al. Risperidone in children with autism and serious behavioral problems. *N Engl J Med.* 2002;347:314-321.

138. Kolevzon A, Mathewson KA, Hollander E. Selective serotonin reuptake inhibitors in autism: a review of efficacy and tolerability. *J Clin Psychiatry.* 2006;67:407-414.

139. Owley T, Walton L, Salt J, et al. An open-label trial of escitalopram in pervasive developmental disorders. *J Am Acad Child Adolesc Psychiatry.* 2005;44:343-348.

140. Hollander E, Phillips AT, Yeh CC. Targeted treatments for symptom domains in child and adolescent autism. *Lancet.* 2003;362:732-734.

141. Namerow LB, Thomas P, Bostic JQ, Prince J, Monuteaux MC. Use of citalopram in pervasive developmental disorders. *J Dev Behav Pediatr.* 2003;24:104-108.

142. Hollander E, Phillips A, Chaplin W, et al. A placebo controlled crossover trial of liquid fluoxetine on repetitive behaviors in childhood and adolescent autism. *Neuropsychopharmacology.* 2005;30:582-589.

143. Sugie Y, Sugie H, Fukuda T, et al. Clinical efficacy of fluvoxamine and functional polymorphism in a serotonin transporter gene on childhood autism. *J Autism Dev Disord.* 2005;35:377-385.

144. Moore ML, Eichner SF, Jones JR. Treating functional impairment of autism with selective serotonin-reuptake inhibitors. *Ann Pharmacother.* 2004;38:1515-1519.

145. Inutsuka M, Kobayashi K, Oka M, Hattori J, Ohtsuka Y. Treatment of epilepsy with electrical status epilepticus during slow sleep and its related disorders. *Brain Dev.* 2006;28:281-286.

146. Ballaban-Gil K, Tuchman R. Epilepsy and epileptiform EEG: association with autism and language disorders. *Ment Retard Dev Disabil Res Rev.* 2000;6:300-308.

147. Mikati MA, Shamseddine AN. Management of Landau-Kleffner syndrome. *Paediatr Drugs.* 2005;7:377-389.

148. Nass R, Gross A, Wisoff J, Devinsky O. Outcome of multiple subpial transections for autistic epileptiform regression. *Pediatr Neurol.* 1999;21:464-470.

149. Anselm IA, Alkuraya FS, Salomons GS, et al. X-linked creatine transporter defect: a report on two unrelated boys with a severe clinical phenotype. *J Inherit Metab Dis.* 2006;29:214-219.

150. Verbruggen KT, Sijens PE, Schulze A, et al. Successful treatment of a guanidinoacetate methyltransferase deficient patient: findings with relevance to treatment strategy and pathophysiology. *Mol Genet Metab.* 2007; 91:294-296.

151. Mindell JA, Emslie G, Blumer J, et al. Pharmacologic management of insomnia in children and adolescents: consensus statement. *Pediatrics.* 2006;117:e1223-e1232.

152. Dosman CF, Brian JA, Drmic IE, et al. Children with autism: effect of iron supplementation on sleep and ferritin. *Pediatr Neurol.* 2007;36:152-158.

153. Stigler KA, Posey DJ, McDougle CJ. Ramelteon for insomnia in two youths with autistic disorder. *J Child Adolesc Psychopharmacol.* 2006;16:631-636.

154. Garstang J, Wallis M. Randomized controlled trial of melatonin for children with autistic spectrum disorders and sleep problems. *Child Care Health Dev.* 2006;32: 585-589.

155. Giannotti F, Cortesi F, Cerquiglini A, Bernabei P. An open-label study of controlled-release melatonin in treatment of sleep disorders in children with autism. *J Autism Dev Disord.* 2006;36:741-752.

156. Weiskop S, Richdale A, Matthews J. Behavioural treatment to reduce sleep problems in children with autism or fragile X syndrome. *Dev Med Child Neurol.* 2005;47: 94-104.

CHAPTER 28

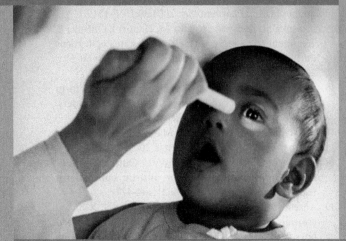

Newborn Neurology

Michael D. Weiss

The neonatal intensive care unit and newborn nursery are often chaotic and noisy environments with a whirlwind of activity and a unique language of acronyms. The goal of this chapter is to provide a systematic, concise, and clinically usable approach to guide the bedside practitioner through this sea of chaos by first reviewing the normal neurological examination of the neonate with an emphasis on normal findings at different gestational ages and possible etiologies of abnormal findings. It will then cover in more detail several neurological abnormalities that are found in the neonatal period, including hypoxic-ischemic encephalopathy (HIE), intraventricular hemorrhage (IVH), and seizures in the newborn. Although there is overlap among these abnormalities, each will be covered individually, with a brief emphasis on the incidence, pathophysiology, pertinent clinical findings, the differential diagnosis, and a brief overview of clinical management.

NEUROLOGICAL EXAMINATION

The neurological examination of the neonate presents the clinician with numerous challenges. First, it tests the examiner's powers of observation. Most of the neurological examination is carried out by observing the neonate's baseline state. The baseline state changes based on the gestational age of the neonate, level of arousal, and recent experiences (eg, postmedical procedures such as IV placement). Second, the patient is unable to respond to verbal commands. And, last, the examiner uses subjective methods of evaluating the neonate's response to various stimuli and cues. This necessitates a high level of experience and knowledge to obtain a thorough and accurate assessment of the neonate's neurological status. This section is

This work was supported by NIH 5R21NS052583-02.

designed to briefly review the complete neurological examination of the neonate. The rationale for each portion of the examination will be reviewed, as will the potential differential diagnosis for abnormal findings. The examination is laid out in a systematic manner beginning with simple observation and proceeding to active evaluation of tone and responses to various stimuli. The examination is performed in this manner to maximize the clinician's time at the bedside while thoroughly examining the neonate's neurological status (Figure 28-1).

Review of History

The first step to a thorough examination is to review the maternal history (age, gravity, parity, pregnancy health status, fetal growth) and the history of the neonate's birth (route of delivery, anesthesia/analgesia, APGAR scores, need for resuscitation) and hospital course from the neonate's chart. Particular attention should be focused on the gestational age of the neonate (as measured by examination—see Figure 28-1). The examiner should also review the neonate's weight, head circumference, and length. It is very important to start with these physical parameters to have the proper context for the remainder of the examination. For example, infants of diabetic mothers will typically be large for gestational age for weight and length with a normal head circumference. These infants may have problems associated with hypocalcemia and hypoglycemia, which may be evident on the neurological examination with findings of jitteriness, agitation, and seizures.[1] The head circumference may also present the examiner with clues to underlying neuropathology. Neonates with microcephaly may have a congenital infection (CMV, rubella, toxoplasmosis), genetic abnormality (trisomy 13, 18, 21), somatic anomalies or syndromes (CHARGE association, Meckel-Gruber syndrome, Smith-Lemli-Opitz

Systematic Approach to the Newborn Neurological Exam

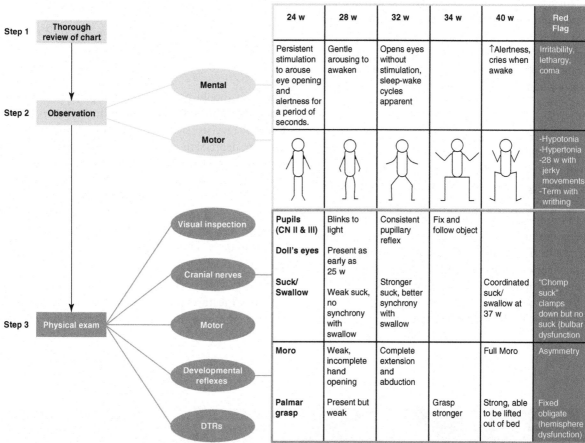

FIGURE 28-1 ■ The neonatal neurological examination. A summary of the neurological examination is illustrated using a flow chart. Step 1 involves a thorough review of the neonate's chart, including the maternal history, birth history, and hospital course. Step 2 involves observation of the neonate and addresses the neonate's mental and motor status. Normal and abnormal findings for both the mental and motor examination are found in the yellow grid square connected to the respective circle. The third step involves the physical examination, which includes visual inspection, examination of the cranial nerves, the motor examination, developmental reflexes, and deep tendon reflexes (DTRs). Normal and abnormal findings for both the cranial nerve and developmental reflex examinations are found in the blue grid square connected to their respective circle.

syndrome, Cornelia de Lange syndrome, Prader-Willi syndrome), in utero drug exposure (cocaine, heroin, ethanol, inhalation of mixed solvent vapor), hormonal disorders (congenital hypothyroidism), congenital developmental abnormality (holoprosencephaly, lissencephaly, polymicorgyria, shizencephaly), or microcephaly vera. Conversely, neonates with macrocephaly may have an underlying ventricular enlargement (aqueductal stenosis, Dandy-Walker syndrome, Arnold-Chiari malformation, vein of Galen malformation) or other etiologies (Soto syndrome, Beckwith-Wiedemann syndrome, fragile X syndrome, cranial mass, familial macrocephaly).

Observation

After completing a thorough review of the history, the examiner should simply observe the neonate. With keen observation, the examiner can gain many details about the neonate's neurological status without disturbing the neonate.

Mental status

The level of alertness is perhaps the most sensitive of all neurological functions since it is dependent on the integrity of several different levels of the central nervous system.[2] Before 28 weeks gestation, the newborn states of wakefulness and sleep are difficult to distinguish, and the neonate requires persistent stimulation to arouse eye opening and alertness for a period of seconds. At 28 weeks, a change occurs, and the neonate is aroused with gentle shaking with periods of alertness lasting several minutes. By 32 weeks, stimulation is no longer necessary; the eyes remain open for long periods of time with observed sleep–waking alterations. By 36 weeks, increased alertness is observed, with vigorous crying during periods of wakefulness. By term, the infant exhibits periods of attention to visual and auditory stimuli. It is important to note that the level of alertness varies depending on the time of the neonate's last feed, environmental stimuli, and recent experiences (such as placement of IV). Several disturbances of arousal can be noted on the examination. An irritable neonate is one who is agitated and cries with minimal stimulation and is unable to be comforted.[3] A lethargic or stuporous neonate will have a sluggish response to sensory stimuli, while a comatose neonate will not be arousable and will have no response to sensory input.

Motor

The examiner should focus on the resting posture of the unswaddled neonate. This observation can reveal the symmetry and maturity of the passive tone with the tone changing as a function of gestational age (Figure 28-1). Flexor tone first develops in the lower extremities and proceeds cephalad correlating with increasing myelination of the subcortical motor pathways, which originate in the brainstem.[3] The examiner should also note any abnormal movements, such as choreathetoid movements, that may indicate an underlying structural or metabolic problem.[3] The normal term neonate displays fisting of the hand (adduction and infolding of the thumbs [cortical thumbs]) with intermittent hand opening.

Physical Examination

Visual inspection and palpation

The head should be visualized and palpated for ridges along the sutures, the size and fullness of the anterior fontanel, excessive head molding or cephalohematomas, and any depressions in the skull. The spine should be carefully inspected for any patches or tufts of hairs, pits, hemangiomas, or lipomas. The entire body should be observed for birthmarks, port wine stains, ash leaf spots, or macules (Figure 28-2). Each of these findings may lead the examiner to consider underlying pathology associated with these skin findings.

Motor

The major features to be evaluated in the motor examination are muscle tone and motility. Development of

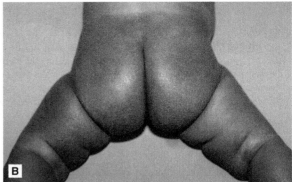

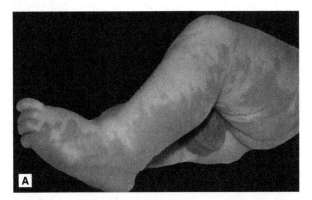

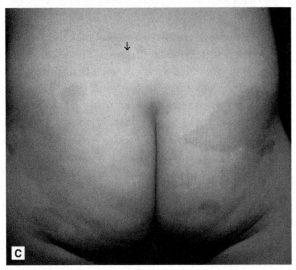

FIGURE 28-2 ■ Various birthmarks and skin lesions in the newborn. Salmon patches, also called "stork bites" **(A)** and Mongolian spots **(B)** are among the most common birthmarks. Café au lait spots **(C)** may be benign, but can also be a sign of neurofibromatosis. Port wine stains **(D)** and hemangiomas **(E, F)** may be located anywhere on the skin. Papules **(G, H)** and macules **(I, J)** may be benign as in the case of neonatal acne **(G)**, erythema toxicum **(I)**, or transient neonatal pustular melanosis **(J)**, but may also be an indication of serious infection such as herpes simplex **(H)**. (A, C, E, F, G, I, J *reproduced with permission from Wolff K, et al., eds. Fitzpatrick's Dermatology in General Medicine. 7th ed. New York; McGraw-Hill; 2008.* **B** *reproduced with permission from Wolff K, et al., eds. Fitzpatrick's Color Atlas & Synopsis of Clinical Dermatology. 5th ed. New York: McGraw-Hill; 2005.* **D** *reproduced with permission from Wolff K, et al., eds. Fitzpatrick's Dermatology in General Medicine. 7th ed. New York: McGraw-Hill; 2008:online edition.* **H** *used with permission from Alvin H. Jacobs, MD.*)

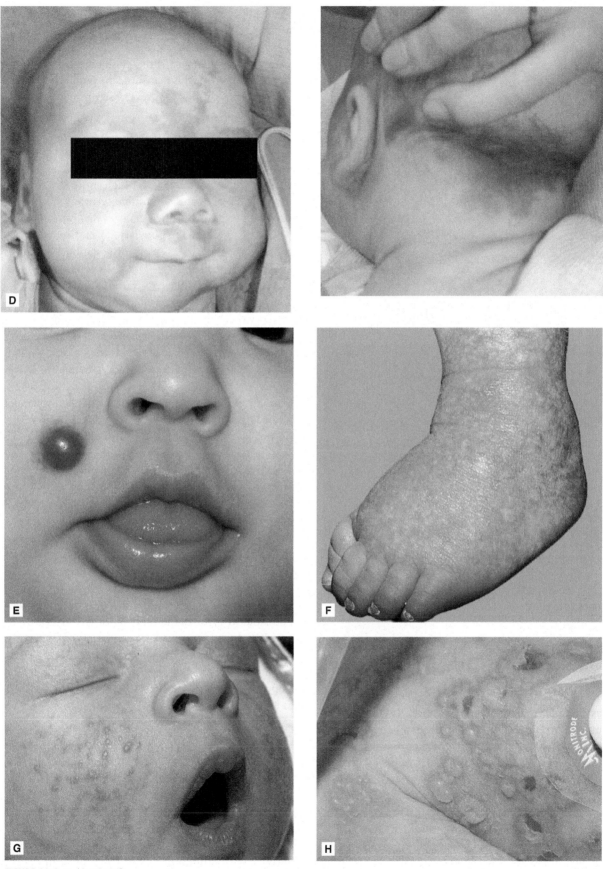

FIGURE 28-2 ■ (Continued)

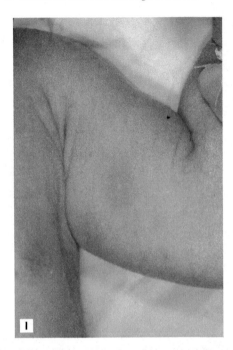

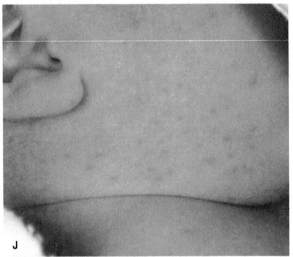

FIGURE 28-2 ■ *(Continued)*

of the upper extremities are appreciated. At 40 weeks, the neonate moves all limbs in an alternating manner. Neck flexor power also becomes apparent. This is illustrated by pulling the neonate to a sitting position using the upper extremities. During this maneuver, the head is held in the same plane as the body for several seconds.[2,4]

Cranial nerves

Even though the neonate's interaction with the examiner is limited, essentially all the cranial nerves can be evaluated. Cranial nerve (CN) I, given its rare involvement in diseases and the difficulty in evaluating the neonate's response, is not usually evaluated. CN II and III can be tested by the pupillary reflex, which appears consistently at 32 to 35 weeks of gestation.[3] Shining a light in the neonate's eyes will elicit a blink response, first appreciated at 28 weeks, testing CN II and VII. By 34 weeks, 90% of infants will fix and follow a fluffy ball of red wool, thus testing CN II, III, IV, and VI.[5] The doll's-eye maneuver can be elicited as early as 25 weeks of gestation and further tests CN III, IV, and VI. It is important to note that spontaneous roving eye movements are common at 32 weeks of gestation, as are dysconjugate eye movement in the term infant when not fixing on an object.[3] Smooth visual tracking movements do not become present until 3 months of life.[6] Facial sensation (CN V) can be tested with a pinprick to different areas of the face with the neonate responding with a facial grimace or change in sucking. CN VII can be tested by observing the face at rest with particular attention to the vertical width of the palpebral fissures, the nasolabial fold, and the position of the corner of the mouth. Changes in these structures should then be observed during crying. With a facial nerve palsy, the corner of the mouth on the affected side droops and the mouth is drawn to the normal side. A coordinated suck and swallow involves the function of CN V, VII, IX, X, and XII. A suck and swallow can be noted as early as 28 weeks, but the synchrony with breathing and feeding is not well developed. As the brain matures, coordination improves at 32 to 34 weeks but is not fully achieved until at least 37 weeks.[7]

Reflexes

Deep tendon reflexes. Deep tendon reflexes (DTRs) in the neonate are elicited in a manner similar to the older pediatric patients. During testing of the DTRs, the head should be maintained in a neutral position to prevent the induction of an asymmetrical tonic neck response, which can produce asymmetrical reflex activity with stimulation. The examiner can readily elicit reflexes in the biceps, brachioradialis, and ankle, although the upper extremity reflexes are often more difficult to elicit than the lower extremities. Testing of

tone proceeds in a caudal-rostral progression, particularly flexor tone, with maturation.[2,4] A 28-week neonate has minimal resistance to passive movement in all limbs, but by 32 weeks, there is distinct flexor tone in the lower extremities. At 36 weeks, flexor tone is prominent in the lower extremities and resistance to movement is present in the upper extremities, while at term, there is strong flexor tone in all extremities.

Parallel to development of tone described above, the quality of neonatal movements advances. The 28-week neonate will have writhing movements of the extremities, while the 32-week neonate will have predominately flexor movement of the hips and knees. At 36 weeks, the active flexor movements in the lower extremities are stronger and prominent flexor movements the DTRs in the neonate can also induce clonus, which is physiologically normal (5-10 beats) if unsustained.[2] The plantar response is considered of limited value since four competing reflexes lead to movement of the toes, depending on how the examination is performed.[2]

Developmental reflexes. The developmental reflexes (Figure 28-3) are a set of reflexes that are found in the neonate and disappear at regular developmental periods as the neonatal brain develops. Volpe has commented that these reflexes are more valuable in assessment of disorders of the lower motor neuron, nerve, and muscle than of the upper motor neuron.[2]

The Moro reflex (Figure 28-3A) consists of bilateral hand opening with upper extremity extension and abduction followed by anterior flexion ("embracing") of the upper extremities, then an audible cry. The reflex is elicited by dropping the head in relation to the neonate's body. The Moro reflex can be first appreciated in a rudimentary form at 28 weeks of gestation with the neonate responding with hand opening. The reflex disappears by 6 months of age.

The tonic neck response (Figure 28-3B) can be elicited by rotating the head to one side. The neonate responds to this action with what has been described as a fencing posture: an extension of the upper extremity on the side to which the face is rotated, and flexion of the upper extremity on the side of the occiput. The response first appears at 35 weeks of gestation and disappears by approximately 6 to 7 months of age.

The palmar grasp (Figure 28-3C) is elicited by stimulating the palm of the neonate's hand with an object. The reflex is present at 28 weeks of gestation, strong at 32 weeks, and strong enough to lift the neonate off the bed by 37 weeks. This reflex disappears by 2 months of age, which coincides with the development of voluntary grasp.

The placing and stepping reflexes (Figure 28-3D) are elicited by contacting the dorsum of the foot against a flat surface. The neonate will respond by flexing the hip and knee and will appear to be taking a step. This reflex is useful if asymmetry occurs and may indicate a lesion in the basal ganglia, brainstem, or spinal cord, although it is difficult to perform in a sick neonate.

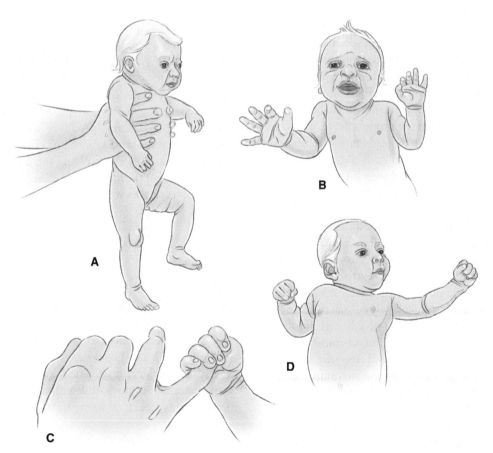

FIGURE 28-3 ■ The neonatal developmental reflexes are **(A)** the Moro or startle reflex, **(B)** the asymmetric tonic neck reflex, **(C)** the grasp reflex, and **(D)** the stepping reflex.

HYPOXIC ISCHEMIC ENCEPHALOPATHY

Definition and Epidemiology

Hypoxic-ischemic encephalopathy (HIE) is the brain manifestation of systemic asphyxia or hypoxia-ischemia,[8] which occurs in about 20 of 1000 full-term infants and in nearly 60% of very low birth weight (premature) newborns.[9-11] Between 20% and 50% of neonates who exhibit HIE die during the newborn period.[12] Of the survivors, up to 25% have permanent neuropsychological handicaps in the form of cerebral palsy, with or without associated mental retardation, learning disabilities, or epilepsy.[13-15]

Pathogenesis

The etiologies of HIE can be grouped into the three epochs in which they occur. The first epoch occurs during the prepartum period. This time interval pertains to problems with either placental perfusion, secondary to maternal diseases or drug use, or with the placenta itself. The second epoch occurs during the delivery process and is associated with a difficult delivery, including an abnormal presentation, prolonged labor, a precipitous delivery, and a difficult delivery requiring forceps. Finally, a time interval not often associated with HIE occurs during the neonatal period. Problems occurring during the neonatal period include severe prematurity, respiratory distress, cardiopulmonary anomalies such as congenital heart disease and diaphragmatic hernia, and infectious diseases, which can produce septic shock.

Hypoxia-ischemia (HI) leads to a complex cascade of events producing cellular damage and destruction.[16,17] Globally, cerebral perfusion is reduced secondary to decreasing cardiac output, depleting the cells in the brain of both oxygen and energy substrates. At the cellular level, ATP is rapidly depleted as a result of the inefficient shift to anaerobic metabolism, which is further compounded by a decrease in glucose delivery. The rapid depletion of ATP results in severe compromise in the basic metabolic processes of the cells, leading to a series of secondary intracellular events that result in cellular damage. These events can be grouped into three major categories: excitatory neurotransmitter toxicity, intracellular calcium overload, and free radical formation. All three categories overlap and are summarized in Figure 28-4. During HIE, there is an excessive release of the excitatory amino acid glutamate from the presynaptic terminal.[18-20] This leads to overstimulation of the glutamate receptors (AMPA, KA, NMDA) located on the postsynaptic neuron, which leads to excitotoxicity, a term coined by Lucas and Olney.[21,22] Please note that neonates are at particular risk for excitotoxicity because the distribution, electrophysiology, and molecular characteristics of excitatory amino acid receptors change markedly throughout normal brain development.[23] The excitatory amino acid receptors have been linked to a variety of physiologic processes during normal neurodevelopment including synaptogenesis and synaptic plasticity.[24] The changes in the excitatory amino acid receptors discussed earlier strongly influence the brain's vulnerability to HIE. Overstimulation of the KA and AMPA receptors leads to the entry of sodium and chloride into the cell, which increases cell osmality, leading to the influx of water. The increase in water influx results in subcellular edema, which if severe enough results in lysis of the cell. Overstimulation of the NMDA receptor triggers the influx of calcium.[25] Calcium is the main second messenger in the cell and, when present in pathologic amounts, activates a series of enzymes, which results in the destruction of the cell (Figure 28-4). Calcium also contributes to the generation of free radicals, such as nitric oxide.[25] Free radicals are chemical species with one or more unpaired electrons in their outer orbital. Free radicals also are generated from fatty acid and prostaglandin metabolism, leading to the formation of damaging amounts of superoxide and hydrogen peroxide.[8] The three aberrant cellular processes lead to both apoptosis and necrosis. HIE pathologically produces several distinct injury patterns.[2] A diffuse pattern involving the cerebral cortex, hippocampus, and deep nuclear structures can be seen with a severe, prolonged insult. Another pattern involves the cerebral cortex, basal ganglia, and thalamus, and is associated with moderate to severe, prolonged hypoxia-ischemia. Severe, abrupt hypoxia-ischemia produces injury to the basal ganglia, thalamus, and brainstem. Finally, an isolated pontosubicular pattern involving the basis pontis and the subiculum of the hippocampus can be seen. The etiology of this pattern is unknown.

Clinical Presentation and Diagnosis

Physical exam

After stabilizing a neonate with HIE (see the "Treatment" section below), attention should be focused on the neurological examination. Clinical acuity can be staged using the system developed by Sarnat and Sarnat[15] (Table 28-1). This staging system should be performed in a serial fashion since a neonate may not remain at one stage but rather improve or deteriorate over time. Volpe describes this process as occurring in defined time intervals in neonates with severe injury.[2] During the first time interval (0-12 hours), the injured neonate will have a depressed level of consciousness, usually deep stupor or coma, intact pupillary and oculomotor responses,

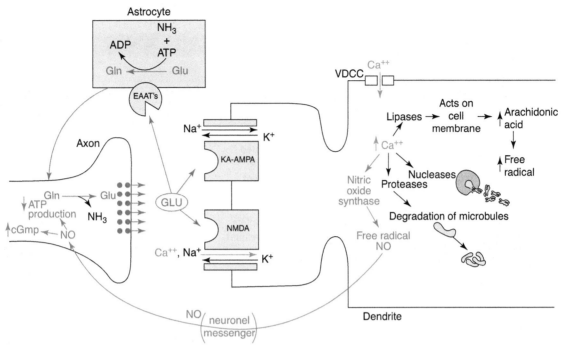

FIGURE 28-4 ■ A summary of the pathophysiology of HIE is presented graphically. Glutamate (GLU) is packaged into vesicles in the presynaptic terminal. Upon depolarization, glutamate is released into the neurosynaptic junction and binds to glutamate receptors on the postsynaptic dendrite. Binding to the kainate (KA) and AMPA receptors triggers the influx of sodium (Na), resulting in the depolarization of the postsynaptic neuron. Binding to NMDA receptors triggers the influx of calcium and sodium into the postsynaptic dendrite. Glutamate is then removed from the neurosynaptic junction via the excitatory amino acid transporters (EAATs) located on the atrocyte. It is then converted into glutamine by the enzyme glutamine synthetase. The glutamine is exported from the astrocyte into the presynaptic neuron, and then converted into glutamate via the action of glutaminase, thus recycling the neurotransmitter. This process is known as the glutamine–glutamate cycle (shown in *yellow*). During HIE, there is a massive release of the excitatory amino acid glutamate from the presynaptic terminal. This leads to overstimulation of the glutamate receptors (AMPA, KA, NMDA) located on the postsynaptic neuron, leading to neuronal death, a process termed excitotoxicity. Overstimulation of the KA and AMPA receptors leads to the entry of sodium and chloride into the cell, which increases cell osmality. The increased influx of sodiums leads to the influx of water, which results in subcellular edema, which if severe enough results in lysis of the cell. Overstimulation of the NMDA receptor triggers the influx of calcium (*green*). In addition, calcium also enters via the voltage-dependent calcium channels (VDCC). Calcium is the main second messenger in the cell and, when present in pathologic amounts, activates a series of enzymes (proteases, nucleases, lipases), which results in the destruction of the cell. Calcium also contributes to the generation of free radicals by activating nitric oxide synthase (*orange*), forming excessive amounts of nitric oxide, which acts as a free radical. Nitric oxide also serves as a second messenger, affecting the presynaptic neuron by activating cyclic GMP (cGMP) and decreasing ATP production. cGMP in excessive amounts affects protein phosphorylation and gating of cation channels adversely.

hypotonia, and possibly seizures. If the pupillary and oculomotor responses are not intact during this time, a severe injury to the brainstem is likely.[2] At 12 to 24 hours, neonates will have a variable change in the level of alertness, more seizures, and apneic spells. Weakness will be noted in the proximal extremities, with the upper more than lower extremities in term neonates and the lower more than upper extremities in premature neonates. Twenty-four to seventy-two hours post-injury, the neonate may have stupor or coma, respiratory arrest, and a lack of pupillary or oculomotor responses. After 72 hours, the neonate may have persistent yet diminishing stupor, hypotonia, and disturbances of suck, swallow, gag, and tongue movement.

Neuroimaging

Neuroimaging allows injured brain regions to be visualized, adding information to the clinician's bedside assessment.

The information can then be used to predict potential long-term disabilities in neonates with HIE. The first imaging technique that can be used is ultrasound (US). Ultrasound has the advantage of being a rapid bedside test, but it provides limited anatomic information. The resistive index obtained with US may be helpful in predicting long-term outcomes.[26] CT is the second imaging option. A low attenuation in the basal ganglia and or thalami indicates severe injury.[26] The CT scan must be repeated 2 to 6 weeks after the initial imaging study to see if the neuronal injury has progressed since the original scan. The final test, MRI, provides very good anatomic differentiation of the region of injury following HIE but has the disadvantage of requiring a relatively long time (compared with CT) for data acquisition. Diffusion-weighted imaging may detect areas of injured brain regions before changes are noted on standard T1- and T2-weighted image studies (Figure 28-5).[26]

Table 28-1.

The Sarnat Classification System

Variable	Stage 1	Stage 2	Stage 3
Level of consciousness	Alert	Lethargic	Coma
Muscle tone	Normal or hypertonia	Hypotonia	Flaccidity
Tendon reflexes	Increased	Increased	Depressed or absent
Myoclonus	Present	Present	Absent
Seizures	Absent	Frequent	Frequent
Complex reflexes			
Suck	Active	Weak	Absent
Moro	Exaggerated	Incomplete	Absent
Grasp	Normal or exaggerated	Exaggerated	Absent
Oculocephalic (doll's-eye)	Normal	Overactive	Reduced or absent
Autonomic reflexes			
Pupils	Dilated, reactive	Constrictive, reactive	Variable or fixed
Respirations	Regular	Variations in depth, rate, periodic	Apneic
Heart rate	Normal or tachycardia	Bradycardia	Bradycardia
EEG	Normal	Low voltage, periodic or paroxysmal	Periodic or Isoelectric

The classification system divides neonates into mild (stage 1), moderate (stage 2), and severe (Stage 3) HIE based on the variables shown in the table.
(Table generated from Vannucci R. Hypoxia ischemia: pathogenesis and neuropathology. In: Fanaroff A, ed. Neonatal-Perinatal Medicine: Diseases of the Fetus and Infant. St. Louis: Mosby; 1997:856-891, which was based on the original work by Sarnat HB, Sarnat MS. Neonatal encephalopathy following fetal distress. A clinical and electroencephalographic study. Arch Neurol. 1976;33:696-705)

EEG

The EEG may provide valuable information on the severity of injury.[15] More recently, amplitude integrated EEG has been used as a method to continuously monitor neonates and predict outcomes based on the background pattern.[27,28]

Treatment

The neonate suffering from HIE should be systemically stabilized. The basic concepts for stabilization are presented in the flow diagram in Figure 28-6. There currently is no specific treatment for HIE that addresses the ongoing neuronal injury. However, hypothermia appears to be the most promising therapy in decades, as demonstrated by two recent clinical trials. The hypothermia studies used either head cooling with mild systemic hypothermia (34-35°C) or whole-body cooling (33.5°C). Both studies used hypothermia for 72 hours. The systemic hypothermia study demonstrated a decrease in death and moderate or severe disability in the hypothermia group compared with a matched control.[29] The head cooling study with mild systemic hypothermia demonstrated that the therapy could safely improve survival without severe

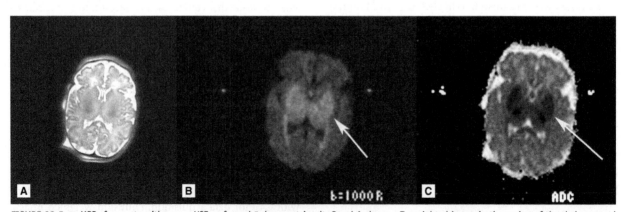

FIGURE 28-5 ■ MRI of neonate with severe HIE performed 5 days post-insult. Panel **A** shows a T_2-weighted image in the region of the thalamus and basal ganglia. Panels **B** and **C** are diffusion weighted and ADC maps similar to the brain region shown on the T_2-weighted image. Although there are subtle changes on the T_2-weighted image, the areas of injury are much more apparent as bright areas in the region of the thalamus and basal ganglia (arrows, panel B) on the diffusion-weighted image and the corresponding dark areas in the same brain region on the ADC map (arrows, panel C).

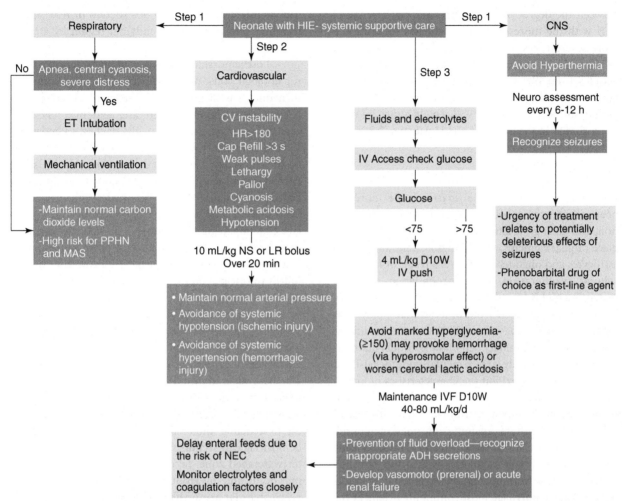

FIGURE 28-6 ■ A suggested schema for the basic steps to stabilize and initially systemically manage a patient with HIE is presented in flow diagram format. The flow diagram uses a systems-based approach common to intensive care medicine (ABCs). Step 1 is establishment of a stable airway. The main goals for management of a neonate on a ventilator are shown in the gray box and involve the maintenance of normal carbon dioxide levels. Normal carbon dioxide levels will prevent increases or decreases in CBF associated with hypercarbia and hypocarbia, respectively. Parallel to the establishment of an airway, the clinician should avoid hyperthermia, as it may worsen the neurological injury. Step 2 is the establishment and maintenance of adequate circulation with the goals of cardiovascular support illustrated in the gray box. Step 3 is the establishment of IV access, preferably central, depending on the acuity of the patient. Normoglycemia should be maintained to minimize further neurological injury. Maintenance fluids should be started at the suggested range and titrated based on the presence of hypotension, syndrome of inappropriate antidiuretic hormone secretion, or renal failure due to hypoxic-ischemic renal injury. Finally, electrolytes should be monitored closely for hyperkalemia and hypocalcemia. A coagulopathy may exist as a result of hypoxic-ischemic injury to the liver, and feeds should be started slowly and with caution after an initial period of NPO due to intestinal hypoxic-ischemic injury.

neurodevelopmental disabilities in neonates with moderate encephalopathy, as defined by amplitude-integrated EEG criteria.[30] Based on these results and ongoing follow-up studies of the enrolled patients, hypothermia will most likely become widespread in clinical practice.

Outcome

Based on a large cohort of neonates with HIE,[14,31] neonates with mild HIE (Sarnat 1) had no long-term deficits at 8 years of age. Six percent of neonates with moderate HIE (Sarnat 2) died, and of the survivors, 20% developed handicaps (seizures, cerebral palsy, mental

retardation, deafness, blindness) at 8 years of age. In the severe category (Sarnat 3), 80% died and 100% of the survivors at 8 years of age had severe handicaps.

INTRAVENTRICULAR HEMORRHAGE

Definition and Epidemiology

Intraventricular hemorrhage (IVH) is an injury primarily associated with prematurity, with an incidence ranging between 40% and 60% in very low birth weight (VLBW) neonates.[2,32] There is an inverse relationship between the degree of prematurity and the severity of IVH with the more premature neonates suffering the more severe types of hemorrhage.[33] The incidence of IVH in VLBW neonates has decreased over recent decades, from 49% to less than 20%.[2] However, the survival of VLBW neonates has improved over the same period, suggesting that IVH will remain a major source of morbidity in the tiniest of NICU patients.[34,35]

Pathogenesis

The subependymal germinal matrix is the source of neuronal precursors between 10 and 20 weeks of gestation, and during the latter half of gestation is the birthplace of glial elements, which migrate and mature into astrocytes and oligodendroglia. As a result of the active cellular proliferation, the subependymal germinal matrix is a highly vascularized structure with a capillary bed that is a vascular end zone of its arterial supply. This makes this region very susceptible to ischemic injury. Furthermore, the capillary bed in the germinal matrix is composed of relatively large, irregular, endothelial-lined vessels that do not exhibit the characteristics of arterioles or venules, making these vessels thin-walled and fragile. The subependymal germinal matrix is the site of origin of IVH. With this anatomic information in mind, the principal mechanism by which an IVH occurs is the rupture of the fragile capillaries within the germinal matrix resulting from fluctuations of blood flow in this region. The hemorrhage most commonly occurs at the head of the caudate nucleus at the level of the foramen of Monro in neonates less than 28 weeks. And, in 80% of the cases, the hemorrhage will rupture through the adjacent ependymal wall into the lateral ventricle with spread of blood throughout the ventricular system.[36]

The subependymal germinal matrix begins to involute following 34 weeks of gestation. Therefore, it is important to note that IVH in the term neonate originates primarily from the choroid plexus.[37]

Several neuropathological processes occur as a result of or accompany IVH. IVH is associated with destruction of the germinal matrix and the glial precursor cells, which are located in the germinal matrix. Roughly 15% of the neonates with IVH will develop a periventricular hemorrhagic infarction.[2] This lesion has a fan-shaped appearance that closely follows the medullary veins in the periventricular cerebral white matter.[2] The incidence of periventricular hemorrhagic infarction is associated with prematurity, with one-third of the cases occurring in neonates between 500 and 800 g. It also is associated with a large IVH in 80% of cases.[36] Careful anatomic studies have demonstrated that periventricular hemorrhagic infarction is not simply an extension of the IVH from the ventricular system into the surrounding parenchyma, but rather is a result of a venous infarction caused by obstruction of flow in the terminal vein in the subependymal region by a large ipsilateral IVH.

Posthemorrhagic hydrocephalus is another neuropathologic consequence of IVH and is more common in neonates with the highest grades of IVH (see the "Diagnosis" section, for grading system).[33] Hydrocephalus is a progressive ventricular dilation secondary to a disturbance in CSF dynamics. Hydrocephalus may occur acutely over a period of days (associated with larger IVH) or subacutely evolving over a period of weeks (associated with smaller IVH). Acute hydrocephalus results from an obstruction of the arachnoid villi by the particulate clot impairing CSF absorption, whereas subacute hydrocephalus is caused by an obliterative arachnoiditis in the posterior fossa, resulting in obstruction of the fourth ventricle or aqueductal obstruction by blood clot, disrupted ependyma, or reactive gliosis.

Periventricular leukomalacia (PVL) is generally a symmetric injury of the periventricular white matter, located at the arterial border zones of the trigone of the lateral ventricles, and occurs more frequently in neonates who have suffered from IVH. The association is believed to occur because of decreases in cerebral blood flow that accompany IVH. The periventricular region is susceptible to ischemia; thus PVL can be considered the nonhemorrhagic infarction of the periventricular white matter watershed zone. Secondary hemorrhage into PVL may occur, and this lesion is difficult to distinguish from periventricular hemorrhagic infarction.

IVH is the end consequence of many factors that may act alone or in concert with each other and may differ over time. These factors can be broken down into three major areas: intravascular, vascular, and extravascular factors.

Intravascular

Intravascular factors involve changes in cerebral blood flow (increase, decrease, fluctations), increases in cerebral venous pressures, and coagulation abnormalities.

Cerebral autoregulation is the mechanism ensuring that cerebral blood flow remains constant over a wide range of systemic pressures by means of compensatory cerebral arteriolar dilation or constriction.[36] The principle etiology of the changes in cerebral blood flow relate to impairment of cerebral autoregulation in the sick premature neonate[38] and the stable premature neonate.[39] When cerebral autoregulation is impaired, the cerebral circulation becomes pressure-passive and fluctuates according to changes in systemic blood pressure, with decreases during periods of hypotension and increases during periods of hypertension. Fluctuations in blood pressure are associated with rapid volume administration, the presence of a patent ductus arteriosus, respiratory distress syndrome, pneumothorax, hypercarbia, seizures, and routine bedside care (eg, suctioning of endotracheal tube). When these fluctuations do occur, injury to the vulnerable capillary bed may occur, resulting in IVH.

Vascular

Vascular factors relate to the fragility of the immature, endothelium-lined microvasculature of the germinal matrix, its rapid rate of oxidative metabolism, and its location in a vascular border zone between the thalamic and striate arteries, rendering it vulnerable to hypoxic-ischemic injury.[36] These anatomic vulnerabilities can be amplified by such conditions as chorioamnionitis and neonatal sepsis, independent of these entities' effects on hemodynamics.

Extravascular

Extravascular factors relate to the space surrounding the germinal matrix capillaries and include deficient vascular support for the germinal matrix capillaries and increased fibrinolytic activity, which may allow minor capillary disruptions to evolve into a large IVH.

Clinical Presentation

Neonates with IVH have been described as having three potential clinical presentations: a catastrophic deterioration, a salutatory deterioration, and a "clinically silent" syndrome.[2]

Neonates who present with a catastrophic deterioration will have a very dramatic presentation that consists of a sudden change in the neonate's baseline status over a period of minutes to hours. Neurological symptoms include deep stupor or coma, respiratory abnormalities (hypoventilation, apnea), generalized tonic

seizures, decerebrate posturing, and pupils fixed to light (depends on gestational age—see the "Physical Examination" section earlier in the chapter for more details). Systemic symptoms may also be present in the form of hypotension, bradycardia, a sudden metabolic acidosis, a dropping hematocrit, temperature instability, hypoglycemia, and a bulging fontanel. Experts have speculated that the described symptoms occur because of movement of blood through the ventricular system with sequential regions of the brain (diencephalon, midbrain, pons, medulla) being affected.[2]

A salutatory deterioration is much more subtle in clinical presentation. The clinical appearance includes an alteration in the level of consciousness, a change in the quantity and quality of spontaneous and elicited motility, hypotonia, and subtle abnormalities of eye position and movement (skew deviation, vertical drift [usually down], incomplete horizontal movement with doll's-eye maneuver).[2] The salutatory syndrome evolves over many hours and may show signs of cessation only to reappear for several more hours. This waxing and waning clinical course may continue for a day or more.

The final presentation is a clinically silent syndrome. These neonates may have little in the way of neurological abnormalities and may only demonstrate an unexplained drop in hematocrit or failure of the hematocrit to rise post-transfusion.[2]

Diagnosis

Ultrasound scan is effective in the diagnosis of IVH, with a 76% to 100% accuracy of detecting grade 1 lesions larger than 5 mm and grade 3 and 4 hemorrhages.[40-43] The scan can be used to visualize the location and severity of the hemorrhage (Figure 28-7). Two major systems are

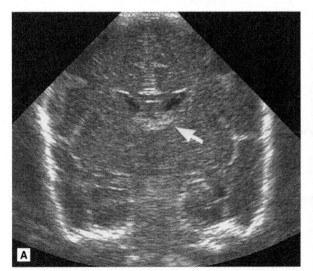
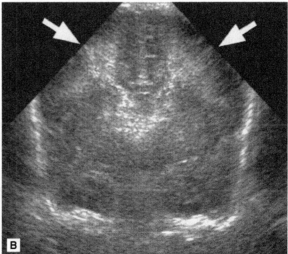

FIGURE 28-7 ■ Ultrasound of prematurely born infant (28 weeks gestation) with intraventricular hemorrhage that was imaged 4 weeks postnatally **(A)** and again 3 days later **(B)**. (*Reprinted with permission from path.upmc.edu/cases/cas85.html. Courtesy of Robert Hevner and Raymond Sobel.*)

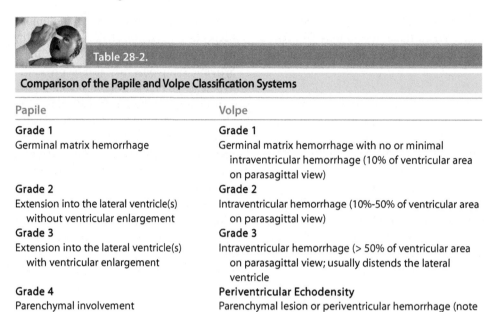

Table 28-2.

Comparison of the Papile and Volpe Classification Systems

Papile	Volpe
Grade 1	**Grade 1**
Germinal matrix hemorrhage	Germinal matrix hemorrhage with no or minimal intraventricular hemorrhage (10% of ventricular area on parasagittal view)
Grade 2	**Grade 2**
Extension into the lateral ventricle(s) without ventricular enlargement	Intraventricular hemorrhage (10%-50% of ventricular area on parasagittal view)
Grade 3	**Grade 3**
Extension into the lateral ventricle(s) with ventricular enlargement	Intraventricular hemorrhage (> 50% of ventricular area on parasagittal view; usually distends the lateral ventricle)
Grade 4	**Periventricular Echodensity**
Parenchymal involvement	Parenchymal lesion or periventricular hemorrhage (note location and extent)

Note that the Volpe system does not include a grade IV hemorrhage. Parenchymal involvement in this classification system is instead categorized as a separate entity because these lesions are not simply an extension of the matrix or intraventricular hemorrhage into the brain parenchyma.

used to gauge the severity of the IVH. The first system was developed by Papile[32] and the second, more recently, by Volpe.[2] Both systems are compared in Table 28-2. As mentioned earlier in the "Clinical Presentation" section, IVH may present with minimal clinical symptoms in the preterm neonate. Therefore, screening procedures are in place in the NICU nationally to detect the presence of IVH in preterm neonates; however, there is no consensus on the target population for screening, the number of examinations, or the timing of the studies. Although there is no treatment for IVH, screening provides the clinician with useful prognostic information for counseling parents about potential long-term neurodevelopmental disabilities.

At the University of Florida, we have developed a screening protocol in our institute (Figure 28-8) that represents a review of the current literature, practice parameters, and a review of our patient demographics over a recent 5-year span. It is presented here as a template that may be used as a starting point for the development of a screening protocol and as a means to discuss the current literature concerning the timing, number of scans, and ages to scan patients. We chose to screen neonates who weighed 1350 g or less with routine screening. Several studies from the literature have demonstrated that 12% to 51% of neonates with a birth weight lesser than 1500 g and/or 33 weeks of gestation will have cranial abnormalities with major abnormalities such as grade 3 or 4 IVH or bilateral cystic PVL occurring in less than 20% of these neonates. Major abnormalities such as grade 3 or 4 IVH, cystic PVL, and ventriculomegaly associated with

posthemorrhagic hydrocephalus, which might alter treatment or provide prognostic information, are considerably more common (20%-25%) in infants with a gestational age lesser than 30 weeks.[26] Based on this information, a consensus group recommended screening all neonates lesser than 30 weeks. We modified our protocol to an older gestational age based on our past patient data because several neonates who had a grade 3 or 4 IVH would not have been screened. We also chose to use a risk-based strategy to screen for neonates between 1350 and 1500 g since neonates in this weight range in our institution usually had an IVH associated with a known risk factor. This allowed our screening protocol to fit our patient population with respect to which neonates to screen. Multiple studies before 1990 suggested that more than 90% of IVHs occurred during postnatal days 4 to 5. More recent studies have shown that approximately 65% of the cases occur within the first week, with hemorrhages detected on later scans between 10 and 14 days. We therefore chose the time interval 7 to 14 days to obtain our initial screening scan. If bedside clinicians detect symptoms consistent with an IVH, they may obtain a scan earlier based on clinical indications. Our time period for the initial screening examination is consistent with that set forth by a consensus panel.[26] Finally, a screening US is performed at 6 weeks in our protocol to detect PVL. MRI provides much better anatomic information with respect to white matter injury, but currently there are insufficient follow-up studies to indicate whether the increased findings on MRI provide any additional information about the neurodevelopmental prognosis. As these studies become available, MRI will

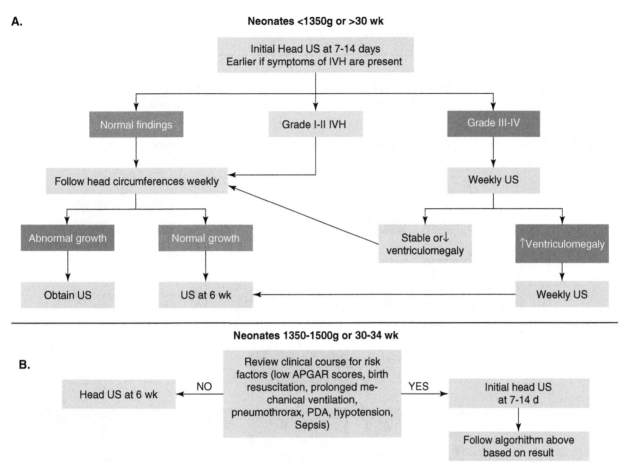

A.

Neonates <1350g or >30 wk

Initial Head US at 7-14 days
Earlier if symptoms of IVH are present

Normal findings → Grade I-II IVH → Grade III-IV

Follow head circumferences weekly ← Weekly US

Abnormal growth | Normal growth | Stable or↓ ventriculomegaly | ↑Ventriculomegaly

Obtain US | US at 6 wk | Weekly US

Neonates 1350-1500g or 30-34 wk

B.

Head US at 6 wk ← NO — Review clinical course for risk factors (low APGAR scores, birth resuscitation, prolonged mechanical ventilation, pneumothrorax, PDA, hypotension, Sepsis) — YES → Initial head US at 7-14 d

Follow algorhithm above based on result

FIGURE 28-8 ■ **A.** Screening protocol used at our institute at the University of Florida for neonates less than 1350 g or more than 30 weeks of gestation. The algorithm is meant to serve as a guide for discussion in the text and has been modified to fit our patient demographics (see text). Neonates with grade III-IV hemorrhages are closely observed with weekly head ultrasounds for 4 weeks. Neonates who continue to have increasing ventriculomegaly will continue with weekly observations and possibly medical interventions (see Figure 28-1). Neonates with a stable or decreasing ventricular size after 4 weeks will have weekly head circumferences measured. Both groups will receive a 6-week head ultrasound to screen for periventricular leukomalacia. **B.** Risk-based strategy that our institute at the University of Florida uses for neonates between 1350 and 1500 g or 30 to 34 weeks.

most likely become the screening tool of choice in the future. Although the consensus panel recommends screening neonates at 36 to 40 weeks post-menstrual age, we chose to have a fixed time point of 6 weeks to decrease the chance of missing a screening examination. It should also be noted that the protocol from our institute uses ultrasound to closely monitor neonates who have grade III or IV IVHs. The rationale for the use of US for this screening purpose pertains to the anatomic information—the ventricles in the neonate may dilate to an impressive degree before the development of rapid head growth and signs of increased intracranial pressure. This is due to the paucity of cerebral myelin, the relative excess of water in the centrum semiovale, and the relatively large subarachnoid space.[2]

Treatment

The ideal treatment for IVH is the prevention of premature births and the prevention of hemorrhages in

neonates. Indomethicin-administered prophylatically in neonates has been shown to be effective in preventing grades 3 and 4 IVH.[44] This short-term benefit may not have long-lasting consequences; follow-up studies in neonates treated with indomethicin prophylatically have not revealed a clear benefit or harm in long-term neurodevelopmental outcomes.[45]

The postnatal management of neonates who have IVH currently centers on the detection and treatment of posthemorrhagic hydrocephalus. Posthemorrhagic hydrocephalus has been shown to cause secondary injury by axonal stretching, periventricular vascular distortion, and compression that may decrease cerebral blood flow, causing ischemic injury and producing alterations in synaptogenesis that may result in abnormal organization of the cerebral cortex. A schema for potential management of posthemorrhagic hydrocephalus is shown in Figure 28-8.

As illustrated in Figure 28-9, several techniques may be used to decrease the progression of hydrocephalus,

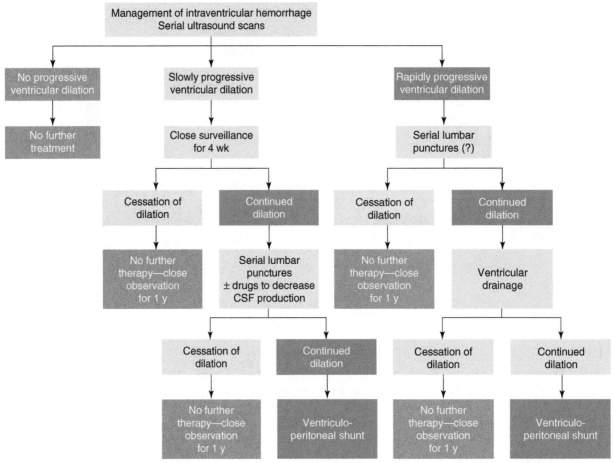

FIGURE 28-9 ■ A proposed schema for managing patients with posthemorrhagic hydrocephalus is presented in flowchart form. Slowly progressive ventricular dilation is defined as moderate dilation with appropriate head growth and stable intracranial pressure. Rapidly progressive ventricular dilation is defined as moderate to severe dilation, excessive rate of head growth, and rising intracranial pressure. See text for further discussion of drug therapy and serial lumbar punctures. (*Reproduced with permission from Volpe JJ. Neurology of the Newborn. 4th ed. Philadelphia: Saunders; 2001.*)

including medications and serial lumbar punctures. Medications that decrease CSF production include acetazolamide and furosemide. Although still employed in the clinical setting, a recent metanalysis concluded that the use of these medications did not reduce the need for a ventriculoperitoneal shunt. Serial lumbar punctures are used to mechanically remove CSF. A recent metanalysis from the Cochrane Collaboration concluded that routine use of serial lumbar punctures could not be supported by the current literature; however, one would find it hard to argue against the use of lumbar punctures in neonates who developed signs of symptomatic raised intracranial pressure (deterioration in neurological signs with a tense fontanelle, decreasing diastolic velocities on cerebral artery Doppler waveforms, deteriorating sensory evoked potentials, directly measured CSF pressure over 12 mm Hg).[46]

Outcomes

Ultrasound findings of a grade 3 or 4 IVH, cystic PVL, and moderate to severe ventriculomegaly at 36 to 40 weeks post-menstruation, have all been significantly associated with cerebral palsy at 2 to 9 years of age in VLBW preterm neonates.[26] Similarly, grade 4 IVH and ventriculomegaly at 36 to 40 weeks post-menstruation have been significantly associated with mental retardation and neuropsychiatric disorders at the same time points.

SEIZURES

Definition and Epidemiology

Neonatal seizures are poorly classified, under-recognized, especially in sick neonates, and often difficult to

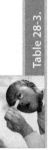

Table 28-3.

Seizures That Occur in the Neonate Based on Patient Demographics, Clinical Presentation, and EEG Correlations

	Subtle	Tonic	Clonic	Myoclonic
Subgroups	May represent clinical subcortical or "brainstem release phenomona"	Two subgroups: Focal tonic seizures Generalized tonic seizures	Two subgroups: Focal clonic seizures Multifocal clonic seizures	Three subgroups: Focal myoclonic seizures Multifocal myoclonic seizures Generalized myoclonic seizures
Patient demographics	Occur both in the full term and premature neonate but are more common in the premature	Frequently associated with IVH	More common in the term neonate.	Seen both in the term and preterm neonate.
Clinical presentation	Bicycling movements, lip smacking, roving eyes, sustained eye opening with ocular fixation, and apnea	**Focal tonic seizures consist of** sustained posturing of a limb or asymmetrical posturing of the trunk or neck. **Generalized tonic seizures are** characterized by tonic extension of both upper and lower extremities (mimicking "decerebrate posturing") or by tonic extension of upper extremities with extension of lower extremities (mimicking "decorticate" posturing).	Rhythmic and usually slow (1-3 jerks/second) **Focal clonic seizures**—involves the face, upper or lower extremeties on 1 side of the body. Infants usually conscious. **Multifocal clonic**—seizures involve several body parts. Neonates do not exhibit the electrical evolution associated with the classical Jacksonian march or a partial seizure with secondary generalization due to insufficient cortical neuronal connections.	Myoclonic movements are distinguished from tonic movements by the more rapid speed of myoclonic jerks and the predilection of the flexor group to be involved in myoclonic seizures. **Focal and multifocal myoclonic** seizures well localized, single or multiple, migrating jerks usually of flexor muscles usually of limbs. Generalized myoclonic seizures involve bilateral jerks of flexion of upper and occasionally of lower extremities.
EEG findings	Typically contain no EEG correlate	Generalized tonic seizures are not commonly associated with EEG correlates while focal tonic seizures are consistently associated with EEG seizure discharges.	Associated with surface EEG rhythmic electrographic seizure activity.	Generalized myolclonic seizures are more likely to associated with EEG discharges than focal or multifocal myoclonic seizures.

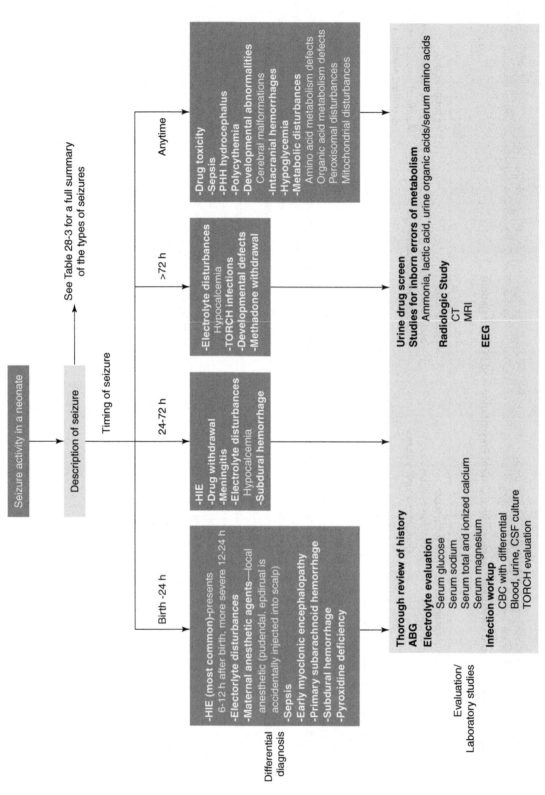

FIGURE 28-10 ■ The differential diagnosis for neonatal seizures is illustrated as a function of the time interval post birth at which the seizure first appears. The etiologies are shown in bold with subcategories and facts about the etiologies shown in plain text. Tests to narrow the differential diagnosis are illustrated in the last box. The clinician should choose the appropriate test to aid in the narrowing of the differential diagnosis.

treat.[47] Neonatal seizures are often the presenting clinical manifestation of underlying neurological conditions such as hypoxia-ischemic encephalopathy, stroke, intraventricular or intraparenchymal hemorrhages, meningitis, sepsis, or metabolic disorders. Of these, hypoxic ischemic encephalopathy is the most common etiology, accounting for 50% to 60% of patients with neonatal seizures.[47]

Pathophysiology

A seizure is the occurrence of an abnormal synchronous electrical discharge (depolarization) of a group of neurons within the central nervous system.[47] During the normal state, the neuron depolarizes as a result of sodium influx into the cell with repolarization occurring when potassium ions are pumped out of the neuron, creating the normal baseline negative electrical potential across the cell membrane. Seizures are generally felt to be the result of excessive depolarization. Electrolyte abnormalities, such as hypocalcemia, can alter the normal membrane potential by increasing the influx of sodium, thereby promoting depolarization. Hypoxia-ischemia and hypoglycemia result in a sharp decrease in energy substrate, which produces failure of the energy-dependent sodium–potassium pump, shifting the membrane potential to a more positive state and promoting depolarization.[2,47] The neonatal brain is particularly vulnerable to seizure activity as a result of an imbalance of excitatory to inhibitory circuitry. The imbalance favors excitation and does so to facilitate important developmental processes that occur during the neonatal period (synaptogenesis, apoptosis, progressive integration of circuitry, synaptic pruning). The imbalance occurs anatomically and physiologically by an overexpression of NMDA receptor in the hippocampus and neocortical regions of the neonatal brain, a delay in the maturation of the inhibitory system, and neurons in such regions as the hippocampus are excited rather than inhibited by the neurotransmitter GABA (normally the primary inhibitory neurotransmitter in the brain).

Clinical Presentation

The various types of seizures in the neonate and the clinical presentation are presented in Table 28-3.

Differential Diagnosis

The differential diagnosis and suggested laboratory tests to narrow the differential are illustrated in Figure 28-10.

Treatment

The clinician should first search for underlying etiologies producing the seizures and treat (hypoglycemia, hypocalcemia, sepsis). If the clinician cannot find a readily identifiable and treatable etiology, the front-line agent of choice for treating seizures is phenobarbital. Phenobarbital as a single agent will stop seizure activity in 42% of patients.[48] When the seizure does not respond to a single agent, phenytoin is added with an increase in efficacy to 65%. Currently, fosphenytoin, the salt ester of phenytoin, is preferred in the neonate because it is an aqueous solution that is soluble in glucose-containing solutions, can be administered more quickly than phenytoin, and will not cause "purple glove syndrome."[49] Purple glove syndrome is necrosis or injury of the soft tissue that can occur with intravenous infusion of the highly alkaline phenytoin. The drug of choice for neonates in status is lorazapam. This agent has several properties that make it ideal—a long half-life and a small volume of distribution, which prolongs its retention at high levels in the brain.[50,51]

REFERENCES

1. Nold JL, Georgieff MK. Infants of diabetic mothers. *Pediatr Clin North Am.* 2004; 51:619-637, viii.
2. Volpe JJ. *Neurology of The Newborn.* Philadelphia: Saunders; 2001.
3. Yang M. Newborn neurologic examination. *Neurology.* 2004;62:E15-17.
4. Saint-Anne Dargassies S. Neurological development in the full-term and premature neonate. New York: *Excerpta Medica*; 1977.
5. Dubowitz LM, Mushin J, De Vries L, Arden GB. Visual function in the newborn infant: is it cortically mediated? *Lancet.* 1986;1:1139-1141.
6. Peiper A. *Cerebral Function in Infancy and Childhood.* Consultants Bureau; 1963.
7. Bu'Lock F, Woolridge MW, Baum JD. Development of coordination of sucking, swallowing and breathing: ultrasound study of term and preterm infants. *Dev Med Child Neurol.* 1990;32:669-678.
8. Vannucci R. Hypoxia ischemia: pathogenesis and neuropathology. In: Fanaroff A, ed. *Neonatal-Perinatal Medicine: Diseases of the Fetus and Infant.* St. Louis: Mosby; 1997:856-891.
9. Giffard RG, Monyer H, Choi DW. Selective vulnerability of cultured cortical glia to injury by extracellular acidosis. *Brain Res.* 1990;530:138-141.
10. Low JA, Lindsay BG, Derrick EJ. Threshold of metabolic acidosis associated with newborn complications. *Am J Obstet Gynecol.* 1997;177:1391-1394.
11. Mulligan JC, Painter MJ, O'Donoghue PA, MacDonald HM, Allan AC, Taylor PM. Neonatal asphyxia. II. Neonatal mortality and long-term sequelae. *J Pediatr.* 1980; 96: 903-907.
12. MacDonald HM, Mulligan JC, Allen AC, Taylor PM. Neonatal asphyxia. I. Relationship of obstetric and neonatal complications to neonatal mortality in 38,405 consecutive deliveries. *J Pediatr.* 1980;96:898-902.
13. Finer NN, Robertson CM, Richards RT, Pinnell LE, Peters KL. Hypoxic-ischemic encephalopathy in term neonates: perinatal factors and outcome. *J Pediatr.* 1981;98:112-117.
14. Robertson CM, Finer NN, Grace MG. School performance of survivors of neonatal encephalopathy associated with birth asphyxia at term. *J Pediatr.* 1989;114:753-760.

15. Sarnat HB, Sarnat MS. Neonatal encephalopathy following fetal distress. A clinical and electroencephalographic study. *Arch Neurol.* 1976;33:696–705.

16. Delivoria-Papadopoulos M, Mishra OP. Mechanisms of cerebral injury in perinatal asphyxia and strategies for prevention. *J Pediatr.* 1998;132:S30-S34.

17. Johnston MV. Excitotoxicity in neonatal hypoxia. *Ment Retard Dev Disabil Res Rev.* 2001;7:229-234.

18. Hagberg H, Thornberg E, Blennow M, et al. Excitatory amino acids in the cerebrospinal fluid of asphyxiated infants: relationship to hypoxic-ischemic encephalopathy. *Acta Paediatr.* 1993;82:925-929.

19. Silverstein FS, Naik B, Simpson J. Hypoxia-ischemia stimulates hippocampal glutamate efflux in perinatal rat brain: an in vivo microdialysis study. *Pediatr Res.* 1991;30:587-590.

20. Andine P, Thordstein M, Kjellmer I, et al. Evaluation of brain damage in a rat model of neonatal hypoxic-ischemia. *J Neurosci Methods.* 1990;35:253-260.

21. Lucas D, Newman SM. The toxic effect of sodium L-glutamate on the inner layers of the retina. *Arch Opthalmol.* 1957:193-201.

22. Olney JW. Brain lesions, obesity, and other disturbances in mice treated with monosodium glutamate. *Science.* 1969;164:719-721.

23. Johnston MV. Neurotransmitters and vulnerability of the developing brain. *Brain Dev.* 1995;17:301-306.

24. McDonald JW, Johnston MV. Physiological and pathophysiological roles of excitatory amino acids during central nervous system development. *Brain Res Rev.* 1990;15:41-70.

25. Johnston MV, Trescher WH, Ishida A, Nakajima W. Neurobiology of hypoxic-ischemic injury in the developing brain. *Pediatr Res.* 2001;49:735-741.

26. Ment LR, Bada HS, Barnes P, et al. Practice parameter: neuroimaging of the neonate: report of the Quality Standards Subcommittee of the American Academy of Neurology and the Practice Committee of the Child Neurology Society. *Neurology.* 2002;58:1726-1738.

27. de Vries LS, Toet MC. Amplitude integrated electroencephalography in the full-term newborn. *Clin Perinatol.* 2006;33:619-632, vi.

28. Hellstrom-Westas L, Rosen I, Svenningsen NW. Predictive value of early continuous amplitude integrated EEG recordings on outcome after severe birth asphyxia in full term infants. *Arch Dis Child Fetal Neonatal Ed.* 1995;72:F34-F38.

29. Shankaran S, Laptook AR, Ehrenkranz RA, et al. Whole-body hypothermia for neonates with hypoxic-ischemic encephalopathy. *N Engl J Med.* 2005;353:1574-1584.

30. Gluckman PD, Wyatt JS, Azzopardi D, et al. Selective head cooling with mild systemic hypothermia after neonatal encephalopathy: multicentre randomised trial. *Lancet.* 2005; 365:663-670.

31. Robertson C, Finer N. Term infants with hypoxic-ischemic encephalopathy: outcome at 3.5 years. *Dev Med Child Neurol.* 1985;27:473-484.

32. Papile LA, Burstein J, Burstein R, Koffler H. Incidence and evolution of subependymal and intraventricular hemorrhage: a study of infants with birth weights less than 1,500 gm. *J Pediatr.* 1978;92:529-534.

33. Vohr B, Ment LR. Intraventricular hemorrhage in the preterm infant. *Early Hum Dev.* 1996; 44:1-16.

34. Hamilton BE, Minino AM, Martin JA, Kochanek KD, Strobino DM, Guyer B. Annual summary of vital statistics: 2005. *Pediatrics.* 2007;119:345-360.

35. McIntire DD, Bloom SL, Casey BM, Leveno KJ. Birth weight in relation to morbidity and mortality among newborn infants. *N Engl J Med.* 1999;340:1234-1238.

36. Roland EH, Hill A. Germinal matrix-intraventricular hemorrhage in the premature newborn: management and outcome. *Neurol Clin.* 2003; 21:833-851, vi-vii.

37. Armstrong DL, Sauls CD, Goddard-Finegold J. Neuropathologic findings in short-term survivors of intraventricular hemorrhage. *Am J Dis Child.* 1987;141:617-621.

38. Muller AM, Morales C, Briner J, Baenziger O, Duc G, Bucher HU. Loss of CO_2 reactivity of cerebral blood flow is associated with severe brain damage in mechanically ventilated very low birth weight infants. *Eur J Paediatr Neurol.* 1997;1:157-163.

39. Boylan GB, Young K, Panerai RB, Rennie JM, Evans DH. Dynamic cerebral autoregulation in sick newborn infants. *Pediatr Res.* 2000;48:12-17.

40. Trounce JQ, Fagan D, Levene MI. Intraventricular haemorrhage and periventricular leucomalacia: ultrasound and autopsy correlation. *Arch Dis Child.* 1986;61:1203-1207.

41. Pape KE, Bennett-Britton S, Szymonowicz W, Martin DJ, Fitz CR, Becker L. Diagnostic accuracy of neonatal brain imaging: a postmortem correlation of computed tomography and ultrasound scans. *J Pediatr.* 1983;102:275-280.

42. Mack LA, Wright K, Hirsch JH, et al. Intracranial hemorrhage in premature infants: accuracy in sonographic evaluation. *AJR Am J Roentgenol.* 1981;137:245-250.

43. Babcock DS, Bove KE, Han BK. Intracranial hemorrhage in premature infants: sonographic-pathologic correlation. *AJNR Am J Neuroradiol.* 1982;3:309-317.

44. Ment LR, Oh W, Ehrenkranz RA, et al. Low-dose indomethacin and prevention of intraventricular hemorrhage: a multicenter randomized trial. *Pediatrics.* 1994; 93:543-550.

45. Fowlie PW, Davis PG. Prophylactic indomethacin for preterm infants: a systematic review and meta-analysis. *Arch Dis Child Fetal Neonatal Ed.* 2003;88:F464-F466.

46. Whitelaw A. Repeated lumbar or ventricular punctures in newborns with intraventricular hemorrhage. *Cochrane Database Syst Rev.* 2001:CD000216.

47. Zupanc ML. Neonatal seizures. *Pediatr Clin North Am.* 2004;51:961-978, ix.

48. Painter MJ, Scher MS, Stein AD, et al. Phenobarbital compared with phenytoin for the treatment of neonatal seizures. *N Engl J Med.* 1999;341:485-489.

49. Morton LD. Clinical experience with fosphenytoin in children. *J Child Neurol.* 1998;13(suppl):S19-S22; discussion S30-S32.

50. Maytal J, Novak GP, King KC. Lorazepam in the treatment of refractory neonatal seizures. *J Child Neurol.* 1991;6:319-323.

51. Deshmukh A, Wittert W, Schnitzler E, Mangurten HH. Lorazepam in the treatment of refractory neonatal seizures. A pilot study. *Am J Dis Child.* 1986;140:1042-1044.

CHAPTER 29

Disorders of Vision and Ocular Motility

Jonathan Etter, M. Tariq Bhatti,
Mays El-Dairi, and David Wallace

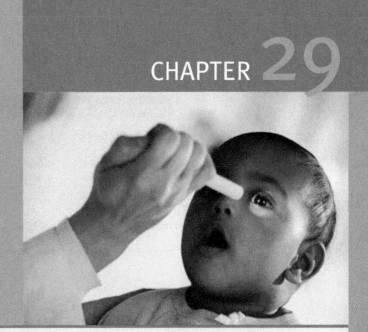

DISORDERS OF VISION

Normal Visual Development

The visual system is immature at birth. Achievement of normal vision is dependent on key anatomic changes during development that involve both the retina and the visual pathways. At the level of the retina, connections between the photoreceptors and the inner retinal cells are not fully formed until a few months after birth.[1] At the level of the brain, myelination of the optic radiations takes place in the first year of life. Normal visual development also depends on well-focused input from the anterior segment of the eye. Hubel and Wiesel found that, if this normal input is not present, then visual deprivation leads to maldevelopment in the cerebral cortex.[2]

Vision Testing in Children

Estimates of visual acuity at birth range from 20/2000 to 20/400. A newborn starts fixating and regarding the mother's face by 2 weeks of age. Between 8 and 10 weeks of age, a normal infant can generally fix and follow a large object over an arc of 180°. A visual problem exists if an infant cannot fix and follow a lighted toy by 3 months of age.

Normal ranges of visual acuity in children vary based on age. Methods to measure visual acuity are also age-dependent. In general, recognition acuity measures are favored over other methods (see "Recognition acuity tests: Allen pictures, HOTV and Snellen letters," p. 380). To assess visual acuity in a preverbal child, motor behavioral responses can be used, such as optokinetic nystagmus or preferential looking tests. When needed, a visual evoked potential test can quantify the visual sensory response. Table 29-1 lists normal ranges of visual acuity by age using the preferential looking test or visual evoked potentials. When children are old enough to verbalize their responses, visual acuity is done by recognition acuity testing. If a child is too shy to talk, he or she can be asked to match pictures or letters with a hand-held card.

Examination Procedures and Guidelines for Referral

Optokinetic nystagmus

This test consists of a cylindrical drum with alternating black and white rectangular stripes. The drum is rotated in the infant's visual field while the examiner observes for smooth pursuit eye movements in the direction of the rotating drum followed by saccadic eye movements in the opposite direction. Horizontal saccades can be elicited at birth in a full-term child, but vertical saccades do not develop until 4 to 6 weeks of age.

Visual evoked potentials

Using scalp electrodes, electroencephalographic activity can be assessed while showing a child a specific visual pattern. Waveforms are compared to age-matched controls.

Preferential looking test

Infants prefer to look toward a pattern stimulus over a nonpattern homogenous single color (Figure 29-1). For this test, an operator holds a large card that carries a pattern on one side and is blank on the other. Through a central viewer the infant's fixation movement can be observed—higher the grating (thinner the stripes of the pattern), the better the visual acuity measured.

	Table 29-1.			
Estimates of Visual Acuity by Age				
Test	Age 2 mo	Age 6 mo	Age 12 mo	Attainment of 20/20 vision (mo)
Forced choice preferential looking test	20/400	20/200	20/50	18-24
Visual evoked response test	20/200	20/60-20/20	20/40-20/20	6-12

Finding and following objects

A simple way of assessing visual function is to show a child a small toy or a familiar object such as a colorful piece of cereal. The examiner elicits the child's determination to reach for the object of regard as well as the child's ability to fix and follow the object as it is moved about in space. Fixation behavior can be assessed separately for each eye by using an eye patch.

Recognition acuity tests: Allen pictures, HOTV, and Snellen letters

Generally beginning at 2 to 3 years of age, a child can name or point to a matching card of familiar pictures (Lea symbols or Allen pictures). Older children can do this with the letters H, O, T, and V (Figure 29-2). Once children learn the alphabet, their vision can be assessed with the Snellen visual acuity chart. A visual acuity of 20/30 signifies that a child can identify a letter at 20 feet that a normal child, or adult, could identify at 30 feet.

Reasons for Referral to an Ophthalmologist

The basic eye examination for the non-ophthalmologist should include gross vision testing, external ocular examination, assessment of the red reflex, and the position of the corneal light reflex. Any abnormality of these tests should prompt a referral to an ophthalmologist. Checking for a red reflex is best performed with the examiner holding a direct ophthalmoscope about 30 cm away from the baby's face and setting the dial on the ophthalmoscope at +8. The infant can be rocked gently or given a bottle to encourage opening of the eyes. Setting the ophthalmoscope to a slit beam sometimes gives a reflex that is easier to evaluate. A normal red reflex is bright orange in a blond infant and brownish-orange in a darkly pigmented infant. If the reflex is difficult to see because of a small pupil, the instillation of dilating drops can facilitate the examination.

Assessment of the corneal light reflex is done by holding a light source (preferably next to a toy to attract the child's attention) and looking at the position of the light reflexes on the cornea. In a normal child the light will fall symmetrically on the nasal border of the pupil in each eye. If there is a strabismus present (see "Disorders of Ocular Motility" later in the chapter), the corneal light reflex will be asymmetrically located between the two eyes.

A particular condition that warrants referral to an ophthalmologist is nystagmus—an involuntary, rhythmic oscillatory movement of the eyes. The most benign form

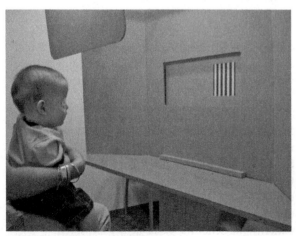

FIGURE 29-1 ■ Preferential looking test.

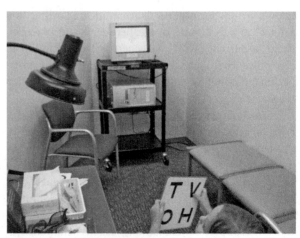

FIGURE 29-2 ■ Child matching the letter H on the screen with one on the card.

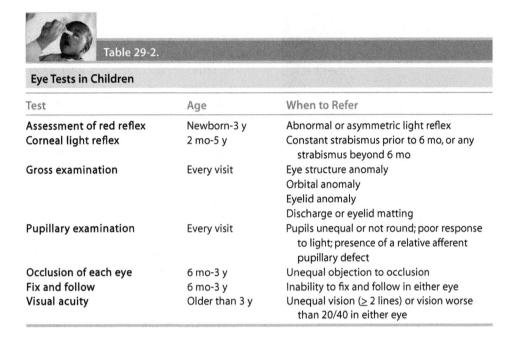

Table 29-2.

Eye Tests in Children

Test	Age	When to Refer
Assessment of red reflex	Newborn-3 y	Abnormal or asymmetric light reflex
Corneal light reflex	2 mo-5 y	Constant strabismus prior to 6 mo, or any strabismus beyond 6 mo
Gross examination	Every visit	Eye structure anomaly
		Orbital anomaly
		Eyelid anomaly
		Discharge or eyelid matting
Pupillary examination	Every visit	Pupils unequal or not round; poor response to light; presence of a relative afferent pupillary defect
Occlusion of each eye	6 mo-3 y	Unequal objection to occlusion
Fix and follow	6 mo-3 y	Inability to fix and follow in either eye
Visual acuity	Older than 3 y	Unequal vision (≥ 2 lines) or vision worse than 20/40 in either eye

is congenital motor nystagmus that begins soon after birth and is not associated with a visual or neurological disorder. A sensory nystagmus is due to a visual pathway dysfunction, usually due to an abnormality of the retina or optic nerve as detected by a dilated eye examination. In the rare cases where the dilated eye examination is normal, an electroretinogram (ERG) may assist in the diagnosis. New-onset nystagmus requires neuroimaging.[3]

General aspects of the eye examination that can be performed by a non-ophthalmologist are outlined in Table 29-2.

Ocular Causes of Decreased Visual Acuity in Children

Based on data from the American Schools for the Blind, in the United States the most common causes of poor vision in children are cortical visual impairment (19%), retinopathy of prematurity (13%), and optic nerve hypoplasia (5%). In developing countries, the World Health Organization estimates that 500,000 people are born blind each year, of which 50% to 90% die mostly due to malnutrition. Thirty percent to seventy percent of childhood blindness is preventable, and the leading causes are corneal opacities or other anterior segment anomalies due to systemic diseases such as measles, congenital rubella, ophthalmia neonaturum, vitamin A deficiency, or side effects from traditional eye medications.[4]

Anomalies of the anterior segment of the eye

The anterior segment of the eye consists of the cornea, anterior chamber, iris, and crystalline lens. The main function of these structures is to focus light onto the

retina. Refractive errors or opacities in the media result in a blurred image. It is important to diagnose and treat these problems at an early age to prevent amblyopia. A congenital cataract that is visually significant should be surgically treated in the first few months of life to prevent severe visual loss and nystagmus. An excellent screening test for media opacities in children is assessing the red reflex (Table 29-3, Figure 29-3). Corneal infections, such as with herpes simplex virus, or trauma resulting in corneal scarring can also result in decreased

Table 29-3.

Causes of Abnormal Red Reflex

Anterior Visual System
Cloudy cornea: congenital glaucoma, metabolic abnormalities, anterior segment dysgenesis
Cataract: idiopathic, familial, associated with genetic or metabolic syndromes (Figure 29-3).

Retinal Disorders
Retinal detachment
Intraocular tumors (eg, retinoblastoma)
Retinopathy of prematurity
Coloboma
Retinal scars

Refractive Errors
High myopia
High hyperopia
Anisometropia

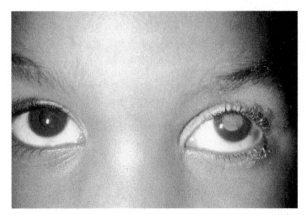

FIGURE 29-3 ■ Cataract in the left eye, showing leucokoria and exotropia.

visual acuity in children, and these problems can be compounded by amblyopia (see section entitled "Amblyopia," p. 384).

Congenital cataracts

A cataract is an opacification of the crystalline lens. It occurs in 1 in 4000 to 10,000 live-born infants. It may be unilateral or bilateral, and may be part of an ocular or systemic syndrome. Surgical removal is warranted when the cataract is visually significant (ie, when the opacity is central and larger than 3 mm in size). Smaller partial cataracts may be managed with pharmacologic pupillary dilation. The visual outcome of congenital cataracts has significantly improved over the past few decades with the advent of newer surgical techniques. Surgery should be performed as soon as the diagnosis is made to prevent irreversible, severe amblyopia. Congenital cataracts may be a familial condition; therefore screening the proband's family members (especially young siblings) for an asymptomatic cataract is recommended. Screening for galactosemia, a treatable systemic disease, is advisable in cases of a congenital cataract. However, routine testing for toxoplasmosis, other agents, rubella, cytomegalovirus, and herpes simplex (TORCH) is controversial and recommended by some only if there are systemic findings suggestive of an infection.[5]

Congenital glaucoma

Glaucoma is an increase in the intraocular pressure causing damage to the optic nerve. Untreated it may cause irreversible vision loss. The most common type of pediatric glaucoma is primary congenital glaucoma, which has an incidence of 1 in 10,000. The primary pathology in congenital glaucoma is intrinsic disease of the aqueous outflow system. A child with congenital glaucoma will present with a large and cloudy cornea, tearing (epiphora), and photophobia. However, the symptoms may vary in severity ranging from pure tearing and photophobia to a very large, cloudy cornea (bupophthalmos).[5,6]

Coloboma

A coloboma is caused by a failure of the embryonic fissure to close. It may involve the eyelid, anterior segment, retina, or optic nerve. Not all colobomas lead to visual impairment. For example, an iris coloboma results in a keyhole-shaped pupil with no reduction in vision. In comparison, a coloboma of the fundus will often have associated visual impairment because of retinal dysplasia, particularly if the macula is involved. Patients with retinal colobomas are advised to have a dilated eye examination twice a year because of an increased risk for retinal holes and detachments. Colobomas may be part of the CHARGE syndrome (coloboma, heart anomalies, choanal atresia, retardation of growth and development, and genital and ear anomalies), an autosomal dominant disorder.[5]

Other rare anterior segment anomalies

Anomalies of the anterior segment of the eye can be isolated or accompanied by systemic abnormalities. There will be a blunted red reflex similar to a congenital cataract. **Persistant hyperplastic primary vitreous** can be seen in children born of mothers who have consumed cocaine. It often presents as a small eye with a unilateral cataract, microcephaly, and mental retardation. **Anterior segment dysgenesis** is a spectrum of abnormalities involving the cornea, iris, and lens due to dysembryogenensis associated with systemic findings such as facial dysmorphism, skin and dental abnormalities, and chromosomal anomalies. A **dermoid** is a white, elevated lesion that can encroach on the cornea, causing astigmatism or occlusion of the visual axis. It may be a manifestation of Goldenhar syndrome (oculo–auricular–vertebral syndrome), consisting of vertebral anomalies, small ears with skin tags, and facial dysmorphism. **Aniridia** (absence of the iris) may be associated with multiple ocular anomalies including glaucoma, macular hypoplasia, and nystagmus. It can have a familial autosomal dominant or sporadic inheritance pattern. The sporadic type may be associated with Wilms tumor, genitourinary anomalies, and mental retardation (WAGR syndrome). **Microphthalmia** is defined as a small eyeball with no structural defect. Vision is often affected because of the presence of other ocular anomalies. Microphthalmia can be a manifestation of an intrauterine infection or trisomy 13 or 18.[5]

Anomalies of the vitreous and retina

The main chamber of the eye is the vitreous cavity, which is filled with a jelly-like substance called the vitreous. The retina is the neurosensory structure of the eye that captures light and transmits a signal to the brain through the optic nerves.

Vitreous hemorrhage

There are multiple causes of a vitreous hemorrhage, but in children the most common causes are retinopathy of prematurity, retinal vessel pathology, ocular trauma, shaken baby syndrome, or an intracranial hemorrhage (Terson syndrome). A vitreous hemorrhage becomes visually significant when it blocks the visual axis. It often resolves spontaneously over several months, but observation is warranted to prevent amblyopia. In persistent cases a vitrectomy is performed. The final visual outcome is dependent on the extent of the disease, with penetrating eye trauma carrying the worst prognosis.[7]

Retinal dystrophies

Retinitis pigmentosa (RP) is a term used for a broad category of diseases affecting the retinal photoreceptor cells (rods and cones). The incidence of primary photoreceptor cell anomalies is 1 in 3000 to 5000. More than 100 genes have been implicated in RP. Of the inherited RP syndromes, recessive X-linked RP is the most common inheritance pattern seen.[8] Typically, visual dysfunction begins with night blindness (nyctalopia) and visual field constriction progressing to decreased central visual acuity. Pigment deposits in a "bone spicule" formation are often seen in the peripheral retina. An ERG can help establish the diagnosis and monitor disease progression. Although there is no cure, vitamin A, palmitate, and omega-3-rich fish may slow the progression of the disease. Systemic diseases associated with RP include Usher syndrome, Laurence-Moon-Bardet-Biedl syndrome, and Kearns-Sayre syndrome. Usher syndrome is characterized by sensorineural hearing loss of variable severity and onset. Patients with Laurence-Moon-Bardet-Biedl syndrome have truncal obesity, renal dysfunction, polydactyly, and short stature. Kearns-Sayre syndrome is a mitochondrial myopathy characterized by external ophthalmolplegia, ptosis, and cardiac conduction block.[8] Congenital stationary night blindness (CSNB) is a retinal dystrophy characterized by decreased vision at night. It is associated with high myopia and fundus pigmentation that is similar to RP; however, CSNB is a nonprogressive disorder.[9]

Leber congenital amaurosis (LCA) is an autosomal recessive disorder characterized by blindness before 6 months of age. It is the cause of approximately 10% to 18% of cases of congenital blindness. The ERG is severely attenuated. Final visual acuity in LCA patients ranges from no light perception to 20/200. Systemic findings in children with LCA include polycystic kidneys, osteoporosis, cleft palate, and skeletal and brain anomalies.[9,10]

Retinopathy of prematurity

Retinopathy of prematurity (ROP) affects premature and low birth weight babies of less than 32 weeks gestation or less than 1251 g, respectively. It is a complex disorder of prematurity caused by the disruption of the normal intrauterine growth of the retina. Management of ROP starts in the nursery with a screening examination to monitor the growth of the retinal vessels. In appropriate cases, treatment is initiated with laser photoablation to the peripheral retina to decrease the probability of a retinal detachment. A vitrectomy is often indicated in cases of severe disease and retinal detachment.

Genetic and metabolic disorders causing a decrease in vision

Sometimes, clinical symptoms and findings on ocular examination may provide clues to the presence of a genetic or metabolic disease. Many metabolic diseases can manifest with accumulation of toxic by-products in the cornea, lens, or retina.

Corneal disorders

The cornea may become opacified in a variety of genetic disorders. In mucopolysaccharidoses (MPS), the cornea is cloudy due to the deposition of glycosaminoglycans in the corneal stroma. Corneal transplant may be required in MPS IV (Morquio), MPS VI (Maroteaux-Lamy), and less commonly in MPS III (Sanfilippo).[11] Other disorders known to cause deposits in the cornea include mucoliposes, Gaucher disease, cystinosis, tyrosinemia, and sphingolipidoses including the juvenile form of metachromatic leukodystrophy. In Wilson disease, alkaptonuria and dyslipoproteinemias deposits occur at the corneal limbus with no effect on vision.

Corneal opacification can be seen in a number of hereditary corneal dystrophies that do not have systemic manifestations (eg, congenital hereditary corneal dystrophies). They usually manifest in late childhood and are characterized by deposits in the cornea that progressively affect vision.

Enlargement of the cornea (megalocornea) can be seen in Marfan syndrome or Ehlers-Danlos syndrome. An abnormally shaped cornea (keratoconus) causing severe astigmatism and scarring is associated with osteogenesis imperfecta and Ehlers-Danlos syndrome.

The cornea is a very sensitive structure and disorders causing corneal exposure or dryness must be managed very carefully to prevent excessive corneal dryness and subsequent infections, scarring, and vision loss.

Lenticular disorders

The lens may opacify due to a variety of metabolic disorders, such as diabetes mellitus, galactosemia, galactokinase deficiency, and Fabry syndrome. Marfan syndrome and homocystenuria is associated with subluxation of the lens.

Retinal disorders

The macular area is devoid of ganglion cells; therefore, in cases of lipid accumulation or edema of the ganglion cell layer, the macula still displays a red choroidal color, giving the look of a red spot surrounded by white retina—clinically described as a cherry red spot. A cherry red spot is most commonly seen following an ischemic or vaso-occlusive event in both adults and children but may also be seen in Tay-Sachs or Sandhoff disease, metachromatic leukodystrophy, and Niemann-Pick disease. Mucopolysccharidoses, mucolipidosis, gangliosidoses, and peroxisomal disorders can also show retinal pigment changes similar to RP.[12]

Congenital optic nerve anomalies

Congenital optic nerve disorders include but are not limited to optic nerve hypoplasia, autosomal dominant optic atrophy, hereditary optic neuropathy of Leber, and morning glory disc anomaly. Children with an optic nerve anomaly may have vision ranging from normal to complete blindness. Anomalies of the optic nerve may be associated with anterior segment, retinal, brain, or other systemic abnormalities.

Optic nerve hypoplasia

Optic nerve hypoplasia (ONH) is the most common congenital optic nerve anomaly. In addition to the appearance of a small nerve, signs of ONH on examination include a "double ring" sign (with the larger ring being the scleral canal and the smaller ring the actual nerve tissue) and anomalous vascular branching pattern. Patients might be asymptomatic in mild cases or they may present with poor vision, nystagmus, strabismus, or a combination of these. Bilateral cases, more commonly than unilateral cases, are associated with congenital malformation of the central nervous system and pituitary axis (septo-optic dysplasia). In these cases, magnetic resonance imaging (MRI) may show an absent infundibular stalk, ectopic bright spot in the hypothalamus, and an absent corpus callosum and septum pellucidum. A particular syndrome associated with ONH is DeMorsier syndrome, which is characterized by a combination of septo-optic dysplasia, facial dysmorphism, and an open anterior fontanel. Patients with DeMorsier syndrome may present with pituitary axis disruption including sudden death due to corticotropin deficiency.[5,13]

Morning glory disc anomaly

Usually a unilateral condition, a morning glory disc is an enlarged optic nerve in the shape of a funnel with an indistinct border surrounded by depigmented areas, giving the appearance of the morning glory flower. It may be associated with a basal encephalocele in patients with midline defects, Moyamoya vascular disorder,[14] and papillorenal disorder. The presentation and management of morning glory disc is similar to ONH.[5,13]

Autosomal dominant optic atrophy

Autosomal dominant optic atrophy (ADOA) presents with vision loss in the first or second decade of life.

Visual acuity may range from 20/20 to 20/200, with some affected individuals visually asymptomatic. Patients with ADOA may have a concomitant blue-yellow color blindness (tritanopia) and visual field testing showing a centrocecal or paracentral scotoma.[5]

Autosomal recessive optic atrophy

Autosomal recessive optic atrophy (AROA) is a more severe condition than ADOA. It presents in infancy with rapid, progressive vision loss followed by a stabilization of visual acuity. Although it can be isolated, AROA is usually associated with other neurological disorders such as Behr and Costeff syndromes. Behr syndrome manifests with AROA associated with ataxia, spinocerebellar degeneration, and mental retardation. Costeff optic atrophy syndrome or type III 3-methyglucaconic aciduria presents with bilateral optic atrophy, spasticity, extrapyramidal dysfunction, and cognitive dysfunction.[5]

Amblyopia

The causes of amblyopia are ocular but pathophysiology is within the central nervous system. Amblyopia is defined as a decrease in visual acuity despite best refractive correction with no organic ocular abnormality seen on examination. Amblyopia can be unilateral or bilateral, and is caused by the lack of a clear image directed onto the retina during visual development. Image blur can be refractive, strabismic, or anatomic in origin. Refractive amblyopia is due to an uncorrected refractive error in one or both eyes, or a difference in refractive error between the two eyes (anisometropia). Strabismic amblyopia is due to early-onset strabismus (see "Disorders of Ocular Motility" later in the chapter) resulting in visual suppression. Deprivational amblyopia is due to ptosis or media opacity of the cornea, lens, or vitreous.

Young children (under the age of 8) are the most susceptible to amblyopia. Congenital media opacities should be treated as early as possible to prevent severe visual loss. Children usually do not complain of decreased vision, especially when it is unilateral; therefore, amblyopia can be overlooked and only detected when there is a noticeable strabismus or during a screening eye examination.

Treatment of amblyopia begins by removing any media opacity and providing the appropriate refractive correction in spectacles. The mainstay of amblyopia treatment is penalization of the fellow eye, either by patching or by cycloplegia with atropine eye drops (Figure 29-4). One large study showed that children with amblyopia may still respond to treatment up to age 17 years, especially if they have not been previously treated.[15] However, results are generally better when treatment is started at younger ages.[16]

One should keep in mind that early-onset eye trauma or infection causing a disturbance to the visual axis (eg, corneal scar or cataract) can be a cause of amblyopia. Prompt referral to an ophthalmologist with close follow-up is indicated in these cases.

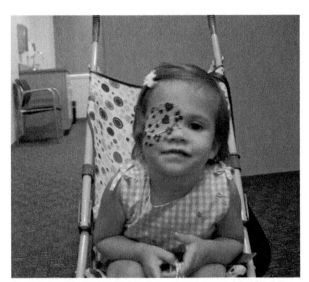

FIGURE 29-4 ■ Child wearing an eye patch for amblyopia treatment.

Neurological Causes for Decreased Visual Acuity

Cortical visual impairment

Cortical visual impairment (CVI) is defined as a decrease in visual function due to an insult to the cerebral cortex. It can be congenital or acquired. The two most common causes of CVI are perinatal hypoxia and prematurity.[17] CVI can also be due to an intrauterine infection, brain malformation, seizure, intracranial bleeding, hydrocephalus, meningitis, encephalitis, and accidental or non-accidental trauma. Children with CVI often have other associated neurological abnormalities due the primary insult extending beyond the affected visual pathways. Visual impairment in patients with CVI can vary in severity.

One common behavior in children with CVI is intermittent visual attention demonstrated by a child reacting positively to visual cues on some occasions and not on others. It has been hypothesized that the main visual disturbance in CVI is not central vision but rather visual difficulties in perception, integration, orientation, focusing on more than one object at a time, facial recognition, tracking moving targets, color discrimination, and depth perception. In CVI, the ocular examination may be normal if the condition is isolated, but neuroimaging often shows damage to the geniculate or extrageniculate visual pathways. The neurological damage is usually permanent and stable but children can show improved visual behavior with age.[18] Commonly, these patients also have associated ocular abnormalities including strabismus, optic atrophy, and significant refractive errors, although the ocular problems are not at a significant level to explain the severity of the visual loss.[17]

Delayed visual maturation

Sometimes a child fails to fix and follow by 3 months of age and has a normal eye examination without a specific cause for visual cortical dysfunction. In most cases this finding is due to delayed visual maturation (DVM). It is hypothesized that DVM results from a delay in the myelination of the visual pathways despite the fact that there is no evidence that the primary visual pathway is involved. Some experts believe that the disorder might be a primary visual inattention disorder. Usually fixation behavior starts to improve between 4 and 12 months of age, and final visual outcome is excellent. If visual attentiveness is not normal by 12 months of age, then CVI should be suspected. Children with DVM have a higher rate of learning disabilities, attention deficit disorders, seizures, autism, and other psychiatric disorders.[19]

Optic nerve glioma

Optic nerve glioma is a low-grade pilocytic astrocytoma representing 5% of all intracranial tumors in children. It can involve the optic nerve, optic chiasm, or both. Clinical presentation is prior to 12 years of age. Approximately 50% of optic nerve gliomas are associated with neurofibromatosis type I. Fifteen percent of patients with neurofibromatosis type I will develop an optic nerve glioma at some point in their life. Children with optic nerve gliomas usually present with decreased visual acuity, proptosis, and a relative afferent pupillary defect. Chemotherapy has evolved over the past decade to become the treatment of choice. Radiotherapy or surgical excision is reserved for chemoresistant cases.[20]

Optic neuritis

Optic neuritis is an inflammatory demyelinating condition of the optic nerve. Presentation is acute in onset with rapidly progressive loss of vision associated with pain on eye movement, decreased color perception, poor contrast sensitivity, and a relative afferent pupillary defect. Retrobulbar optic neuritis refers to a normal appearing optic nerve with the pathologic process affecting the posterior or retrobulbar portion of the optic nerve. Neuroretinitis, commonly seen in cat scratch disease, refers to optic nerve edema associated with macular exudates in a star-like pattern.

Optic neuritis may occur in children or adults as an isolated condition or part of a systemic demyelinating disorder such as multiple sclerosis or Devic disease (neuromyelitis optica). Other optic neuropathies in the differential diagnosis of optic neuritis include viral or bacterial infection (cat scratch disease, toxoplasmosis, toxocara, Lyme disease, and syphilis), postimmunization, exposure to an exogenous toxin such as lead, or prolonged treatment with medications such as chloramphenicol or vincristine.

The initial evaluation of a child with an acute inflammatory demyelinating optic neuritis includes a MRI of the brain and spine, lumbar puncture with opening pressure, and cerebrospinal fluid analysis. Visual symptoms generally start improving spontaneously 1 to 4 weeks after onset, and recovery is usually almost complete. Intravenous corticosteroids can improve the rate of visual recovery but have been shown to have no affect on the final visual outcome. It has been stated that children who present with optic neuritis are at less risk of developing multiple sclerosis than adults. This premise is controversial and has not been well studied, in part because optic neuritis is relatively uncommon in children.[21,22]

Papilledema

Papilledema is swelling of the optic nerve head secondary to increased intracranial pressure. Clinical signs and symptoms include headaches, transient visual obscurations, or a sixth-nerve palsy. Visual acuity is not acutely affected by papilledema although the visual field may show an enlarged blind spot. On fundus examination the optic nerve is edematous, elevated, congested, and hyperemic. The disc margins are blurred and there is loss of spontaneous venous pulsations and obliteration of the optic cup. Severe papilledema may also show disc hemorrhages, peripapillary exudates, or macular swelling with exudates. Untreated chronic papilledema results in optic nerve damage as manifested by a pale atrophic optic disc, severe peripheral vision loss, and reduced central visual acuity.

Common etiologies of papilledema in children include intracranial tumors, idiopathic intracranial hypertension, obstructive hypdrocephalus, trauma, venous sinus thrombosis, intracranial hemorrhage, and encephalopathy.

Management of papilledema involves treating the underlying cause and decreasing the intracranial pressure either pharmacologically with acetazolamide, or surgically with a cerebrospinal fluid diversion procedure. Optic nerve sheath fenestration is reserved for cases of vision loss unresponsive to intracranial pressure reduction.[23]

Visual field defects

Homonymous hemianopia can occur in children and has the same clinical features as in adults. However, in children the most common causes are traumatic brain injuries and brain tumors. Following trauma, visual fields have been found to improve in 33% to 50% of cases, generally within the first 3 months after the injury.[24]

Children usually do not complain of visual field loss and formal visual field testing can be very challenging at a young age. The examiner may grossly assess the status of the peripheral vision by using a toy or a familiar object (like a bottle) for fixation, and then slowly bringing into the child's field of view another object of equal interest. Older children can perform standardized visual field tests (static or dynamic perimetery). These tests require the child to sit behind a screen and signal when the incoming light from the screen is seen. Standardized visual field testing is usually not reliable before the age of 8 years. The pattern of visual field loss can indicate the location of the lesion along the visual pathway (Figure 29-5).

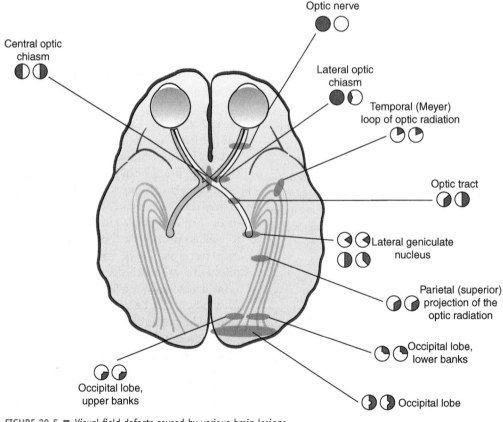

FIGURE 29-5 ■ Visual field defects caused by various brain lesions.

DISORDERS OF OCULAR MOTILITY

Definition

Strabismus—derived from the Greek word "strabismus," meaning the condition of squinting—may be a primary disorder with no definitive etiology or a secondary condition due to disease of the brain, brainstem, ocular motor cranial nerves, orbit, neuromuscular junction, or extraocular muscles. This section discusses some of the more common conditions of strabismus or ocular motility disorders in children. The description of strabismic conditions is associated with a language of its own that is often unfamiliar to non-ophthalmologists (Tables 29-4 and 29-5). Heterotropia is a term that implies an ocular deviation that cannot be controlled by fusion (the ability of the brain to unify images perceived by corresponding retinal areas) and is present under binocular conditions. Heterotropia can be a constant or intermittent phenomenon. It implies an ocular deviation masked or controlled by fusion manifest only when fusion is disrupted. Heterophoria is a normal physiologic state.

Relevant Anatomy

Extraocular muscles

There are six extraocular muscles that directly control eye movements: four recti muscles (inferior, superior, lateral, and medial) and two oblique muscles (superior and inferior) (Figure 29-6). The levator palpebrae superioris is the seventh extraocular muscle needed for eyelid elevation. Each extraocular muscle is responsible for movement of the eye in a specific direction or *primary action* (Table 29-6, Figure 29-7). The superior rectus, inferior rectus, superior oblique, and inferior oblique muscles also have secondary actions that vary depending on the position of the eye in the orbit.

Cranial nerve III (CN III)

Located in the midbrain, the nucleus of CN III consists of six subnuclei: levator complex (innervates the two levator

Table 29-4.

Nomenclature of Ocular Deviations

Orthotropia: no misalignment of the eyes
Esotropia: misalignment created by an in-turning eye
Exotopia: misalignment created by an out-turning eye
Hypertropia: misalignment created by an eye deviated superiorly
Hypotropia: misalignment created by an eye deviated inferiorly[a]

[a] By convention, when one eye is said to be lower compared to its fellow eye, the fellow eye is often referred to as the hypertropic eye.

Table 29-5.

Abbreviations of Ocular Deviations

Esodeviations:	ET—esotropia; E(T)—intermittent esotropia; E—esophoria
Exodeviations:	XT—exotropia; X(T)—intermittent exotropia; X—exophoria
Hyperdeviations:	RHT—right hypertropia; LHT—left hypertropia RH(T)—right intermittent hypertropia; LH(T)—intermittent left hypertropia RH—right hyperphoria; LH—left hyperphoria

palpebrae superioris muscles), superior rectus subnucleus (innervates the contralateral superior rectus muscle), and the inferior oblique, inferior rectus, and medial rectus subnuclei (innervate their respective ipsilateral extraocular muscles).[25] The Edinger-Westphal nucleus is located rostral to all the other subnuclei and provides parasympathetic input to the pupillary constrictor muscle of the iris. Fascicles from the nuclear complex of CN III travel ventrally exiting the midbrain into the interpeduncular fossa. As the trunk of CN III leaves the brainstem, it travels between the posterior cerebral and superior cerebellar arteries running parallel with the posterior communicating artery. Because of the intimate anatomic proximity of these vessels to CN III, aneurysms located at the basilar tip, superior cerebellar artery, and posterior communicating arteries may all result in CN III paresis. After traveling in the subarachnoid space, the nerve enters the lateral cavernous sinus above CN IV (Figure 29-13). In the anterior cavernous sinus, CN III splits into a superior and inferior division. The two divisions then enter the orbit via the superior orbital fissure through the annulus of Zinn (Figure 29-8).

Cranial nerve IV

The nucleus of cranial nerve IV (CN IV) is located caudal to the CN III nuclear complex. Its course within the brainstem is very short, with the fibers decussating in the anterior medullary vellum. CN IV is the only CN to exit the brainstem dorsally. It has a long subarachnoid course before it arrives to the cavernous sinus. It enters the orbit via the superior orbital fissure above the annulus of Zinn (Figure 29-8).

Cranial nerve VI

The nucleus of cranial nerve IV (CN VI) is located in the pons on the floor of the fourth ventricle under the facial colliculus (Figure 29-8). CN VI contains two sets of neurons: primary motor neurons that form the peripheral nerve, and interneurons that form the medial longitudinal fasciculus (MLF). The primary

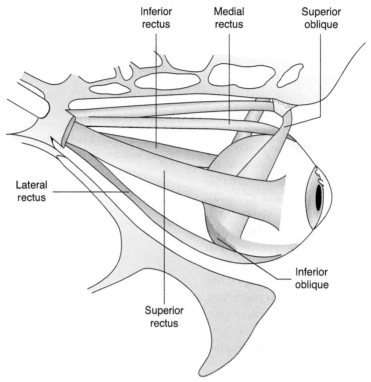

Inferior rectus   Medial rectus   Superior oblique

Lateral rectus

Inferior oblique

Superior rectus

FIGURE 29-6 ■ Superior view of the six extraocular muscles.

motor neurons travel within the brainstem to exit the pons caudally. Once in the subarachnoid space, the nerve climbs up the clivus to the petrous apex and turns under the petroclinoid ligament to arrive at the cavernous sinus. Within the cavernous sinus CN VI is the only CN to run within, rather than along, the lateral wall of the cavernous sinus. CN VI terminates in the lateral orbit after going through the superior orbital fissure and the annulus of Zinn. The interneurons of the CN VI nucleus travel in the MLF to synapse on the CN III subnucleus (Figure 29-9).

Non-Neurogenic Strabismic Disorders

An important early step in the evaluation of a child with strabismus is to determine whether the deviation is similar in all directions of gaze (comitant) and if the excursions of the eye(s) are limited. Comitance with normal eye movements often suggests a non-neurogenic strabismic disorder. Another important step is determining whether the eye is esotropic, exotropic, hypertropic, or hypotropic. This section will provide an overview of some of the major non-neurogenic strabismic disorders.

Table 29-6.

Ocular Motor Cranial Nerve Innervation and Action of Extraocular Muscles

Extraocular Muscle	Cranial Nerve Innervation	Action(s)
Lateral rectus	Cranial nerve VI	Abduction
Medial rectus	Cranial nerve III (inferior division)	Adduction
Superior rectus	Cranial nerve III (superior division)	Primary action: elevation
		Secondary actions: adduction, intorsion
Inferior rectus	Cranial nerve III (inferior division)	Primary action: depression
		Secondary actions: adduction, intorsion
Superior oblique	Cranial nerve IV	Primary action: intorsion
		Secondary actions: depression, abduction
Inferior oblique	Cranial nerve III (inferior division)	Primary action: extorsion
		Secondary actions: elevation, abduction

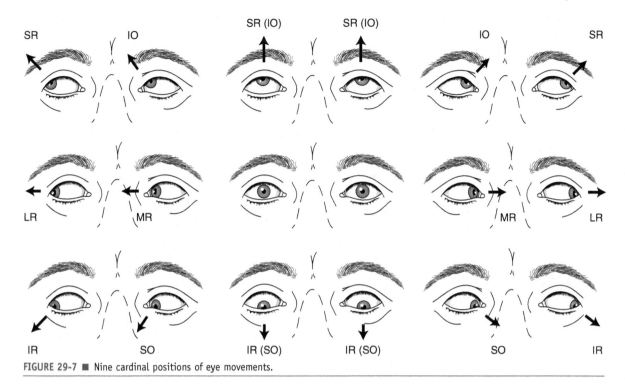

FIGURE 29-7 ▧ Nine cardinal positions of eye movements.

Ocular motility disorders with limited eye movements, which are often of neurogenic etiology, will be discussed in a separate section later.

Non-neurogenic esotropia

Congenital esotropia. Congential esotropia is a condition of unknown etiology that occurs prior to 6 months of age. Typically there is a large-angle deviation. The esotropia in later infancy is constant but prior to 12 weeks of age it may be variable or intermittent. Often there is a family history of strabismus. Children with congenital esotropia may exhibit alternate fixation (in horizontal gaze the contralateral eye will be used to fixate on an object), which can give the impression of limited abduction of the ipsilateral eye. Full eye movements in such cases can be demonstrated by the doll's-head maneuver or eliciting the vestibular ocular reflex by rotating the child.

Accommodative esotropia. Accomodative esotropia is the most common type of eso deviation in children presenting between 6 months and 7 years of age. It can be subdivided into two broad categories: hyperopic refractive error and excess convergence with accommodation.

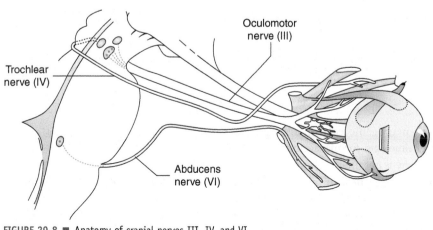

FIGURE 29-8 ▧ Anatomy of cranial nerves III, IV, and VI.

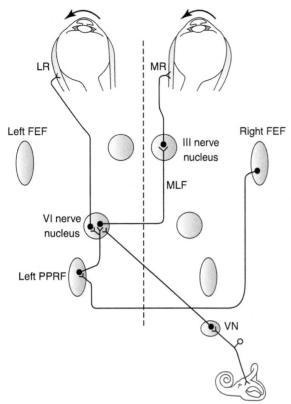

FIGURE 29-9 ■ Anatomy of horizontal eye movements. Interneurons from CN VI are contained in the medial longitudinal fasciculus (MLF) and travel to the contralateral CN III nucleus to initiate adduction of the opposite eye.

With the refractive error variant there is an uncorrected hyperopia (far-sightedness) that requires accommodation and convergence to view objectives of regard. The excess convergence variant is independent of an uncorrected refractive error.

Acquired esotropia. Acquired esotropia generally occurs after 6 months of age. Its etiology is typically idiopathic but can occur in the setting of central nervous system (CNS) disease such as an intracranial tumor, meningitis, or structural malformation.[26-28] Any cause of reduced vision in one eye may result in an acquired esotropia. Rarely, acquired esotropia may present in an intermittent pattern cycling between orthotropia and esotropia over a 24-hour period of time. This entity, called cyclic esotropia, may evolve into a constant esotropia.[29]

Management of non-neurogenic esotropia

Children with non-neurogenic esotropia should be referred to an ophthalmologist for management. Amblyopia is a concern if there is not timely restoration of normal ocular alignment or the institution of amblyopic treatment (see section "Amblyopia," p.384). The primary management of congenital esotropia involves correcting any existing refractive error and amblyopia. Once optimal

visual rehabilitation has been established, strabismus surgery is warranted. Treatment for refractive accommodative esotropia is spectacles with a hyperopic correction. Treatment for convergence-related accommodative esotropia is varied and can involve bifocal spectacles, miotic therapy, and strabismus surgery.[30] Acquired esotropia may present in the setting of CNS disease; therefore neuroimaging is needed.

Non-neurogenic exotropia

Intermittent exotropia. Intermittent exotropia is the most common type of exotropia in children occurring before 6 years of age. The deviation, initially intermittent, may evolve later into a constant misalignment.

Constant exotropia. Constant exotropia may occur in a newborn and often resolves by 6 months of age. An exotropia persisting beyond 4 months of age is indicative of a craniofacial anomaly, trauma, cerebral palsy, or structural defect of the eye.[31] A constant exotropia presenting in an older child is often the result of sensory deprivation to one eye caused by a media opacity, retinal disease, or optic nerve dysfunction.

Management of non-neurogenic exotropia

A complete neurological evaluation is necessary for infants with a constant exotropia. Neuroimaging should be performed given the potential for CNS disease, as mentioned above.[31] For both intermittent and constant exotropia, referral to an ophthalmologist is indicated for correction of any existing refractive error, amblyopia treatment, or strabismus surgery.

Ocular Motor Cranial Nerve Abnormalities

Definition

Children with dysfunction of CN III, IV, or VI will demonstrate limitation of eye movements in a specific pattern, with deviation measurements revealing an incomitant strabismus. Some children may not complain of double vision because of the phenomenon of suppression. If an ocular motor cranial nerve palsy is suspected, the first step is to determine which CN is affected by recognizing the pattern of the ocular motility abnormality.

Differential diagnosis and physical examination

CN III palsy. A complete CN III palsy results in an eye that is turned down and out in primary gaze and upper eyelid ptosis, with or without a dilated pupil (mydriasis; Figure 29-10). A child with an incomplete CN III palsy may present with partial ptosis and residual ability to elevate, depress, and adduct the eye. Aberrant regeneration

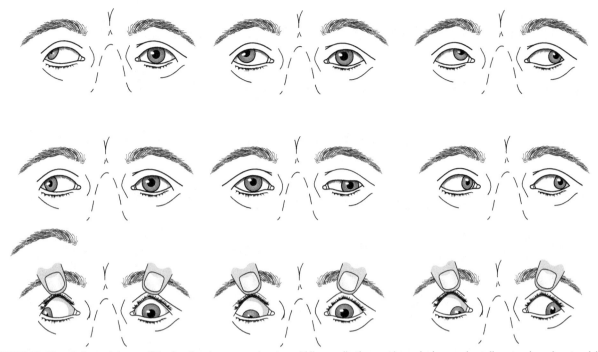

FIGURE 29-10 ■ Left cranial nerve III palsy. In primary gaze (center, middle panel), the paretic eye is down and out (hypotropia and exotropia). Note the dilated left pupil and ptotic left upper eyelid. The left eye has limited elevation, depression, and adduction.

or synkinesis of CN III should be suspected in a child who demonstrates any of the following:

1. Eyelid retraction during adduction
2. Pupillary miosis during adduction, elevation, or depression
3. Adduction during attempted elevation or depression

Aberrant regeneration is often indicative of a congenital CN III palsy.

CN IV palsy. CN IV palsy results in a hypertropia in primary gaze (Figure 29-11). Depending on the degree of dysfunction, there may or may not be a visible limitation of depression of the eye in the adducted position. Children with CN IV palsy will often compensate with a head tilt to the opposite side of the palsy. This finding may often be revealed by reviewing old pictures. The diagnosis of a CN IV palsy is based on the Parks-Bielschowsky three-step test.[32] A positive test is indicated by a hypertropia in primary gaze that increases in contralateral gaze and ipsilateral head tilt to the eye with the palsy.

CN VI palsy. CN VI palsy will present with a limitation of abduction associated with an esotropia in primary gaze from the unbalanced activity of the medial rectus muscle (Figure 29-12). The esotropia will increase in the field of action of the palsy. Children may be inclined to adopt a face turn towards the side of the palsy to resolve the double vision. When evaluating a child

with an abduction deficit other causes should be considered (Table 29-7).

Evaluation and treatment

The evaluation of a patient suspected of an ocular motor cranial neuropathy should include an assessment for other CN involvement and neurological deficits. Because a lesion can occur anywhere from the nucleus to the branches of the peripheral nerve, the location of the lesion can often be suspected based on the "company that it keeps".

CN III palsy. Congenital CN III palsy is the most common cause of an isolated CN III palsy in a child and is often the result of birth trauma.[33] On occasion a congenital CN III palsy may be seen in concert with other neurological findings and developmental delays.[34] The palsy is typically unilateral, incomplete, and displays synkinesis.[34] Congenital CN III palsy may also be accompanied by cyclic spasms (alternating spasm and paresis of muscles innervated by CN III), which typically present with pupillary constriction, adduction, and lid elevation. Other causes of isolated CN III palsy include trauma, infection, and neoplasm. Intracranial aneurysms, in particular posterior communicating artery aneurysms, are an infrequent cause of CN III palsy in children.[35,36] Ophthalmoplegic migraine is a rare syndrome marked by headache, nausea, vomiting, and eye pain. The palsy most often sets in as the headache is resolving. Occasionally, an

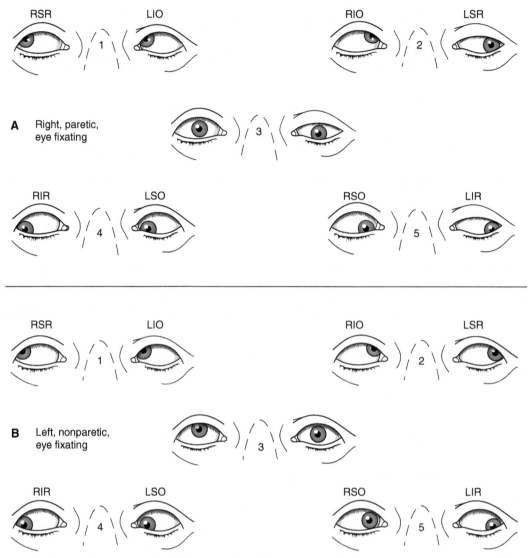

FIGURE 29-11 ■ Right cranial nerve IV palsy. Whether the right or left eye is fixating, the paretic eye will always be hypertropic in primary gaze. In left and upgaze (2), there is an increase in the hypertropia from overaction of the inferior oblique muscle. In left and downgaze (5), there is an increase in the hypertropia from underaction of the superior oblique muscle.

acquired CN III palsy can occur without an identifiable cause. There are several specific brainstem syndromes involving CN III (Table 29-8).

Some authors recommend an MRI and magnetic resonance angiography in all patients under 50 years of age presenting with a CN III palsy with or without pupil involvement.[37] Performing a conventional catheter angiography in children with a CN III palsy is controversial, given the rarity of an intracranial aneurysm as the underlying cause. Once the etiology of the CN III palsy is determined and appropriately treated, and if the child continues to have an ocular motility deficit, it is advisable to consult an ophthalmologist for amblyopia treatment and consideration of strabismus surgery. The surgical correction of CN III can be difficult to achieve.[38]

Table 29-7.

Differential Diagnosis of Abduction Deficit

Duane syndrome
Medial orbital wall trauma[a]
Myasthenia gravis
Postsurgical (iatrogenic)
Spasm of near reflex
Thyroid eye disease

[a]*Orbital disease is an important cause of ophthalmoparesis in adults and children. Full discussion of orbital disease is beyond the scope of this chapter; however, strabismus accompanied by exophthalmos, enophthalmos, or other stigmata of orbital disease should raise suspicion of conditions such as thyroid ophthalmopathy, orbital wall trauma, or orbital mass.*

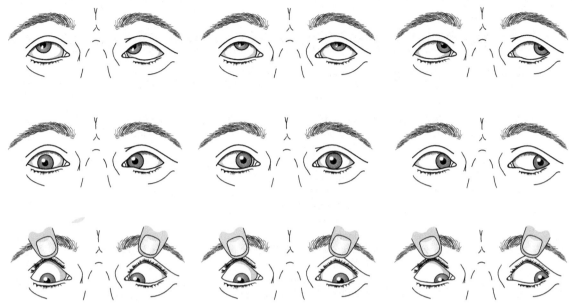

FIGURE 29-12 ■ Right cranial nerve VI palsy. In primary gaze, there is an esotropia of the right eye. Note the limitation of abduction of the right eye (*middle left panel*).

CN IV palsy. The two most common causes of CN IV palsy in children are congenital and trauma.[39,40] Less often, CN IV palsy may be idiopathic or the result of hydrocephalus. Congenital CN IV palsy is marked by large vertical fusional amplitudes (typically greater than 3 prism diopters), a head tilt opposite the side of the palsy, and facial asymmetry with vertical sloping of the mouth on the side of the head tilt.[41] Because the CN IV nucleus lies near the oculosympathetic axons, a lesion within the brainstem in this area will result in an ipsilateral Horner syndrome and contralateral superior oblique palsy.[42]

Cases of congenital CN IV palsy do not require radiologic evaluation. However, if there is any concern for a structural lesion, neuroimaging should be obtained.

Traumatic CN IV palsy is often observed for several months prior to surgical repair. Congenital CN IV palsy may be operated on sooner to avoid an abnormal head position.

CN VI palsy. CN VI palsy in children is frequently due to either trauma or an intracranial neoplasm.[39,43] Brainstem glioma is a common tumor associated with CN VI palsy.[44] Isolated CN VI palsy may also be seen in a viral or postimmunization setting.[45] Any cause of raised intracranial pressure can lead to a CN VI palsy—a "false localizing sign." Several well-defined syndromes associated with CN VI palsy have been described with localizing anatomic value (Table 29-9).

Expectant observation is recommended for a CN VI palsy presumed to be of viral or postimmunization

Table 29-8.		
Major Brainstem Syndromes Involving CN III		
Syndrome	Signs	Territory (Other Tracts Affected)
Benedikt syndrome	Ipsilateral CN III palsy	Midbrain (red nucleus)
	Contralateral extremity tremor	
Weber syndrome	Ipsilateral CN III palsy	Anterior midbrain (cerebral peduncle or corticospinal tract)
	Contralateral extremity weakness or paralysis	
Nothnagel syndrome	Unilateral bilateral CN III palsy	
	Cerebellar ataxia	Midbrain tectum (superior cerebellar peduncles)

Table 29-9.

Localization of CN VI Palsy Based on Symptoms and Signs

Anatomic Localization	Symptoms/Signs	Causes
Pons (lesion may affect CN VI nucleus or fascicle)	CN VI palsy with a combination of: ■ CN V or CN VII palsy[a] ■ Horner syndrome[a] ■ Decreased sense of taste[a] ■ Contralateral hemiplegia[b]	Infarction Hemorrhage Neoplasm Multiple sclerosis
Cerebellopontine angle	CN VI palsy with a combination of: ■ CN V or CN VII palsy ■ CN VIII palsy (deafness, vertigo, tinnitus)	Neoplasm
Petrous pyramid (apex)	CN VI palsy with a combination of : ■ CN VII palsy ■ Ipsilateral hearing loss ■ Ipsilateral ear or facial pain ■ Leakage of CSF from ear	Inflammation of petrous temporal bone from mastoiditis or otitis media (Gradenigo syndrome)

[a] *Components of Foville syndrome.*
[b] *Component of Millard-Gubler syndrome.*

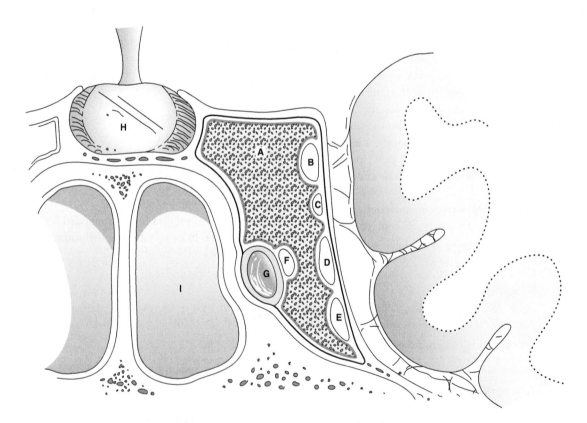

FIGURE 29-13 ■ Cavernous sinus anatomy. **A.** Cavernous sinus. **B.** Cranial nerve III. **C.** Cranial nerve IV. **D.** Ophthalmic division of cranial nerve V. **E.** Maxillary division of cranial nerve V. **F.** Cranial nerve VI. **G.** Carotid artery. **H.** Pituitary gland. **I.** Sphenoid sinus.

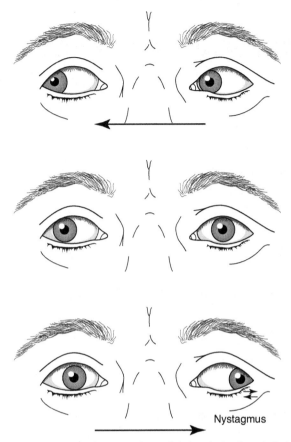

FIGURE 29-14 ■ Right internuclear ophthalmoplegia. There is limitation of adduction of the right eye with an abducting nystagmus of the fellow eye (*bottom panel*). Note the slight exotropia of the right eye in primary gaze (*center panel*).

etiology. In these situations, the child is closely followed for the development of any other neurological signs or symptoms. If the abduction deficit fails to improve after a few months, or if it improves followed by a recurrence, a cranial MRI, serologic testing, and lumbar puncture are indicated. Referral to an ophthalmologist for a child with CN VI palsy is suggested for amblyopia management and possible surgery. Injection of botulinum toxin into the antagonist muscle (medial rectus muscle) can correct the esotropia.[46]

Multiple ocular motor nerve palsies (CN II, CN III, CN IV, CN V and CN VI). Dysfunction of more than one ocular motor cranial nerve is strongly indicative of pathology within the cavernous sinus or orbit (Figure 29-13). Optic neuropathy in the setting of external ophthalmoplegia should prompt an investigation for a lesion within the orbital apex.

Internuclear Ophthalmoplegia

Definition

Internuclear ophthalmoplegia (INO) is the result of a lesion to the MLF.

Differential diagnosis and physical examination

In young adults there is a strong association between INO and multiple sclerosis. The etiologies of INO in children include multiple sclerosis, inborn errors of metabolism, brainstem tumors, encephalitis, structural malformations, trauma, and stroke.[47-49] Myasthenia gravis (Figure 29-10) can cause a pseudo-INO.

Clinically, an INO will have the following features (Figure 29-14):
1. Limitation of abduction of the eye ipsilateral to the lesion
2. Nystagmus of the contralateral abducting eye.
3. Hypertropia or skew deviation.

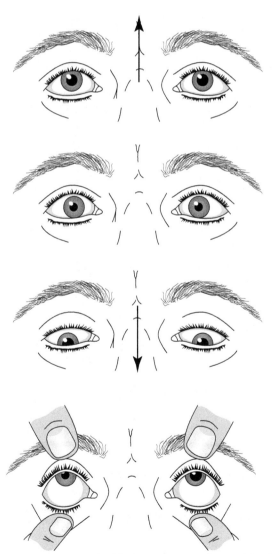

FIGURE 29-15 ■ Dorsal midbrain syndrome. Upgaze paresis with normal downgaze (*left panel*). The upgaze palsy is overcome with Bell phenomenon, indicating a supranuclear palsy (*right panel*). Note bilateral lid retraction and dilated pupils.

Table 29-10.

Miscellaneous Ocular Motility Disorders of Particular Interest

Disorder	Summary
Duane syndrome	Clinical features ■ Commonly unilateral ■ Limitation of abduction ■ Globe retraction on attempted adduction ■ Affected eye will exhibit characteristic upshoot or downshoot with attempted adduction Subclassification ■ Abduction deficit (type 1)—most common ■ Adduction deficit (type 2) ■ Abduction and adduction deficit (type 3) Pathophysiology: absence of CN VI nucleus.[50]
Myasthenia gravis	Onset: third to fifth decade of life[51] Prevalence: 0.3 per 100,000 in children under 14 years of age[52] Common clinical and ancillary features ■ Limited extraocular movements that may occur in any pattern ■ Fatigable ptosis ■ Normal pupil reactions ■ Cogan lid twitch (an upward movement of the eyelid after eyes have moved from downgaze to the primary position) ■ Positive ice pack test ■ Positive edrophonium test ■ Characteristic EMG findings ■ Anti-acetylcholinesterase receptor antibodies (50% sensitive in ocular myasthenia gravis) ■ Ocular myasthenia frequently progresses to generalized myasthenia[51] Variants 1. Autoimmune—most common 2. Transient neonatal myasthenia occurs in neonates born to mothers with myasthenia in the first few days of life resolving within weeks to months 3. Congenital myasthenia encompasses a group of myasthenic disorders in children born to mothers without myasthenia. Not immune mediated and with various pathology at the acetylcholine synapse[48] Note: Botulism, a disorder of the neuromuscular junction, can be confused with myasthenia. In contrast to myasthenia, pupils are dilated and poorly reactive in botulism
Congenital ocular motor apraxia (COMA)	Clinical features ■ Inability to initiate horizontal saccades with relatively intact vertical saccades ■ Horizontal head thrust in the direction of attempted fixation; as the eyes fixate, the head continues to rotate and overshoots; head rotates opposite its initial movement so that the fixated eyes are in primary gaze Associated neurological and systemic conditions[53] ■ Gaucher disease ■ Joubert syndrome ■ CNS lesions ■ CNS development disorders ■ Hydrocephalus ■ Encephalitis Neuroimaging recommended
Spasm of the near reflex	Clinical features ■ Intermittent miosis ■ Accommodation ■ Convergence ■ Induced myopia and miosis during episodes differentiate spasm of near reflex from bilateral CN VI palsies Etiology is psychiatric in most cases although neurological disease has been noted in rare cases[54] Careful history and examination required to help elucidate any potential organic pathology

Table 29-10. (*Continued*)

Miscellaneous Ocular Motility Disorders of Particular Interest

Disorder	Summary
Mobius syndrome	Clinical features ■ CN VI and CN VIII palsies ■ Limb abnormalities ■ Tongue and palate malformations ■ Poland syndrome ■ Other CN deficits[55]
Parinaud or dorsal midbrain syndrome	Clinical features ■ Supranuclear vertical gaze palsy (Figure 29-15) ■ Convergence retraction nystagmus ■ Eyelid retraction ■ Light-near dissociation of pupil ■ Skew deviation ■ Excessive or limited convergence Etiologies[56] ■ Hydrocephalus ■ Intracranial tumors (pineal region) ■ Drug intoxication ■ Metabolic disease ■ Stroke

Evaluation and treatment

Cranial MRI is recommended in cases of INO. Treatment involves management of the underlying etiology. If the INO is persistent, referral to an ophthalmologist can be considered for prism therapy or surgical correction.

Miscellaneous Disorders of Ocular Motility Dysfunction

Miscellaneous disorders of ocular motility dysfunction are summarized in Table 29-10.

REFERENCES

1. Hollenberg MJ, Spira AW. Human retinal development: ultrastructure of the outer retina. *Am J Anat.* 1973; 137:357-385.
2. Wiesel TN, Hubel DH. Effects of visual deprivation on morphology and physiology of cells in the cats lateral geniculate body. *J Neurophysiol.* 1963;26:978-993.
3. Sergot R Denise H. Pediatric neuro-ophthalmology. In: Harley RD, et al., eds. *Harley's Pediatric Ophthalmology.* Philadelphia, PA: Lippincott Williams & Wilkins; 2005.
4. Steinkuller PG, Du L, Gilbert C, et al. Childhood blindness. *J Aapos.* 1999;3:26-32.
5. Levin AV. Congenital eye anomalies. *Pediatr Clin North Am.* 2003;50:55-76.
6. Freedman S, Walton D. Glaucoma in infants and children. In: Harley RD, et al., eds. *Harley's Pediatric Ophthalmology.* Philadelphia, PA: Lippincott Williams & Wilkins; 2005.
7. Spirn MJ, Lynn MJ, Hubbard GB III. Vitreous hemorrhage in children. *Ophthalmology.* 2006;113:848-852.
8. Bhatti MT. Retinitis pigmentosa, pigmentary retinopathies, and neurologic diseases. *Curr Neurol Neurosci Rep.* 2006; 6:403-413.
9. Thompson L, Kaufman LM. The visually impaired child. *Pediatr Clin North Am.* 2003; 50:225-239.
10. Fazzi E, Signorini SG, Scelsa B, et al. Leber's congenital amaurosis: an update. *Eur J Paediatr Neurol.* 2003;7:13-22.
11. Ashworth JL, Biswas S, Wraith E, et al. Mucopolysaccharidoses and the Eye. *Surv Ophthalmol.* 2006;51:1-17.
12. Poll-The BT, Maillette de Buy Wenniger-Prick LJ, Barth PG, et al., The eye as a window to inborn errors of metabolism. *J Inherit Metab Dis.* 2003;26:229-244.
13. Brodsky MC. Congenital optic disk anomalies. *Surv Ophthalmol.* 1994;39:89-112.
14. Krishnan C, Roy A, Traboulsi E. Morning glory disk anomaly, choroidal coloboma, and congenital constrictive malformations of the internal carotid arteries (Moyamoya disease). *Ophthal Genet.* 2000;21:21-24.
15. Kowal L. PEDIG study on amblyopia; vision therapy by atropine penalization versus occlusion. *Binocul Vis Strabismus Q.* 2002;17:275.
16. Scheiman MM, Hertle RW, Beck RW, et al. Randomized trial of treatment of amblyopia in children aged 7 to 17 years. *Arch Ophthalmol.* 2005;123:437-447.

17. Khetpal V, Donahue SP. Cortical visual impairment: etiology, associated findings, and prognosis in a tertiary care setting. *J AAPOS*. 2007 Jun;11:235-239.

18. Good WV, Jan JE, DeSa L, et al. Cortical visual impairment in children. *Surv Ophthalmol*. 1994;38:351-364.

19. Hoyt CS. Delayed visual maturation: the apparently blind infant. *J AAPOS*. 2004;8:215-219.

20. Jahraus CD, Tarbell NJ. Optic pathway gliomas. *Pediatr Blood Cancer*. 2006;46:586-596.

21. Brady KM, Brar AS, Lee AG, et al. Optic neuritis in children: clinical features and visual outcome. *J AAPOS*. 1999;3:98-103.

22. Wilejto M, Shroff M, Buncic JR, et al. The clinical features, MRI findings, and outcome of optic neuritis in children. *Neurology*. 2006;67:258-262.

23. Thuente DD, Buckley EG. Pediatric optic nerve sheath decompression. *Ophthalmology*. 2005;112:724-727.

24. Kedar S, Zhang X, Lynn MJ, et al. Pediatric homonymous hemianopia. *J AAPOS*. 2006; 10:249-252.

25. Porter J, Guthrie B, Sparks D. Innervation of monkey extraocular muscles: localization of sensory and motor neurons by retrograde transport of horseradish peroxidase. *J Comp Neurol*. 1983;218:208-219.

26. Williams A, Hoyt C. Acute comitant esotropia in children with brain tumors. *Arch Ophthalmol*. 1989;107:376-378.

27. Liu GT, Quinn GE, Schaffer DB. Comitant esodeviation resulting from neurologic insult in children. *J AAPOS*. 1997;1:143-146.

28. Biousse V, Newman N, Petermann S, et al. Isolated comitant esotropia and Chiari I malformation. *Am J Ophthalmol*. 2000;130:216-220.

29. Helveston E. Cyclic strabismus. *Am Orthopt J*. 1973;23:48-51.

30. Berk A, Kocak N, Ellidokuz H. Treatment outcomes in refractive accommodative esotropia. *J AAPOS*. 2004;8:384-388.

31. Biglan A, Davis J, Cheng K, et al. Infantile exotropia. *J Pediatr Ophthalmol Strabismus*. 1996;33:79-84.

32. Parks M. Isolated cyclovertical muscle palsy. *Arch Ophthalmol*. 1958;60:1027-1035.

33. Ing E, Sullivan T, Clarke M, et al. Oculomotor nerve palsies in children. *J Pediatr Ophthalmol Strabismus*. 1992;26:331-336.

34. Balkan R, Hoyt C. Associated neurologic abnormalities in congenital third nerve palsies. *Am J Ophthalmol*. 1984;97:315-319.

35. Gabianelli E, Klingele T, Burde R. Acute oculomotor nerve palsy in childhood. Is arteriography necessary? *J Clin Neuroophthalmol*. 1989;9:33-36.

36. Miller N. Solitary oculomotor nerve palsy in childhood. *Am J Ophthalmol*. 1977;83:106-111.

37. Burde R, Savino P, Trobe J. *Clinical Decisions in Neuro-Ophthalmology*. 3rd ed. St. Louis, MO: Mosby; 2002.

38. Mudgil A, Repka M. Ophthalmologic outcome after third cranial nerve palsy or paresis in childhood. *J AAPOS*. 1999;3:2-8.

39. Holmes J, Mutyala S, Maus T, et al. Pediatric third, fourth, and sixth nerve palsies: a population-based study. *Am J Ophthalmol*. 1999;127:388-392.

40. Kodsi S, Younge B. Acquired oculomotor, trochlear, and abducent cranial nerve palsies in pediatric patients. *Am J Ophthalmol*. 1992;114:568-574.

41. Wilson M, Hoxie J. Facial asymmetry in superior oblique muscle palsy. *J Pediatr Ophthalmol Strabismus*. 1993;30:315-318.

42. Guy J, Day A, Mickle J, et al. Contralateral trochlear nerve paresis and ipsilateral Horner's syndrome. *Am J Ophthalmol*. 1989;107: 73-76.

43. Harley R. Paralytic strabismus in children. Etiologic incidence and management of the third, fourth, and sixth nerve palsies. *Ophthalmology*. 1980;87:24-43.

44. Robertson D, Hines J, Rucker C. Acquired sixth-nerve paresis in children. *Arch Ophthalmol*. 1970;83:574-579.

45. Werner D, Savino P, Schatz N. Benign recurrent sixth nerve palsies in childhood. Secondary to immunization or viral illness. *Arch Ophthalmol*. 1983;101:607-608.

46. Wagner R, Frohman L. Long-term results: botulinum for sixth nerve palsy. *J Pediatr Ophthalmol Strabismus*. 1989;26:106-108.

47. Steinlin M, Blaser S, MacGregor D, et al. Eye problems in children with multiple sclerosis. *Pediatr Neurol*. 1995;12:207-212.

48. Brodsky M, Baker R, Hamed L. *Pediatric Neuro-Ophthalmology*. New York: Springer; 1996:279.

49. Arnold AC, Baloh RW, Yee RD, et al. Internuclear ophthalmoplegia in the Chiari type II malformation. *Neurology*. 1990;40:1850-1854.

50. Hotchkiss M, Miller N, Clark A, et al. Bilateral Duane's retraction syndrome. A clinical-pathologic case report. *Arch Ophthalmol*. 1980;98:870-874.

51. Weinberg D, Lesser R, Vollmer T. Ocular myasthenia: a protean disorder. *Surv Ophthalmol*. 1994;39:169-210.

52. Kalb B, Matell G, Pirskanen R, et al. Epidemiology of myasthenia gravis: a population-based study in Stockholm, Sweden. *Neuroepidemiology*. 2002;21:221-225.

53. Harris C, Shawkat F, Russell-Eggitt I, et al. Intermittent horizontal saccade failure ("ocular motor apraxia") in children. *Br J Ophthalmol*. 1996;80:151-158.

54. Dagi L, Chrousos G, Cogan D. Spasm of the near reflex associated with organic disease. *Am J Ophthalmol*. 1987;103:582-585.

55. Miller M, Stromland K. The mobius sequence: a relook. *J AAPOS*. 1999;3:199-208.

56. Maybodi M, Richard W, Bachynski B. Ocular motility disorders. In: Wright KH, Spiegel PH, eds. *Pediatric Ophthalmology and Strabismus*. New York: Springer Verlag; 2003:876-917.

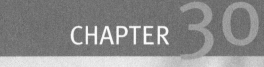

CHAPTER 30

The Floppy Infant Syndrome

Paul R. Carney, James D. Geyer, and Edgard Andrade

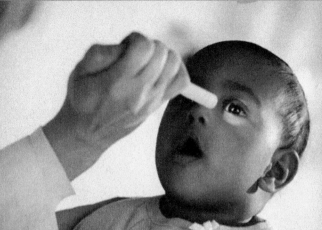

DEFINITIONS AND EPIDEMIOLOGY

Hypotonia is a condition of abnormally low muscle tone (the amount of tension or resistance to movement in a muscle), often involving reduced muscle strength.[1] Hypotonia is not a specific neurological disorder, but a potential manifestation of many different diseases and disorders that affect motor nerve control by the brain or muscle strength (Table 30-1). Recognizing hypotonia, even in early infancy, is usually relatively straightforward, but diagnosing the underlying cause can be difficult and often unsuccessful. The long-term effects of hypotonia on a child's development and later life depend primarily on the severity of the muscle weakness and the nature of the cause. Some disorders have a specific treatment but the principal treatment for most hypotonia of idiopathic or neurological cause is physical therapy and/or occupational therapy to help the child compensate for the neuromuscular disability.

SIGNS AND OBJECTIVE MANIFESTATIONS

Floppy Infant Syndrome

Since hypotonia is most often diagnosed during infancy, it is also known as "floppy infant syndrome" or "infantile hypotonia" (Figure 30-1). Hypotonic patients may display a variety of objective manifestations that indicate decreased muscle tone. Infants with hypotonia have

Table 30-1.

Normal Major Developmental Milestones

Age (mo)	Motor	Language	Adaptive Behavior
4-6	Head lift from prone position	Cries	Smiles
4	No head lag when pulled to sitting position	Sounds of pleasure	Smiles, laughs aloud
5	Voluntary grasp with both hands	"Ah, goo"	Smiles at self
6	Grasps with one hand; rolls, sits with support	Increasing sounds	Food preference
8	Sits with support; transfers objects with hands; rolls from supine to prone positions	Combines syllables	Responds to "No"
10	Creeps, stands holding, finger-thumb apposition in picking up objects	Increasing sounds	Waves "bye-bye," plays "peek-a-boo"
12	Stands holding, walks with support	Says 2 to 3 words with cueing	Acknowledges names of objects
15	Walks alone	Several words	Points, imitates
18	Walks up and down stairs	Many well words	Follows simple commands
24	Runs	2- to 3-word phrases	Points to body parts

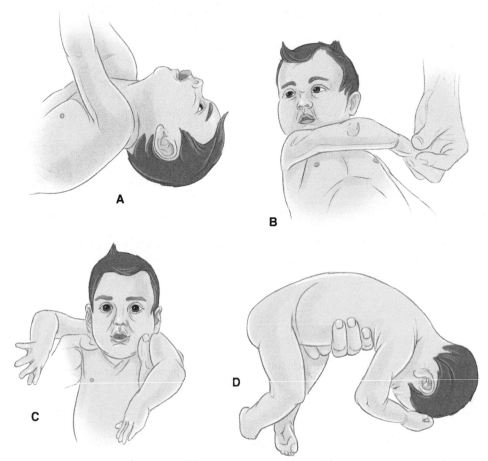

FIGURE 30-1 ■ Measures of hypotonia. **(A)** Pull to sit. **(B)** Scarf sign. **(C)** Shoulder suspension. **(D)** Ventral suspension.

a floppy or "rag doll" appearance because their arms and legs hang by their sides and they have little or no head control. Motor skills delay is often observed, along with hypermobile or hyperflexible joints, drooling and speech difficulties, poor reflexes, decreased strength, decreased activity tolerance, rounded shoulder posture, with leaning onto supports, and poor attention and motivation. The extent and occurrence of specific objective manifestations depends upon the age of the child, the severity of the hypotonia, the specific muscles affected, and sometimes the underlying cause. Hypotonic infants often have difficulty feeding, as their mouth muscles cannot maintain a proper suck-swallow pattern, or a good breast-feeding latch. Hypotonia does not affect intellect. However, depending on the underlying condition, some children with low tone may develop language and social skills later in childhood.

Developmental Delay

Children with normal muscle tone are expected to achieve certain physical abilities within an average timeframe after birth (Tables 30-1 and 30-2). Most low-tone infants have delayed developmental milestones, but the length of delay can vary widely. Motor skills are particularly susceptible to the low-tone disability. They can be divided into two areas, gross motor skills and fine motor skills, both of which are affected. Hypotonic infants are late in lifting their heads while lying on their stomachs, rolling over, lifting themselves into a sitting position, remaining seated without falling over, balancing, crawling, and walking. Fine motor skills delays occur in grasping a toy or finger, transferring a small object from hand to hand, pointing out objects, following movement with the eyes, and self-feeding.

Speech difficulties can result from hypotonia. Low-tone children learn to speak later than their peers, even if they appear to understand a large vocabulary, or can obey simple commands. Difficulties with muscles in the mouth and jaw can inhibit proper pronunciation, and discourage experimentation with word combination and sentence-forming. Since the hypotonic condition is actually an objective manifestation of some underlying disorder, it can be difficult to determine whether speech delays are a result of poor muscle tone or some other neurological condition, such as mental retardation, that may be associated with the cause of hypotonia.

Table 30-2.

Summary of the Neurologic Examination with Respect to Gestational Age

	28 Wk	32 Wk	34 Wk	40 Wk	Red Flags
Mental status	Needs gentle rousing to awaken	Opens eyes spontaneously; sleep-wake cycles apparent		At 36 wk ↑alertness, cries when awake	Irritable or lethargic infant
Cranial nerves					
Pupils	Blinks to light	Consistent pupillary reflex	Fix and follow		
Hearing	Pauses, no orientation to sound			Head + eyes turn to sound	No response to auditory stimulus
Suck + swallow	Weak suck, break here no synchrony with swallow	Stronger suck, better synchrony with swallow		Coordinated suck + swallow at 37 wk	"Chomp suck:" clamps down on pacifier but no suck (bulbar dysfunction)
Motor	Minimally flexed	Flexed hips and knees	↑ Flexion at hips + knees	Flexed in all extremities	Hypotonia Hypertonia 28-wk infant with jerky movements Full-term infant with writhing movements
Reflexes					
Moro	Weak, incomplete hand opening	Complete extension + abduction		Full Moro (with ant. flexion)	Asymmetry
ATNR				ATNR appears at 35 wk.	If obligatory or sustained, suggests pyramidal or extrapyramidal motor abnormal
Palmar grasp	Present but weak		Grasp stronger	Strong grasp, able to be lifted out of bed	Fixed obligate grasp (suggests B hemispheric dysfunction)

ATNR, asymmetric tonic neck reflex.

Muscle Tone versus Muscle Strength

The low muscle tone associated with hypotonia must not be confused with low muscle strength. In body building, good muscle tone is equated with good physical condition, with taut muscles, and a lean appearance, whereas an out-of-shape, overweight individual with fleshy muscles is said to have "poor tone." Neurologically, however, muscle tone cannot be changed under voluntary control, regardless of exercise and diet. True muscle tone is the inherent ability of the muscle to respond to a stretch. For example, by straightening the flexed elbow of an unsuspecting child with normal tone, the biceps will quickly contract as a way of protection against possible injury. When the perceived danger has passed, the muscle then relaxes, and returns to its normal resting state. The child with low tone has muscles that are slow to initiate a muscle contraction, contract very slowly in response to a stimulus, and cannot maintain a contraction for as long as his or her "normal" peers. Because these low-toned muscles do not fully contract before they again relax, they remain lax and fail to maintain a full muscle contraction over time.

Diagnosis

Diagnosing hypotonia in a child includes obtaining family medical history and a physical examination (Table 30-3). Symptoms may vary depending on severity and cause (Table 30-4). The initial examination should be focused on determining whether the hypotonia is a result of an upper motor neuron (central) or lower motor neuron (peripheral) disturbance. Tests and laboratory investigations include computerized tomography

Table 30-3.

Diagnosis and Investigations

1. **History and Physical Examination**
   - Determine birth history, age and rapidity of onset, progression of symptoms, and whether all muscles are involved or just one limb.
   - Determine posture of trunk, whether "frog-leg" position is present, muscle bulk, presence of fasciculation, head lag, examine flexion and extension of the joints.
2. **Test and Laboratory**
   - **a. First Line**
     - CT scan
     - Nerve conduction studies and EMG
     - Serum electrolytes, calcium, glucose, CPK
     - Blood culture, lumbar puncture
   - **b. Second Line**
     - TORCH screen
     - Karyotype
     - Serum amino acids
     - Urine amino acids and organic acids
     - Drug screen
     - Biopsy—muscle, liver
3. **Management**
   - Determine whether respiratory status is adequate or intubation is required.
   - Counsel families with afflicted children about management, prognosis, and genetic implications.
   - Develop a management plan that involves the family and community resources.
   - Select patients requiring specialized care.

Table 30-4.

Hypotonia

Symptoms
- Reduced muscle tone
- Muscle weakness
- Weak infant suck
- Weak cry
- Listless
- Reduced spontaneous activity
- Loss of head control

Neurological Manifestations
- Low Dubowitz score
- Posture—square window
- Popliteal angle
- Head lag
- Arm recoil
- Leg recoil
- Ventral suspension
- Scarf sign
- Heel to ear
- Ankle dorsiflexion

Evidence of Upper Motoneuron Lesion
- Dysmorphic features
- Seizures
- Ocular problems
- Minimal weakness (able to move limbs off bed)
- Fisting of hands (after 6 weeks of age)
- Scissoring on vertical suspension
- Hyperreflexia
- Malformation of other organs

Evidence of Lower Motoneuron Lesion
- Weakness (unable to move limbs off bed)
- Normal or decreased reflexes
- Fatigability
- Fasciculation
- Lack of muscle mass (atrophy)
- Social and cognitively age appropriate
- Elevated CPK

(CT) scans, magnetic resonance imaging (MRI) scans, electroencephalogram (EEG), blood tests, genetic testing (chromosome karyotype and tests for specific gene abnormalities), metabolic CSF studies, electromyography muscle tests, or muscle and nerve biopsy in order to determine the cause (Table 30-5). Mild or benign hypotonia is often diagnosed by physical and occupational therapists through a series of exercises designed to assess developmental progress, or observation of physical interactions. Since a hypotonic child has difficulty deciphering spatial location, the child may have some recognizable coping mechanisms, such as locking the knees while attempting to walk. A common sign of low-tone infants is a tendency to observe the physical activity of those around them for a long time before attempting to imitate, due to frustration over early failures. Developmental delay can indicate hypotonia.

Prognosis and Treatment

Hypotonia is a condition that can be helped with early intervention. Treatment begins with a thorough diagnostic evaluation, including an assessment of motor and sensory skills, balance and coordination, mental status, reflexes, and functioning of the nerves. Once a diagnosis has been made, the underlying condition is treated first, followed by symptomatic and supportive therapy for the hypotonia. Physical therapy can improve fine motor control and overall body strength. Occupational and speech-language therapy can help breathing, speech, and swallowing difficulties. Therapy for infants and young children may also include sensory stimulation programs. There is currently no known treatment or cure for most causes of hypotonia, and objective manifestations can be lifelong. The outcome in any

Table 30-5.

Causes of Hypotonia

Amenable to Rapid Treatment
Electrolyte/metabolic (eg, hypokalemia, hypermagnesemia, acidemia, hypoglycemia)
Toxins/drugs
Hypothyroidism

Central Causes
"Benign congenital hypotonia"
Cerebral malformations (holoprosencephaly); neurode generative (leukodystrophy)
Seizures, trauma (subarachnoid or subdural hemorrhage)
Hydrocephalus/increased intracranial pressure
Infectious causes (eg, encephalitis, abscess, meningitis)
Neoplasm
Hypoxic/ischemic encephalopathy

Neural Disease, Peripheral
Anterior horn cell (eg, progressive spinal muscular atrophy, infarction, infection)
Peripheral nerves/polyneuropathies (Guillain-Barré, Charcot-Marie-Tooth, trauma)
Myoneural junction (myasthenia gravis, botulism)

Muscular Disease
Muscular dystrophy
Myotonic dystrophy
Congenital myopathies

Other Genetic Causes
Trisomy 21
Glycogen storage disease
Niemann-Pick disease
Tay-Sachs disease
Prader-Willi syndrome

particular case of hypotonia depends largely on the nature of the underlying disease. In some cases, muscle tone improves over time, or the patient may learn or devise coping mechanisms that enable him or her to overcome the most disabling aspects of the disorder. However, hypotonia caused by motor neuron diseases can be progressive and life-threatening.

Along with normal pediatric care, specialists who may be involved in the care of a child with hypotonia include developmental pediatricians (specialize in child development), neurologists, neonatologists (specialize in the care of newborns), geneticists, occupational therapists, physical therapists, speech therapists, orthopedists, pathologists (conduct and interpret biochemical tests and tissue analysis), and specialized nursing care.

If the underlying cause is known, treatment is tailored to the specific disease, followed by symptomatic and supportive therapy for the hypotonia. In very severe cases, treatment may be primarily supportive, such as mechanical assistance with basic life functions like breathing and feeding, physical therapy to prevent muscle atrophy and maintain joint mobility, and measures to try to prevent opportunistic infections such as pneumonia. Treatments to improve neurological status might involve such things as medication for a seizure disorder, medicines or supplements to stabilize a metabolic disorder, or surgery to help relieve the pressure from hydrocephalus (increased fluid in the brain).

For children with hypotonia, physical therapy to improve motor control and overall body strength is highly recommended. Occupational therapy can assist with fine motor skill development and hand control, and speech-language therapy can help breathing, speech, and swallowing difficulties. Therapy for infants and young children may also include sensory stimulation programs. Ankle/foot orthoses are sometimes used for weak ankle muscles. Toddlers and children with speech difficulties may benefit greatly by using sign language.

SELECTED AND MOST COMMON CAUSES OF CONGENITAL HYPOTONIA

Table 30-6 gives an overview of the most common causes of congenital hypotonia.

Prader-Willi Syndrome

Prader-Willi syndrome is characterized by a deletion of the proximal arm of chromosome 15. Most cases are due to maternal dysomia, a defective inheritance of both chromosomes 15 from the mother. This is the basis of genetic imprinting, a phenomenon also seen in patients with Angelman syndrome. Clinically, the patient presents with hypotonia, hypogonadism, obesity, short stature, and psychomotor slowing. Not uncommonly, patients affected are born with congenial hip dysplasia or club foot. On physical examination, deep tendon reflexes are absent and hypotonia is profound. Usually, the neonate is fed by prolonged period of time through a nasogastric tube because of swallowing difficulties. By the first anniversary, these feeding difficulties are replaced by a voracious appetite. Mental deficiencies of different ranges are a constant throughout the lifespan. Several dysmorphic features are more evident after the second year of life and include almond-shaped eyes and small, puffy hands and feet. Short stature is treated with

Table 30-6.

Etiology and Localization of Hypotonia in Newborns and Infants

Cerebral
Benign congenital hypotonia
Prader-Willi syndrome
Chronic nonprogressive encephalopathy
Lowe syndrome
Refsum disease
Neonatal adrenoleukodystrophy
Familial dysautonomia
GM1 gangliosidosis

Spinal Cord
Spinal cord injury
Hypoxic ischemic myelopathy

Motor Unit
Spinal muscular atrophies: types 1, 2, 3
Arthrogryposis congenital
Cytochrome-c oxidase deficiency
Polyneuropathies

Neuromuscular Transmission
Botulism
Congenital myasthenia

Myopathies
Central core disease
Minicore disease
Nemalin myopathy
Myotubular myopathy
Congenital fiber-type disproportion myopathy
Congenital muscular dystrophy
Congenital myotonic dystrophy

growth hormone[2] and the patients are usually enrolled in a judicious dietary therapy.

Congenital Muscular Dystrophy

Congenital muscular dystrophy (CMD) is a group of disorders characterized by the presence of hypotonia, joint contractures, diffuse muscle weakness, and atrophy. There are two recognized forms: merosin positive and negative. This protein is located in the extracellular matrix and is the bridging protein for the dextroglycan complex. The deficiency is considered primary or secondary. Patients with primary merosin deficiency have symptoms localizing only to muscle. In secondary merosin deficiency, muscle and brain are affected.

There is a subset of patients with congenital muscular dystrophy with clinical symptoms affecting only the muscle but with a muscle biopsy positive for the presence of merosin, which demonstrates the genetic heterogeneity of this disorder. Examples of this subtype are rigid spine syndrome and Ullrich disease. Serum creatine kinase (CK) levels are elevated and muscle biopsy demonstrates fiber necrosis and regeneration. Typically, the brain MRI is normal. Other than prevention of contractions with physical therapy, no other specific therapies are available for the treatment of this disorder.

A different subset of patients with primary merosin deficiency and a CMD phenotype has been described. The abnormal gene is located on chromosome 6. In addition to hypotonia and arthrogryposis, severe respiratory insufficiency and contractures are present at birth. Clubfoot and bilateral congenital hip dislocation are associated features. The cause of death is related to pulmonary hypoventilation. CK is high and electromyogram (EMG) demonstrates a myopathic pattern. Muscle biopsy typically demonstrates variation in fiber size and replacement of normal muscle tissue by extensive fibrosis and adipose tissue. A mononuclear infiltrate surrounding the scarce muscle fibers is typically present. Brain MRI would demonstrate abnormal myelination patterns, particularly of the occipital lobes. Genetic testing is available. Therapy is limited to aggressive physical therapy to prevent contractions.

Patients with CMD affecting both brain and muscle may have one of the following three disorders: Fukuyama disease, muscle–eye–brain disease, or Walker-Warburg syndrome. The distinguishing feature of these three disorders is an abnormality in neuronal migration, which may result in liscencephaly, polymicrogyria, and heterotopic tissue. Fukuyama disease occurs almost universally in Japanese descendents and there is a reduction on merosin activity. Most mothers with an affected child have a history of spontaneous abortions. Diffuse hypotonia, facial weakness, weak cry, and poor sucking are accompanying features. Deep tendon reflex are absent. Seizures occurring early in life are a common manifestation of cerebral involvement. The degree of developmental delay is severe and global. Severe handicaps and caquexia are progressive, and patients usually do not survive the first decade of life.

Muscle–eye–brain disease occurs mainly in Finland and patients usually have a normal merosin activity. Congenital hypotonia and several types of congenital eye malformations are present, including glaucoma, myopia, retinal atrophy, and cataracts. Mental retardation is also present.

Although Walker-Warburg syndrome is characterized by a reduction of merosin activity, this syndrome shares similar phenotypic brain and muscle abnormalities of patients with muscle–eye–brain disease. Ocular abnormalities present in this disorder are cataracts, retinal dysplasia, detachment, and optic nerve hypoplasia. The diagnosis of these three entities is suspected by an elevated CK level, myopathic EMG features, and muscle biopsy showing proliferation of adipose and collagen tissue that replaces muscle tissue. The MRI shows exvacuo hydrocephalus and lucency of white matter. Despite the advances in the understanding of this disorder, treatment is supportive.

Congenital Myotonic Dystrophy

Congenital myotonic dystrophy is a multisystemic autosomal dominant disorder characterized by a triplet repeat of the DMPK gene on chromosome 19. Genetic anticipation has been reported and the number of repeats can be increased in successive generations. Hence, symptoms can be more severe and of earlier onset in younger affected siblings. Mothers are usually affected because the repeat changes from mother to child are greater. Typically, pregnancy is characterized by polyhydramnios and reduced fetal movements. Premature difficult labor follows due to weak uterine contractions. Respiratory muscles such as the diaphragm and the intercostal muscles could be affected, requiring prompt ventilatory assistance. Several typical dysmorphic features are present, which include a prominent mouth in which the upper lip forms an inverted "V," facial hypotonia, arthrogryposis, and bilateral clubfoot. Several gastrointestinal complications such as swallowing difficulties, aspiration, and regurgitation are present. Deep tendon reflexes are usually absent. Percussion maneuvers and EMG are unreliable tests for evaluation of CMD in the newborn. Other complications include congenital cataracts, cardiomyopathy, and diabetes mellitus. Hence, screening for these potentially treatable disorders is recommended. Nonetheless, severe mental retardation is the rule. The diagnosis of CMD is suspected by examining the mother. Genetic testing is available. Prevention of contractures includes physical therapy and casting. Yearly blood glucose monitoring and formal eye examination is recommended.

Acid Maltase Deficiency (Pompe Disease)

A multisystemic autosomal recessive lysosomal disorder, acid maltase deficiency is characterized by the abnormal storage of glycogen in the cell, due to a deficient acid maltase activity. The mutation is linked to chromosome 17. There are three recognized forms according to the age of onset: infantile, childhood, and adult. Symptoms in the infantile form usually appear at 2 months of age. Hypotonia and congestive heart failure are presenting symptoms and the ECG typically shows short PR intervals and high QRS complexes. Signs of nervous system dysfunction are altered mental status and hyporeflexia.

The muscle biopsy shows large vacuoles packed with glycogen and diminished acid maltase activity. Enzyme replacement therapy with the recombinant human alpha glycosidase (rhGAA) drug (Myozime) seems to be a long-term effective therapy. Respiratory insufficiency, maintenance of normal cardiac function, improvement of skeletal function, and decrease of initially raised laboratory parameters such as creatine kinase, lactic dehydrogenase, and transaminases are potential benefits.[3] However, nearly all infants with Pompe disease develop antibodies, some of which inactivate the enzyme. Alternatives of care under investigation include the use of immunosuppressant agents to curb this antibody response and suppress the production of anti-rhGAA antibodies.

Spinal Muscular Atrophy

There are three different types of spinal muscular atrophy (SMA), of which type I is described in this chapter. Invariable, symptoms are evident in the first 6 months of life. Normal individuals have two almost identical copies of the survival motor gene (SMN1 and SMN2). Affected individuals have a missing copy and usually the SMN1 on chromosome 5 is the primary SMA disease-causing gene. Reduced fetal movements due to early neuronal degeneration may occur. The affected newborns are diffusely weak, hypotonic, hyporeflexic, and may even have respiratory compromise leading to hypoxic encephalopathy. Intercostal muscle paralysis and thoracic collapse may occur and patients may develop paradoxical breathing. Others may have diaphragmatic paralysis as the initial presenting feature. Most patients adapt well to extra uterine life and the respiratory drive is not compromised. Facial expression and extraocular movements are in general intact. Progressive weakness, tongue atrophy, or tongue fasciculations are evident in older infants. Once gag reflex is lost the risk of aspiration and pneumonia is increased. Death may occur in the first 6 months of life. However, prediction of survival is not possible and the infant may be able to sit but not to walk. CK levels are usually normal but may be mildly elevated in severe cases. EMG shows fibrillations and fasciculations at rest. Nerve conduction velocities are typically normal. Muscle biopsy demonstrates combinations of small and hypertrophied fibers. Genetic testing is available. Hence, muscle biopsy is not any longer needed to confirm the diagnosis. Most individuals are homozygous for the point mutation of the SMN1 gene. Five percent could be compound heterozygotes for the point mutation. Treatment is supportive. Compassionate clinical trials with histone deacetylase inhibitors such as valproic acid or hydroxyurea have shown trend to improvement in some clinical outcome measures.[4]

Cytochrome-c Oxidase Deficiency

The mitochondrial disorder cytochrome-c oxidase deficiency is a clinically heterogeneous multi-phenotypic disorder, ranging from isolated myopathy to severe systemic disease. In normal subjects, the electron transfer chain and the oxidative phosphorilation are the principal sources of ATP. Deficiencies of this group of mitochondrial enzymes may cause several upper and lower motor neuron symptoms. Isolated cytochrome-c oxidase deficiency is autosomal recessive and most cases are sporadic. However, clinical manifestations depend on the number of deficient enzymes, the percentage of reduction, and the genetic heterogeneity of this group of disorders. Onset of symptoms is usually in the first 6 months of life and those include diffuse weakness, respiratory failure, severe lactic acidosis, glycosuria, proteinuria, phosphaturia, and aminoaciduria. The prognosis is poor and survival usually is not longer than 6 months of age. CK levels are high and EMG is usually normal. Muscle biopsy reveals enlarged vacuoles that stain positive for glycogen and lipids. Ragged red fibers are also present. No effective treatment is available.

Clinical trials utilizing dichloroacetate blunted the postprandial increase in circulating lactate. However, it did not improve neurological or other measures of clinical outcome.[5]

REFERENCES

1. Bodensteiner JB. The evaluation of the hypotonic infant. *Semin Pediatr Neurol*. 2008 Mar;15(1):10-20.
2. Saito T, Yamamoto Y, Matsumura T, Fujimura H, Shinno S. Serum levels of vascular endothelial growth factor elevated in patients with muscular dystrophy. *Brain Dev*. 2009 Sep;31(8):612-7.
3. Merk T, Wibmer T, Schumann C, Kruger S. Glycogen storage disease type II (Pompe disease)—influence of enzyme replacement therapy in adults. *Eur J Neurol*. Dec 9, 2008. E-pub.
4. Liang WC, You CY, Chang JG, et al. The effect of hydroxyurea in spinal muscular atrophy cells and patients. *J Neurol Sci*. 2008;268:87-94.
5. Stacpoole PW, Kerr DS, Barnes C, et al. Controlled clinical trial of dichloroacetate for treatment of congenital lactic acidosis. *Pediatrics*. 2006;117:1519-1531.

Appendix

ORGANIZATIONS

Muscular Dystrophy Association

3300 East Sunrise Drive
Tucson, AZ 85718-3208
mda@mdausa.org
http://www.mda.org
Tel: 520-529-2000, 800-344-4863
Fax: 520-529-5300

March of Dimes Foundation

1275 Mamaroneck Avenue
White Plains, NY 10605
askus@marchofdimes.com
http://www.marchofdimes.com
Tel: 914-428-7100, 888-MODIMES (663-4637)
Fax: 914-428-8203

National Organization for Rare Disorders (NORD)

P.O. Box 1968
55 Kenosia Avenue
Danbury, CT 06813-1968
orphan@rarediseases.org
http://www.rarediseases.org
Tel: 203-744-0100, Voice Mail 800-999-NORD (6673)
Fax: 203-798-2291

CHAPTER 31

Coma

Ikram Ul Haque

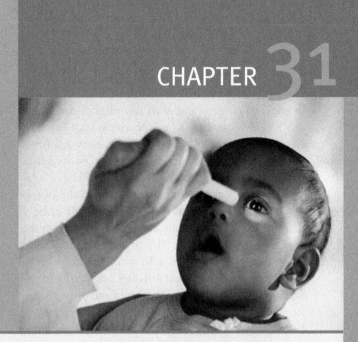

DEFINITIONS AND EPIDEMIOLOGY

Coma is a common neurological emergency seen in critically ill children. Coma is not a disease per se but instead an acute state of disordered consciousness clinically manifested due to a wide variety of medical and surgical disease processes that affect the central nervous system (CNS). It is usually described as "a state of unarousable unresponsiveness in which the eyes remain continuously closed and there is no understandable response to environmental or intrinsic stimulation."[1] In contrast to the sleep state, during coma a person cannot be aroused by appropriate intense stimuli, there is no evidence of sleep–wake cycles on the electroencephalogram (EEG), and the behavioral responses mostly consist of reflex activity.

There is a lack of comprehensive large studies evaluating the overall incidence of coma in children. Most studies have a small number of subjects, are affected by the segregation of studies into traumatic and nontraumatic causes, and use a variety of definitions to define coma. This is further complicated by the fact that coma is seen in an extremely wide range of disease processes.

A number of studies report different epidemiologic rate and outcomes for coma in children. For example, a prospective, population-based, epidemiologic study from the United Kingdom of nontraumatic coma in 278 children aged between 1 month and 16 years defined coma as a Glasgow Coma Scale (GCS) score below 12 for more than 6 hours. They reported an incidence of 30.8 per 100,000 children per year, and 6.0 per 100,000 per year in the general population. In this study, age-specific incidence was significantly higher in the first year of life (ie, 160 per 100,000 children per year). CNS specific presentations became more common with increasing age, but in infants nearly two-thirds of cases

presented with nonspecific systemic signs. Infection was the most common overall etiology and the etiology remained unknown in 14% of cases despite extensive investigation and/or autopsy. Mortality was highly dependent on etiology; at approximately 12 months after coma onset, overall series mortality was 46%.[2] Another prospective observational study from a tertiary care teaching/referral hospital in India followed 100 children with all causes of coma from 2 months to 12 years of age. Overall mortality was 35%; CNS infection was the most common etiology followed by toxic/metabolic causes of coma in this study population.[3]

A recent analysis of children from 0 to 14 years of age who suffered from traumatic brain injury (TBI) in 2003 estimated that 1,565,000 TBIs in the United States resulted in 1,224,000 emergency department visits, 290,000 hospitalizations, and 51,000 deaths.[4] Although many of these children sustained severe TBI (defined as GCS ≤ 8), it is not clear how many of these children were actually in coma after the injury. A previous study reported the rate of coma from TBI was 140 per 100,000 children per year in the United States.[5] Kraus and associates calculated an incidence of severe TBI in children up to 14 years of age of 27 per 10,000 children per year.[6] A 9-year prospective study from a pediatric trauma center in France followed 585 children from 1 month to 15 years of age with a presenting GCS lower than 8. Mortality rate was 22%; Glasgow Outcome Scale (GOS) score was lesser than 3 in 53% of the cases at discharge and 60% at 6-month follow-up.[7] Most of the studies in children with coma or TBI also suggest that younger children are at higher risk of developing nontraumatic coma, with the lowest risk between 5 and 8 years of age, while the risk of traumatic coma increases with mobility with the highest rates seen in older-age children.

PATHOGENESIS

To understand coma and other disorders of consciousness it is important to define consciousness. Currently, there is no universally acceptable, satisfactory definition of consciousness. For medical purposes, normal consciousness is thought to be a product of two basic neurophysiologic functions of the brain: arousal and awareness. **Arousal** or wakefulness is used to describe a behavior change that occurs during transition from the sleep state to wakeful state. This brain function is linked to the ascending reticular activating system (ARAS), which is a network of neural tissues originating in the tegmentum of the pons and midbrain and projecting to the hypothalamus, thalamus, and cerebral cortex.[8,9] **Awareness** of self and environment encompasses multiple brain functions including attention to environment and perception to various stimuli, memory, executive function, and motivation.[10] In children, the concept of consciousness requires understanding the child's developmental level and age-appropriate response.

Impaired consciousness can result from derangement in arousal, awareness, or both in varying depths. In general, awareness cannot occur without arousal, but arousal can be seen without awareness, as seen in patients with vegetative states. A wide range of terms have been used to describe the altered consciousness spectrum from normal consciousness to coma and brain death. Terms such as somnolence, stupor, obtundation, and lethargy lack precision and their use should be discouraged. Since impaired consciousness may be brief, lasting only a few minutes, as with syncope, hypoglycemic episodes, and seizures, this should not be confused with coma. Hence, coma is characterized by a complete absence of both arousal and awareness for more than or equal to 1 hour duration.[11]

Coma is a manifestation of a wide variety of medical and surgical conditions in which CNS involvement may result from a direct insult to the CNS, or may result from secondary brain involvement due to systemic disease. These conditions can be broadly categorized into two groups: (1) those with structural causes or (2) those with metabolic/toxic causes (Table 31-1). Structural conditions affecting the CNS can be further subdivided based on the location into (1) supratentorial and (2) subtentorial. In general, the following rules apply for structural lesions of CNS to induce coma:

1. Cerebral cortex lesions have to involve both hemispheres.
2. Unilateral cortical lesion must be large enough to cause displacement of midline brain structures.[1]
3. Smaller brainstem and diencephalic lesions have to involve bilateral structures.
4. Compartment shifts needs to be of significant magnitude to cause compression or disruption of ARAS.[12]

Table 31-1.

Etiologies of Coma

1. **Central Nervous System**
   a. Supratentorial lesions
      i. Cerebral hemorrhage
      ii. Large cerebral infarction
      iii. Epidural/subdural hematoma
      iv. Brain tumor/abscess
      v. Meningitis/encephalitis
   b. Subtentorial lesions
      i. Pontine/cerebellar hemorrhage
      ii. Midbrain infarction
      iii. Cerebellar tumor/abscess
      iv. Acute demyelination
   c. Generalized or complex partial seizures, status epilepticus, post-ictal state
   d. Hydrocephalus/raised intracranial pressure
   e. Traumatic brian injury
2. **Metabolic/Toxic**
   a. Metabolic
      i. Hypoxia/hypercarbia
      ii. Hypothermia/hyperthermia
      iii. Hypoglycemia/severe hyperglycemia
      iv. Hyponatremia/hypernatremia
      v. Systemic inflammatory response syndrome/shock states
      vi. Hepatic encephalopathy
      vii. Renal failure
      viii. Hypertensive encephalopathy
      ix. Urea cycle defects
   b. Toxic
      i. Medication ingestion (opioids, tricyclics, neuroleptics, aspirin, acetaminophen, anticonvulsants, benzodiazepines, etc.)
      ii. Drug abuse (alcohol, cocaine, amphetamines, etc.)
      iii. Inhalation (carbon monoxide)
   c. Endocrine
      i. Panhypopituitarism
      ii. Thyroid dysfunction
      iii. Adrenal insufficiency
3. **Psychogenic Unresponsiveness**
4. **Pharmacologically Induced**

Metabolic and Toxic causes usually result in secondary injury to the CNS related to the pathophysiology of the disease process itself and may include hypoxia, hypoglycemia, seizures, toxicity, change in brain volume due to altered electrolytes, and toxins as listed in Table 31-1. Two other causes of coma in children are worth mentioning here. Although not very common, in some clinical situations coma can be pharmacologically induced as a therapeutic maneuver, such as for the treatment of refractory status epilepticus or increased intracranial pressure. Finally, coma rarely can be imitated by some psychological disease processes, but this should be differentiated from actual coma and should be termed "psychogenic unresponsiveness."

CLINICAL PRESENTATION

Diseases that cause a reduced level of consciousness in children present with similar overlapping clinical signs and symptoms and are difficult to differentiate from one another. For CNS structural lesions, one important clinical pattern to recognize is termed the "herniation syndrome." This term describes signs and symptoms resulting from compression of brain tissue by the pressure forces generated by intracranial space-occupying lesions, whether blood, edema, or tumor. The total volume of the cranial cavity is limited; therefore any space-occupying lesions must initially shift cerebrospinal fluid and then brain tissue itself from one intracranial compartment to another or toward the foramen magnum. Coma can result when the pressure on the brainstem disrupts the reticular activating system (RAS). In general, there are slight differences in presentation among the broad categories of causes of coma that are summarized in the following section.

Patients with supratentorial lesions usually present with focal neurological signs like contralateral hemiparesis, aphasia, sensory deficit, behavioral changes related to frontal lobe dysfunction, headache, and/or focal seizures. Abnormal signs usually are confined to a single or adjacent anatomic level. Motor dysfunction tends to move from a rostral to caudal direction. Brainstem functions are usually spared until herniation develops and coma ensues.

Patients with subtentorial lesions usually present with brainstem localizing signs. These include pupillary size and response abnormalities, absent or disconjugate caloric eye response, ataxic breathing, bilateral motor deficits, or signs of cerebellar dysfunction. These signs may precede coma, but the onset of coma in these cases could be sudden.

In contrast, patients with metabolic/toxic causes commonly present with delirium preceding coma. Signs and symptoms of systemic disease process are present. Pupillary reaction is generally symmetrical and usually preserved except for specific cases of poisoning. Abnormal motor signs, if present, are symmetrical and sensation is usually intact. Hypothermia is common and other signs like tremors, myoclonus, or asterixis may be present. Often these patients will have brain dysfunction at multiple anatomic levels simultaneously.

DIFFERENTIAL DIAGNOSIS

Coma must be differentiated from other conditions that mimic the clinical picture of coma. These conditions include locked-in syndrome, akinetic mutism, minimally conscious state, vegetative state, brain death, psychogenic unresponsiveness, and pharmacologically induced coma. These conditions are briefly described here and summarized in Table 31-2.

Locked-in syndrome is a rare condition, especially in children, but can occur with brainstem injuries sparing the midbrain. Patients have mostly intact arousal and awareness but a severely limited ability to communicate their awareness due to paralysis of voluntary muscles and anarthria. This has been seen in patients with trauma,[13] pontine glioma,[14] basilar artery occlusion[15] with profound neuromuscular dysfunction from Guillain-Barré syndrome,[16] spinal muscular atrophy,[17] botulism, and organophosphate toxicity.[18] The diagnosis can be substantiated with the help of EEG or functional MRI imaging.[19,20]

Akinetic mutism is a state of profound apathy with intact awareness, revealed by attentive visual pursuit, but a paucity and slowness of voluntary movements without evidence of paralysis. These patients seem on the verge of initiating speech or motor activity but that never seems to happen. It is seen with bilateral injuries within the paramedian midbrain, basal diencephalon, or inferior frontal lobes, occurring with traumatic brain injury,[21] hydrocephalus,[22] central nervous system (CNS) infection,[23] tumors, and tumor resection.[24,25]

Table 31-2.

Differential Diagnosis of Coma-Like Conditions

	Arousal	Awareness	Motor Function	Breathing Activity	Sleep–Wake Cycles
Locked-in syndrome	Present	Present	Absent/eye blinking/vertical eye movement	Present	Present
Akinetic mutism	Present	Partially present	Decreased movements	Present	Present
Minimally conscious state	Present	Partially present	Nonpurposeful	Present	Present
Vegetative state	Present	Absent	Nonpurposeful	Present	Present
Coma	Absent	Absent	Nonpurposeful	Present	Absent
Brain death	Absent	Absent	None/spinal reflexes	Absent	Absent

Minimally conscious state is a relatively new term used to describe patients who have some intermittent evidence of reproducible and purposeful (even if severely limited) nonreflexive motor movements or affective behaviors, such as simple command following, gestural or verbal responses to questions, intelligible verbalizations, smiling or crying in response to the emotional content of stimuli, reaching accurately toward the location of an object, or visual pursuit or fixation in response to visual stimuli.[26] This condition is most commonly confused with vegetative state.

Vegetative state is a state in which the patient demonstrates arousal but self- and environmental awareness is absent. These patients have intact hypothalamic and brainstem (vegetative) functions, which are sufficient to allow for prolonged survival with supportive care.[11, 27] They have preservation of both respiratory function and sleep–wake cycles including periods of spontaneous eye opening. These patients demonstrate some irreproducible reflex movements in response to external stimuli, which may be interpreted by some observers as being purposeful and voluntary. A vegetative state is considered permanent if it lasts longer than 12 months after traumatic brain injury or longer than 3 months after nontraumatic brain injury.[11]

Brain death is a complete and irreversible loss of brain and brainstem function characterized by loss of consciousness, cranial nerve functions, and motor functions, and loss of breathing activity.

Psychogenic unresponsiveness can on rare occasion mimic coma in psychological conditions like schizophrenia, catatonia, hysteria, and malingering. These patients otherwise usually have normal neurological examinations. This can often be identified by the resistance offered during the examination such as resisting eye opening for eye examination or presence of bizarre motor responses during motor reflex assessment. The EEG pattern is usually normal.

DIAGNOSIS

Diagnosis of coma is purely clinical. Current diagnostic criteria for diagnosis of coma are mostly based on absence rather than presence of certain neurobehavioral actions seen in normal consciousness. All of the following are required.

- No spontaneous or stimulus-induced eye-opening
- No age-appropriate command following
- No intelligible age-appropriate speech or verbal response
- No purposeful movement
- No discrete defensive movements or capacity to localize noxious stimuli
- Duration of more than 1 hour
- Duration lasting rarely for more than 2 to 4 weeks

Defining Depth of Coma

Objective scoring systems have been used to uniformly define level of consciousness, such as the widely accepted Glasgow Coma Scale (GCS) originally published by Jennette and Bond in the 1970s.[28] Although originally designed to assess depth of coma after head injury in adults, the GCS has been applied widely in the assessment of pediatric neurological status. This scale was subsequently modified for use in children less than 5 years of age and includes age-appropriate verbal and motor responses, although overall scoring remains the same as shown in Table 31-3.[29,30] Children with normal consciousness have a GCS of 15; a GCS of 12 to 14 is considered "mild," GCS of 9 to 11 is considered "moderate," and GCS lesser than 8 is considered "severe" alteration of

Table 31-3.

Modified Glasgow Coma Scale for Pediatrics

Score	0-1 y	> 1 y	
1. Eye Opening			
4	Spontaneous	Spontaneous	
3	To shout	To verbal command	
2	To pain	To pain	
1	No response	No response	

Score	0-1 y	>1 y	
2. Best Motor Response			
6	Spontaneous and purposeful movements	Obeys commands	
5	Localizes pain	Localizes pain	
4	Flexion withdrawal	Flexion withdrawal	
3	Decorticate	Decorticate	
2	Decerebrate	Decerebrate	
1	No response	No response	

Score	0-2 y	2-5 y	> 5 y
3. Best Verbal Response			
5	Appropriate cry, smiles, coos	Appropriate words and phrases	Oriented, converses
4	Cries	Inappropriate words	Disoriented, converses
3	Inappropriate cry	Cries/screams	Inappropriate words
2	Grunts	Grunts	Incomprehensible sound
1	No response	No response	No response

A score is given in each category. The individual scores are then added to give a total, with a minimal score of 3 and a maximum of 15.
From Reilly PL, Simpson DA, Sprod R, Thomas L. Assessing the conscious level in infants and young children: a pediatric version of the Glasgow Coma Scale. Childs Nerv Syst. 1988;4:30-33.

consciousness. GCS has its limitations with issues related to interobserver reliability and assessment of depth of coma, but it is widely accepted and is commonly used by health care providers. Other scoring system have been suggested, but are not commonly applied.[31]

History and Physical Examination

Evaluation of coma requires a rapid assessment and simultaneous initiation of therapies to avoid delays in treatment for potentially reversible causes that may resolve without long-term disability. Coma may present as progression of a known illness or without any precedent illness. Acute onset of coma *within a few minutes* suggests cerebrovascular disease or cardiac arrhythmia, while a subacute course of *minutes to a few hours* suggests a postictal state after seizure, infection, or drug intoxication. History of recent head injury should raise suspicion of intracranial bleeding (eg, subdural or epidural hematoma). A slower onset over *hours to days* of deterioration of mental status suggests the possibility of CNS tumor or metabolic causes.

The general physical examination may also render clues toward the underlying cause of coma. This should include complete examination of the head, scalp, skin, and back of the patient as initial stabilization is being done. Some helpful diagnostic clues on physical examination are listed in Table 31-4. Disordered breathing patterns have been described in patients with altered consciousness either due to injury involving brainstem respiratory centers or interference with higher regulation centers.[32,33] Although sometimes helpful diagnostically, altered breathing can be seen in a variety of other conditions like hemodynamic shock, metabolic disorders, after giving drugs used for sedation or analgesia, and mechanical ventilation, which may limit the usefulness of these patterns in most patients. **Cheyne-Stokes respiration** is a cyclical pattern of alternating hyperpnea and apnea seen in patients with a bilateral hemispheric or diencephalic injury, but may also be present in congestive heart failure and sleep apnea. **Hyperventilation** is seen in injuries to pontine or midbrain tegmentum; however, it is also widely seen in various conditions including respiratory failure, hemodynamic shock, fever, sepsis, metabolic disarray, and psychiatric disease. **Apneustic breathing** is characterized by a prolonged pause at the end of inspiration and indicates lesions at the mid- and caudal portions of the pons. **Ataxic breathing** is irregular in both rate and tidal volume and suggests damage to the medulla.

The neurological examination is focused on assessing the etiology of coma with the basic goal of determining if the coma is due to a bilateral cortical hemispheric issue or a RAS problem. Pupillary size and

Table 31-4.

Helpful Symptoms and Signs Providing Clues for Identification of Coma Etiology

Fever	Meningitis, encephalitis, post-ictal states, anticholinergic poisoning
Hypothermia	Drug poisoning, hypoglycemia, hypothyroidism, brainstem lesion
Hypotension	Septic shock, hypovolemia, ongoing occult bleeding
Hypertension (severe)	Hypertensive encephalopathy, intracranial bleeding
Hypoventilation	Drug toxicity, pulmonary disease, brainstem lesion
Hyperventilation	Metabolic acidosis, uremia, hepatic disease, salicylate poisoning
Stiff neck	Acute meningitis, subarachnoid hemorrhage
Petechiae	Meningococcemia, idiopathic thrombocytopenic purpura, bacterial endocarditis
Cardiac arrhythmia	Tricyclic poisoning, myocardial infarction
Pupil size and light response	
Bilateral large and fixed	Anticholinergic poisoning, midbrain lesion, brain death
Bilateral pinpoint reactive	Narcotic poisoning, pontine lesions, cholinergic poisoning
Unilateral large sluggish	Third cranial nerve lesion
Unilateral pinpoint	Horner syndrome
Midpoint and fixed	Midbrain lesion
Eye position	
Conjugate lateral gaze	Ipsilateral hemispheric lesion, contralateral pontine lesion
Downward gaze	Acute hydrocephalus, midline thalamic bleeding
Upward gaze	Bilateral hemispheric lesion

response to light should be examined with bright light and preferably in a dark room. The pupillary reflex requires intact parasympathetic and sympathetic systems to constrict or dilate, and most midbrain lesion not only affect the RAS but also the pupil reactivity while metabolic causes of coma may spare these reflexes. Some abnormal responses are noted in Table 31-4.

Eye gaze and movements are coordinated by the following cranial nerves: oculomotor nerve (III), trochlear nerve (IV), abducens nerve (VI) and nuclei in the midbrain and pons. Conjugate horizontal eye movements require connections between the ipsilateral abducens (lateral rectus muscle) and contralateral oculomotor (medial rectus muscle) nuclei along the medial longitudinal fasciculus. Rapid eye movements (saccades) initiate from the frontal eye fields, whereas the smooth pursuit of a moving stimulus arises from the occipitoparietal visual area. Eye movements are modulated by proprioceptive (spinocerebellar tract) and vestibular nerve (VIII) inputs from the medulla and coordinated by the cerebellum. All of these help to maintain visual fixation despite movement of the head, and create the oculocephalic or "doll's-eye" reflex. An oculocephalic reflex is abnormal in a comatose patient when one or both eyes do not move in the opposite direction of head rotation or vertical movement. If neck movement is contraindicated, as with the cervical spine injury, the caloric response (oculovestibular reflex) is used to test the same pathways. Irrigation of one external ear canal with warm or cold water induces convection currents in the endolymph of the semicircular canals. When higher-level brain function is impaired, warm water stimulation leads to slow horizontal deviation of the eyes away from the irrigated ear, whereas cold water will effect slow deviation toward the irrigated ear. In conscious patients, saccades back toward the initial point of fixation attempt to counter these slow deviations. This could be memorized by the familiar mnemonic **COWS** (Cold water Opposite, Warm water Same). No saccadic responses are seen in comatose patients.

Corneal reflexes test the sensory input pathway along the ophthalmic branch of the trigeminal nerve (V) to its nucleus in the medulla, which communicates with the facial nerve (VII) nuclei in the pons to effect direct and consensual eyelid closure. An asymmetric response is suggestive of a structural lesion interrupting the reflex arc. Bilateral absence of the corneal reflex can be seen with metabolic disorders, but can be altered by use of sedation and paralysis. Gag and cough reflexes can be elicited if there is intact functioning of the glossopharyngeal nerve (IX) and vagal nerve (X) afferents. Although commonly assessed by manipulation of the endotracheal tube, this can be a less specific way of testing because it stimulates additional spinal cord-mediated reflexes.

Motor and verbal responses are a crucial part of neurological assessment of comatose patients as reflected by their inclusion in the GCS (Table 31-3). The patient should be observed for spontaneous motor activity and if not present, response to various stimuli should be elicited. Comatose patients may show purposeful movements sometimes, such as reaching for the endotracheal tube or localizing to pain stimuli at the notch of the supraorbital nerve. An asymmetric motor pattern represents contralateral lesions of the cerebral cortex, while localization suggests intact sensory pathways. Decorticate "flexor" posturing consist of flexion of arms and extension of legs; in contrast, both arms and legs are extended in decerebrate "extensor" posturing. Although decerebrate posturing carries a worse prognosis than decorticate posturing, both can result from hemispheric and brainstem lesions.

Finally, extreme care in interpreting motor responses is needed to avoid confusing reflex activity with other responses that may look like spontaneous activity. For example, the triple flexion response, which is flexion of lower extremity to tactile or pain stimuli of the lower extremity, can be seen in deep coma or brain-dead patients.[34] This reflex response is recognized by a very rapid and stereotyped response.

Diagnostic Tests

Coma may require immediate lifesaving treatment before a conclusive diagnosis of the underlying etiology can be made. There are no studies validating the utility of any specific laboratory study in children with decreased mental status. In general, diagnostic tests are ordered based on clinical suspicion of the specific etiology, but certain routine laboratory studies should be obtained in all cases upon presentation. These tests are summarized in Table 31-5. Some of these tests may provide diagnostic clues while tests like arterial blood gas analysis and urine and blood toxicology could possibly help with acute management of the patient, such as use of antidotes if appropriate. It is important to remember that children often present with unfamiliar or atypical clinical features of specific drugs or toxins.[35,36]

Neuroimaging by computed tomography (CT) is routinely recommended in children with coma since it is the quickest study with sufficient sensitivity for detecting structural pathology that needs immediate intervention, such as cerebral edema, tumor, hemorrhage, and herniation. A diagnostic study of CT scan detection of raised intracranial pressure (ICP) as measured by ICP monitoring found a sensitivity of 84% with specificity of 44%. Thus, CT scanning is helpful, but it is important to remember that CT findings may be absent even in the presence of raised ICP.[37] Abnormal head CT scans are more common in patients who have focal neurological signs, unfortunately some times structural lesion in children may not produce focal signs. Patients without a surgically

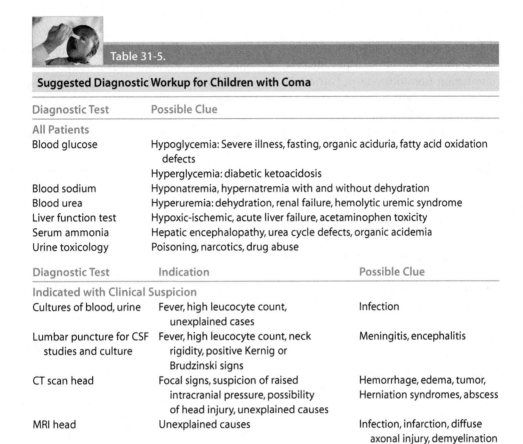

Table 31-5.

Suggested Diagnostic Workup for Children with Coma

Diagnostic Test	Possible Clue	
All Patients		
Blood glucose	Hypoglycemia: Severe illness, fasting, organic aciduria, fatty acid oxidation defects	
	Hyperglycemia: diabetic ketoacidosis	
Blood sodium	Hyponatremia, hypernatremia with and without dehydration	
Blood urea	Hyperuremia: dehydration, renal failure, hemolytic uremic syndrome	
Liver function test	Hypoxic-ischemic, acute liver failure, acetaminophen toxicity	
Serum ammonia	Hepatic encephalopathy, urea cycle defects, organic acidemia	
Urine toxicology	Poisoning, narcotics, drug abuse	

Diagnostic Test	Indication	Possible Clue
Indicated with Clinical Suspicion		
Cultures of blood, urine	Fever, high leucocyte count, unexplained cases	Infection
Lumbar puncture for CSF studies and culture	Fever, high leucocyte count, neck rigidity, positive Kernig or Brudzinski signs	Meningitis, encephalitis
CT scan head	Focal signs, suspicion of raised intracranial pressure, possibility of head injury, unexplained causes	Hemorrhage, edema, tumor, Herniation syndromes, abscess
MRI head	Unexplained causes	Infection, infarction, diffuse axonal injury, demyelination syndromes and tumors
EEG	Known seizure disorder, patients with neuromuscular paralysis, subtle paroxysmal activity, unexplained causes	Status epilepticus, herpetic encephalitis

remediable lesion on initial CT scan should not undergo serial examinations at 24 and 48 hours unless there is a clear deterioration of the clinical course.[38] Magnetic resonance imaging (MRI) can provide greater structural detail as well as better early evidence of infection, infarction, diffuse axonal injury, and demyelination.[39,40] Therefore, an MRI should be obtained in comatose children when the child can safely withstand the longer acquisition times.

Lumbar puncture is an invasive test but considered as a gold standard for microbiologic cultures and polymerase chain reaction studies to confirm CNS infection.[41,42] Performing lumbar puncture in patients with raised intracranial pressure carries a risk of worsening impending herniation, as reported in adult patients.[43] No pediatric studies have evaluated the risk of performing a lumbar puncture during increased intracranial pressure, but if clinical suspicion of raised intracranial pressure is high, a CT scan should be obtained before the procedure. Antimicrobial therapy

should not be delayed to obtain a CSF sample if the clinical suspicion of CNS infection is strong.

Electroencephalography (EEG) is frequently indicated in patients with known seizure disorder and prolonged coma after seizure activity to rule out nonconvulsive status epilepticus or in cases of unexplained coma. Although diagnostic yield and specificity are low during coma, some helpful features have been suggested. In patients with metabolic coma, a generic pattern of diffusely decreased frequency and increased amplitude has been described, often in association with "triphasic waves."[44] Some comatose patients have an EEG that superficially resembles an awake (alpha) pattern. This is called "alpha-coma," and is most commonly seen in patients with extensive damage or dysfunction involving the brainstem or cerebral cortex and generally carries a poor prognosis.[45] Herpesvirus encephalitis has been associated with changes such as periodic sharp waves or epileptiform discharges called "PLEDS" (periodic lateralized epileptiform discharges).[46,47]

Consultation or Referral

Coma in pediatrics is an emergency and often requires a multidisciplinary approach for optimal patient care. Appropriate consultation from different pediatric subspecialists should be emergently obtained and transfer to an appropriate facility should be done quickly after initial stabilization. There is some evidence that outcome of severely injured children is better at specialized centers.[48] Some suggested reasons for seeking immediate subspecialty consults are listed in Table 31-6. In general, referral should be considered in the following situations:

1. There is uncertainty regarding the diagnosis or management.
2. The clinician does not have privileges to provide the type of care needed (eg, surgery).
3. The clinician is ethically opposed to providing care (eg, hospice care, or alternatively, definitive care at the patient's/family's request when it would be futile).
4. When there is a conflict (eg, personality conflict or the patient is a close friend or family member) and the clinician feels he or she cannot be objective.
5. Consultation as a second opinion may be wise when the diagnosis is unexpected (eg, a young person with severe injury) and the prognosis is grim or the patient is not getting better.

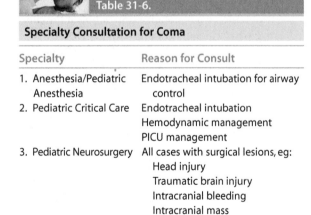

Table 31-6.

Specialty Consultation for Coma

Specialty	Reason for Consult
1. Anesthesia/Pediatric Anesthesia	Endotracheal intubation for airway control
2. Pediatric Critical Care	Endotracheal intubation Hemodynamic management PICU management
3. Pediatric Neurosurgery	All cases with surgical lesions, eg: Head injury Traumatic brain injury Intracranial bleeding Intracranial mass Intracranial pressure monitor placement
4. Pediatric Neurology	All unexplained medical coma EEG monitoring Status epilepticus requiring general anesthesia Prognostication in prolonged coma state

TREATMENT

Coma in many cases is a symptom of a potentially life-threatening condition that requires swift and prompt assessment and intervention simultaneously. No single algorithm is currently available for clinician to follow because of the wide spectrum of conditions causing coma. A basic sequential approach is suggested, consisting of initial stabilization, emergent diagnostic evaluation and intervention if needed, and then focusing on detailed evaluation and etiology-specific management as summarized in Figure 31-1.

Initial Stabilization

Regardless of the etiology, any child presenting with decreased level of consciousness should receive **A**irway, **B**reathing, **C**irculation, **D**isability, and **E**xposure (ABCDE) evaluation. Intervention should be done as quickly as possible for initial stabilization. No studies have evaluated the risk of airway obstruction and decreased rate of breathing with decreased mental status in children. In a pediatric near-drowning case series, 50% of children were apneic when their GCS was 3 or 4.[49] The airway should be opened for signs of obstruction and oxygen should be provided if oxygen saturation is less than 95%. Bag-mask ventilation should be done for persistent hypoxemia, decreasing breathing rate, ineffective breathing, or apnea. Cervical spine injury should be assumed, especially in trauma patients because neck pain and tenderness are difficult to assess in patients with decreased mental status. Immobilization of the cervical spine should be done until definitive diagnosis is established. Endotracheal (ET) intubation should be considered with apnea, oxygen saturation below 92% despite airway positioning and bag-mask ventilation, GCS lower than 8 and loss of airway protective (cough and gag) reflexes, signs of raised intracranial pressure, shock state, and need for ongoing resuscitation. ET intubation should be done by the most experienced person available, especially in cases of trauma with possible C-spine injury or raised intracranial pressure. Hypotension and signs of poor perfusion (eg, capillary refill > 2 s, mottled extremities, diminished peripheral pulses, and decreased urine output) should be promptly treated with rapid IV normal saline boluses or blood depending upon presentation; hypotonic IV fluids should be avoided.[50] A majority of patients with traumatic brain injury with intracranial hemorrhage, brain edema, or raised intracranial pressure will have hypertension on presentation most likely due to a stress response to maintain cerebral perfusion pressure. In the setting of traumatic or nontraumatic brain injury, hypertension should not be treated emergently except in patients with hypertensive encephalopathy coma.

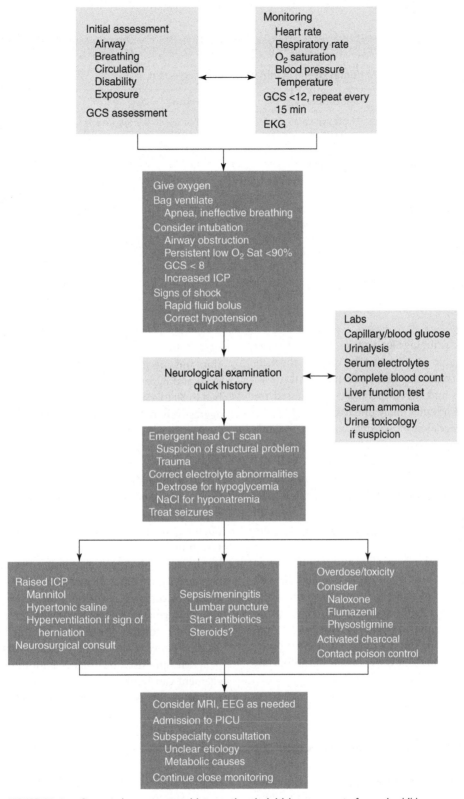

FIGURE 31-1 ■ Suggested assessment and interventions in initial management of coma in children.

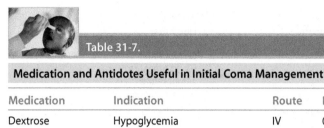

Table 31-7.

Medication and Antidotes Useful in Initial Coma Management

Medication	Indication	Route	Dose
Dextrose	Hypoglycemia	IV	0.5 g/kg/dose
Naloxone	Opiate CNS toxicity	IV	0.1 mg/kg/dose (max 2 mg/dose)
Flumazenil	Benzodiazepine CNS toxicity	IV	0.01 mg/kg/dose (max 1 mg)
Physostigmine	Anticholinergic CNS toxicity	IV	0.02 mg/kg/dose
Mannitol	Increased intracranial pressure	IV	0.5-1 g/kg/dose
3% Saline	Increased intracranial pressure	IV	3-5 mL/kg infusion over 15-30 min
Lorazepam	Active seizure	IV	0.1 mg/kg/dose
Fosphenytoin	Active seizure	IV	20 mg/kg loading dose
Activated charcoal	Ingestion of significantly toxic poison	PO	1-2 g/kg/dose

Laboratory tests, including blood glucose and electrolytes mentioned in Table 31-5, should be quickly checked. Complete patient exposure should be done to evaluate for signs of injuries and the GCS should be assessed for changes every 15 minutes in the initial few hours.

Narcotic ingestion or overdose and hypoglycemia are common findings in children with coma of an unknown etiology, and their immediate reversal can improve consciousness quickly. If raised intracranial pressure is suspected, mannitol or 3% saline should be given during stabilization. Doses and indications of some helpful initial medications for coma patients are listed in Table 31-7.

Immediately after hemodynamic stabilization, a head CT scan should be obtained in all children with coma and suspicion of structural cause or in otherwise unclear cases. Subsequently, a detailed history and physical examination should be obtained, and etiology-specific workup, including but not limited to lumbar puncture, EEG, or MRI, should be done along with appropriate consultation and transfer arrangements.

Specific Etiology Management

It is impossible to discuss the management of all the specific etiologies of coma in this chapter. There are a few common and important situations that clinicians managing pediatric patients with coma need to know. These are briefly discussed here.

Patients with increased ICP

If raised ICP is suspected with traumatic or nontraumatic cause, treatment should be started immediately, especially if signs of herniation are identified. Detailed guidelines for traumatic brain injury management have been published.[51] General measures include ET intubation and mechanical ventilation and avoiding hypoxemia and hyperventilation, elevation of the head of the bed to 30 to 45°, maintaining neutral neck position, and aggressively reducing fever. In cases of impending herniation, hyperventilation can be used for short duration until other measures are taken to decrease intracranial pressure. Since hyperventilation raises intrathoracic pressure and may impair venous return, it is important to avoid hypotension, hence blood pressure should be frequently monitored. Bolus fluid administration will often restore venous return to maintain a cerebral perfusion pressure greater than 50 mm Hg.[52] Hyperosmolar therapy with either mannitol or 3% saline[53] should be started immediately and subsequently continued guided by cerebral perfusion pressure and ICP, if available. Immediate neuroimaging with CT scan and neurosurgical consult should be obtained for surgical lesions. Patients should be subsequently managed in pediatric intensive care units. ICP monitoring and management can improve outcome following TBI, but has not been effective in improving outcome in patients with brain edema and raised ICP due to hypoxic ischemic brain injury.[54]

Patients with meningitis and/or severe sepsis

In patients with strong suspicion of CNS infection or severe systemic infection, in addition to the general measures discussed above, emergent broad-spectrum antimicrobial administration is crucial. Although lumbar puncture is considered the gold standard to confirm the diagnosis of meningitis, antibiotic therapy should never be delayed for obtaining a CSF sample. Clinical decision rules have been published to help clinicians manage children with meningeal signs.[41] Patients with meningitis and low GCS, abnormal pupillary reflexes, focal neurological signs, or posturing should undergo a CT scan to rule out increased ICP before lumbar puncture. Steroid therapy with dexamethasone, 0.15 mg/kg, before or with the first dose of antibiotics decreases mortality and neurological sequelae in bacterial meningitis in adults but its utility in children is still debated.[55]

Patients with convulsive or nonconvulsive status epilepticus

Patients with convulsive status are easy to identify and require prompt management with anticonvulsants. In refractory cases, emergent neurologist consultation and an EEG should be obtained. Electrolytes like serum sodium, calcium, and magnesium should be checked, especially in infants, and corrected if abnormal. Often patients will remain unconscious due to a post-ictal state for up to 1 hour. In general, if consciousness is not recovered by 30 minutes after seizure activity ends without any apparent reason, nonconvulsive status should be ruled out by obtaining an urgent EEG along with other neuroimaging. Children with refractory status epilepticus should be admitted to the PICU for induction of general anesthesia and EEG burst suppression.

Patients with coma due to toxins

Patients with suspicion of drug ingestion or intoxication and coma should be stabilized with general measures first. If signs and symptoms of narcotics, benzodiazepines, or anticholinergics are present, antidotes like naloxone, flumazenil, or physostigmine respectively, could be used to improve consciousness. Sodium bicarbonate is suggested in cases of tricyclic antidepressent toxicity. Activated charcoal should be given to decrease systemic absorption, although this should be done only after securing the airway in the comatose child. Doses of these medications are given in Table 31-7.

Patients with coma due to metabolic causes

Although the list of metabolic diseases resulting in coma is very long, some common ones are hypoglycemia, diabetic ketoacidosis, hyperammonemia (eg, from hepatic failure, organic acidurias, urea cycle defects, amino acid transport defects, or Reye syndrome), and nonhyperglycemic ketacidosis (eg, from organic acidopathies, amino acidopathies, fatty acid oxidation defects, and mitochondrial diseases). After initial patient stabilization with general measures, emergent consult with endocrine and metabolic disease experts should be obtained. Patients with severe hyperammonemia may require emergent dialysis for correction. Special laboratory test like plasma lactate levels, plasma amino acids profile, urinary amino acid, and organic acid profile should be sent to delineate the diagnosis.

PROGNOSIS

Outcome of children in coma is highly dependent on the cause, location, severity, and extent of brain injury caused by the disease process. In general, studies suggest that children with traumatic brain injury do much better as a group compared to adults.[56] Traumatic brain injury is one of the most common causes of neurological morbidity and mortality during childhood.[57] A large population-based study of nontraumatic coma in children reported 46% mortality and 30% neurological morbidity.[58] A significant number of coma survivors require extensive support and rehabilitation care, especially if the recovery from coma results in a vegetative state.[59]

REFERENCES

1. Plum F, Posner JB. The diagnosis of stupor and coma. *Contemp Neurol Ser.* 1972;10:1-286.
2. Wong CP, Forsyth RJ, Kelly TP, Eyre JA. Incidence, aetiology, and outcome of non-traumatic coma: a population based study. *Arch Dis Child.* 2001;84:193-199.
3. Bansal A, Singhi SC, Singhi PD, Khandelwal N, Ramesh S. Non traumatic coma. *Indian J Pediatr.* 2005;72:467-473.
4. Rutland-Brown W, Langlois JA, Thomas KE, Xi YL. Incidence of traumatic brain injury in the United States, 2003. *J Head Trauma Rehabil.* 2006;21:544-548.
5. Michaud LJ, Rivara FP, Grady MS, Reay DT. Predictors of survival and severity of disability after severe brain injury in children. *Neurosurgery.* 1992;31:254-264.
6. Kraus JF, Rock A, Hemyari P. Brain injuries among infants, children, adolescents, and young adults. *Am J Dis Child.* 1990;144:684-691.
7. Ducrocq SC, Meyer PG, Orliaguet GA, et al. Epidemiology and early predictive factors of mortality and outcome in children with traumatic severe brain injury: experience of a French pediatric trauma center. *Pediatr Crit Care Med.* 2006;7:461-467.
8. Parvizi J, Damasio AR. Neuroanatomical correlates of brainstem coma. *Brain.* 2003;126:1524-1536.
9. Moruzzi G, Magoun HW. Brain stem reticular formation and activation of the EEG. 1949. *J Neuropsychiatry Clin Neurosci.* 1995;7:251-267.
10. Young GB, Pigott SE. Neurobiological basis of consciousness. *Arch Neurol.* 1999;56:153-157.
11. Medical aspects of the persistent vegetative state (1). The Multi-Society Task Force on PVS. *N Engl J Med.* 1994;330:1499-1508.
12. Wijdicks EFM, Wijdicks EFM. *Neurologic Complications of Critical Illness.* 2nd ed. Oxford: Oxford University Press; 2002.
13. Landrieu P, Fromentin C, Tardieu M, Menget A, Laget P. Locked in syndrome with a favourable outcome. *Eur J Pediatr.* 1984;142:144-145.
14. Masuzawa H, Sato J, Kamitani H, Kamikura T, Aoki N. Pontine gliomas causing locked-in syndrome. *Childs Nerv Syst.* 1993;9:256-259.
15. Rosman NP, Adhami S, Mannheim GB, Katz NP, Klucznik RP, Muriello MA. Basilar artery occlusion in children:

misleading presentations, "locked-in" state, and diagnostic importance of accompanying vertebral artery occlusion. *J Child Neurol.* 2003;18:450-462.

16. Bakshi N, Maselli RA, Gospe SM, Jr., Ellis WG, McDonald C, Mandler RN. Fulminant demyelinating neuropathy mimicking cerebral death. *Muscle Nerve.* 1997;20:1595-1597.

17. Echenberg RJ. Permanently locked-in syndrome in the neurologically impaired neonate: report of a case of Werdnig-Hoffmann disease. *J Clin Ethics.* 1992;3:206-208.

18. Golden GS, Leeds N, Kremenitzer MW, Russman BS. The "locked-in" syndrome in children. *J Pediatr.* 1976;89:596-598.

19. Laureys S, Owen AM, Schiff ND. Brain function in coma, vegetative state, and related disorders. *Lancet Neurol.* 2004;3:537-546.

20. Laureys S, Pellas F, Van Eeckhout P, et al. The locked-in syndrome : what is it like to be conscious but paralyzed and voiceless? *Prog Brain Res.* 2005;150:495-511.

21. van Mourik M, van Dongen HR, Catsman-Berrevoets CE. The many faces of acquired neurologic mutism in childhood. *Pediatr Neurol.* 1996;15:352-357.

22. Abekura M. Akinetic mutism and magnetic resonance imaging in obstructive hydrocephalus. Case illustration. *J Neurosurg.* 1998;88:161.

23. Mellon AF, Appleton RE, Gardner-Medwin D, Aynsley-Green A. Encephalitis lethargica-like illness in a five-year-old. *Dev Med Child Neurol.* 1991;33:158-161.

24. Shinoda M, Tsugu A, Oda S, et al. Development of akinetic mutism and hyperphagia after left thalamic and right hypothalamic lesions. *Childs Nerv Syst.* 1993;9:243-245.

25. Kadota Y, Kondo T, Sato K. Akinetic mutism and involuntary movements following radical resection of hypothalamic glioma—case report. *Neurol Med Chir (Tokyo).* 1996;36:447-450.

26. Ashwal S. Medical aspects of the minimally conscious state in children. *Brain Dev.* 2003;25:535-545.

27. Zeman A. Persistent vegetative state. *Lancet.* 1997;350:795-799.

28. Jennett B, Bond M. Assessment of outcome after severe brain damage. *Lancet.* 1975;1:480-484.

29. Gordon NS, Fois A, Jacobi G, Minns RA, Seshia SS. The management of the comatose child. *Neuropediatrics.* 1983;14:3-5.

30. Reilly PL, Simpson DA, Sprod R, Thomas L. Assessing the conscious level in infants and young children: a paediatric version of the Glasgow Coma Scale. *Childs Nerv Syst.* 1988;4:30-33.

31. Kirkham FJ, Newton CR, Whitehouse W. Paediatric coma scales. *Dev Med Child Neurol.* 2008;50:267-274.

32. Bang A, Gustavsson M, Larsson C, Holmberg S, Herlitz J. Are patients who are found deeply unconscious, without having suffered a cardiac arrest, always breathing normally? *Resuscitation.* 2008;78:116-118.

33. Gifford RR, Plaut MR. Abnormal respiratory patterns in the comatose patient caused by intracranial dysfunction. *J Neurosurg Nurs.* 1975;7:57-61.

34. Saposnik G, Maurino J, Saizar R, Bueri JA. Spontaneous and reflex movements in 107 patients with brain death. *Am J Med.* 2005;118:311-314.

35. Abbruzzi G, Stork CM. Pediatric toxicologic concerns. *Emerg Med Clin North Am.* 2002;20:223-247.

36. Lifshitz M, Shahak E, Sofer S. Carbamate and organophosphate poisoning in young children. *Pediatr Emerg Care.* 1999;15:102-103.

37. Hirsch W, Beck R, Behrmann C, Schobess A, Spielmann RP. Reliability of cranial CT versus intracerebral pressure measurement for the evaluation of generalised cerebral oedema in children. *Pediatr Radiol.* 2000;30:439-443.

38. Figg RE, Burry TS, Vander Kolk WE. Clinical efficacy of serial computed tomographic scanning in severe closed head injury patients. *J Trauma.* 2003;55:1061-1064.

39. Tong KA, Ashwal S, Holshouser BA, et al. Hemorrhagic shearing lesions in children and adolescents with post-traumatic diffuse axonal injury: improved detection and initial results. *Radiology.* 2003;227:332-339.

40. Sundgren PC, Reinstrup P, Romner B, Holtas S, Maly P. Value of conventional, and diffusion- and perfusion weighted MRI in the management of patients with unclear cerebral pathology, admitted to the intensive care unit. *Neuroradiology.* 2002;44:674-680.

41. Oostenbrink R, Moons KG, Derksen-Lubsen AG, Grobbee DE, Moll HA. A diagnostic decision rule for management of children with meningeal signs. *Eur J Epidemiol.* 2004;19:109-116.

42. Feigin RD, McCracken GH, Jr., Klein JO. Diagnosis and management of meningitis. *Pediatr Infect Dis J.* 1992;11:785-814.

43. Hasbun R, Abrahams J, Jekel J, Quagliarello VJ. Computed tomography of the head before lumbar puncture in adults with suspected meningitis. *N Engl J Med.* 2001;345:1727-1733.

44. Kaplan PW. The EEG in metabolic encephalopathy and coma. *J Clin Neurophysiol.* 2004;21:307-318.

45. Kaplan PW, Genoud D, Ho TW, Jallon P. Etiology, neurologic correlations, and prognosis in alpha coma. *Clin Neurophysiol.* 1999;110:205-213.

46. Ch'ien LT, Boehm RM, Robinson H, Liu C, Frenkel LD. Characteristic early electroencephalographic changes in herpes simplex encephalitis. *Arch Neurol.* 1977;34:361-364.

47. Smith JB, Westmoreland BF, Reagan TJ, Sandok BA. A distinctive clinical EEG profile in herpes simplex encephalitis. *Mayo Clin Proc.* 1975;50:469-474.

48. Potoka DA, Schall LC, Ford HR. Improved functional outcome for severely injured children treated at pediatric trauma centers. *J Trauma.* 2001;51:824-832; discussion 832-834.

49. Jacobsen WK, Mason LJ, Briggs BA, Schneider S, Thompson JC. Correlation of spontaneous respiration and neurologic damage in near-drowning. *Crit Care Med.* 1983;11:487-489.

50. Yu PL, Jin LM, Seaman H, Yang YJ, Tong HX. Fluid therapy of acute brain edema in children. *Pediatr Neurol.* 2000;22:298-301.

51. Guidelines for the acute medical management of severe traumatic brain injury in infants, children, and adolescents. *Crit Care Med.* 2003;31(suppl):S407-S491.

52. Hackbarth RM, Rzeszutko KM, Sturm G, Donders J, Kuldanek AS, Sanfilippo DJ. Survival and functional outcome in pediatric traumatic brain injury: a retrospective review

and analysis of predictive factors. *Crit Care Med.* 2002;30:1630-1635.

53. Georgiadis AL, Suarez JI. Hypertonic saline for cerebral edema. *Curr Neurol Neurosci Rep.* 2003;3:524-530.

54. Bohn DJ, Biggar WD, Smith CR, Conn AW, Barker GA. Influence of hypothermia, barbiturate therapy, and intracranial pressure monitoring on morbidity and mortality after near-drowning. *Crit Care Med.* 1986;14:529-534.

55. van de Beek D, de Gans J, McIntyre P, Prasad K. Corticosteroids for acute bacterial meningitis. *Cochrane Database Syst Rev.* 2007:CD004405.

56. Boyer MG, Edwards P. Outcome 1 to 3 years after severe traumatic brain injury in children and adolescents. *Injury.* 1991;22:315-320.

57. Arias E. United States life tables, 2004. *Natl Vital Stat Rep.* 2007;56:1-39.

58. Forsyth RJ, Wong CP, Kelly TP, et al. Cognitive and adaptive outcomes and age at insult effects after non-traumatic coma. *Arch Dis Child.* 2001;84:200-204.

59. Heindl UT, Laub MC. Outcome of persistent vegetative state following hypoxic or traumatic brain injury in children and adolescents. *Neuropediatrics.* 1996;27:94-100.

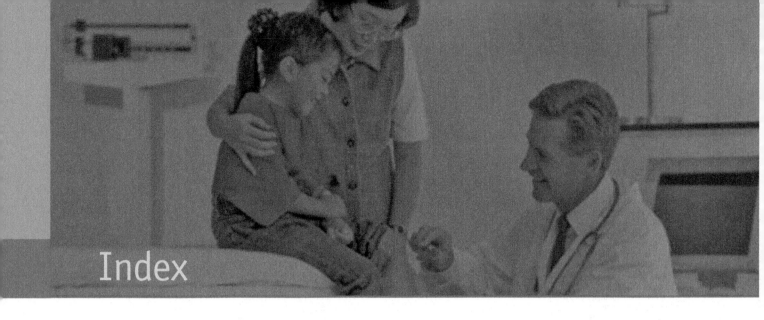

Index